Insurance Handbook for the Medical Office

Get Connected to Content Updates, Study Tools, and More!

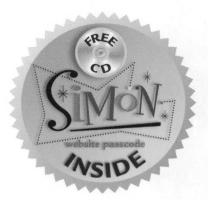

Meet SIMON;

Your free online Website companion.

Sign on at:

http://www.wbsaunders.com/SIMON/Fordney/Handbook/
 Enter your unique passcode and get ready to experience a whole new learning environment!

What you'll receive:

Whether you're a student or an instructor, you'll find information just for you. Things like: ▪ Content updates ▪ Links to related Websites ▪ Author information . . . and more!

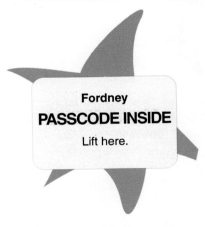

Fordney
PASSCODE INSIDE
Lift here.

If passcode tab is removed, this textbook cannot be returned to W.B. Saunders

Plus: WebLinks

Use your unique passcode to access active Websites keyed specifically to the contents of this book. The WebLinks are updated continually, with new ones added as they develop.

Plus, FREE CD in back!

This student software challenge is designed especially to support Fordney's **Insurance Handbook for the Medical Office, 7th edition.**

▪ An interactive program featuring the HCFA-1500 claim form along with 10 scored patient case studies with related insurance form information.

▪ This hands on tool will help you master the complexities of the HCFA-1500 and understand how insurance billing works. Assignments increase in difficulty to help you gain confidence throughout the course.

W. B. Saunders Company

Insurance Handbook for the Medical Office

SEVENTH EDITION

Marilyn Takahashi Fordney, CMA-AC, CMT

Formerly Instructor of Medical Insurance, Medical Terminology,
Medical Machine Transcription, and Medical Office Procedures

Ventura College
Ventura, California

Technical Collaborator and Contributing Author:

Linda L. French, CMA-C, NCICS

Business Consultant and Instructor of Medical Insurance Procedures
and Medical Terminology

Simi Valley Adult School and Career Institute
Simi Valley, California;

Ventura College
Ventura, California;

Oxnard College
Oxnard, California

Visit us at: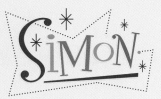

http://www.wbsaunders.com/SIMON/Fordney/handbook.

W.B. Saunders Company

An Imprint of Elsevier Science

Philadelphia   London   New York   St. Louis   Sydney   Toronto

W.B. SAUNDERS COMPANY
An Imprint of Elsevier Science

The Curtis Center
Independence Square West
Philadelphia, Pennsylvania 19106

Library of Congress Cataloging-in-Publication Data

Fordney, Marilyn Takahashi

Insurance handbook for the medical office/ Marilyn Takahashi Fordney.—7th ed

p.; cm.
Includes bibliographical references and index.

ISBN 0–7216–9518–3

1. Insurance, Health—United States—Handbooks, manuals, etc. 2. Medical offices—
   Management—Handbooks, manuals, etc. 3. Medical claims processing industry.
   Insurance handbook for the medical office

HG9396 .F67 2002

368.38'0024'61—dc21   2001020299

Editor-in-Chief:	Andrew Allen
Senior Acquisitions Editor:	Adrianne Williams
Developmental Editor:	Rae L. Robertson
Project Manager:	Tina Rebane
Illustration Specialist:	John S. Needles, Jr.
Book Designer:	Gene Harris

INSURANCE HANDBOOK FOR THE MEDICAL OFFICE   ISBN 0–7216–9518–3

Printed in the United States of America.

Last digit is the print number: 9   8   7   6   5   4   3   2

This book is dedicated to insurance billing and coding specialists throughout the nation, to insurance billing and coding instructors, and new and former students who motivate me to continue writing in this challenging and ever-changing career field.

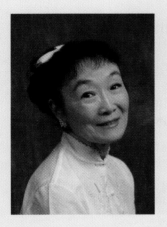

Welcome to the 25th Silver Anniversary Edition.

When this book made its first appearance in 1977, few people were aware of how important the subject of health insurance would become. *Insurance Handbook for the Medical Office* now celebrates its 25th year and through the years has gained wide acceptance across the nation. A considerable number of changes have occurred since the previous edition, making major revision and expansion necessary. It has been challenging and exciting to put the seventh edition together because of the incorporation of full color, addition of icons, and color enhancements to existing and new figures. Because changes take place in the insurance industry on a daily basis, *Insurance Handbook for the Medical Office* will be revised every two years to keep the information current.

Purpose

The goals of this text are to increase efficiency and streamline administrative procedures for one of the most complex tasks of the physician's business: insurance coding and billing.

In recent years, the community and health care professionals have witnessed emergence of an administrative medical specialty known either as insurance billing specialist, medical biller, or reimbursement specialist. Certification is being offered by several national organizations, and the career is quickly achieving recognition and professionalism. Thus, the *Handbook* has been written to address this as another profession that has branched from the administrative medical assistant career. Health care reform means an explosion of jobs in the medical field, especially for those trained in coding and processing insurance claims, manually as well as electronically. Training in this area is necessary because it is common to find medical practices either undercharging or not charging for billable services due to lack of knowledge by office personnel.

Insurance claims are being submitted for patients on recommendation of management consultants to control cash flow, obtain correct reimbursement amounts, honor insurance contracts, compete with other medical practices, and maintain a good relationship with patients. Even offices that do not routinely complete insurance claims for patients will make exceptions for the aged or those patients who suffer from mental incompetence, illiteracy, diminished eyesight, or a poor command of the English language. When the bill is for hundreds or thousands of dollars or when a surgical report is required, the physician's office should submit the bill to obtain maximum reimbursement. Those who administer the federal government's Medicare program increasingly promote electronic transmission of insurance claims. Because of these factors, as well as the requirement to document care, the amount of paperwork has increased by leaps and bounds, becoming burdensome and unwieldy. This text addresses all clerical functions of the medical biller, and illustrations throughout the text feature generic forms created to help simplify billing procedures.

A number of schools and colleges have established one-year certificate programs for those interested in a career as an insurance billing specialist, and many existing programs offer medical insurance as a full-semester, 18-week course. Community college extension divisions also offer community service classes and short courses in this subject. Some schools include this as part of a medical assisting program's curriculum so the individual is knowledgeable in all administrative aspects of a physician's office. The text may be used as a learning tool and resource guide in all of those programs as well as in vocational or commercial training institutes and welfare-work programs. It also serves as a text for in-service training in the private medical office. It may be used for independent home study if no formal classes are available in the community. The lay reader not pursuing a career in the medical field will find it useful when working with a claims assistance professional or for billing his or her insurance plans. Insurance companies and their agents have found this a valuable reference book when answering clients' questions.

The text is designed primarily for the student who plans to seek employment in an outpatient setting (physician's office or clinic) or wishes to establish an independent billing business and needs a good understanding of the reimbursement process. Since many types of insurance coverage are available in the United States, those types most commonly encountered in physicians' offices and clinics have been emphasized in this text in simple, nontechnical explanations and tables. Documentation in the medical record is the key to substantiating procedure and diagnostic code selections for proper reimbursement. Thus this seventh edition is enhanced with a chapter entitled Medical Documentation. In recent years, the federal government targeted this issue with the introduction of Medicare compliance policies related to documentation; such issues are therefore covered to help physicians comply with possible reviews or audits of their billing practices. Finally, it may be used as a stand-alone reference source or as an educational tool to increase the knowledge of someone presently working as an insurance billing specialist in a private medical office.

Content

New Features

▶ Each chapter has been updated to reflect 2001 policies and procedures.
▶ All chapters have been completely restructured for better organization and flow of content, with legal information appearing in those chapters where it applies to insurance billing and coding. The information presented is not a substitute for legal advice, and the physician and his or her insurance billing specialist should always seek the counsel of an attorney about specific questions of law as they relate to medical practice.
▶ Chapter 3, Medical Documentation, has been added.
▶ Chapter 6 contains a special color-coded icon feature that denotes and helps clarify information by using a block-by-block approach specific to each different payer and templates illustrating placement of information on the HCFA-1500 insurance claim form. These icons are as follows:

All Payers: All payer guidelines including all private insurance companies and all federal and state programs.

All Private Payers: All private insurance companies.

Medicaid: State Medicaid programs.

Medicare: Federal Medicare programs, Medicare/Medicaid, Medicare/Medigap, and Medicare Secondary Payer (MSP).

TRICARE: TRICARE Standard (formerly CHAMPUS), TRICARE Prime, TRICARE Extra.

CHAMPVA: Civilian Health and Medical Program of the Department of Veterans Affairs.

Workers' Compensation: State workers' compensation programs.

▶ The chapter in the previous edition emphasizing the Blue Plans has been deleted because most Blue Plans have been bought by private insurance companies and operate similarly to other private plans and managed care contracts.

General Features

The chapters of the previous edition were reviewed by experts so that improvements in content, clarity of topics, and deletions could be considered. Objectives are presented at the beginning of each chapter to guide the instructor in preparing lecture material and inform the reader about what will be presented. By reviewing the key terms introducing each chapter, the student is alerted to important words for the topic. The text is leavened with amusing approaches and quotes from insurance scenarios.

Basic health insurance information and coding examples are shown for the person who needs to study for a certification examination. Special emphasis is placed on correct and incorrect procedural codes and appropriate documentation—the keys to obtaining maximum reimbursement. Chapter 7, Electronic Data Interchange, explains electronic claims transmission and computer claim systems, carrier direct or clearinghouse. Many specific quick-action solutions for insurance problems, tracing delinquent claims, and appealing denied claims are mentioned. A separate chapter on managed care systems and how to administer them is presented. Thorough up-to-date information is presented for Medicare, Medicaid, TRICARE, private plans, workers' compensation, managed care plans, disability income insurance, and disability benefit programs. Helpful billing tips and guidelines for submitting insurance claims are given for each type of insurance program covered. Chapter 16, Hospital Billing, is intended especially for those students interested in pursuing a career in the hospital setting. A final chapter provides information pertinent to seeking a position as an insurance billing specialist, a self-employed claims assistance professional, or an electronic claims processor.

Appendix A lists addresses of insurance claims offices and insurance commissioners by state, territory, or Canadian province. Appendix B is a comprehensive reference resource of available audiotapes, books, newsletters, periodicals, software, and videotapes designed to assist the insurance billing specialist. Addresses, toll-free telephone numbers, and websites are listed at the end to assist the reader in locating a special item, if desired. At the back of the book is an extensive glossary of basic medical and insurance terms and abbreviations.

Supplements

Workbook

New Features

▶ Self-study review questions for each chapter, with answers in Appendix D
▶ Expansion of the test section at the end of the *Workbook*

General Features

For the learner, the *Workbook* that accompanies the text is a practical approach to learning insurance billing. It progresses from easy to more complex issues within each chapter and advances as new skills are learned and integrated. Chapter outlines serve as a lecture guide. Each chapter has performance objectives for assignments that indicate to students what will be accomplished. Key terms are repeated for quick reference when studying. Patients' medical records, ledgers, and encounter forms are presented as they might appear in the doctor's files, so the student may learn how to abstract information to complete claim forms properly and accurately. For this edition, the patient records and ledgers have been updated and reworded to correspond with the 2001 procedural and diagnostic code books. Easily removable insurance claim forms and other sample documents are included in the *Workbook* for completion and to enhance typing skills. Some assignments give students hands-on experience in typing forms for optical character recognition (OCR) computer equipment, which is used in many states for insurance claims processing and payment. Current procedural and diagnostic code exercises are used throughout the *Workbook* to facilitate and enhance coding skills for submitting a claim or posting to a patient's ledger. Critical thinking problems are presented in certain sections. Special appendices are at the end of the *Workbook*. These include a simulated practice, the college clinic, with a group of physicians who employ the student, a mock fee schedule with codes and fees (including Medicare), and an abbreviated Medicare Level II HCPCS alphanumeric code list. The appendices may be used as reference tools to complete the procedural code problems.

Handbook learning objectives, *Workbook* performance objectives for all assignments, use of the text with reinforcement by *Workbook* assignments and the test section at the end of the *Workbook*, and incorporation of classroom activities and suggestions from the *Instructor's Electronic Resource Guide on CD-ROM* provide a complete competency-based educational program.

Software

Because many medical practices use computer technology to perform financial operations, a user-friendly computer software tutorial program has been developed to accompany the *Handbook* and *Workbook*. The goal is to give the learner a hands-on, realistic approach as though working in a medical setting by selecting appropriate patient files to obtain needed information to complete the HCFA-1500 insurance claim form. These files include a patient information form for each case and either an encounter form or patient medical record. Key terms and abbreviations are integrated into the medical records of the last five cases, and definitions may be accessed from a linked glossary. The skill of extracting data from these documents and inserting data accurately, as well as assigning diagnostic and procedural code numbers to the HCFA-1500 claim form, is developed.

The tutorial allows the user to complete the HCFA-1500 insurance claim form by entering data in a "free form" manner. This means it is possible to move freely around the claim form, skipping unnecessary blocks and returning to blocks previously filled in. Claim form blocks with incorrect information are highlighted for immediate feedback, and a second attempt is offered to correct errors. If an error is repeated on a second try, correct information is filled in by the computer in italicized font. On printout, this emphasizes all blocks where more than one attempt was needed. Detailed score reports may be printed so that the instructor has access to the information.

The instructor may wish the student to work through basic cases one through four strictly for learning and to use case five for testing and grading. The last five cases, which are advanced and insurance specific (e.g., Medicare, TRICARE, Medicaid), may be used for practice or testing.

A section of the software designed for "Other patients" allows the user to complete and print all *Workbook* assignments in which the HCFA-1500 insurance claim form is required. This simulated learning methodology makes possible an easier transition from classroom to workplace.

Instructor's Electronic Resource Guide on CD-ROM

The instructor's manual has gone from a paperback book to *Instructor's Electronic Resource Guide on CD-ROM* and features the following:

1. Assists in development of a course in medical insurance
2. Renders ideas on how to use the text as an adjunct to a medical office procedures course
3. Gives classroom and suggested activities
4. Provides answer keys to the *Workbook* assignments and tests with rationale, optional codes, and further explanations for the majority of the code problems
5. Furnishes lecture slides for all chapters for use in overhead projection or in a Power Point presentation.
6. Contains a computerized test bank of over 1,000 questions to assist the instructor in test construction. It gives a variety of testing formats, such as multiple choice, true or false, mix and match,

completion of blanks, and labeling of illustrations. Questions are rated, i.e., Difficulty: easy, moderate, or hard, to help the instructor with test construction to the course being taught.

If an instructor is interested in establishing a one-year certificate program for insurance billing specialists and wishes networking and other information on how other schools have set up a program for this career field, write to or e-mail the author, using the mailing address in the resource.

Website

Shortly after the publication of this edition there will be a companion website established for instructors and students. Errors, corrections, and important technical updates will be available, as well as additional exercises for students. Many other features will be made available as the months progress—so go to the web site *http://www.wbsaunders.com/SIMON/Fordney/Handbook/* and experience it.

> An important update as this book was going to press that affects almost all chapters is that in June 2001 the Bush Administration gave a new name to the Health Care Financing Administration (HCFA). It is now known as the Centers for Medicare and Medicaid Services (CMS).

Summary

Escalating costs of medical care, the impact of technology, and the explosion of managed care plans have affected insurance billing procedures and claims processing and have required new legislation for government and state programs. Therefore, it is essential that all medical personnel handling claims continue to update their knowledge. This may be accomplished by reading bulletins from state agencies and regional insurance carriers, speaking with insurance representatives, or attending insurance workshops offered at local colleges or local chapters of professional associations, such as those mentioned in Chapters 1 and 17. It is hoped that this text will resolve any unclear issues pertaining to current methods and become the framework on which the insurance billing specialist builds new knowledge as understanding and appreciation of the profession are attained.

Marilyn Takahashi Fordney, CMA-AC, CMT
Oxnard, California

Acknowledgments

During my 14 years as a medical assistant, 19 years of teaching, and 26 years of writing, hundreds of students, physicians, friends, colleagues, and instructors have contributed valuable suggestions and interesting material for this book. I wish to express my thanks to all of them, with special emphasis on the following:

Lois C. Oliver, retired Professor, Pierce College, Woodland Hills, California, helped me organize my first medical insurance class in 1969 and offered assistance and encouragement throughout the preparation of the first edition of the *Handbook*.

Marcia O. "Marcy" Diehl, CMA-A, CMT, co-author and retired instructor, Grossmont Community College, El Cajon, California, generously shared her knowledge, ideas, and class materials.

Members of the *California Association of Medical Assistant Instructors (CAMAI)* contributed suggestions for improving the text and gave me motivation from time to time to continue the project.

Mary E. Kinn, CPS, CMA-A, author and retired Assistant Professor, Long Beach City College, Long Beach, California, provided a perspective review of my syllabus. Without her positive endorsement, the first edition of this book might not have been published.

Overwhelming thanks to my technical collaborator and contributor, Linda L. French, CMA-C, NCICS, who helped with the tremendous overhaul and restructuring of each chapter and lent technical and editorial assistance for the entire project. Writing has its ups and downs, and she gave me support during many of the difficult periods. Special thanks to the students of Linda's classes at the Simi Valley Adult School and Career Institute in Simi Valley, California, who contributed their criticisms, lent technical subject matter, offered suggestions, and through voluntary participation helped to enhance and create *Workbook* assignments. A note of appreciation to my assistant, Nina Janis, who did many tasks to allow me free time to research and write.

I gratefully acknowledge the artist involved with the design of the cover and full-color format, Gene Harris, Design Department, W. B. Saunders Company. The photograph for the Preface was taken by Jim Woods of Camarillo, California, and the photographs throughout the text were taken by Jack Foley, photographer, and Nick Kaufmann Productions, whom I wish to acknowledge and thank.

I also wish to thank the Print Shop Staff, Publications Department, Ventura College, Ventura, California, who printed the first California syllabus of this text.

I am indebted to many individuals on the staff of the W. B. Saunders Company for encouragement and guidance. I express particular appreciation to Adrianne Williams, Senior Acquisitions Editor, and her assistant, Rae Robertson, Developmental Editor; Tina Rebane, Production Editor, and Jeanne M. Carper, Copy Editor, for expert editing and coordination of the entire project. My thanks go also to Norman Stellander, Senior Production Manager, and John Needles, Jr., Illustrations Specialist.

Numerous supply companies were kind enough to cooperate by providing forms and descriptive literature of their products, and their names will be found throughout the text and workbook figures.

But colleagues, production staff, and editors working as a team do not quite make a book; there are others to whom I must express overwhelming debt and enduring gratitude, and these are the consultants who reviewed some of the chapters or who provided vital information about private, state, and federal insurance programs. Without the knowledge of these advisers, the massive task of compiling an insurance text truly national in scope might never have been completed. Although the names of all those who graciously assisted me are too numerous to mention, I take great pride in listing my principal consultants for this seventh edition.

Principal Consultants and Reviewers

Contents

Unit 5
Employment

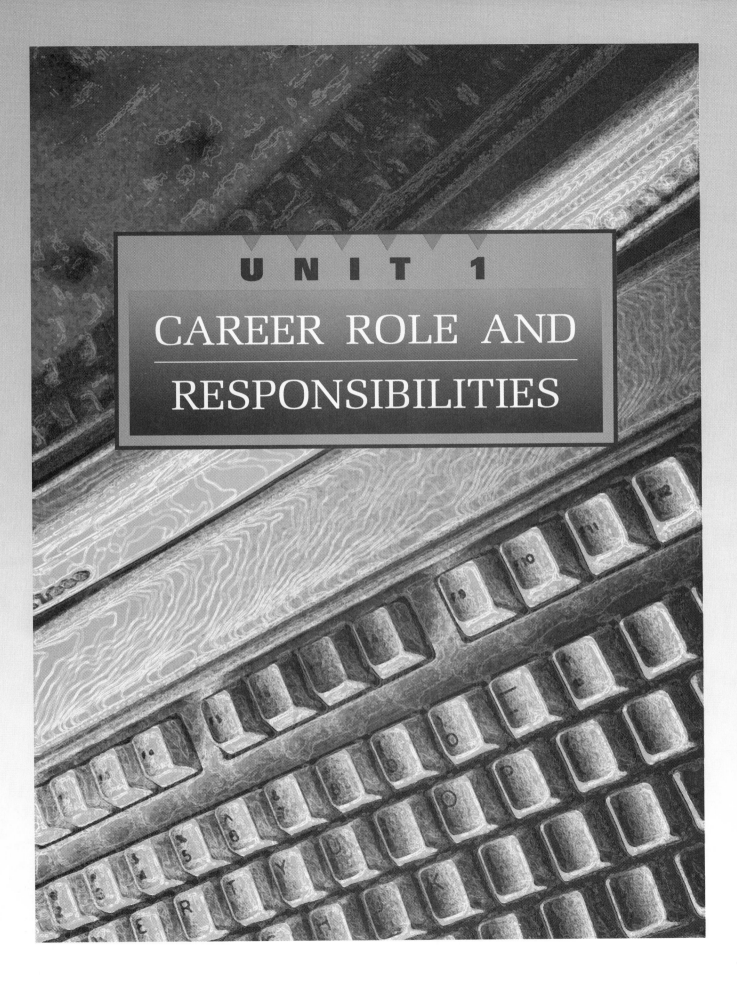

UNIT 1

CAREER ROLE AND RESPONSIBILITIES

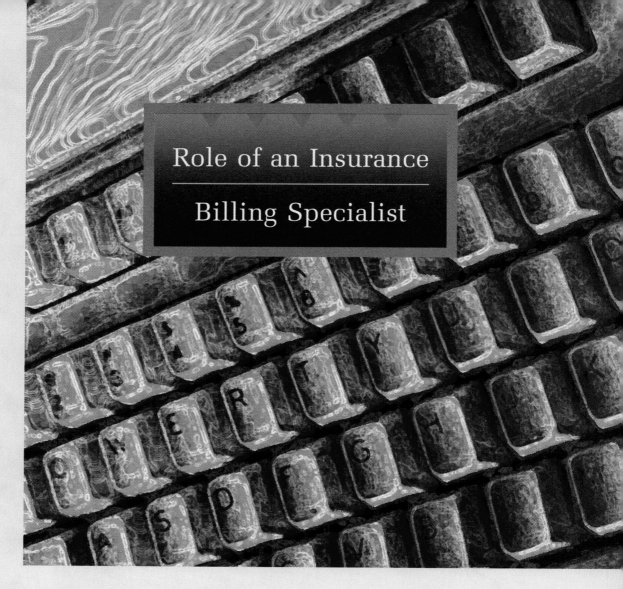

Role of an Insurance
Billing Specialist

1

CHAPTER OUTLINE

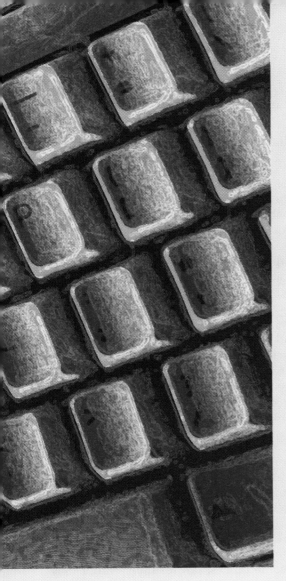

- List personal qualifications and skills to be acquired by an insurance billing specialist.
- State the personal image to be projected as an insurance billing specialist.
- Specify the educational requirements for a job as an insurance billing specialist and as a coder.
- Explain how insurance knowledge and medical knowledge can be kept current.
- Differentiate the differences between medical ethics and medical etiquette.
- Define confidential communication.
- Illustrate the difference between privileged and non-privileged information.
- Translate the Latin phrase *respondeat superior*.
- List various types of insurance fraud.
- Define abuse as it relates to the subject of insurance claims.
- State some precautions to take for financial protection.

OBJECTIVES*

After reading this chapter you should be able to:

- Identify the background and importance of insurance claims completion, coding, and billing.
- Name at least three skills possessed by insurance billing specialists.
- Describe the variety of career possibilities and areas of specialization open to those trained as insurance billing specialists.

KEY TERMS

abuse

American Health Information Management Association (AHIMA)

American Medical Association (AMA)

blanket-position bond

bonding

cash flow

churning

claims assistance professional (CAP)

confidential communication

embezzlement

ethics

etiquette

fraud

insurance billing specialist

list service (listserv)

multiskilled health practitioner (MSHP)

nonprivileged information

personal bond

phantom billing

ping-ponging

position-schedule bond

privileged information

reimbursement specialist

respondeat superior

yo-yoing

---

*Performance objectives and exercises for hands-on practical experience for this chapter appear in the *Workbook*.

Role of the Insurance Billing Specialist

Welcome to the world of insurance billing, an exciting, ever-changing, and fast growing career field. To help you focus on important terms and definitions, some of the basic words in this and subsequent chapters appear boldfaced or italicized. See the Glossary at the end of this textbook for a comprehensive list of key terms, with detailed definitions to broaden your knowledge.

In the past, a medical assistant working in a physician's office performed both administrative and clinical duties. Then, as decades passed, he or she performed either one or the other. Now, due to changes in government regulations and standards for the insurance industry, specific medical assisting job tasks have become specialized. In a medical practice, it is commonplace to find administrative duties shared by a number of employees (e.g., administrative medical assistant, bookkeeper, file clerk, insurance billing specialist, office manager, receptionist, transcriptionist). In some work settings, an **insurance billing specialist** may be known as an electronic claims processor, a medical biller, or a **reimbursement specialist.** In clinics and large practices, it is common to find a billing department made up of many people, and within the department each position is a specialist, such as Medicare billing specialist, Medicaid billing specialist, coding specialist, insurance counselor, collection manager, and medical and financial records manager.

Some medical practices and clinics contract with management services organizations (MSOs), which perform a variety of business functions, such as accounting, billing, coding, collections, computer support, legal advice, marketing, payroll, and management expertise. An insurance billing specialist may find a job working for an MSO as a part of this team.

Cost pressures on health care providers are forcing employers to reduce personnel costs by hiring **multiskilled health practitioners** (MSHPs). An MSHP is a person cross-trained to provide more than one function, often in more than one discipline. Knowledge of insurance claims completion and coding enhances skills so that he or she can offer more flexibility to someone hired in a medical setting.

There are also people called **claims assistance professionals** (CAPs), who work for the consumer and help patients organize, file, and negotiate health insurance claims of all types. Their primary goals are to assist the consumer in obtaining maximum benefits and to tell the patient what checks to write to providers to make sure there is no overpayment. A medical insurance billing specialist may also function in this role.

Job Responsibilities

Administrative front office duties have gained in importance for the following reasons. Documentation is vital to good patient care. It must be done comprehensively for proper reimbursement. Diagnostic and procedural coding must be reviewed for its correctness and completeness. Insurance claims must be promptly submitted manually or transmitted electronically (ideally within 48 hours) to ensure continuous cash flow. **Cash flow** is the amount of actual money available to the medical practice. Without money coming in, overhead expenses cannot be met and a practice would fold. Data required for billing must be collected from hospitals, laboratories, and other physicians involved in a case.

In large medical practices, an insurance billing specialist may act as an insurance counselor, taking the patient to a private area of the office to discuss the patient's treatment plan and insurance coverage and negotiate a reasonable payment plan. This is done to ensure the physician will be paid for services rendered and to develop good communication lines. The counselor learns the deductible amount and verifies with the insurance company whether any preauthorization, precertification, or second-opinion requirements exist. Counseling helps obtain payment in full when expensive procedures are necessary. In some offices, the insurance biller may act as a collection manager who answers routine inquiries related to account balances and insurance submission dates, assists patients in budgeting, follows up on delinquent accounts, and traces denied, "adjusted," or unpaid claims (Fig. 1-1).

In 1997 the American Association of Medical Assistants (AAMA) developed a role delineation study analyzing the many job functions of the medical assistant. Table 1-1 shows the Medical Assistant Role Delineation Chart, with highlighted areas indicating material covered in this textbook. The topics shown on the role delineation chart must be studied to pass the certification examination offered by the AAMA. Further information about many types of certification and registration are shown in Chapter 17.

Educational and Training Requirements

Generally, a high school diploma or general equivalency diploma (GED) is required for entry into an insurance billing and/or coding specialist accredited program. The accredited program usually offers additional education in medical terminology,

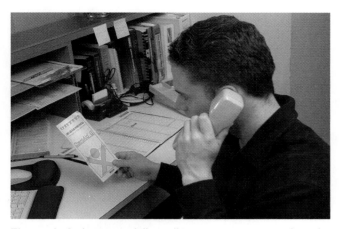

Figure 1–1. Insurance biller talking to a patient on the telephone about copayment required for an office visit under the patient's insurance plan.

insurance claims completion, procedural and diagnostic coding, anatomy and physiology, computer skills, ethics and medicolegal knowledge, and general office skills. For one who seeks a job as a coder, completion of an accredited program for coding certification or an accredited health information medical record technology program is necessary.

For one who seeks a job as an insurance billing specialist, experience in coding and insurance claims completion and/or completion of a 1-year insurance specialist certificate program at a community college is usually required. The curriculum that might be offered in a 1-year certificate program is shown in Figure 1–2. Since the information contained in that figure is specifically from a community college in Pennsylvania, you might find that the courses in your locale may be labeled with different titles and time frames. Courses should cover medical terminology, anatomy and physiology, introduction to computer technology, procedural and diagnostic coding, and a comprehensive course on medical insurance billing. A 2-year educational course can result in obtaining an associate degree. Training prepares an individual for a wide range of employment opportunities. If you are planning to become an electronic claims processor, then knowledge of computer hardware and software, electronic data transmission requirements, and health care claim reimbursement is recommended. Many accredited programs include an externship (on-the-job) period of training that may be paid or unpaid.

The **American Health Information Management Association** (AHIMA) published diagnostic and procedure coding competencies for outpatient services and diagnostic coding and reporting requirements for physician billing. Refer to these competencies for a more inclusive list of educational and training requirements (Fig. 1–3).

If your goal is to become a claims assistance professional, it is necessary to have a moderate to high degree of knowledge of the health insurance business. In addition to insurance terminology, claims procedures, and coding, you must know commercial insurance carriers' requirements and Medicare policies and regulations. You will also need human relations skills and proficiency in running a business, including marketing and sales expertise.

To reach a professional level, certification is available from many national associations, depending on the type of certification desired. Refer to Chapter 17 for more information on this topic.

Career Advantages

Jobs are available in every state, ranging from non-management to management positions. Insurance billing specialists can receive a salary of $8,000 part time to $40,000 full time or more per year depending on knowledge, experience, duties, responsibilities, locale, and size of the employing institution. Jobs are available in consulting firms, insurance and managed care companies, clinics, hospitals, multispecialty medical groups, and private physicians' practices and as instructors or lecturers. You can be your own boss by either setting up an in-home billing service or establishing an office service for billing.

Many people establish self-owned and self-operated businesses within their communities as medical insurance billing specialists, coders, claim assistance professionals, or collectors. However, the responsibilities are greater in this area, because you have to set up the business, obtain clients, and advertise and market the business (see Chapter 17).

Another advantage of this career field is the opportunity to have flexible hours. Most employees in the physician's office must adhere to the physician's schedule. However, the medical insurance billing specialist may want to come in early to transmit electronic claims during nonpeak hours or stay late to make collection calls. It may be advantageous to both the physician and the insurance specialist to vary his or her schedule according to the needs of the practice. In-home or office billing services save a medical practice valuable time, money, and overhead costs because the physician does not have to cover benefits or equipment.

A great asset to a medical practice is a collector of delinquent accounts. This job is for individuals who have current knowledge of state and federal collection laws and interact well with people in

TABLE 1–1   **Medical Assistant Role Delineation Chart**

ADMINISTRATIVE

Administrative Procedures
- Perform basic clerical functions
- Schedule, coordinate, and monitor appointments
- Schedule inpatient/outpatient admissions and procedures
- Understand and apply third party guidelines
- Obtain reimbursement through accurate claims submission
- Monitor third party reimbursement
- Perform medical transcription
- Understand and adhere to managed care policies and procedures
- Negotiate managed care contracts (adv*)

Practice Finances
- Perform procedural and diagnostic coding
- Apply bookkeeping principles
- Document and maintain accounting and banking records
- Manage accounts receivable
- Manage accounts payable
- Process payroll
- Develop and maintain fee schedules (adv*)
- Manage renewals of business and professional insurance policies (adv*)
- Manage personal benefits and maintain records (adv*)

CLINICAL

Fundamental Principles
- Apply principles of aseptic technique and infection control
- Comply with quality assurance practices
- Screen and follow up patient test results

Diagnostic Orders
- Collect and process specimens
- Perform diagnostic tests

Patient Care
- Adhere to established triage procedures
- Obtain patient history and vital signs
- Prepare and maintain examination and treatment areas

- Prepare patient for examinations, procedures, and treatments
- Assist with examinations, procedures, and treatments
- Prepare and administer medications and immunizations
- Maintain medication and immunization records
- Recognize and respond to emergencies
- Coordinate patient care information with other health care providers

GENERAL (TRANSDISCIPLINARY)

Professionalism
- Project a professional manner and image
- Adhere to ethical principles
- Demonstrate initiative and responsibility
- Work as a team member
- Manage time efficiently
- Prioritize and perform multiple tasks
- Adapt to change
- Promote the CMA credential
- Enhance skills through continuing education

Communication Skills
- Treat all patients with compassion and empathy
- Recognize and respect cultural diversity
- Adapt communications to individual's ability to understand
- Use professional telephone technique
- Use effective and correct verbal and written communications
- Recognize and respond to verbal and nonverbal communications
- Use medical terminology appropriately

Legal Concepts
- Maintain confidentiality
- Practice within the scope of education, training, and personal capabilities
- Prepare and maintain medical records
- Document accurately
- Use appropriate guidelines when releasing information
- Follow employer's established policies dealing with the health care contract
- Follow federal, state, and local legal guidelines
- Maintain awareness of federal and state health care legislation and regulations
- Maintain and dispose of regulated substances in compliance with government guidelines
- Comply with established risk management and safety procedures
- Recognize professional credentialing criteria
- Participate in the development and maintenance of personnel, policy, and procedure manuals
- Develop and maintain personnel, policy, and procedure manuals (adv*)

Instruction
- Instruct individuals according to their needs
- Explain office policies and procedures
- Teach methods of health promotion and disease prevention
- Locate community resources and disseminate information
- Orient and train personnel (adv*)
- Develop educational materials
- Conduct continuing education activities (adv*)

Operational Functions
- Maintain supply inventory
- Evaluate and recommend equipment and supplies
- Apply computer techniques to support office operations
- Supervise personnel (adv*)
- Interview and recommend job applicants (adv*)
- Negotiate leases and prices for equipment and supply contracts (adv*)

continued

Table 1-1 *continued*		
GENERAL (TRANSDISCIPLINARY)		

Communication Skills

■ Receive, organize, prioritize, and transmit information

■ Serve as liaison

■ Promote the practice through positive public relations

Green colored blocks represent skills taught in this textbook.

White colored blocks are additional skills an insurance billing specialist may need.

* Denotes advanced skills.

Reprinted by permission of the American Association of Medical Assistants from the AAMA Role Delineation Study. Occupational Analysis of the Medical Assisting Profession.

person and by telephone. This aspect of financial management and other jobs involving telephone communications are an opportunity for someone visually impaired because when properly and specifically trained he or she is usually a good listener. However, special equipment may be necessary to enhance job performance (e.g., Braille keyboard, magnified computer screen, audible

Figure 1–2. Example of a 1-year medical insurance specialist certificate program offered at a community college. Basic coding is taught as a part of the course in Administrative Medical Office Management, and advanced coding is covered in Principles and Applications of Medical Insurance. Human Biology may be titled Anatomy and Physiology in some colleges. (Reprinted with permission from Community College of Allegheny County, Pittsburgh, PA.)

MEDICAL INSURANCE SPECIALIST CERTIFICATE PROGRAM

PROGRAM DESCRIPTION: The Medical Insurance program prepares you for employment in the area of medical insurance and health care claims processing. This program also serves the needs of health care personnel interested in upgrading their professional skills. Training in computerized medical billing, CPT-4 and ICD-9-CM coding, and processing medical insurance claims are included in the curriculum. Students may be enrolled on a full-time or part-time basis, and may complete the program by attending either day or evening classes. Accelerated or fasttrack courses are also available for those wishing to complete this program within a short time period. The program graduates students with marketable skills that will be in demand well into the 21st century. They are employed in hospitals, insurance companies, private medical laboratories, billing bureaus, and doctors' offices. Graduates may apply credits toward other certificate or associate degree programs.

The following courses are included in this program:

First Semester

Medical Terminology	3 Credits
Administrative Medical Office Management	4 Credits
Human Biology	5 Credits
Typewriting I or Keyboarding	3 Credits
	TOTAL 15 Credits

Second Semester

Principles and Applications of Medical Insurance	3 Credits
Current Issues of Medical Insurance	3 Credits
Medical Financial Management	3 Credits
Word Processing	3 Credits
Basic Principles of Composition	3 Credits
	TOTAL 15 Credits

AMERICAN HEALTH INFORMATION MANAGEMENT ASSOCIATION
ICD-9-CM AND CPT-HCPCS AMBULATORY CARE CODING COMPETENCIES

ICD-9-CM - *International Classification of Diseases - 9th Revision, Clinical Modification, Volumes 1 and 2,*
Superintendent of Documents, US Government Printing Office, P. Box 371954,
Pittsburgh, PA 15250-7954, (202) 783-3238.
Volume 3, American Health Information Management Association, 919 N. Michigan Avenue,
Suite 1400, Chicago, IL 60611, (312) 787-2672.
CPT - Current Procedural Terminology, American Medical Association
515 N. State St., Chicago, IL 60610, (800) 621-8335.
HCPCS - HCFA *[Health Care Financing Administration] Common Procedure Coding System-Level Two*
Superintendent of Documents, US Government Printing Office,
Washington, DC 20402. (202) 783-3238

ICD-9-CM DIAGNOSTIC CODING

1. Read and interpret medical record documentation to identify all diagnoses, conditions, problems, or other reasons for the ambulatory care encounter/visit.

2. Assess the adequacy of medical record documentation to ensure that it supports the diagnoses, conditions, problems, or other reasons for an ambulatory care encounter/visit assigned codes.

3. Clarify conflicting or ambiguous information appearing in a medical record by consulting the appropriate physician.

4. Apply the Basic Coding Guidelines for Outpatient Services* and Diagnostic Coding and Reporting Requirements for Physician Billing* to select and sequence diagnoses, conditions, problems, or other reasons which require coding in an ambulatory care encounter/visit.

5. Exclude from coding diagnoses, conditions, and problems which are no longer being treated or which have no bearing on the management of the current ambulatory care encounter/visit.

6. Apply knowledge of ICD-9-CM instructional notations and conventions to locate and assign the correct diagnostic codes and sequence them correctly.

7. Apply knowledge of anatomy, clinical disease process, and diagnostic terminology to assign accurate codes to each individual diagnosis, condition, problem, or other reason for encounter/visit.

8. Apply knowledge of disease processes to assign non-indexed medical terms to the appropriate class in the classification system.

9. Conduct quality assessment to ensure continuous improvement in ICD-9-CM coding and collection of quality health data.

CPT-HCPCS PROCEDURAL CODING

1. Read and interpret medical record documentation to identify all sevices and procedures performed during the ambulatory care encounter/visit.

2. Assess the adequacy of medical record documentation to ensure that it supports the procedures and services assigned codes.

3. Clarify conflicting, ambiguous, or non-specific information appearing in a medical record by consulting the appropriate physician.

4. Apply knowledge of CPT format, guidelines, and notes, to locate the correct codes for all services and procedures performed during the encounter/visit and sequence them correctly.

5. Apply knowledge of the HCPCS-Level Two (alphanumeric) coding system, if applicable, to locate the correct procedural codes and sequence them correctly.

6. Apply knowledge of anatomy and procedural terminology to assign accurate codes to procedures.

7. Apply knowledge of procedural terminology to recognize when an unlisted procedure code must be used in CPT.

8. Refuse to unfairly maximize reimbursement by unbundling services and codes that do not conform to CPT basic coding principles and payer reimbursement guidelines.

9. Apply knowledge of payer reimbursement guidelines to ensure optional reimbursement.

10. Conduct quality assessment to ensure continuing improvement in CPT/HCPCS-Level Two coding.

*Diagnostic Coding Guidelines for Outpatient Services and Diagnostic Coding and Reporting Requirements for Physician Billing were published in the First Quarter 1990 Coding Clinic for ICD-9-CM (Vol. 7, No. 1), a quarterly publication of the Central Office on ICD-9-CM at the American Hospital Association and the October 1990 Journal of the American Medical Association. January 1, 1992

Figure 1–3. Diagnostic and procedural coding competencies for outpatient services and diagnostic coding and reporting requirements for physician billing. (Reprinted with permission from the American Health Information Management Association, Chicago, IL, as published in the First Quarter 1990 Coding Clinic for ICD-9-CM [Vol. 7, No. 1].)

scanner, tape recorder). You may contact the American Collectors Association (ACA) in Minneapolis, Minnesota, which has developed a training program for the visually impaired. Chapter 9 is devoted entirely to the topic of collections.

Qualifications

Attributes

There are many characteristics or qualities that an individual should have to function well as an insurance billing specialist. Strong critical thinking and reading skills with good comprehension are a must. It is important to be a logical and practical thinker as well as creative in solving problems. Being meticulous and neat makes it easier to get the job done at the work station. A person with good organizational skills and who is conscientious and loyal is always an asset to the employer. To have a curious nature means he or she will dig deeper into an issue and is simply not satisfied with an answer unless the whys and whats are defined. This also helps one to grow while on the job and not become stagnant. This list is by no means complete, and maybe you can think of some additional attributes that might lead to a more successful career.

Skills

Completing insurance claims encompasses many skills and to be proficient, one needs the following:

▶ Solid foundation and working knowledge of medical terminology, including anatomy and physiology and disease and treatment terms as well as meaning of abbreviations.

  Application: Interpretation of patient's chart notes and code manuals.

  Incorrect: Final diagnosis: ASHD.
  Correct: Final diagnosis: Arteriosclerotic heart disease.

  It would be difficult to locate the diagnostic code using an abbreviation so you must be able to translate it.

▶ Expert use of procedural and diagnostic code books and other related resources

  Application: Code manuals and other reference books are used to assign accurate codes for each case billed.

▶ Precise reading skills

  Application: Differentiate between a technical description of two different but similar procedures.

  Procedure (CPT) Code No. 43352 Esophagostomy *(fistulization of esophagus, external; cervical approach)*

Procedure (CPT) Code No. 43020 Esophagotomy *(cervical approach, with removal of foreign body)*

  Note that the additional letter "s" to the surgical procedure in part one of the example changes the entire procedure.

▶ Basic mathematics

  Application: Total fees on the insurance claim forms and adjust and total accounts. It is essential that these figures be accurate.

▶ Knowledge of medicolegal rules and regulations of various insurance programs

  Application: Avoid filing of claims considered fraudulent or abusive because of code selection and program policies.

▶ Basic typing or keyboarding and computer skills

  Application: Good keyboarding skills and knowledge of computer software programs is essential because the industry increasingly involves electronic claims submission; handwritten claims are a format of the past.

▶ Proficiency in accessing information through the Internet

  Application: Obtain federal, state, and commercial insurance regulations and current information as needed through the Internet. Sign on as a member of a **list service (listserv)** which is a service run from a web site where questions may be posted. Find one composed of working coders to obtain answers on how to code complex, rare, or difficult medical cases.

▶ Knowledge of billing and collection techniques

  Application: Use latest billing and collection ideas to keep cash flow constant and to avoid delinquent accounts.

▶ Expertise in the legalities of collection on accounts

  Application: Avoid lawsuits by knowing state and federal collection laws as they apply to medical collection of accounts receivable.

▶ Generate insurance claims with speed and accuracy

  Application: If you develop your own business as a medical claims and billing specialist, you may be paid according to how many claims you can generate in an hour. You may charge less for claims that can be done quickly and more for claims that take longer to complete. The faster you become, the more money you earn. Therefore, accuracy in selecting the correct codes and speed in completing claims also become marketable skills. Measure your claim productivity for speed and time when you complete the insurance claim forms for this course and see how progressively fast you can get.

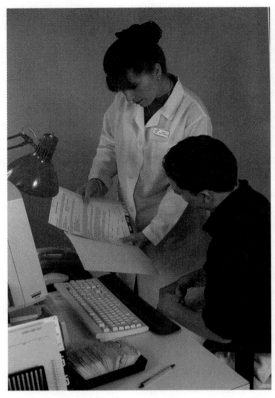

Figure 1–4. Illustration of male and female medical personnel projecting a clean, fresh, and professional image with hairstyling in good taste.

Personal Image

To project a professional image, be attentive to apparel and grooming (Fig. 1–4). If a person works at home, the tendency is to dress casually (e.g., blue jeans, sneakers, shorts, tank tops). However, in a work setting, a uniform may be required or business attire that is conservative and stylish but not trendy is acceptable. For women, this includes a business suit, dress, or skirts of appropriate length; slacks; sweaters; blouses; and dress shoes. For men, a business suit, or dress slacks and jacket, shirt, tie (optional), and dress shoes are appropriate.

It is important that hair be clean and in a style that flatters. Because fragrances can be offensive or cause allergies to some clients and patients, so they should not be used. Fingernails should be carefully manicured. Long artificial nails are not considered to be part of a professional image; clear or muted pleasant colored polish without glued-on designs or rhinestones is acceptable. For a woman, subdued eye makeup is appropriate for day use.

For either gender, jewelry should be simple and dangling earrings avoided. A professional pin is frequently worn in an office setting and at professional functions. Consult the employer for office policy regarding body piercing and tattoos.

Behavior

There are many aspects to what makes an individual a true professional. Getting along with people rates high on the list, as does maintaining confidentiality of patients' medical histories and ongoing medical treatment. An insurance billing specialist depends on many coworkers for information needed to bill claims (e.g., the receptionist who collects the patient information). It is therefore necessary to be a team player and treat patients and coworkers with courtesy and respect. Consider all coworkers' duties as important because they are part of the team helping you obtain the goal of processing the billing and obtaining maximum reimbursement for the patient and physician. Communicate effectively. Be honest, dependable, and on time. Never take part in office gossip or politics. Be willing to do the job and be efficient in how you carry it out.

Medical Etiquette

Before beginning work as an insurance billing specialist, it is wise to have a basic knowledge of medical etiquette as it pertains to the medical profession, the insurance industry, and the medical coder (Fig. 1–5). Medical **etiquette** has to do with how medical professionals conduct themselves. Customs, courtesy, and manners of the medical profession can be expressed in three simple words—*consideration for others.*

Several points about medical etiquette bear mentioning:

1. Never keep another physician waiting longer than necessary in the reception room. Usher him or her into the physician's office as soon as it is free.

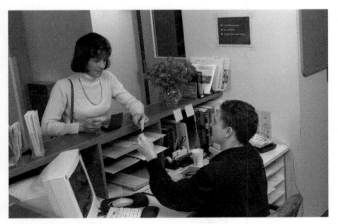

Figure 1–5. Interaction of insurance billing specialist with patient depicting medical etiquette.

2. Always connect another physician on the telephone to your physician immediately, asking as few questions as possible. The only exception to this is if you know the physician calling is treating one of your patients and you wish to verify the name to pull the chart for your physician.

3. Follow the basic rules of etiquette with coworkers while working in the office, such as acknowledging people who enter your office or come to your desk by saying "I'll be with you in a moment."

4. Identify yourself to callers and to those you call.

5. Do not be too casual by using first names until you know it is appropriate to do so.

6. Keep a professional demeanor and maintain a certain amount of formality when interacting with others. Remember to be courteous and always project a professional image.

Medical Ethics

Medical **ethics** are not laws but are standards of conduct generally accepted as a moral guide for behavior by which an insurance billing or coding specialist may determine the propriety of his or her conduct in a relationship with patients, the physician, coworkers, the government, and insurance companies. Acting with ethical behavior means to carry out responsibilities with integrity, decency, honesty, competence, consideration, respect, fairness, trust, and courage.

The earliest written code of ethical principles and conduct for the medical profession originated in Babylonia about 2500 BC and is called the Code of Hammurabi. Then in about the fifth century BC, Hippocrates, a Greek physician who is known as the Father of Medicine, conceived the Oath of Hippocrates.

In 1980 the **American Medical Association** (AMA) adopted a modern code of ethics called the Principles of Medical Ethics for the benefit of the health professional and to meet the needs of changing times. The Principles of Medical Ethics of the AMA shown in the following box guide physicians' standards of conduct for honorable behavior in the practice of medicine.

It is the coder's responsibility to inform administration or his or her immediate supervisor if unethical or possibly illegal coding practices are taking place. Illegal activities are subject to penalties, fines, an/or imprisonment and can result in loss of morale, reputation, and the goodwill of the community.

Preamble

The medical profession has long subscribed to a body of ethical statements developed primarily for the benefit of the patient.

As a member of the profession, a physician must recognize responsibility not only to patients, but also to society, to other health professionals, and to self. The following Principles adopted by the American Medical Association are not laws, but standards of conduct which define the essentials of honorable behavior for the physician.

I. A physician shall be dedicated to providing competent medical service with compassion and respect for human dignity.

II. A physician shall deal honestly with patients and colleagues, and strive to expose those physicians deficient in character or competence, or who engage in fraud or deception.

III. A physician shall respect the law and also recognize a responsibility to seek changes in those requirements which are contrary to the best interests of the patient.

IV. A physician shall respect the rights of patients, of colleagues, and of other health professionals, and shall safeguard patient confidences within the constraints of the law.

V. A physician shall continue to study, apply and advance scientific knowledge, make relevant information available to patients, colleagues, and the public, obtain consultation, and use the talents of other health professionals when indicated.

VI. A physician shall, in the provision of appropriate patient care, except in emergencies, be free to choose whom to serve, with whom to associate, and the environment in which to provide medical services.

VII. A physician shall recognize a responsibility to participate in activities contributing to an improved community.

Some principles of ethics for the medical assistant and insurance billing specialist are as follows:

▶ Never make critical remarks about a physician to a patient or anyone else.

▶ Maintain dignity; never belittle patients.

▶ Notify your physician if you discover that a patient of your practice may have questionable issues of care, conduct, or treatment with your office or another physician's practice. In certain circumstances, it may be unethical for two physicians to treat the same patient for the same condition.

▶ Maintain a dignified, courteous relationship with all persons in the office—patients, staff, and the physician—as well as with insurance adjusters, pharmaceutical representatives, and others who come into or telephone the office.

▶ Do not make critical statements about the treatment given a patient by another physician.

It is *illegal* to report incorrect information to government-funded programs, such as Medicare, Medicaid, and TRICARE. However, private insurance carriers operate under different laws and it is *unethical, not illegal*, to report incorrect information to private insurance carriers. Incorrect information can possibly damage the individual and the integrity of the database, may allow reimbursement for services that should be paid by the patient, or can deny payment that should be made by the insurance company.

Some examples of illegal or unethical coding are

1. Violating guidelines by using code numbers or modifiers to increase payment when the case documentation does not warrant it
2. Coding procedures for payment that were not performed
3. Unbundling services provided into separate codes when one code is available
4. Failure to code a relevant condition or complication when it is documented in the medical record
5. Coding a service in such a way that it is paid when it usually is not covered
6. Coding another condition as the principal diagnosis when the majority of the patient's treatment is for the preexisting condition

Because some insurance billing specialists also have medical assistant responsibilities, the American Association of Medical Assistants, Inc. (AAMA) has established a code of ethics. This code is appropriate for all medical assistants, members and nonmembers, regardless of whether they are performing administrative or clinical duties (Fig. 1–6).

In the final analysis, most ethical issues can be reduced to right and wrong with the main focus— not to lose sight of the moral dictum to do no harm.

Confidential Communication

When working with patients and their medical records, the insurance billing specialist must be responsible for maintaining confidentiality of communication. **Confidential communication** is a privileged communication that may be disclosed only with the patient's permission. Everything you see, hear, or read about patients remains confidential and does not leave the office. Never talk about patients or data contained in medical records where others may overhear. Some employers require employees to sign a confidentiality agreement (Fig. 1–7). Such agreements should be updated periodically to address issues raised by the use of new technologies.

Privileged Information

Privileged information is related to the treatment and progress of the patient. The patient must sign an authorization to release this information or selected facts from the medical record. Some states have passed laws allowing certain test results (e.g., disclosure of the presence of the human immunodeficiency virus [HIV] or alcohol or substance

Figure 1–6. Principles of medical ethics for medical assistants as established by the American Association of Medical Assistants, Inc., Chicago, IL. Reprinted with permission.

AMERICAN ASSOCIATION OF MEDICAL ASSISTANTS, INC.
PRINCIPLES OF MEDICAL ETHICS

Members of this association dedicated to the conscientious pursuit of their profession, and thus desiring to merit the high regard of the entire medical profession and the respect of the general public which they serve, do pledge themselves to strive always to:

1. Render service to humanity with full respect for the dignity of person.

2. Respect confidential information gained through employment unless legally authorized or required by responsible performance of duty to divulge such information.

3. Uphold the honor and high principles of the profession and accept its disciplines.

4. Seek to continually improve the knowledge and skills of medical assisting for the benefit of patients and professional colleagues.

5. Participate in additional service activities which aim toward improving the health and well-being of the community.

EMPLOYEE CONFIDENTIALITY STATEMENT

As an employee of _____ ABC Clinic, Inc. _____ (employer), and having been trained as an insurance billing specialist with employee responsibilities and authorization to access personal medical and health information, I recognize that violation of confidentiality statutes and rules may lead to immediate dismissal from employment and, depending on state laws, criminal prosecution. I understand that such violation may cause irreparable damage to my employer, and the employer and any other injured party may seek legal action against me. I acknowledge that this signed document will be placed in my personnel file at this facility.

Mary Doe   _Brenda Shield_
Signature   Witness signature

_____Mary Doe_____
Print name

___September 14, 2000___
Date

Figure 1–7. An example of an employee confidentiality agreement that may be used by an employer when he or she is hiring an insurance billing specialist.

abuse) and other information to be placed separate from the patient's medical record. A special authorization form to release this information is used.

Nonprivileged Information

Nonprivileged information consists of ordinary facts unrelated to treatment of the patient. This might include the patient's name, city of residence, and dates of admission or discharge. The patient's authorization is not needed unless the record is in a specialty hospital (e.g., alcohol treatment) or in a special service unit of a general, hospital (e.g., psychiatric unit). Professional judgment is required. The information is disclosed on a legitimate "need-to-know" basis, meaning the medical data needs to be revealed to the attending physician because this may have some effect on the treatment of the patient.

Right to Privacy

All patients have a right to privacy. It is important never to discuss patient information other than with the physician, an insurance company, or individual who has been authorized by the patient. If a telephone inquiry is made about a patient, ask the caller to put the request in writing and include the patient's signed authorization. If the caller refuses, have the physician return the call. If a relative telephones asking about a patient, have the physician return the call. When you telephone a patient about an insurance matter and reach voice mail, use care in the choice of words when leaving the message in the event the call was inadvertently received at the wrong number. Leave your

name, the office name, and return telephone number. Never attempt to interpret a report or provide information regarding the outcome of laboratory or other diagnostic tests to the patient. Let the physician do it (Fig. 1–8).

Do not discuss a patient with acquaintances—yours or the patient's. Do not leave patients' records or appointment books exposed on your desk. If confidential documents are on your desk that patients can easily see as they walk by, either turn the documents over or lock them in a secure drawer when you leave your desk, even if you are gone for only a few moments. If patient information is on your computer, either turn the screen off or save it on disk, lock the disk away, and clear the information from the screen. Never leave a computer screen with patient information visible,

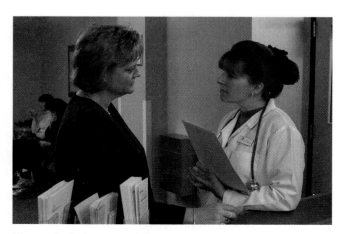

Figure 1–8. Insurance billing specialist consulting with the supervisor/office manager discussing office policies regarding release of a patient's medical record.

even for a moment, if another patient may see the data. Properly dispose of notes, papers, and memos by using a shredding device. Be careful when using the copying machine because it is easy to forget to remove the original insurance claim or medical record from the document glass. Use common sense and follow the guidelines mentioned in this chapter to help you keep your professional credibility and integrity.

Exceptions to the Right to Privacy

The few exceptions to the right of privacy and privileged communication are patient records of industrial cases (i.e., workers' compensation), reports of communicable diseases, child abuse, gunshot wounds and stabbings resulting from criminal actions, and diseases and ailments of newborns and infants. Also, any medical information obtained by a Medicare insurance carrier is subject to disclosure to the beneficiary to whom that information pertains. Medical information cannot be accepted by a Medicare insurance carrier from physicians on a confidential basis without the patient's knowledge, either expressed or implied. Expressed and implied contracts are defined in detail in the next chapter. Even if medical information is marked "Confidential," the Medicare insurance carrier must still disclose it to the beneficiary or his representative on request, either directly or through designated professional medical personnel.

Professional Liability

Employer Liability

As mentioned earlier, insurance billing specialists can be either self-employed or employed by physicians, clinics, or hospitals. Physicians are legally responsible for their own conduct and for any actions of their employees performed within the context of their employment. This is referred to as vicarious liability, also known as ***respondeat superior***, which literally means "let the master answer." However, this does not mean that an employee cannot be sued or brought to trial. Actions of the insurance biller may have a definite legal ramification on the employer depending on the situation. For example, if an employee knowingly submits a fraudulent Medicare or Medicaid claim at the direction of the employer and subsequently the business is audited, the employer and the employee can be brought into litigation by the state or federal government. An insurance biller should always check with his or her physician-employer to see whether he or she is included in the medical professional liability insurance policy otherwise known as malpractice insurance. If not included, he or she could be sued as individuals. It is the physician's responsibility to make certain all staff members are protected.

Fraud

Fraud is *knowing* and *intentional* deception (lying) or misrepresentation that could result in some unauthorized benefit to the deceiver or some other person. It is a felony, and if detected, financial or prison penalties can be imposed, depending on the laws of the state. It is important to tell the patient how services will be billed to avoid possible fraud and abuse audits. For example, a hospitalized patient is not always aware that the attending physician has requested a consultation, which will result in a separate bill, or that a simple invasive procedure done in the physician's office may be referred to as a surgical procedure on the monthly statement because the code number is obtained from the surgical section of the procedure code book. If a Medicare or TRICARE case is involved, then fraud becomes a federal offense and federal laws apply. Claims are audited by state and federal agencies as well as private insurance companies.

Usually fraud involves careful planning. Some examples are shown in Table 1–2. Two types of intent must be proved; intent to agree to practice a fraudulent act and intent to commit a major offense. When an insurance billing specialist completes the insurance claim form with billing information that does not reflect the true situation, then he or she may be found guilty of conspiring to commit fraud. It is not necessary to receive monetary profit from a fraudulent act to be judged guilty in participating in a criminal conspiracy.

Unintentional fraud may occur when completing the HCFA-1500 insurance claim form. For example, in a Medicare case, if benefits are assigned to the physician and the statement "signature on file" is inserted in Block 12 and the records do not contain the patient's authorization to file the claim on his or her behalf, this is a federal violation. The insurance billing specialist must verify that the authorization is for the insurance company in question. To prevent this problem from occurring in Medicare cases, obtain lifetime authorizations for the Medicare fiscal intermediary and for the patient's supplemental (Medigap) insurance company.

TABLE 1–2	**Examples of Fraud**
▶ Bill for services or supplies not provided (**phantom billing** or invoice ghosting) or for an office visit if a patient fails to keep an appointment and is not notified ahead of time that this is office policy ▶ Alter fees on a claim form to obtain higher payment ▶ Forgive the deductible or copayment ▶ Alter medical records to generate fraudulent payments ▶ Leave relevant information off a claim (e.g., failing to reveal whether a spouse has health insurance coverage through an employer) ▶ Upcode (e.g., submitting a code for a complex fracture when the patient had a simple fracture) ▶ Shorten (e.g., dispensing less medication than billed for) ▶ Split billing schemes (e.g., billing procedures over a period of days when all treatment occurred during one visit) ▶ Use another person's insurance card in obtaining medical care ▶ Change a date of service ▶ Post adjustments to generate fraudulent payments	▶ Solicit, offer, or receive a kickback, bribe, or rebate in return for referring a patient to a physician, physical therapist, or pharmacy or for referring a patient to obtain any item or service that may be paid for in full or in part by Medicare or Medicaid ▶ Restate the diagnosis to obtain insurance benefits or better payment ▶ Apply deliberately for duplicate payment (e.g., billing Medicare twice, billing Medicare and the beneficiary for the same service, or billing Medicare and another insurer in an attempt to get paid twice) ▶ Unbundle or explode charge (e.g., billing a multichannel laboratory test as if individual tests were performed) ▶ Collusion between a physician and a carrier employee when the claim is assigned (if the physician deliberately overbilled for services, overpayments could be generated with little awareness on the part of the Medicare beneficiary) ▶ Bills based on gang visits (e.g., a physician visits nursing home and bills for 20 visits without furnishing any specific service to, or on behalf of, individual patients)

A coder or biller who has knowledge of fraud or abuse should take the following measures:

1. Notify the provider both personally and with a dated, written memorandum.
2. Document the false statement or representation of the material fact.
3. Send a memorandum to the office manager or employer stating your concern if no change is made.
4. Keep a written audit trail with dated memoranda.
5. Do not discuss the problem with anyone who is not immediately involved.

Abuse

Abuse means incidents or practices by physicians, not usually considered fraudulent, that are inconsistent with accepted sound medical business or fiscal practices. Some examples are shown in Table 1–3.

In subsequent chapters about various insurance programs, additional information about fraud and abuse pertinent to each program is given.

Employee Liability

Errors and omissions insurance is protection against loss of monies due to failure through error or unintentional omission on the part of the individual or service submitting the insurance claim. Some physicians contract with a billing service to handle claims submission, and some agreements contain a clause stating that the physician will hold the company harmless from "liability resulting from claims submitted by the service for any account." This means the physician is responsible for mistakes made by the billing service. Thus, an errors and omissions insurance would not be needed in this instance. If a physician asks the insurance biller to do something that is in the least bit ques-

TABLE 1-3	**Examples of Medical Billing Abuse**

- Refer excessively to other providers for unnecessary services, also called **ping-ponging**
- Charge excessively for services or supplies
- Perform a battery of diagnostic tests when only a few are required for services, also called **churning**
- Violate Medicare's physician participating agreement
- Call patients back for repeated and unnecessary follow-up visits, also called **yo-yoing**
- Bill Medicare beneficiaries at a higher rate than other patients
- Submit bills to Medicare instead of to third party payers (e.g., claims for injury from an automobile accident, in a store, or the workplace)
- Breach assignment agreement
- Fail to make required refunds when services are not reasonable and necessary

- Require patients to contract to pay their physician's full charges, in excess of the Medicare charge limits
- Require a patient to waive rights to have the physician submit claims to Medicare and obligate a patient to pay privately for Medicare-covered services
- Require patients to pay for services not previously billed, including telephone calls with the physician, prescription refills, and medical conferences with other professionals
- Require patients to sign a global waiver agreeing to pay privately for all services that Medicare will not cover, and using these waivers to obligate patients to pay separately for a service that Medicare covers as part of a package or related procedures

tionable, such as write off patient balances for certain patients automatically, then make sure you have a legal document or signed waiver of liability relieving you of the responsibility for such actions.

Scope of Practice

When working as a claims assistance professional (CAP), he or she acts as an informal representative of patients (policyholders and Medicare beneficiaries) helping to obtain insurance reimbursement. CAPs review and analyze existing or potential policies, render advice and offer counseling, recommendations, and information. A CAP may not interpret insurance policies or act as an attorney. The legal ability of a CAP to represent a policyholder is limited. When a claim cannot be resolved after a denied claim has been appealed to the insurance company, the CAP must be careful in rendering a personal opinion or advising clients that they have a right to pursue legal action. In some states, a CAP could be acting outside the scope of the law (scope of practice) by giving advice to clients on legal issues even if licensed as an attorney but not practicing law full time. If the client wishes to take legal action, it is his or her responsibility to find a competent attorney specializing in contract law and insurance. In some states, giving an insured client advice on purchase or discontinuance of insurance policies is construed as being an insurance agent.

A number of states require CAPs to be licensed, depending on the services rendered to clients. CAPs who perform only the clerical function of filing health insurance claims do not have to be licensed except in Florida. Check with your state's Department of Insurance and insurance commissioner (see Chapter 8 and Appendix A) to determine whether you should be licensed.

If working as a CAP who does not handle checks or cash, inquire about an errors and omissions insurance policy by contacting the Alliance of Claims Assistance Professionals (ACAP).[*] When employed as a medical assistant who is submitting insurance claims, information on professional liability insurance may be obtained from the American Association of Medical Assistants, Inc.[†]

---

[*]c/o Susan A. Dressier, CCAP, 731 South Naperville Road, Wheaton, IL 60187-6407.
[†]20 North Wacker Drive, Chicago, IL 60606.

Embezzlement

Embezzlement means stealing money that has been entrusted in one's care. In many cases of insurance claims embezzlement, the physician is held as the guilty party and has to pay huge sums of money to the insurance carrier when false claims are submitted by an employee. If an undiscovered embezzler leaves the employer and you are hired to replace that person, you could be accused some months down the line of doing something that you did not do. Take precautions as an employee and to protect the medical practice.

Precautions for Financial Protection

To prevent stealing from a medical practice, these office policies should be routinely practiced. Ask the physician or supervisor to initial all entries about adjustments, discounts, and write-offs on either the ledger cards or day sheets. If a patient owes money to the physician that is uncollectable and adjusted off, be sure the physician dates and initials the ledger that shows the closed account. Ask the physician to occasionally check an entire day's records (the patient sign-in log and appointment schedule) with the day sheet, ledger cards, encounter forms, and cash receipt slips. A daily trial balance of accounts receivable including daily deposit of checks and cash can assist in reviewing monthly income and aid in discovering embezzlement. Review the monthly bank statement to verify that all deposits tally with the receipts for each business day (Fig. 1−9). If poor bookkeeping and record keeping are noticed, bring this to your employer's attention.

All insurance payment checks should be immediately stamped within the endorsement area on the back "For Deposit Only," called a *restrictive endorsement*. The bank should be given instruc-

tions never to cash a check made payable to the physician.

Encounter forms, transaction slips, and cash receipts should be prenumbered. If a mistake is made when completing one, void it and keep the slip as part of the financial records. It is especially imperative to have prenumbered insurance forms if the physician's practice allows the use of a signature stamp when submitting claims. Thus, filing of fictitious insurance claims can be totally eliminated.

As a precautionary measure, always type your initials at the bottom left or top right corner of the insurance claim forms that you submit. This will indicate to office personnel who did the work. Always retain the Explanation of Benefits or Remittance Advice documents that accompany checks from insurance companies.

Only a few of the many precautions for protection are mentioned here; embezzlement can occur in accounts receivable, accounts payable, with petty cash, use of computers, and in various other aspects of a medical practice.

Bonding

Insurance billers, CAPs, or anyone who handles checks or cash should be bonded or insured. A practice that carries a fidelity or *honesty bond* means that an insurance company will prosecute any guilty employees. **Bonding** is an insurance contract by which a bonding agency guarantees payment of a certain sum to a physician in case of a financial loss caused by an employee or some contingency over which the payee has no control. Bonding methods for a practice with three or more office employees are

▶ **Position-schedule bond** covers a designated job, such as a bookkeeper or nurse, rather than a named individual. If one employee in a category leaves, the replacement is automatically covered.

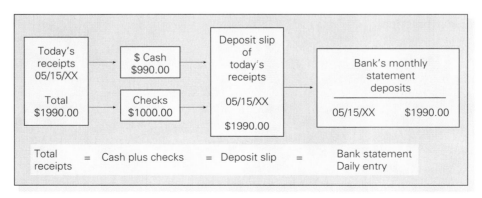

Figure 1−9. Explanation of an audit trail to review monies received by a medical practice and monies deposited into a bank account.

- **Blanket-position bond** provides coverage for all employees regardless of job title.
- **Personal bond** provides coverage for those who handle large sums of money. A thorough background investigation is required.

Such bonding contracts may be obtained from a casualty insurance agent or broker. Bond coverage should be reviewed periodically with the insurance agent to ensure that coverage is keeping pace with the expansion of the business.

Future Challenges

As you begin your study to become an insurance billing specialist remember that you are expected to profitably manage a medical practice's financial affairs or patient accounts; otherwise, you will not be considered qualified for this position. In subsequent chapters you will learn the important information and skills to help you achieve this goal. You will be expected to:

- Know billing regulations for each insurance program and managed care plan in which the practice is a participant.
- State various insurance rules regarding treatment and referral of patients.
- Become proficient in computer skills and various medical software.
- Learn electronic billing software and the variances of each payer.
- Develop diagnostic and procedural coding expertise.
- Know how to interpret remittance advice summary reports and/or explanation of benefit documents.
- Attain bookkeeping skills necessary to post, interpret, and manage patient accounts.
- Keep up to date by reading the latest journals and newsletters and attending seminars on billing and coding.
- Cross-train so you become familiar with other spects of the medical practice.

RESOURCES ON THE INTERNET

 For up-to-date information on fraud alerts, visit the Office of the Inspector General and Federal Bureau of Investigation web site:

www.hcfa.gov

The national hotline of the Office of the Inspector General is 1-800-HHS-TIPS. To obtain current information on fraud in the Medicaid program, visit the web site:

http://www.hcfa.gov/medicaid/mbfraud.htm

STUDENT ASSIGNMENT LIST

✔ Read Introduction in the *Workbook*, which explains how you will be working as an insurance billing specialist during this course.

✔ Study Chapter 1.

✔ Answer the review questions in the *Workbook* to reinforce the theory learned in this chapter and to help prepare you for a future test.

✔ Complete the assignments in the *Workbook* to help develop critical thinking and writing skills. As you proceed through the assignments in the *Workbook*, you will broaden your knowledge of medical terminology as well as gain an entry-level skill in diagnostic and procedural coding and insurance claim completion.

✔ Turn to the Glossary at the end of this textbook for a further understanding of the Key Terms used in this chapter.

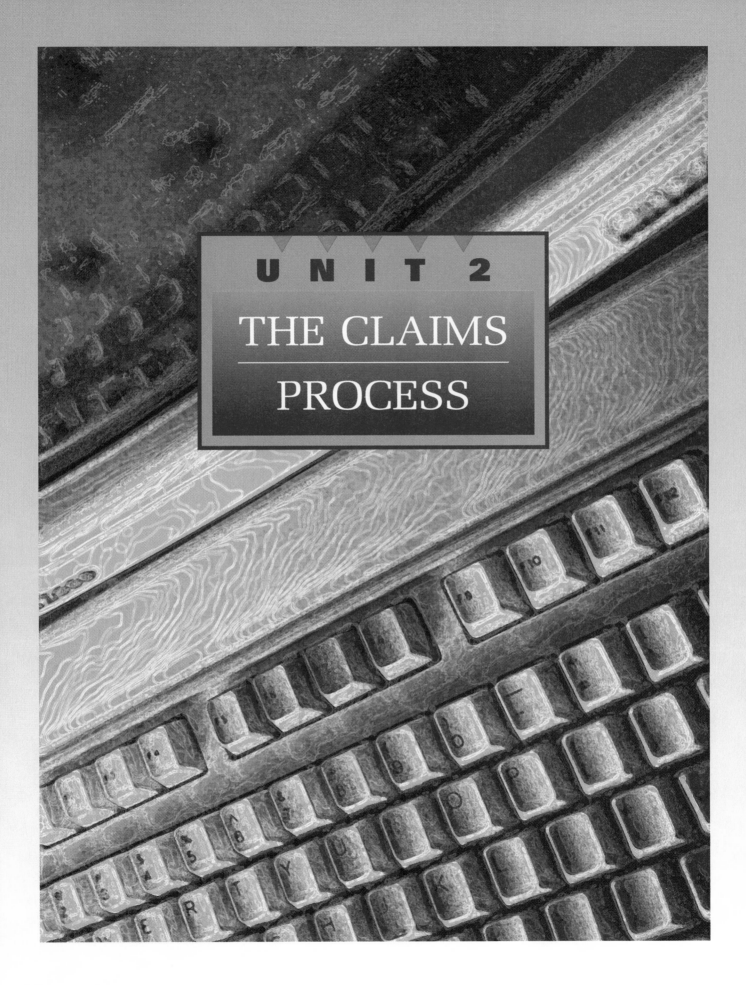

UNIT 2

THE CLAIMS

PROCESS

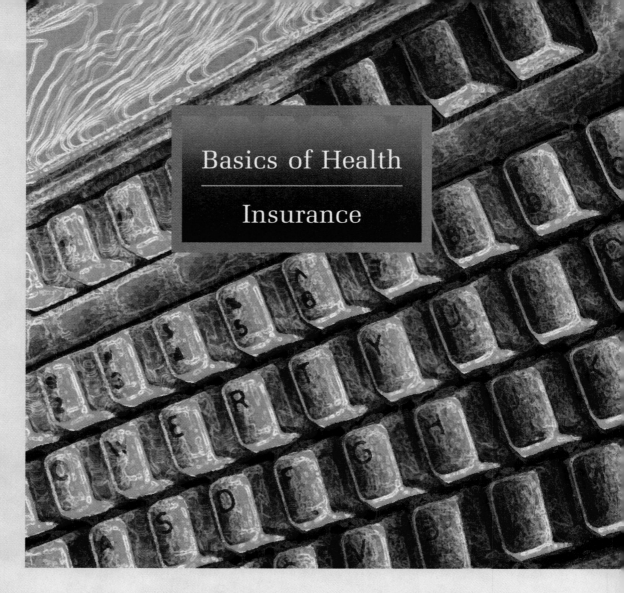

Basics of Health Insurance

2

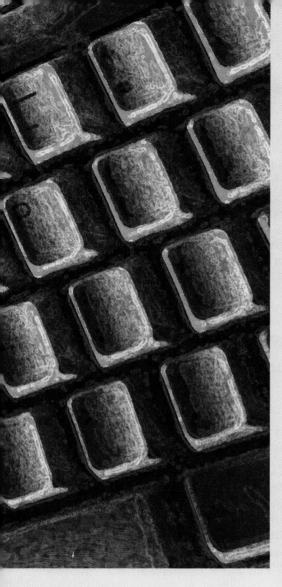

Encounter Form

Physician's Signature

Determine Fees

Bookkeeping—Ledger Card

Insurance Form

Provider's Handwritten
Signature

Office Pending File and
Insurance Claims Register

Mailing the Claim Form

Insurance Payments

Monthly Statement

*Procedure: Posting to a
Patient's Ledger*

Keeping Up to Date

OBJECTIVES*

After reading this chapter,
you should be able to:

■ Describe the history of insurance in the United
States.

■ Distinguish between the
three major classes of
health insurance contracts.

■ State four concepts of a
valid insurance contract.

■ Explain the difference
between an implied and an
expressed physician/patient
contract.

■ Describe in general terms
the important federal, state,
and private health insur-
ance plans.

■ Define common insurance
terms.

■ List four actions to prevent
problems when given sig-
nature authorization for insurance claims.

■ Handle insurance claims in
the physician's office to obtain payment and minimize
their rejection by insurance
carriers.

■ Explain the process of a
physician-based insurance
claim from obtaining pa-
tient data, claim form completion, insurance carrier
processing, and payment
received.

■ Establish an insurance
claims register or log.

■ Determine the appropriate
questions to ask a patient
for a complete patient
record.

■ List the functions of a tickler file.

■ Record proper information
and post to the patient's
ledger after claims submission and payment received.

KEY TERMS

applicant

assignment

blanket contract

capitation

CHAMPVA

claim

coinsurance

Competitive Medical Plan
(CMP)

conditionally renewable

contract

day sheet

deductible

disability income insurance

electronic signature

eligibility

emancipated minor

encounter form

exclusions

exclusive provider
organization (EPO)

expressed contract

extend

foundation for medical
care (FMC)

guaranteed renewable

guarantor

health insurance

health maintenance
organization (HMO)

high risk

implied contract

indemnity

independent or individual
practice association (IPA)

continued

History

The insurance industry is among the world's largest businesses. In the 1800s, life insurance came to be widely offered. Because anyone can have an accident or become ill unexpectedly, leading to large expenses, health insurance began to be available in the early part of this century. **Health insurance** is a contract between a policyholder and an insurance carrier or government program to reimburse the policyholder for all or a portion of the cost of medically necessary treatment or preventive care rendered by health care professionals. Its main purpose was to help offset some of the high costs accrued during sickness or when an injury occurred.

During the Renaissance, when Italian traders insured valuable cargo to be shipped across the Mediterranean, they recorded the insurance agreement on a piece of folded paper called a *polizza*. English merchants adapted the term to their insurance practices, modifying the pronunciation to suit the Anglo-Saxon tongue, resulting in the word "policy."

Insurance in the United States

In 1850, the Franklin Health Assurance Company of Massachusetts began offering insurance for nonfatal injury. Then about 10 years later, the Travelers Insurance Company of Hartford marketed a plan that is similar to today's health insurance. Many other companies began writing health insurance policies, and in 1911 Montgomery Ward and Company offered benefits to its ill or injured employees. This was the first group plan. These commercial plans paid only when an individual was sick or received an injury.

By the 1960s, most private insurance companies sold policies that included hospital care, surgical fees, and physicians' services. In addition to those benefits, many plans now offer catastrophic health insurance coverage, preventive care, dental insurance, disability income insurance, and long-term care and home health care insurance for the chronically ill, disabled, and developmentally disabled. State insurance laws regulate the way policies are written and minimum requirements of coverage.

In the past decade, medical care costs have escalated, forcing insurance companies to reduce their forms of coverage and the federal government to adopt cost-containment policies for the Medicare, Medicaid, and TRICARE programs. Although managed care began in the 1930s when Kaiser Industries provided health care to their employees, it was not until the 1980s that many types of plans sprung up across the nation to control the cost of medical care and to help those who could not afford health insurance. Because individual needs vary, each patient may have a different type of health insurance policy with various benefits. Patients may be covered under different types of private, state, or federal programs.

Legal Principles of Insurance

The role of a medical insurance billing specialist is to complete the insurance claim accurately and to facilitate claims submission so reimbursement is received quickly. However, before developing the skill of coding and completing insurance claim forms, it is necessary to know frequently encountered legal problems and how to handle them. Legal situations occur daily in the performance of these job duties and involve confidentiality of medical records, accurate insurance claim completion, fraud and abuse issues, credit and collection laws, and so on. An insurance biller cannot escape liability by pleading ignorance. It cannot be overemphasized that keeping up to date on health care plan policies and procedures is essential. Most legal issues of health insurance claims fall under civil law. Insurance is regulated by state laws and is not considered a federally regulated industry.

It is important for an insurance billing specialist to know some basic insurance terms, understand basic insurance concepts, and have a working knowledge of medical terminology.

Insurance Contracts

The first legal item in the business of handling medical insurance is the insurance contract (also known as a policy). There is no standard health insurance contract. Individuals who take out a policy receive an original document composed by the insuring company.

There are four considerations involved in drawing up a valid insurance contract:

1. The person must be a mentally competent adult and not under the influence of drugs or alcohol.
2. The insurance company must make an offer (the signed application), and the person must accept the offer (issuance of the policy), without concealment or misrepresentation of facts on the application.
3. An exchange of value (the first premium payment) submitted with the application, known as a *consideration*, must be present.
4. A legal purpose must exist, which, in the case of a health insurance policy, is an insurable interest. This means the policyholder expects to continue in good health, but if an accident or illness strikes, then the insurance policy provides something of value.

When a fraudulent statement is made by the subscriber, a policy can be challenged. A *challenged policy* means that coverage may not be in effect. After a policy has been in force for 2 years (3 years in some states), a policy becomes *incontestable* (may not be challenged). If the time limit has passed and a policy is guaranteed renewable, the policy becomes incontestable even if false statements were made on the application. Further information and additional insurance terminology concerning contracts are provided in detail in Chapter 3.

Physician/Patient Contracts and Financial Obligation

Implied or Expressed Contracts

A physician and his or her staff must be aware of the physician's obligations to each patient, the physician's liabilities in regard to his or her service, and the patient's obligations to the physician. The physician/patient contract begins when the physician accepts the patient and agrees to treat the patient. This action can be either an implied or expressed contract. An **implied contract** is defined as not manifested by direct words but implied or deduced from the circumstance, the general language, or the conduct of the patient. For example, if Mary Johnson goes to Dr. Doe's office and Dr. Doe gives Ms. Johnson professional services that she accepts, this is an implied contract. If the patient is unconscious when treatment is rendered, treatment is based on an implied-in-fact contract. An **expressed contract** can be verbal or written. However, most physician/patient contracts are implied.

Private Patients

Although a patient carries medical insurance, the contract for treatment is between the physician and the patient. The patient is liable for the entire bill. The insurance is meant to help offset the expense.

Guarantor

A **guarantor** is an individual who promises to pay the medical bill by signing a form agreeing to pay or who accepts treatment, which constitutes an expressed promise. Usually, a patient is the guarantor and must be of legal age (18 or 21 years, depending on state law). Most laws governing financial responsibility state that a husband is responsible for his wife's debts; a wife is not always responsible for her husband's debts. However, would always depend on the way the co

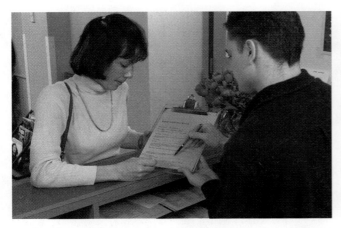

Figure 2–1. Receptionist explaining where a guarantor's signature goes on a patient registration form for the medical services rendered to a family member. ·

application reads and individual state laws. A father is ordinarily responsible for his children's debts if they are minors and are not emancipated (Fig. 2–1). Children may or may not be responsible for the debts of their parents, depending on the circumstances.

Emancipated Minor

An **emancipated minor** is a person younger than 18 years of age who lives independently, is totally self-supporting, is married or divorced, is a parent even if not married, or is in the military and possesses decision-making rights. College students living away from home even when financially dependent on their parents are considered emancipated. Parents are not liable for the medical expenses incurred by an emancipated minor. The patient record should contain the minor's signed statement that he or she is on his or her own.

Managed Care Patients

A physician under contract to a managed care plan periodically receives an updated list of current enrollees. The physician is obligated to see those individuals who are enrolled should one of them call for an appointment. However, the contract for treatment occurs when the patient is first seen. If the physician no longer wishes to treat a patient on a managed care plan, termination is handled according to the same method that is used when discharging patients who are insured under private insurance or state or government programs. The method of how to do this is explained in the next chapter.

An insurance specialist should be able to read and interpret managed care plan contracts, but if the specialist is unable to interpret these matters, professional assistance from the physician's attorney, the medical practice's accountant, or the managed care plan should be sought. He or she should understand billing and collection requirements and track payments made by the managed care plan.

Employment and Disability Examinations

Courts in most jurisdictions have ruled that there is no physician/patient relationship in an employment or disability examination and the doctor does not owe a duty of care to the person being examined, chiefly because the insurance company is requesting the examination and the patient is not seeking the medical services of the physician.

Workers' Compensation Patients

When a person is injured on the job, this becomes a workers' compensation case and may be referred to as an industrial accident or illness. In this type of case, the contract exists between the physician and the insurance company. When there is a dispute as to whether the injured party was hurt at work, a Patient Agreement form (see Chapter 14, Fig. 14–17) must be signed by the patient agreeing to pay the physician's fees if the case is declared not work related.

The Insurance Policy

Insurance policies are complex and contain a great deal of technical jargon. This can cause misunderstanding by patients or anyone trying to obtain information from the policy. Basic health insurance coverage includes benefits for hospital, surgical, and other medical expenses. **Major medical** or *extended benefits* contracts are designed to offset large medical expenses caused by prolonged illness or serious injury. Some of these policies include coverage for *extended care* or *skilled nursing facility* benefits. The **insured** is known as a **subscriber** or, in some insurance programs, a **member**, *policyholder,* or *recipient* and may not necessarily be the patient seen for the medical service. The insured is the individual (enrollee) or organization protected in case of loss under the terms of an insurance policy. In group insurance, the employer is considered the insured, and the employees are the risks. However, when completing an insurance claim form, the covered employee is listed as the insured. A policy might also include *dependents* of the insured. Generally, this term refers to the spouse and children of the insured, but under some contracts, parents, other family members, and domestic partners may be covered as dependents.

Policy Application

Before a policy is issued, the insurance company decides whether it will enter into a contract with the **applicant** who is applying for the insurance coverage. Information is obtained about the applicant so the company can decide whether to accept the risk. Generally, the application form has two sections: part one contains basic information about the application, and part two concerns the health of the individual.

An insurance policy is a legally enforceable agreement, or **contract**. If a policy is issued, the applicant becomes part of the insurance contract or plan. The policy becomes effective only after the company offers the policy and the person accepts it and then pays the initial premium (Fig. 2–2). If a premium is paid at the time the application is submitted, then the insurance coverage can be put into force before the policy is delivered. Depending on the laws in some states, the applicant can also have temporary conditional insurance if the agent issues a specific type of receipt.

Policy Renewal Provisions

Health insurance policies may have renewal provisions written into the policy stating the circumstances when the company may refuse to renew, may cancel coverage, or may increase the premium. There are five classifications: (1) cancelable,

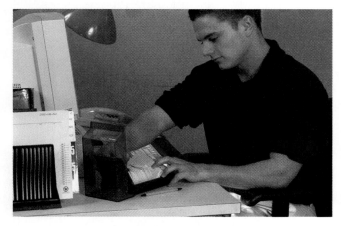

Figure 2–2. Insurance billing specialist searching in an index file for an insurance company's telephone number to inquire about a patient's coverage under an insurance policy.

(2) optionally renewable, (3) conditionally renewable, (4) guaranteed renewable, and (5) noncancelable.

▶ A renewable provision in a *cancelable* policy grants the insurer the right to cancel the policy at any time and for any reason. The company notifies the insured the policy is canceled and refunds any advance premium the policyholder has paid. In some states, this type of policy is illegal.

▶ In an **optionally renewable** policy, the insurer has the right to refuse to renew the policy on a date (premium due or anniversary date) specified in the contract and may add coverage limitations or increase premium rates.

▶ **Conditionally renewable** policies grant the insurer a limited right to refuse to renew a health insurance policy at the end of a premium payment period. Reasons stated in the policy may be due to age and/or employment status but not because of the insured's health status.

▶ The **guaranteed renewable** classification is desirable because the insurer is required to renew the policy as long as premium payments are made. However, these policies may have age limits of 60, 65, or 70 years, or they may be renewable for life.

▶ In a **noncancelable policy**, the insurer cannot increase premium rates and must renew the policy until the insured reaches the age specified in the contract. Some disability income policies have noncancelable terms.

Policy Terms

To keep the insurance in force, a person must pay a monthly, quarterly, or annual fee called a **premium.** If the premium is not paid, a *grace period* of 10 to 30 days is usually given before insurance coverage ceases. In addition, usually a **deductible** (a specific amount of money) must be paid each year before the policy benefits begin. The higher the deductible is, the lower the cost of the policy. Most policies have a **coinsurance** or *cost-sharing* requirement, which means the insured will assume a percentage of the fee (e.g., 20%) or pay a specific dollar amount (e.g., $5 or $10) for covered services. Managed care plans and state and federal programs refer to this as *copayment* (copay). It is not advisable to routinely waive copayments because most insurance companies do not tolerate this practice. If the provider is audited, the federal government can assess penalties for not collecting copayments for patients seen under the Medicare program. However, if copayments are waived on a case-by-case basis, as in a courtesy discount, there should not be any problems with commercial insurance carriers or Medicare. Generally, deductibles and copayments should be collected at the time of service.

Health insurance policies consider an *accident* to be an unforeseen and unintended event. Some policies cover accidents occurring from the first day the policy is in force. Others may contain an *elimination period* or a *waiting period* before benefits for sickness or accident become payable.

It is the patient's responsibility to give a written notice of **claim** to the insurance company within a certain number of days, known as a *time limit.* However, in most cases, the claim is filed for the patient by the provider of professional services. The insurance billing specialist must be able to abstract proper information from the patient record, which is used to code the diagnoses and services rendered; to complete an insurance claim form; to make entries on the patient's ledger card; and to follow up on unpaid claims. If any one of these procedures is not done properly, correct reimbursement or payment (also called **indemnity**) from the insurance *carrier* will not be generated. Follow-up on unpaid claims is made by contacting the claims representative, called an *adjuster.* If the payment is to go directly from the insurance company to the physician, then the patient must sign a document granting permission.

Coordination of Benefits

A *coordination of benefits* statement is included in most policies.

When the patient has more than one insurance policy, this clause requires insurance companies to coordinate the reimbursement of benefits, thus preventing the duplication or overlapping of payments for the same medical expense.

Most state legislatures have adopted the *birthday law,* which is a change in the order of determination of coordination of benefits regarding primary and secondary carriers for dependent children. Rather than the father's insurance being primary, the father's *or* mother's carrier may be primary. The health plan of the person whose birthday (month and day, *not* year) falls earlier in the calendar year will pay first, and the plan of the other person covering the dependent will be the secondary payer. If both mother and father have the same birthday, the plan of the person who has had coverage longer is the primary payer. If one of the two plans has not adopted this birthday rule (i.e., if one plan is in another state), the rules of the plan without the birthday rule determine which plan is primary and which is sec-

ondary. In cases of divorce, the plan of the parent with custody of the children is the primary payer unless the court determines differently and it is so stated in the divorce settlement.

Unions and companies that self-insure their employees do not fall under this birthday law. The states that do not have birthday laws are Georgia, Hawaii, Idaho, Massachusetts, Mississippi, Vermont, Virginia, and Washington, DC.

General Policy Limitations

Health insurance policies contain **exclusions**— some more than others. If a person has an injury or illness that is excluded in his or her policy, then there is no insurance coverage for that injury or illness. These exclusions or limitations of the policy could be such factors as losses resulting from military service, attempted suicide, or self-inflicted injuries; losses due to an injury on the job; pregnancy; and so on. Be aware that some insurance policies may state that a procedure or service is not covered (excluded) when the state law says the procedure is a "mandated benefit." Some examples are reconstructive breast surgery after mastectomy, surgical procedures affecting the upper and lower jawbones, and infertility coverage under group policies. Thus, further investigation is necessary beyond reading the policy.

Many policies do not provide benefits for conditions that existed and were treated before the policy was issued, called *preexisting conditions.* In some instances, such conditions might be covered after a specified period of time after the issuance of the policy. Some policies have a *waiver* or *rider,* which is an attachment to a policy that modifies clauses and provisions of the policy by either adding coverage or excluding certain illnesses or disabilities that would otherwise be covered. Generally, waivers are used to eliminate benefits for specific preexisting conditions.

Case Management Requirements

Preapproval

Many private insurance carriers and prepaid health plans have certain requirements that must be met before they will approve hospital admissions, inpatient or outpatient surgeries, and elective procedures. First **eligibility** requirements must be obtained. These are conditions or qualifying factors that must be met before the patient receives benefits (medical services) under a specified insurance plan, government program, or managed care plan. The carrier can refuse to pay part or all of the fee if these requirements are not met. **Precertification** refers to discovering whether a treatment (surgery, hospitalization, tests) is covered under a patient's contract. **Preauthorization** relates not only to whether a service or procedure is covered but also to finding out whether it is medically necessary. **Predetermination** means discovering the maximum dollar amount that the carrier will pay for surgery, consulting services, radiology procedures, and so on.

Obtain precertification or predetermination when a procedure is tentatively scheduled. The information that may be required to obtain precertification approval by fax or telephone is shown in Figure 2–3. To obtain predetermination by mail, use the form shown in Figure 2–4. For an example of a preauthorization form, see Chapter 10–1, Figure 10–1. This form can also be used to document the information received when verifying the patient's insurance coverage by telephone. It should become part of the patient's record and used for reference when billing future insurance claims.

Figure 2–3. Insurance precertification form. This form can be faxed to the insurance company or used when telephoning to obtain approval for hospitalization under a patient's insurance policy or managed care plan.

COLLEGE CLINIC
4567 Broad Avenue
Woodland Hills, XY 12345-0000

Phone: 013/486-9002   Fax: 013/590-2189

Insurance Precertification Form

Date: _5/4/XX_
To: Insurance Carrier _Cal-Net Care_   From: _Janet_ Office Mgr.
    Address _9900 Baker Street_
            Los Angeles, CA 90067

Check those that apply: Admission certification ✔   Outpatient___ Inpatient ✔
                             Surgery certification ✔   Emergency situation ✔

Patient's name _Ronald Stranton_   Date of Birth: _4-14-49_
Patient's address _639 Cedar Street_   Sex: Male ✔ Female ___
                  Woodland Hills, XY 12345 Social Security No. _527-00-7250_
Insured's Name _Same_   Policy Group ID No. _A59_
Insured's Address _____   Employer: _Aerostar Aviation_

Treating physician _Clarence Cutler, M.D._   NPI #: _430 500 4700_
Primary Care Physician _Gerald Practon, M.D._ NPI #: _462 7889 700_

Name of Hospital _College Hospital_   Admission Date: _5/4/XX_
                                              Estimated Length of Stay: _3-5 d_
Admitting Diagnosis _Volvulus_   Diagnosis Code: _560.2_
Complicating conditions to substantiate need for inpatient hospitalization _____
                  Complete bowel obstruction
Date current illness or injury began _5/2/XX_
Procedure/surgery to be done _Reduction of Volvulus_   Procedure code _44050_

Second opinion needed   Yes ___   No ✔ Date performed _____

Telephone precertification: _Emergency Cert. 5/4/XX_
Name of representative certifying _McKenzie Kwan_
Direct-dial telephone number of representative _1-800-463-9000 ex. 227_

Reason(s) for denial _____
Certification approved   Yes ✔ No ___ Certification approval No. _69874_
Authorization for services Yes ✔ No ___ Authorization No. _69874E_

Note: The information contained in this facsimile message is confidential and privileged information intended only for the use of the individual or entity named above. If the reader of this message is not the intended recipient, you are hereby notified that any dissemination, distribution, or copying of this communication is strictly prohibited. If you have received this communication in error, please immediately notify me by telephone and return the original facsimile to me via the U.S. Postal Service. Thank you.

INSURANCE PREDETERMINATION FORM

Patient: __Jane Doe__   Member # __46215H__

Address: __2 Main Street__   Group # __1207__

City __Woodland Hills__   State __XY__   ZIP __12345-0001__

Tel. No. __013-272-0811__   Date of Birth __11-5-1960__   Soc. Sec. # __421-03-1941__

Insurance Company __ABC Insurance Company__   Relationship to insured: Self __X__

Insurance Co. Address __45 Center Street__   Spouse ____

__Woodland Hills, XY 12345__   Child ____

Telephone No. __013-473-2181__   Other ____

Employer: __Pentel Corporation__

Copy of Insurance card attached? Yes __X__ No ____

Prior Authorization __craniotomy (infratentorial) CPT code 61314__

- -

BENEFITS:

Major medical:	Yes ____	No ____	% Payable:	_____
Deductible:	Yes ____	No ____	Amount: $	_____
Time interval: Year ____		Month ____	Other:	_____
Per family:	Yes ____	No ____	Per person: Yes _____	No _____
Co-Insurance	Yes ____	No ____	Amount: $	_____

COVERAGE:

1. Office visits: Yes ____ No ____   Amount $ _____

2. Office x-rays and lab: Yes ____ No ____   Amount $ _____

3. Hospital surgery: Yes ____ No ____   Limit $ _____ UCR

    Second opinion required: Yes ____ No ____

    Preadmission hospital and

    surgical authorization: Yes ____ No ____

4. Office surgery: Yes ____ No ____   Limit $ _____ UCR

5. General anesthesia: Yes ____ No ____   Per hr. $ _____ Limit $ _____

FEE SCHEDULE:

1. RVS   Yes ____ No ____   1999   2000 conversion factor: _____

2. Other: _____

DEPENDENT COVERAGE:

1. Spouse: Yes ____ No ____   Same? _____

2. Children: Yes ____ No ____   Same? _____

IS YOUR FEE SCHEDULE FOR A   ____Neurosurgeon____   THE SAME AS OTHER

(Physician's specialty)

MEDICAL SPECIALISTS?   Yes ____ No ____

WHEN CAN I EXPECT PAYMENT AFTER SUBMISSION? _____

PERSON VERIFYING: _____   DATE: _____

(Name)

Figure 2–4. Insurance predetermination form. This form can be sent to the insurance company to find out the maximum dollar amount that will be paid for primary surgery, consulting services, postoperative care, and so on.

After the information is received from the insurance carrier, give the patient an estimate of fees for the proposed surgery. An example of suggested wording for a letter is given in Figure 2–5. This written estimate makes collection quicker and easier.

Choice of Health Insurance

There are three ways in which a person can obtain health insurance: (1) take out insurance through a group plan (contract or policy), (2) pay

COLLEGE CLINIC
4567 Broad Avenue
Woodland Hills, XY 12345-0000

Phone: 013/486-9002   **Fax: 013/590-2189**

Current date

Patient's name
Address
City, State, ZIP code

Dear

This letter gives you an estimate of the fees for your proposed surgery. Verification of coverage and benefit information has been obtained from your insurance company. Listed are your benefits for the proposed surgical expenses and the estimated balance after your insurance carrier pays.

Surgical procedure   craniotomy
Date of surgery   February 21, 20XX
Name of hospital   College Hospital
Hospital address   4500 Broad Ave., Woodland Hills, XY 12345

	Insurance pays	Estimated balance
Surgeon's fee	2548.09	1344.24	1203.85
Preoperative visit			
Preoperative tests			

You have a policy deductible of <u>$1000</u> which___ has __✓__ has not been met.

The surgery requires the use of an anesthesiologist, assistant surgeon, and a pathologist. These physicians will bill you separately for their services. The hospital will also bill you separately.

This office will file your insurance claim for the surgical procedure, so the insurance payment should come directly to us. If the insurance carrier sends you the payment, then you are responsible to get the payment to this office within five days. Your balance after surgery should be approximately $1203.85. You are responsible for any remaining balance after our office receives the insurance payment.

Thank you for choosing our medical practice. If you have any questions, please call me.

Sincerely,

Karen Martinez, CMA
Administrative Medical Assistant

Figure 2-5. Sample letter to a patient supplying an estimate of the fees for proposed surgery.

the premium on an individual basis, or (3) enroll in a prepaid health plan.

Group Contract

A *group contract* is any insurance plan by which a group of employees (and their eligible dependents) or other homogeneous group is insured under a single policy issued to their employer or leader, with individual certificates given to each insured individual or family unit. A group policy usually provides better benefits and offers lower premiums. However, the coverage for each person in the group is the same. If a new employee declines enrollment, he or she must sign a waiver stating this fact.

Conversion Privilege

Many physicians can obtain comprehensive group coverage through plans sponsored by the professional organizations to which they belong. Sometimes this is called a **blanket contract.** If the person leaves the employer or organization or the group contract is terminated, the insured may continue the same or lesser coverage under an individual policy if the group contract has a *conversion privilege.*

Usually, conversion from a group policy to an individual policy increases the premium and reduces the benefits. However, if the person has a condition that would make him or her ineligible for coverage or is a case considered at **high risk,** it is advantageous to convert to an individual policy because no physical examination is required; therefore, a preexisting condition cannot be excluded.

Income Continuation Benefits

Under the Consolidated Omnibus Budget Reconciliation Act of 1985 (COBRA), when an employee is laid off from a company with 20 or more workers, federal law requires that the group health insurance coverage be extended to the employee and his or her dependents at group rates for up to 18 months. This also applies to those workers who lose coverage because of reduced work hours. In the case of death of a covered employee, divorced or widowed spouse, or employee entitled to Medicare, the extension of coverage may be for 36 months. However, the employee must pay for the group policy; this is known as *income continuation benefits.* For additional information on this topic, see the section on COBRA in Chapter 11.

Medical Savings Accounts

The Health Insurance Portability and Accountability Act of 1996 (HIPAA) was federal legislation created to (1) expand efforts to combat fraud and abuse, as learned in the previous chapter, (2) protect workers and their families so they can obtain and maintain health insurance if they change or lose their jobs, and (3) establish a medical savings account pilot project. A *medical savings account* (MSA) is a type of tax-free savings account that allows individuals and their employers to set aside money to pay for health care expenses. An employer can set up an MSA for his or her employees and make an annual contribution to the MSA, which is tax deductible for both employer and employee. MSA balances accumulate from year to year tax free, but in a flex account (another type of MSA), unused funds may not be carried over. Earned interest is not taxed. MSAs are portable, allowing individuals to take their MSA with them when they change jobs or relocate.

Individual Contract

Any insurance plan issued to an individual (and dependents) is called an *individual contract.* Usually, this type of policy has a higher premium, and often the benefits are less than those obtainable under a group health insurance plan. Sometimes this is called **personal insurance.**

Prepaid Health Plan

This is a program of health care in which a specified set of health benefits is provided for a subscriber or enrolled group of subscribers who pay a yearly fee or fixed periodic payments. Providers of services are paid by capitation. **Capitation** is a system of payment used by managed care plans in which physicians and hospitals are paid a fixed, per capita amount for each patient enrolled over a stated period of time, regardless of the type and number of services provided. For additional information on this topic, refer to Chapter 10.

Types of Health Insurance Coverage

Many forms of health insurance coverage are currently in effect in the United States. These are referred to as third party payers (private insurance, government plans, managed care contracts, and workers' compensation). A brief explanation of the programs to be discussed in this text is given here, but for an in-depth study, refer to the appropriate chapters that follow.

CHAMPVA

The Civilian Health and Medical Program of the Department of Veterans Affairs is administered by the Department of Veterans Affairs. This federal program shares the medical bills of spouses and children of veterans with total, permanent, service-connected disabilities or of the surviving spouses and children of veterans who died as a result of service-connected disabilities (see Chapter 13).

Competitive Medical Plan

A **Competitive Medical Plan (CMP)** is a type of managed care organization created by the 1982 Tax Equity and Fiscal Responsibility Act (TEFRA). This federal legislation allows for enrollment of Medicare beneficiaries into managed care plans (see Chapter 11).

Disability Income Insurance

Disability income insurance is a form of health insurance that provides periodic payments to replace income when the insured is unable to work as a result of illness, injury, or disease (see Chapter 15). This type of insurance should not be confused with workers' compensation, because those injuries must be work related.

Exclusive Provider Organization

An **exclusive provider organization (EPO)** is a type of managed health care plan in which subscriber members are eligible for benefits only when they use the services of a limited network of providers. EPOs combine features of both HMOs and PPOs. Employers agree not to enter into an agreement with any other plan for coverage of eligible employees. EPOs are regulated under state health insurance laws (see Chapter 10).

Foundation for Medical Care

A **foundation for medical care (FMC)** is an organization of physicians, sponsored by a state or local medical association, concerned with the development and delivery of medical services and the cost of health care (see Chapter 10).

Health Maintenance Organization

A **health maintenance organization (HMO)** is an organization that provides a wide range of comprehensive health care services for a specified group at a fixed periodic payment. The emphasis is on preventive care. Physicians are reimbursed by capitation. An HMO can be sponsored by the government, medical schools, hospitals, employers, labor unions, consumer groups, insurance companies, or hospital medical plans (see Chapter 10).

Independent or Individual Practice Association

An independent or individual practice association (IPA) is a type of managed care plan in which a program administrator contracts with a number of physicians who agree to provide treatment to subscribers in their own offices or clinics for a fixed capitation payment per month. Subscribers to IPA plans have limited or no choice of physician. IPA physicians continue to see their fee-for-service patients (see Chapter 10).

Maternal and Child Health Program

A **Maternal and Child Health Program (MCHP)** is a state and federal program for children who are younger than 21 years of age and have special health care needs. It assists parents with financial planning and may assume part or all of the costs of treatment, depending on the child's condition and the family's resources (see Chapter 12).

Medicaid

Medicaid (MCD) is a program sponsored jointly by federal, state, and local governments to provide health care benefits to indigent persons on welfare (public assistance), aged individuals who meet certain financial requirements, and the disabled. Some states have expanded coverage for other medically needy individuals who meet special state-determined criteria. Coverage and benefits vary widely from state to state. In California, this program is known as *Medi-Cal* (see Chapter 12 and Appendix C).

Medicare

Medicare (M) is a hospital insurance system (Part A), supplementary medical insurance (Part B), and Medicare Plus (+) Choice Program (Part C) for those at 65 years of age, created by the 1965 Amendments to the Social Security Act and operated under the provisions of the act. Benefits are also extended to certain disabled people (e.g., totally disabled or blind) and coverage and payment are provided for those requiring kidney dialysis and kidney transplant services (see Chapters 11 and 12).

Medicare/Medicaid

Medicare/Medicaid (Medi-Medi) is a program that covers those persons eligible for both Medicare and Medicaid (see Chapters 11 and 12).

Point-of-Service Plan

A **point-of-service (POS) plan** is a managed care plan consisting of a network of physicians and hospitals that provides an insurance company or employer with discounts on its services. Patients can refer themselves to a specialist or see a nonprogram provider for a higher copayment (see Chapter 10).

Preferred Provider Organization

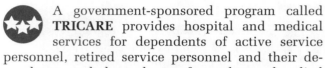 A variation of a managed care plan is a **preferred provider organization (PPO).** This is a form of contract medicine by which a large employer (e.g., hospitals or physicians) or any organization that can produce a large number of patients (e.g., union trusts or insurance companies) contracts with a hospital or a group of physicians to offer medical care at a reduced rate (see Chapter 10).

TRICARE

A government-sponsored program called **TRICARE** provides hospital and medical services for dependents of active service personnel, retired service personnel and their dependents, and dependents of members who died on active duty (see Chapter 13).

Unemployment Compensation Disability

Unemployment Compensation Disability (UCD) or State Disability Insurance (SDI) is insurance that covers off-the-job injury or sickness and is paid for by deductions from a person's paycheck. This program is administered by a state agency (see Chapter 15).

Veterans Affairs Outpatient Clinic

A **Veterans Affairs (VA) outpatient clinic** is where medical and dental services are rendered to a veteran who has a service-related disability (see Chapter 13).

Workers' Compensation Insurance

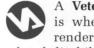 **Workers' compensation (WC) insurance** is a contract that insures a person against on-the-job injury or illness. The employer pays the premium for his or her employees (see Chapter 14).

Examples of Insurance Billing

Sometimes, it is difficult to comprehend the full scale of insurance billing. As an example of total medical billing, six cases are presented to help you understand the entire billing picture from simple to complex.

CASE 1: A new patient comes in with complaints of a sore throat and an infected nail. Evaluation and management (E/M) services are discussed in detail in Chapter 5.
The physician's office bills for:
Evaluation and management services
Penicillin injection
Office surgery for infected nail
Sterile surgical tray (may or may not be billed depending on insurance carrier)

CASE 2: A patient comes in because of an accident and has complaints that require evaluation and management services, x-ray films, and laboratory studies (urinalysis) performed in the physician's office.
The physician's office bills for:
Evaluation and management services
X-ray studies (including interpretation), and laboratory tests (urinalysis) including interpretation

CASE 3: A patient is seen by the family physician after office hours in the hospital emergency department.
The physician's office bills for evaluation and management services.
The hospital bills for hospital (outpatient) emergency department services (use and supplies).

CASE 4: A physician sends a patient's Papanicolaou smear to a private clinical laboratory.
The physician's office bills for evaluation and management services.
The laboratory bills for the Papanicolaou smear.

CASE 5: A patient is sent to a local hospital for an upper gastrointestinal radiographic series. An x-ray technician takes the films in the hospital, and a privately owned radiologic group does the interpretation.
The hospital bills for the technical component of the upper gastrointestinal x-ray series (use of equipment).
The radiologic group bills for the professional component of the upper gastrointestinal x-ray series (the interpretation).

CASE 6: A patient is seen in the office and is immediately hospitalized for surgery.
The physician's office bills for initial hospital admission (evaluation and management ser-

vices) and surgical procedure (e.g., hysterectomy). (The physician is a surgeon.)

The assistant surgeon bills for assisting the surgeon during hysterectomy (some insurance carriers do not allow payment).

The anesthesiologist bills for anesthesia administered during hysterectomy.

The hospital (inpatient) bills for hospital room, operating room, anesthesia supplies, medications, x-ray films, laboratory tests, and medical and surgical supplies (dressings, intravenous lines). The hospital (inpatient) might also bill for blood for transfusions, electrocardiogram, radiation therapy, and respiratory therapy.

A medical assistant or insurance billing specialist in the offices of the attending physician, assistant surgeon, anesthesiologist, radiologic group, and private clinical laboratory will submit an itemized statement and/or insurance claim form or give the patient the necessary information to submit his or her own claim to the insurance company. *Exception:* Generally, Medicare patients may not submit their own claims for physician or hospital services. Exceptions are mentioned in Chapter 11.

In the hospital and hospital emergency department, a member of the hospital staff inputs services into a central computer system that produces an itemized statement and completed insurance claim form via computer to be submitted to the insurance carrier. Hospital billing is explained in Chapter 16.

PROCEDURE: Handling and Processing Insurance Claims

To maintain a harmonious patient/physician relationship, be friendly and courteous when handling insurance claims. If the patient feels free to discuss personal financial problems at any time and is educated regarding the physician's fees, collections can often be significantly improved and simplified.

There are four basic methods of processing insurance claims for a medical practice: (1) manually preparing claims for submission, (2) in-office electronic filing by fax or computer, (3) contracting with an outside service bureau to prepare and submit the claims manually or electronically, or (4) use of a telecommunications networking system. The fourth method is a system in which a computer is networked via modem (telephone line) to another computer at another site so that the patients' insurance information is available to generate the insurance claim. This method may be used by an outside billing service or may be used when a medical practice has two or three offices and all billing is accomplished at one site.

In the use of any of these methods, the basic steps (Fig. 2–6 A and B) in handling and processing insurance claims are as follows:

1. Preregistration—Patient Registration Form: Some medical practices either preregister a new patient during the initial telephone call or a designated staff member may contact the patient before the appointment time. It is a good idea to give instructions on how to get to the office and ask the patient to arrive early. This allows time to collect vital statistics and insurance information and discuss the patient's responsibility with respect to payment policies. The patient may be sent an informative brochure with a patient registration form and a letter confirming the appointment. A **patient registration form** may also be called a *patient information form* or *intake sheet* (Figs. 2–7 and 2–8). It can be one that is developed by the physician and personalized for his or her own use or a generic form purchased from a medical supply company.

If the patient has a medical problem that makes it difficult to complete the form, such as rheumatoid arthritis of the hands or limited vision, then the insurance billing specialist may have to interview the patient and fill in the necessary data. Obtain *complete* information on a new patient by using a form that will contain information pertinent to credit and collections. This information must be *accurate.* Instruct the patient to fill in all spaces and indicate N/A (not applicable) if an item does not apply. If the form is returned with blank spaces, assist the patient in completing them. Verify insurance and all other information that may have changed at each visit, because patients may transfer from one insurance plan to another, move, or change jobs. This may be done by giving the patient either an update form or a copy of the previously completed patient registration form and asking him or her to correct any incorrect data in red (Fig. 2–9). Established patients may have changed employers or gotten married or divorced.

The following facts should be recorded:

▶ Name: first, middle initial, and last. The name should be identical to the one on the insurance identification card. (Some pediatric patients do not have the same last name as their parents or

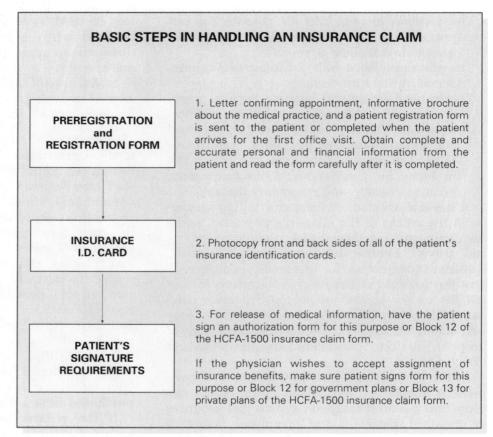

Figure 2–6. (A) Basic steps in handling an insurance claim.

BASIC STEPS IN HANDLING AN INSURANCE CLAIM

| PREREGISTRATION and REGISTRATION FORM | 1. Letter confirming appointment, informative brochure about the medical practice, and a patient registration form is sent to the patient or completed when the patient arrives for the first office visit. Obtain complete and accurate personal and financial information from the patient and read the form carefully after it is completed. |

| INSURANCE I.D. CARD | 2. Photocopy front and back sides of all of the patient's insurance identification cards. |

| PATIENT'S SIGNATURE REQUIREMENTS | 3. For release of medical information, have the patient sign an authorization form for this purpose or Block 12 of the HCFA-1500 insurance claim form.

If the physician wishes to accept assignment of insurance benefits, make sure patient signs form for this purpose or Block 12 for government plans or Block 13 for private plans of the HCFA-1500 insurance claim form. |

stepparents. An insurance check is usually received with the policyholder's name, and it is time consuming to find and give credit to the patient's account. If using a computer system, cross-reference the name or Social Security number so that when you call up the policyholder's name, the patient's name will also appear. If a manual system is used, keep an alphabetical card index of parental or billing names that also lists each patient's name.)

▶ Street address including apartment number and ZIP code and telephone number with area code
▶ Business address, telephone number with extension, and occupation
▶ Date of birth (recorded on insurance forms as eight digits, e.g., January 2, 1936 is written as 01-02-1936)
▶ Person responsible for account (guarantor) or insured's name
▶ Social Security number
▶ Spouse's name and occupation
▶ Referring physician's name or other referral source
▶ Driver's license number

▶ Emergency contact (close relative or friend with name, address, and telephone number)
▶ Insurance billing information: All insurance company names, addresses, and policy and group numbers. This is important because of the coordination of benefits clause written into some health insurance policies. Elderly patients are given the option of joining managed care programs and are allowed to switch every 30 days. Always ask each elderly patient whether he or she is covered by traditional Medicare or a Medicare HMO (health maintenance organization). A good patient information sheet will have space where this information can be written in by the patient.

2. Insurance Identification Card: Always copy front and back sides of the patient's insurance card and date the photocopy (Fig. 2–10). Sometimes the reverse side of the card provides information, such as deductible, copayment, preapproval provisions, and insurance company address and telephone number. A copy produces error-free insurance data and can be used in lieu of completing

BASIC STEPS IN PROCESSING AN INSURANCE CLAIM

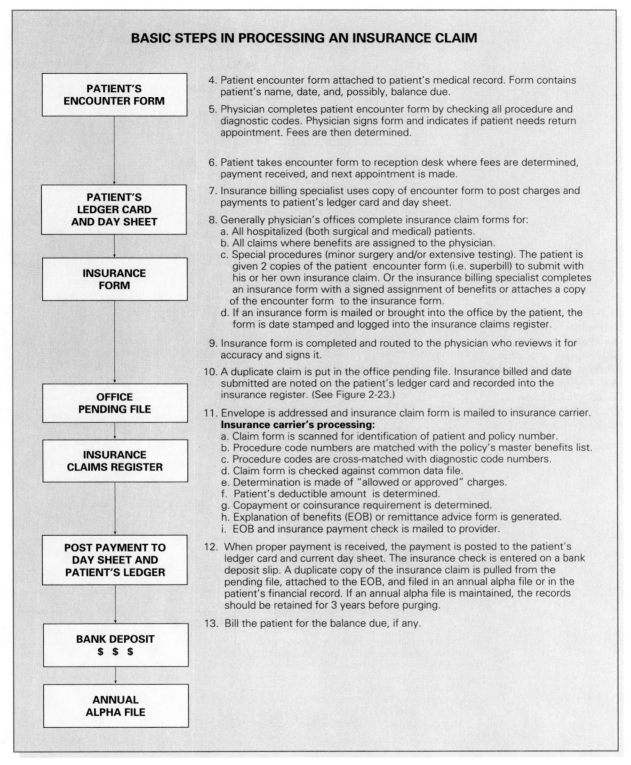

PATIENT'S ENCOUNTER FORM

PATIENT'S LEDGER CARD AND DAY SHEET

INSURANCE FORM

OFFICE PENDING FILE

INSURANCE CLAIMS REGISTER

POST PAYMENT TO DAY SHEET AND PATIENT'S LEDGER

BANK DEPOSIT $ $ $

ANNUAL ALPHA FILE

4. Patient encounter form attached to patient's medical record. Form contains patient's name, date, and, possibly, balance due.

5. Physician completes patient encounter form by checking all procedure and diagnostic codes. Physician signs form and indicates if patient needs return appointment. Fees are then determined.

6. Patient takes encounter form to reception desk where fees are determined, payment received, and next appointment is made.

7. Insurance billing specialist uses copy of encounter form to post charges and payments to patient's ledger card and day sheet.

8. Generally physician's offices complete insurance claim forms for:
   a. All hospitalized (both surgical and medical) patients.
   b. All claims where benefits are assigned to the physician.
   c. Special procedures (minor surgery and/or extensive testing). The patient is given 2 copies of the patient encounter form (i.e. superbill) to submit with his or her own insurance claim. Or the insurance billing specialist completes an insurance form with a signed assignment of benefits or attaches a copy of the encounter form to the insurance form.
   d. If an insurance form is mailed or brought into the office by the patient, the form is date stamped and logged into the insurance claims register.

9. Insurance form is completed and routed to the physician who reviews it for accuracy and signs it.

10. A duplicate claim is put in the office pending file. Insurance billed and date submitted are noted on the patient's ledger card and recorded into the insurance register. (See Figure 2-23.)

11. Envelope is addressed and insurance claim form is mailed to insurance carrier.
    Insurance carrier's processing:
    a. Claim form is scanned for identification of patient and policy number.
    b. Procedure code numbers are matched with the policy's master benefits list.
    c. Procedure codes are cross-matched with diagnostic code numbers.
    d. Claim form is checked against common data file.
    e. Determination is made of "allowed or approved" charges.
    f. Patient's deductible amount is determined.
    g. Copayment or coinsurance requirement is determined.
    h. Explanation of benefits (EOB) or remittance advice form is generated.
    i. EOB and insurance payment check is mailed to provider.

12. When proper payment is received, the payment is posted to the patient's ledger card and current day sheet. The insurance check is entered on a bank deposit slip. A duplicate copy of the insurance claim is pulled from the pending file, attached to the EOB, and filed in an annual alpha file or in the patient's financial record. If an annual alpha file is maintained, the records should be retained for 3 years before purging.

13. Bill the patient for the balance due, if any.

Figure 2–6 Continued. (*B*) Basic steps in processing an insurance claim in a physician's office, to the insurance carrier, by the insurance company, and after payment is received.

Insurance cards copied   ☒   **Patient Registration**   Account #: ___84516___
Date: _Jan. 20, 20XX_   **Information**   Insurance #: _H-550-64-5172-02_
                                                                             Co-Payment : $_OV $10 ER $50_

Please PRINT AND complete ALL sections below!

Is your condition the result of a work injury? YES ⃝NO An auto accident? YES ⃝NO
Date of injury: _____

PATIENT'S PERSONAL INFORMATION Marital status ☐ Single ☒ Married ☐ Divorced ☐ Widowed
                              Sex: ☐ Male ☒ Female
Name: _____FUHR_____LINDA_____L._____
             last name   first name   initial
Street Address: ___3070 Tipper Street___ (Apt # _4_) City: _Oxnard_____ State: _CA_ Zip: _93030_
Home phone:(805)276-0101__ Work phone:(805)372-1151__ Social Security # _550-64-5172_
Date of Birth:_11_/05_/65_ Driver's License: (State & Number) _G0075012_
Employer/Name of School _Electronic Data Systems_____ ☒Full Time ☐Part Time
Spouse's Name: _FUHR_____GERALD_____T.__ Spouse's Work phone:(805)921-0075
               last name   first name   initial
How do you wish to be addressed?___LINDA_____ Social Security # ___545-01-2771___

PATIENT'S/ RESPONSIBLE PARTY INFORMATION
Responsible party: ___GERALD T. FUHR_____ Date of Birth: _06-15-64_
Relationship to patient: ☐ Self ☒Spouse ☐Other   Social Security # _545-01-2771_
Responsible party's home phone:(805) 276-0101____ Work phone:(805) 921-0075
   Address: ___3070 Tipper Street___ (Apt # _4_) City: _Oxnard__ State: _CA_ Zip: _93030_
Employer's Name: _General Electric_____ Phone number:(805) 485-0121
   Address: ___317 East Main_____ City: _Oxnard__ State: _CA_ Zip: _93030_
   Your occupation: _Technician_____
Spouse's Employer's Name: _Electronic Data Systems_ Spouse's Work phone:(805)372-1151
   Address: _2700 West 5th Street_____ City: _Oxnard____ State: _CA_ Zip: _93030_

PATIENT'S INSURANCE INFORMATION Please present insurance cards to receptionist.
PRIMARY insurance company's name: __Aetna Life Insurance Company___
Insurance address: _P.O. Box 12340_____ City: _Fresno___ State: _CA_ Zip: _93765_
Name of insured: _Linda L. Fuhr_____ Date of Birth:_11/05/65_ Relationship to insured: ☒Self ☐Spouse
                                                                                        ☐Other ☐Child
Insurance ID number: _H-550-64-5172-02_ Group number: _17098-020-00004_
SECONDARY insurance company's name: __None____
Insurance address: _____ City: _____ State: ___ Zip: ____
Name of insured: _____ Date of Birth:_____ Relationship to insured: ☐Self ☐Spouse
                                                                              ☐Other ☐Child
Insurance ID number: _____ Group number:_____
Check if appropriate: ☐Medigap policy ☐Retiree coverage

PATIENT'S REFERRAL INFORMATION   (Please circle one)
Referred by: _Margaret Taylor (Mrs. W. T.)_ If referred by a friend, may we thank her or him? ⃝Yes No
Name(s) of other physician(s) who care for you: _Jason Smythe, MD_____

EMERGENCY CONTACT
Name of person not living with you:_Hannah Gildea_____ Relationship: __Aunt____
Address: __4621 Lucretia Avenue_____ City:_Oxnard___ State: _CA_ Zip: _93030_
Phone number (home):(805) 274-0132__ Phone number (work):(__)_____

Assignment of Benefits • Financial Agreement

I hereby give lifetime authorization for payment of insurance benefits be made directly to_____ , and
any assisting physicians, for services rendered. I understand that I am financially responsible for all charges
whether or not they are covered by insurance. In the event of default, I agree to pay all costs of collection, and
reasonable attorney's fees. I hereby authorize this healthcare provider to release all information necessary to
secure the payment of benefits.
I further agree that a photocopy of this agreement shall be as valid as the original.
Date: _Jan 20, 20XX_ Your signature: _Linda L. Fuhr_
Method of payment: ☐ Cash ☒ Check ☐Credit Card

Figure 2–7. Patient registration information form showing a comprehensive listing of personal and financial information obtained from the patient on his or her first visit to the office. (Courtesy of Bibbero Systems, Inc., Petaluma, CA. Phone: 800-242-2376; FAX: 800-242-9330.)

the insurance section of the patient registration form. On a return visit, ask to see the card and check it with the data on file (Fig. 2–11). If it differs, photocopy both sides and write the date on the copy, using this as the base for revising data on file.

3. Patient's Signature Requirements

RELEASE OF INFORMATION

If the physician is submitting an insurance claim for the patient, the patient must sign a release of information form (also known as an authorization

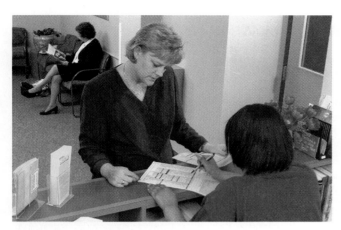

Figure 2–8. Receptionist giving instructions to a patient on how to complete the patient registration form.

or consent form) before information can be given to an insurance company, attorney, or other third party (Fig. 2–12). This often appears on the bottom portion of the patient registration form and may be worded to include an annual or lifetime authorization depending on the type of insurance or federal program.

ASSIGNMENT OF BENEFITS

If the physician wishes to receive the check by accepting assignment, the patient must sign an assignment of benefits form for each insurance company. However, before explaining an assignment, it is important to define the difference between participating and nonparticipating providers. A **participating provider (par)** has a contractual agreement with an insurance plan to render care to eligible beneficiaries and bills the insurance carrier directly. The insurance carrier pays its portion of the allowed amount, and the provider bills the patient for the balance not paid by the insurer after the disallowed portion is adjusted off of the account. However, in Blue Plans, the provider is referred to as a *member physician* and may accept the payment as *payment in full* or may bill the patient for any unpaid balance depending on the contract. Managed care plans also refer to participating providers as member physicians. A **nonparticipating provider (nonpar)** is a physician without a contractual agreement with an insurance plan to accept an allowed amount and to render care to eligible beneficiaries. The provider may or may not file an insurance claim as a courtesy to the patient and usually expects full payment at the time of service.

The general definition of **assignment** is the transfer, after an event insured against, of an individual's legal right to collect an amount payable under an insurance contract. Most of the time an agreement is obtained by having the patient sign an assignment of insurance benefits document directing payment to the physician. However, many health insurance claim forms (e.g., HCFA-1500 form) contain a provision that, when signed by the insured, directs the insurance company to pay benefits directly to the provider of care on whose charge the claim is based. An assignment of benefits becomes a legally enforceable document but must refer to specific hospitalization, course of treatment, or office visits. Each course of treatment needs to have an assignment document executed by the patient unless an annual or lifetime signature authorization is accepted and in the patient's financial file, except when automobile or homeowners' liability insurance is involved.

Private Carriers

For private insurance companies with whom the provider does not have a contractual agreement, accepting assignment means that the insurance check will be directed to the provider's office instead of to the patient. Because there is no signed agreement with the carrier, the difference between the billed amount and the carrier's allowed amount is not written off but collected from the patient as well as any copayment or deductible. In private third party liability cases, the physician needs to negotiate with the insurance company to make sure benefits are paid to him or her directly.

Managed Care

In managed care plans, a participating provider (also called a *preferred provider*) is a physician who has contracted with a plan to provide medical services to plan members. A nonparticipating provider refers to a physician who has not contracted with a managed care plan to provide medical services to plan members. For individuals who have signed with managed care contracts the assignment is automatic.

Medicaid

For Medicaid cases, there is no assignment unless the patient has other insurance in addition to Medicaid.

PATIENT INFORMATION UPDATE

Welcome, we are delighted to see you again!
Please take a few minutes to help us update our records.

Name __Linda_____ L._____ Fuhr_____   Today's Date __6-30-XX__
     FIRST   MIDDLE   LAST

1. Has your name changed since your last visit here? ____Yes __X_No
   If yes, what was your old name? __N/A__
   What name do you use for health insurance if different from above?__N/A_____

2. If you have a new or different address since your initial visit here, please
   indicate below:
   _____2201 West Klein Street_____
   _____Oxnard, CA 93033_____

3. Has your marital status changed? ____Yes __X_No

4. Has your telephone number changed?__X_Yes
   Please indicate your correct telephone number ___805-401-7600_____

5. Has your employment changed? ____Yes __X_No
   Please indicate your new employer name and address:
   _____N/A_____

   New employer telephone #:_____—_____

6. Have you changed health insurance companies? ____Yes __X_No
   If yes, please indicate your new health insurance carrier and address.
   Primary _____N/A_____   Secondary _____N/A____
   _____   _____

   Group Nos. _____   Group Nos. _____
   Subscriber Nos. _____   Subscriber nos. _____

7. Who is responsible for this bill? ___Gerald T. Fuhr_____

8. Please note any change in your health since your last visit?
   Illness _____
   Accident _____
   Allergies _____
   Medications being taken __Thyroid_____

   Other _____

9. Signature ___*Linda L Fuhr*_____

PATIENT INFORMATION UPDATE

Figure 2–9. Patient information update form showing questions to ask the patient for updating a previous patient registration information form. (Courtesy of Professional Filing Systems, Inc., Atlanta, GA.)

Medicare

In the Medicare program, the words participating, nonparticipating, and assignment have slightly different meanings. A physician who accepts assignment on Medicare claims is called a *participating (par) physician* and may not bill, or accept payment for, the amount of the difference between the submitted charge and the Medicare allowed amount. However, an attempt must be made to collect 20% of the allowed charge (coinsurance) and any amount applied to the deductible. A physician who does not participate is called a *nonparticipating (nonpar) physician* and has an option regarding assignment. The physician may not accept assignment for all services or has the option of accepting assignment for some services and collecting from the patient for other services performed at the same time and place. The physician collects the fee from the patient but may bill no more than the Medicare limiting charge. The check is sent to the patient. When treating federal or state government employees or a Medicare recipient, the physician may lose the fee if government guidelines are not followed.

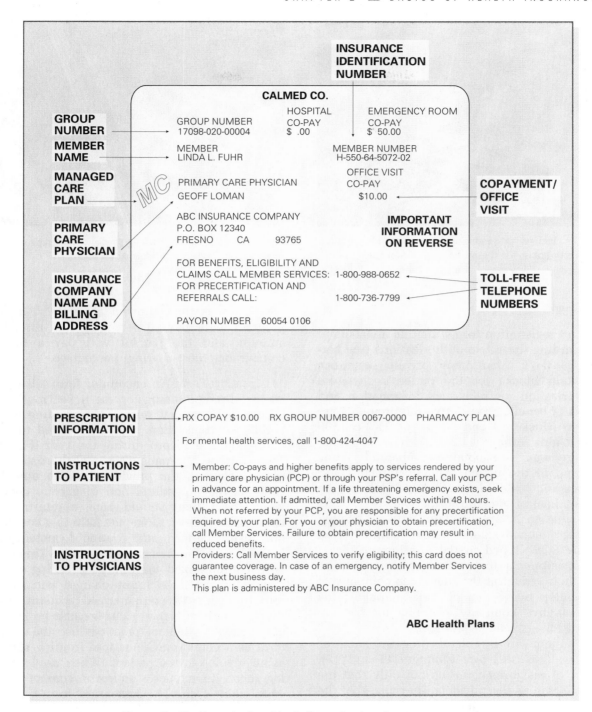

Figure 2–10. Front (*top*) and back (*bottom*) sides of an insurance card.

TRICARE

A provider who accepts TRICARE standard assignment (participates) agrees to accept the allowable charge as the full fee and cannot charge the patient the difference between the provider's charge and the allowable charge.

Workers' Compensation

For industrial cases, there is no assignment. The workers' compensation carrier pays the fee for services rendered according to its fee schedule and the check automatically goes to the physician. The patient is not responsible for payment of services for any work-related injury or illness.

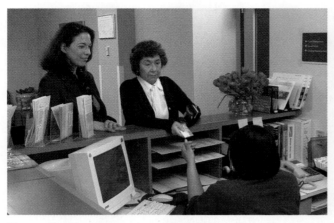

Figure 2–11. Patient presenting an insurance identification card to the receptionist for the purpose of photocopying.

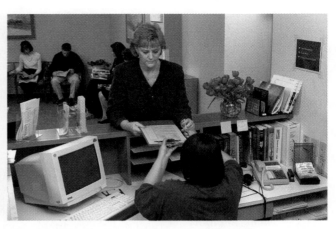

Figure 2–12. Insurance billing specialist obtaining the patient's signature on a release of information form.

SIGNATURE GUIDELINES

Most patient registration forms include a statement to sign regarding these two authorizations (see bottom of Fig. 2–7). Also many private insurance forms contain blocks for the patient's signature with authorization for release of information and assignment of benefits. These two requirements are included in Blocks 12 and 13 of the HCFA-1500 insurance claim form (Fig. 2–13). If these signature requirements are obtained separately, they may be filed in the patient's medical record and the abbreviation "SOF" (signature on file) may be used on the insurance claim form.

When using an insurance claim with no printed assignment, attach a signed patient authorization form with "SOF" typed in the appropriate place. Because attachments to insurance forms may be lost after their arrival at the insurance company, it is wise to make two copies of the assignment (one for the insurance company and one for the patient's file in the physician's office).

For a patient on a federal program such as Medicare or TRICARE (see Chapters 11 and 13), acceptance of assignment means not only that the check will come to the physician but also that the physician will accept what the federal program

designates as the "allowed amount." The federal program will pay a percentage of the allowed amount, and the patient will pay a remaining coinsurance (cost-sharing) percentage.

4. Encounter Form: An **encounter form** (also called a charge slip, communicator, fee ticket, multipurpose billing form, patient service slip, routing form, superbill, or transaction slip) is attached to the patient's medical record during the visit (Fig. 2–14). This contains the patient's name, the date, and, in some instances, the previous balance due. It also contains the procedural and diagnostic codes and when the patient should have a return appointment. This two- or three-part form is a combination bill, insurance form, and routing document used in both computer and pegboard systems. This can also be a computerized multipurpose billing form that may be scanned to input charges and diagnoses into the patient's computerized account. Time is saved and fewer errors occur because no keystrokes are involved. Medical practices use the encounter form as a communications tool (routing sheet) and as an invoice to the patient. When used as a routing sheet, it becomes a *source document* for insurance claim data. The encounter form's procedure and diagnostic code sections should be updated an-

---

READ BACK OF FORM BEFORE COMPLETING & SIGNING THIS FORM.

12. PATIENT'S OR AUTHORIZED PERSON'S SIGNATURE I authorize the release of any medical or other information necessary to process this claim. I also request payment of government benefits either to myself or to the party who accepts assignment below.

SIGNED _____   DATE _____

13. INSURED'S OR AUTHORIZED PERSON'S SIGNATURE I authorize payment of medical benefits to the undersigned physician or supplier for services described below.

SIGNED _____

Figure 2–13. Sections 12 and 13 from the health insurance claim form HCFA-1500, illustrating authorization for release of information and assignment of benefits.

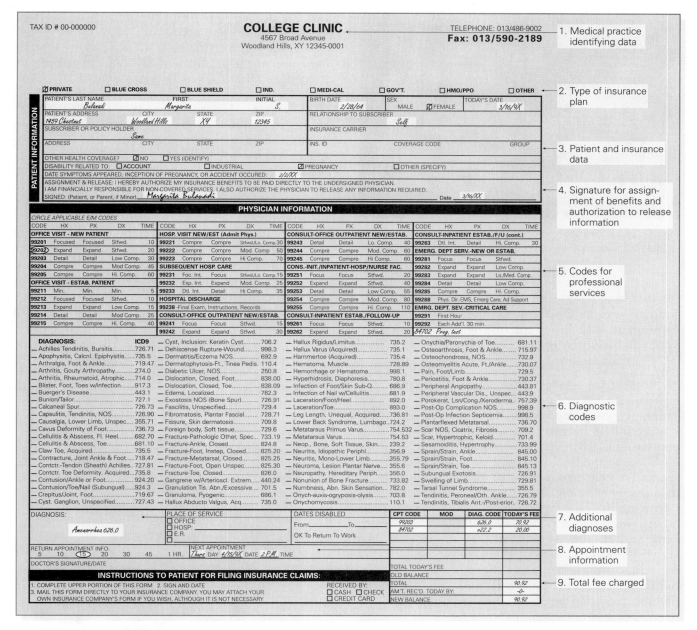

Figure 2–14. Encounter form; procedural codes for professional services are taken from the *Current Procedural Terminology* (CPT) book, and diagnostic codes are taken from the *International Classification of Diseases, 9th revision, Clinical Modification* (ICD-9-CM) book. (Courtesy of Bibbero Systems, Inc., Petaluma, CA. Phone: 800-242-2376; FAX: 800-242-9330.)

nually with correct descriptions because changes, additions, and deletions occur. Remove all codes not used or seldom used and revise and add current valid commonly used codes for the practice. Do not print large quantities because codes change annually. Some practices develop encounter forms for different services (e.g., surgical services, office services [within the facility], and out-of-office service [hospital visits, emergency, outpatient facility, nursing home, or house calls]). Examples of en-

counter forms are shown in Chapter 7, Figure 7–9, and Chapter 9, Figure 9–7.

5. Physician's Signature: After examination and treatment, the physician completes the encounter form by checking off the procedure (services and treatments) codes and diagnostic code(s) (Fig. 2–15). The physician signs the form and indicates whether the patient needs another appointment.

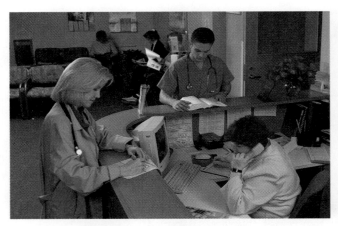

Figure 2–15. Physician checking off procedures on the encounter form at the conclusion of a patient's office visit.

6. Determine Fees: The patient carries the encounter form to the reception desk where fees are determined and input for billing (Fig. 2–16). He or she is given the opportunity to pay and make a future appointment.

7. Bookkeeping—Ledger Card: The value of maintaining careful records of all insurance matters cannot be overemphasized. A financial accounting record or **ledger card** is maintained for each patient who receives professional services (Fig. 2–17). The medical assistant or insurance billing specialist may use a copy of the encounter form to daily **post** (record) professional fees (charges), payments (cash, check, or credit card), adjustments, and balance due to the patient's ledger card and to the day sheet (Fig. 2–18). A **day sheet,** or daily record sheet, is a register for recording daily business transactions. All patients seen in one day will have their charges (debits) recorded on the day sheet, along with all payments and adjustments (credits). Each day the totals are carried forward and a new day sheet is set up to receive posting for that day. The ledger card should show an entry of the date an insurance claim is sent, including the date of services that were billed. Each service must be posted on a single line, and a **running balance** is calculated in the right column. When the ledger is completely filled up, the account balance is brought forward (also known as **extend**) to a new card. If a practice is computerized, all financial transactions are executed using billing software. Patients who are private one month and on the Medicaid program the next month may require two ledgers to keep private and state records separate. An established private patient who is injured on the job would require two ledgers,

one for private care and one for posting workers' compensation insurance.

Step-by-step instructions for completing a ledger card are given at the end of this chapter in the procedure "Posting to a Patient's Ledger."

8. Insurance Form: Generally, the insurance billing specialist in the physician's office completes the insurance claim forms for the following cases: (a) all hospitalized (both surgical and medical) patients, (b) all claims in which the benefits are assigned to the physician, and (c) special procedures (minor surgery or extensive testing). In these cases, the insurance billing specialist completes the HCFA-1500 insurance claim form with accurate procedural and diagnostic codes, including any appropriate documents (operative report or invoice), and mails it to the correct insurance carrier.

The minimum information required by third party payers is

◗ What was done? (services and procedures using procedure codes discussed in Chapter 5)
◗ Why was it done? (diagnoses using diagnostic codes discussed in Chapter 4)

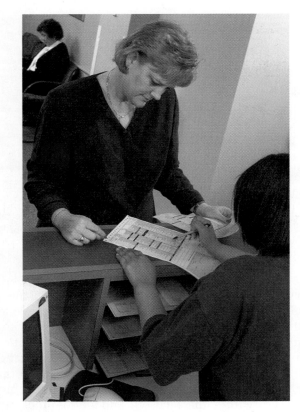

Figure 2–16. Patient carrying the encounter form to the medical office's check-up station.

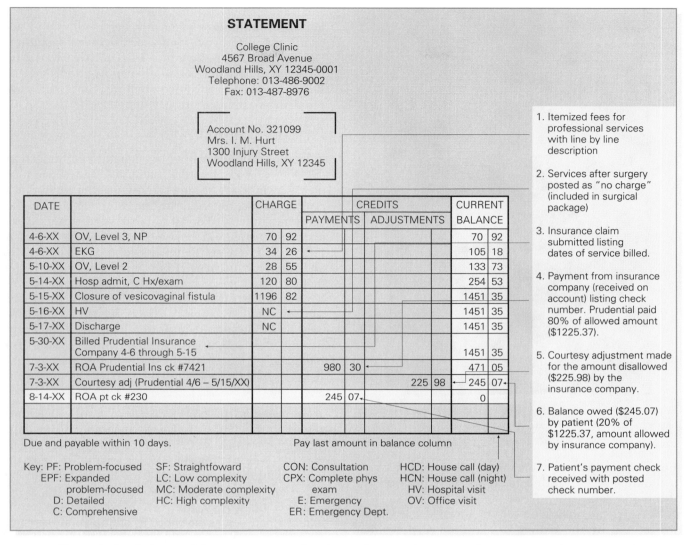

STATEMENT

College Clinic
4567 Broad Avenue
Woodland Hills, XY 12345-0001
Telephone: 013-486-9002
Fax: 013-487-8976

Account No. 321099
Mrs. I. M. Hurt
1300 Injury Street
Woodland Hills, XY 12345

DATE		CHARGE		CREDITS		CURRENT	
---	---	---	---	PAYMENTS	ADJUSTMENTS	BALANCE	
4-6-XX	OV, Level 3, NP	70	92			70	92
4-6-XX	EKG	34	26			105	18
5-10-XX	OV, Level 2	28	55			133	73
5-14-XX	Hosp admit, C Hx/exam	120	80			254	53
5-15-XX	Closure of vesicovaginal fistula	1196	82			1451	35
5-16-XX	HV	NC				1451	35
5-17-XX	Discharge	NC				1451	35
5-30-XX	Billed Prudential Insurance Company 4-6 through 5-15					1451	35
7-3-XX	ROA Prudential Ins ck #7421			980	30	471	05
7-3-XX	Courtesy adj (Prudential 4/6 – 5/15/XX)				225	98	245	07
8-14-XX	ROA pt ck #230			245	07	0	

Due and payable within 10 days.   Pay last amount in balance column

Key: PF: Problem-focused   SF: Straightfoward   CON: Consultation   HCD: House call (day)
EPF: Expanded   LC: Low complexity   CPX: Complete phys   HCN: House call (night)
problem-focused   MC: Moderate complexity   exam   HV: Hospital visit
D: Detailed   HC: High complexity   E: Emergency   OV: Office visit
C: Comprehensive   ER: Emergency Dept.

1. Itemized fees for professional services with line by line description

2. Services after surgery posted as "no charge" (included in surgical package)

3. Insurance claim submitted listing dates of service billed.

4. Payment from insurance company (received on account) listing check number. Prudential paid 80% of allowed amount ($1225.37).

5. Courtesy adjustment made for the amount disallowed ($225.98) by the insurance company.

6. Balance owed ($245.07) by patient (20% of $1225.37, amount allowed by insurance company).

7. Patient's payment check received with posted check number.

Figure 2–17. Ledger card illustrating posting of professional service descriptions, fees, payments, adjustments, and balance due.

▶ When was it performed? (date of service [DOS])
▶ Where was it received? (place of service [POS])
▶ Who did it? (provider name and identifying number)

A helpful hint is to group together all ledgers and charts from patients who have the same type of insurance and bill them all at one time. This cuts down on errors and makes completing the forms easier.

Submit claims as soon as possible after professional services are rendered except for patients receiving care over a continuing period of time when billing is to be sent in at the end of the treatment. There are time limits (30 days to 1½ years) for filing an insurance claim from the date of service. This can vary depending on the commercial carrier, federal or state program, or whether the claim is for an illness or accident. Claims filed after the time limit will be denied. This topic is further discussed within the chapters on Medicare, Medicaid, TRICARE, and workers' compensation.

Financial losses from delay can occur in the following instances. If a patient has had a long-term illness, insurance benefits can expire before a claim is processed. If several physicians treat the same patient, some insurance companies pay only one of the physicians (typically, whoever files the claim first is paid first). In this scenario, the other physicians may have to wait for disbursement by the physician who received the check. Submit

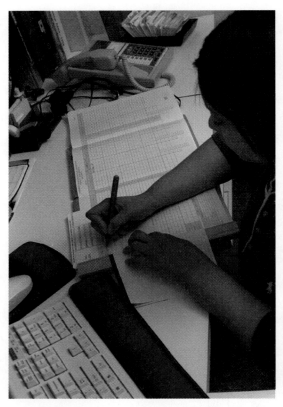

Figure 2–18. Medical office employee posting to a patient's ledger card and/or day sheet.

hospitalized patients' insurance claim forms twice a month (on the 15th and 30th) regardless of the discharge date.

If a private insurance claim form is mailed or brought in by the patient at the time of the office visit, that form is date-stamped and reviewed to be sure the patient has signed the release of information statement. Patients who submit their own insurance claims are given two copies of the encounter form. The patient retains one copy for personal records and attaches the second copy to the insurance claim form and forwards it to the insurance company.

9. Provider's Handwritten Signature: The completed insurance form is reviewed for accuracy and routed to the provider (physician). A *provider* refers to any individual or organization that provides health care services. Providers may be physicians, hospitals, physical therapists, medical equipment suppliers, and pharmacies. Generally when submitting insurance claims, the provider must hand write his or her name attesting to the document. However, there are some exceptions in that most private payers will accept a completed insurance claim with no signature as long as the physician's name is preprinted on the form. In addition, some insur-

ance companies require that the provider have a notarized authorization on file before they will accept a claim form without the provider's signature. However, when a signature is required, it can be accepted in several formats—handwritten, facsimile stamp, and electronic signature. State and government programs require a signature.

PHYSICIAN'S REPRESENTATIVE

Sometimes a physician gives signature authorization to one person on the staff to sign insurance claims, who then becomes known as the physician's representative, referred to in Figure 2–19 as the "attorney-in-fact." For an authorization of this type, a document should be typed and signed before a notary. This means that whoever signs the form is attesting to it because it is a legal document. If the medical practice is ever audited and fraud or embezzlement is discovered, then the person who had signature authorization can be brought into the case as well as the physician. If this involves a Medicare patient, the federal government will prosecute. If a Medicaid patient is involved, the state prosecutes.

SIGNATURE STAMP

Some medical practices use a facsimile signature stamp so the staff can process insurance forms and other paperwork without interrupting the physician or waiting for her or his signature. For an authorization of this type, a document should be typed and signed before a notary (Fig. 2–20).

However, use of this stamp can lead to problems, because it is possible to stamp unauthorized checks, transcribed medical reports, prescriptions, or credit card charge slips. If such a stamp is used infrequently, then discontinue the practice. If one is used regularly, prevent problems by doing the following:

▶ Make only one stamp.
▶ Allow only long-term, trusted, bonded staff members to have access to the stamp.
▶ Keep the stamp in a location with a secure lock.
▶ Limit access to the stamp.

For information on state laws, contact your state legislature at your state capitol. For data about signatures on hospital medical records, see Chapter 16, Hospital Billing.

COMPUTERIZED SIGNATURES

There are two types of computerized signatures, electronic and digital. An **electronic signature** looks like the signer's handwritten signature. The signer authenticates the document by key entry or with a pen pad using a stylus to capture the live signature.

PROVIDER'S NOTARIZED SIGNATURE AUTHORIZATION

State of ___Iowa___)
)ss
County of _Des Moines_)

Know all persons by these presents:

That I, _John Doe, MD_ have made, constituted, and appointed and by these presents do make, constitute and appoint _Mary Coleman_ my true and lawful attorney-in-fact for me and in my name place and stead to sign my name on claims, for payment for services provided by me submitted to the _Blue Cross and Blue Shield of Iowa_ . My signature by my said attorney-in-fact includes my agreement to abide by the full payment concept and the remainder of the certification appearing on all _HCFA-1500_ claim forms. I hereby ratify and confirm all that my said attorney-in-fact shall lawfully do or cause to be done by virtue of the power generated herein.

In witness whereof I have hereunto set my hand this __20th__ day of _January_ 20 XX .

_____
          John Doe, MD
                (Signature)

Subscribed and sworn to before me this _20th_ day of _January_ 20 XX

_____
              Notary Public

My commission expires _____ .

Figure 2–19. Example of a provider's signature authorization form that can be completed, notarized, and sent to the insurance carrier after a copy is retained for the physician's records.

> **Example: David Smith, MD**

It can also be defined as an individualized computer access and identification system (e.g., a series of numbers, letters, electronic writing, voice, computer key, and fingerprint transmission [biometric system]).

A *digital signature* may be lines of text or a text box stating the signer's name, date, and time and a statement indicating a signature has been attached from within the software application.

> **Example: Electronically signed: David Smith, MD**
> **07/12/2000   10:30:08**

10. Office Pending File and Insurance Claims Register: A duplicate of the claim is retained in the office pending file in the event payment is not received and the claim must be followed up. This file may also be referred to as a suspense, follow-up, or tickler file (Figs. 2–21 and 2–22). The term "tickler" came into existence because it tickles or jogs the memory at certain dates in the future.

Establish an insurance claims register (tracing file) to keep track of the status of each case that has been billed (Fig. 2–23). Record to whom the claim was sent and the submission date on the insurance claims register and the patient's ledger card. The insurance billing specialist handling the insurance forms can see at a glance which claims are becoming delinquent and the amounts owed to the physician. This is an efficient method used for 30- to 60-day follow-up.

Keep two copies of each claim for the physician's records, one to be filed by patient name and the other by carrier name. *Or* simply record the name of the insurance company on each patient's ledger card and keep a file for each carrier by date of service. Filing by carrier allows all inquiries to be included in a single letter to the insurance company to eliminate having to write to the same company three or four times.

Ledger cards are referred to as financial records and are always kept separate from the medical

PROVIDER'S NOTARIZED FACSIMILE OR STAMP SIGNATURE AUTHORIZATION

State of ___Florida___)
)ss
County of __Jacksonville__)

___John Doe, MD___ being first duty sworn, deposes and says:

I hereby authorize the ___Blue Cross of Florida___
                                                    (Name of Fiscal Administrator)
to accept my facsimile or stamp signature shown below

_____*John Doe, MD*_____
                    (Facsimile or Stamp Signature)

as my true signature for all purposes under the __Medicare__
                                                                          (Name of Insurance Program)
in the same manner as if it were my actual signature, including
my agreeing to abide by the full payment concept and the
remainder of the certification normally signed by the source of
care as it appears on all <u>HCFA-1500</u> claim forms.

_____*John Doe, MD*_____
                    (Signature)

Subscribed and sworn to before me this _3rd_ day
of __January__ 20XX.

_____
                    Notary Public in and for
_____ County, State of_____
(SEAL)
My commission expires _____.

Figure 2–20. Example of a provider's facsimile or stamp signature authorization form that can be completed, notarized, and sent to the insurance carrier after a copy is retained for the physician's records.

record. For easy and quick access, some practices prefer to keep additional financial records also separate from the patient's medical records. The financial record should contain all billing information, a copy of the completed patient information form, patient authorization or signature-on-file form, copies of insurance identification cards, responsible-party authorization, insurance correspondence, explanation of benefits or remittance advice documents, and a log of all telephone conversations and actions taken regarding insurance disputes or collection activities.

11. Mailing the Claim Form: A large manila envelope is addressed, and the claim form is mailed to the insurance carrier. Mail claims in batches to each carrier to save on postage. Refer to Figure 2−6*B* for the nine phases of processing by the insurance carrier of a claim form for payment.

12. Insurance Payments

BANK DEPOSIT AND ANNUAL ALPHA FILE

A payment (check) from the insurance carrier should be received in 2 to 8 weeks, accompanied by an explanation of benefits/remittance advice

document. The duplicate claim form is pulled from the file to verify the payment received against the amount billed. The payment is posted (credited) to the patient's ledger card and current day sheet indicating the date of posting, name of insurance company, check or voucher number, amount received, and contracted adjustment. The check is then entered on a bank deposit slip and may be deposited at the bank. After proper payment is received, the duplicate copy of the insurance claim is attached to the explanation of benefits form. These are filed in an annual alpha file according to insurance type, date of service, or patients' names. A date file using the posting date as reference is another option. Some medical practices file claim forms at the back section of the patient's medical record after payment is received and accepted; however, this is an optional but not preferred system.

If an annual alpha file is maintained, the records should be retained for 3 years before purging to meet the requirements of the Internal Revenue Service. The Internal Revenue Service can request tax records for the 3 years preceding an audit. The audit can include records for the previous 6 years if taxpayers fail to report more than 25% of their gross

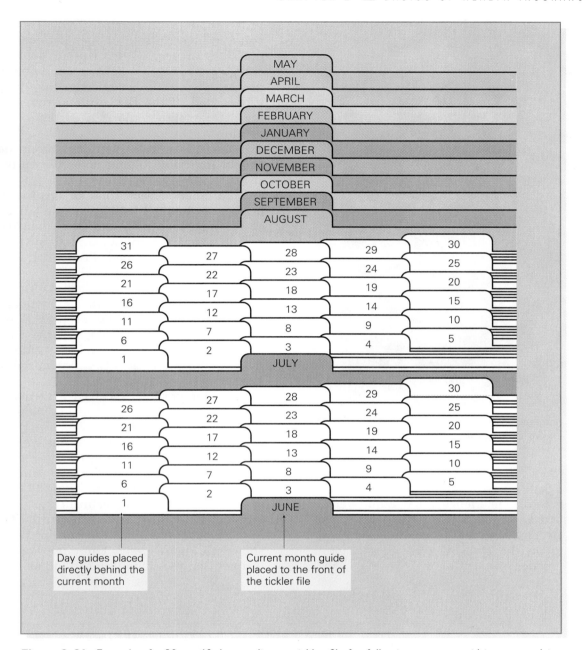

Figure 2–21. Example of a 30- to 60-day pending or tickler file for following up on unpaid insurance claims.

income. There are no time limitations if taxpayers file a fraudulent return or fail to file a return.

For further information on improper payments received and tracing delinquent claims, see Chapter 8.

13. Monthly Statement: The patient who has insurance should be sent a monthly statement for all outstanding charges. A note stating "Your insurance has been billed" should appear on the itemized statement. The patient should always be billed the same fee as that submitted to the insurance company. After the insurance plan has paid, a message should appear on the statement indicating the amount the patient owes.

PROCEDURE: Posting to a Patient's Ledger

Follow these steps to post charges, payments, adjustments, and balances to a patient's ledger/account (see Fig. 2–17).

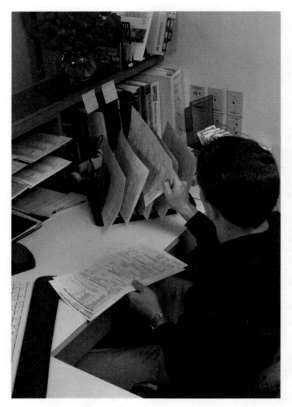

Figure 2–22. Insurance billing specialist using a desk sorter to alphabetize insurance claims to make filing easier in the tickler file.

1. Insert the patient's name and address to prepare the ledger card. Some ledgers may require additional information (attending physician's name, type of insurance, patient's telephone number), depending on the style of card chosen for a medical practice.

2. Post the date of service (DOS) in the date column, description of the services in the professional service description column, and charge amount in the charge column. The posting date is the actual date the transaction is recorded. If the DOS differs from the posting date, reference the DOS in the description column.

3. Add the charge to the running current balance, and in the right column enter the current balance.

4. Enter a notation each time an insurance claim has been submitted listing the date billed, name of the insurance plan, and the inclusive from and to dates of service covered by the claim submission (e.g., Billed Prudential Insurance Company 4–6 through 5–15).

5. Post all amounts paid for each date of service in the payment column, referencing that it was received on account (ROA). List the payer (patient [pt] or name of the insurance company) and check/voucher number (e.g., ROA pt ck #230 or ROA Prudential Ins ck #7421).

6. Subtract the payment received from the amount in the running current balance column and enter the current balance.

7. Post the contracted insurance plan discount in the "Adjustment" column by referencing the DOS, insurance company name, and type of contract discount (e.g., HealthNet PPO discount or Medicare courtesy adjustment).

8. Subtract the adjustment amount from the running balance and enter the current balance as shown in Figure 2–17. Optional: Post the adjustment on the same line as the payment.

Figure 2–23. Insurance claims register. This is an example of how a form can be set up to establish an easy way to follow up on insurance claims.

Patient's Name Group/policy No.	Name of Insurance Company	Claim Submitted		Follow-Up		Claim Paid		Difference
		Date	Amount	Date	Date	Date	Amt	
Davis, Bob	BC/BS	1-7-00	319.37			2/28/00	294.82	24.55
Cash, David	BC	1-8-00	268.08	2-10-00	3-10-00			
Smythe, Jan	Medicaid	1-9-00	146.15	2-10-00				
Phillips, Emma	Medicare	1-10-00	96.28	2-10-00				
Perez, Jose	Medi-Medi	1-10-00	647.09	2-10-00				
Amato, Joe	Tricare	2-1-00	134.78	3-10-00				
Rubin, Billy	Aetna	2-4-00	607.67	3-10-00				
Pfeifer, Renee	Travelers	2-10-00	564.55	3-10-00				
Tam, Chang	Prudential	2-15-00	1515.79					
Brown, Harry	Allstate	2-21-00	121.21					
Park, James	BC	2-24-00	124.99					

INSURANCE CLAIMS REGISTER   Page No. _____

Date	Description	Charge	Payment	Adjustment	Balance
					1346.17
7-3-xx	ROA Prudential Ins #7421		980.30	120.80	245.07

9. Submit an itemized billing statement to the patient for the balance due.

Keeping Up to Date

▶ Make a folder or binder of pertinent insurance information. Obtain information booklets and manuals from the local offices of the various insurance companies. Obtain sample copies of all the forms required for the insurance plans most used in your physician's office. Keep samples of completed claim forms.
▶ Changes occur daily and monthly so keep well informed by reading your Medicaid, Medicare, TRICARE, and local medical society bulletins. Maintain a chronologic file on each of these bulletins for easy reference, always keeping the latest bulletin on top.
▶ Attend any workshops offered in your area on insurance in the medical practice. Network with other insurance specialists to compare policies and discuss common problems. The American Association of Medical Assistants has chapters in many states that feature educational workshops and lectures.
▶ Become a member of the Alliance of Claims Assistance Professionals, American Academy of Professional Coders, American Association of Medical Billers, and/or American Health Information Management Association. Each of these associations distributes journals or newsletters on a monthly basis featuring current information.

For addresses of the professional associations mentioned in this chapter, refer to Chapter 17.

STUDENT ASSIGNMENT LIST

✔ Study Chapter 2.
✔ Answer the review questions in the *Workbook* to reinforce the theory learned in this chapter and to help prepare you for a future test.
✔ Complete the assignments in the *Workbook* to help reinforce the basic steps in submitting an insurance claim form.
✔ Turn to the Glossary at the end of this textbook for a further understanding of the Key Terms used in this chapter.

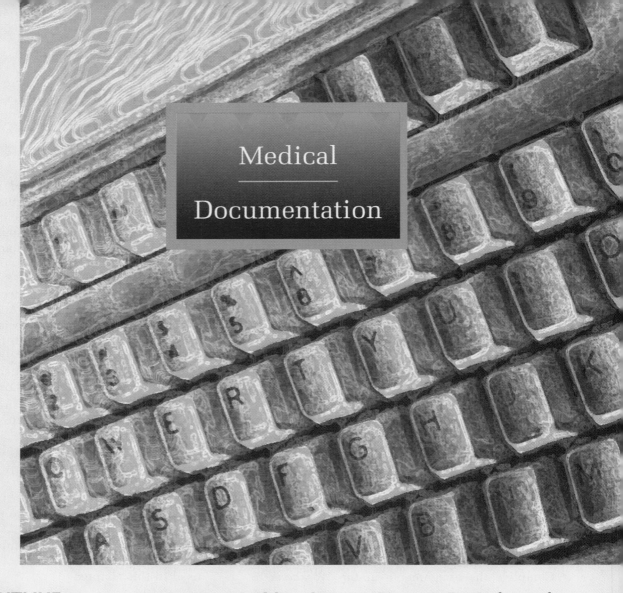

Medical
Documentation

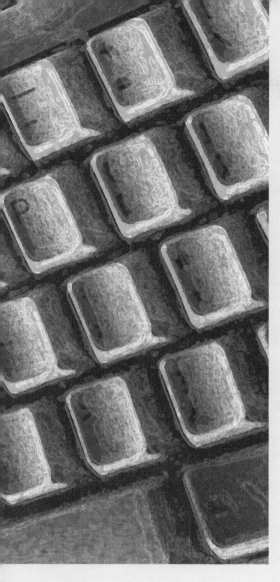

- List documents required for an internal review of medical records.
- Describe the difference between prospective and retrospective review of records.
- State reasons why an insurance company may decide to perform an external audit of medical records.
- Identify principles for release and retention of medical records.
- Explain techniques used for fax confidentiality.
- Respond appropriately to the subpoena of a witness and records.
- Formulate a procedure for termination of a case.
- Prepare legally correct medicolegal forms and letters

Retention of Records

Termination of a Case

Prevention of Legal Problems

OBJECTIVES*

After reading this chapter you should be able to:

- Name steps in the documentation process.
- Explain reasons medical documentation is required.
- Identify principles of documentation.
- State contents of a medical report.
- Define common medical, diagnostic, and legal terms.

---

*Performance objectives and exercises for hands-on practical experience for this chapter appear in the *Workbook*.

KEY TERMS

acute

attending physician

breach of confidential communication

chief complaint (CC)

chronic

comorbidity

compliance program

comprehensive (C)

concurrent care

consultation

consulting physician

continuity of care

counseling

critical care

detailed (D)

documentation

emergency care

eponym

established patient

expanded problem focused (EPF)

external audit

facsimile (fax)

family history (FH)

high complexity (HC)

history of present illness (HPI)

internal review

low complexity (LC)

medical necessity

medical record

medical report

continued

The Documentation Process

Medical Record

The connection between insurance billing and the medical record needs to be explained to better understand the importance of the medical record, the foremost tool of clinical care and communication. A **medical record** can be defined as written or graphic information documenting facts and events during the rendering of patient care. A **medical report** is part of the medical record and is a permanent legal document that formally states the consequences of the patient's examination or treatment in letter or report form. It is this record that provides the information needed to complete the insurance claim form. When billing the insurance company, the date of service (DOS), place of service (POS), type of service (TOS), diagnosis (dx or Dx), and procedures must be recorded. These data are transferred as codes on the claim form for interpretation by the insurance company.

The key to substantiating procedure and diagnostic code selections for appropriate reimbursement is supporting documentation in the medical record. Proper documentation can prevent penalties and refund requests should the physician's practice be reviewed or audited. Some states and/or facilities use different terminology when referring to the medical record, such as medical information, health record, progress or chart note, hospital record, or health care record.

Documenters

All individuals providing health care services may be referred to as documenters because they chronologically record pertinent facts and observations about the patient's health. This process is called **documentation** (charting) and may be handwritten or dictated. It is the physician's responsibility to either hand write the medical information or dictate it for transcription. The receptionist obtains the first document completed by the patient called the patient registration information form as shown in Chapter 2, Figure 2–7. The medical assistant is often the one to record entries for no-show appointments, prescription refills, and telephone calls in the patients' medical records. The insurance billing specialist uses the information in the medical record for billing purposes, and it is his or her responsibility to bring any substandard documentation to the physician's attention.

When referring to guidelines for documentation of the medical record and completion of the insurance claim form, a physician's title may change depending on the circumstances of each patient encounter. This can get confusing at times, so to clarify the physician's various roles, some of these titles are defined as follows:

▶ **Attending physician** refers to the medical staff member who is legally responsible for the care and treatment given to a patient.
▶ **Consulting physician** is a provider whose opinion or advice regarding evaluation and/or management of a specific problem is requested by another physician.

▶ **Ordering physician** is the individual directing the selection, preparation, or administration of tests, medication, or treatment.

▶ **Referring physician** is a provider who sends the patient for tests or treatment.

▶ **Treating or performing physician** is the provider who renders a service to a patient.

Reasons for Documentation

It is of vital importance that every patient seen by the physician have comprehensive legible documentation regarding what occurred during the visit for the following reasons.

1. Avoidance of denied or delayed payments by insurance carriers investigating the medical necessity of services.
2. Enforcement of medical record-keeping rules by insurance carriers requiring accurate documentation that supports procedure and diagnostic codes.
3. Subpoena of medical records by state investigators and/or the court for review.
4. Defense of a professional liability claim.

General Principles of Medical Record Documentation

In the early 1990s, the American Medical Association (AMA) decided to eliminate the terminology "office visits" when coding for those services and adopted the phrase "evaluation and management." This term better reflects the components involved when performing an office visit. The AMA and Health Care Financing Administration (HCFA) then developed documentation guidelines for *Current Procedural Terminology* (CPT) evaluation and management (E/M) services. These were released to Medicare carriers by HCFA in 1995 and then modified and released again in 1997. The guidelines were developed because Medicare has an obligation to those enrolled to ensure that services paid for have been provided and are medically necessary. It was discovered during audits that some medical practices should improve their quality of documentation.

Physicians are not required to use these guidelines but are encouraged to for the four reasons previously stated. Some physicians have adopted the 1995 guidelines, and others use those introduced in 1997. A modification to the 1997 guidelines is under consideration but as of this edition has not been released. Insurance claims processors and auditors may use the 1995 or 1997 guidelines

when doing an internal or external chart audit to determine whether the reported services were actually rendered and the level of service was warranted. A variety of formats of documentation are accepted by Medicare fiscal intermediaries (claims processors) as long as the information is discernible. When significant irregular reporting patterns are detected, a review will be conducted.

Medical Necessity

If a treatment is questioned as to whether it is medically necessary, the payment may be delayed. As a rule, **medical necessity** is criteria used by insurance companies when making decisions to limit or deny payment in which medical services or procedures must be justified by the patient's symptoms and diagnosis. This must be done in accordance with standards of good medical practice, and the proper level of care provided in the most appropriate setting. However, insurers differ on this definition and may or may not cover the services, depending on the benefits of the plan.

External Audit Point System

During the performance of an audit, a point system is used while reviewing each patient's medical record. Points are awarded only if documentation is present for elements required in the medical record. Because every medical record is documented differently by each provider of service, a patient's history may contain details for more than one body area. Thus, when gathering points, it is possible the auditor may shift the points from the history of present illness to those required for the review of the patient's body systems. In addition, when sufficient points have been reached within a section for the level of code used in billing, then no further documentation is counted for audit purposes even though there may be additional comments for other body systems. This point system is used to show where deficiencies occur in medical record documentation. It is also used to evaluate and substantiate proper use of diagnostic and procedural codes.

Health maintenance organizations (HMOs), preferred provider organizations (PPOs), and all private carriers have the right to claim refunds in the event of accidental (or intentional) miscoding. However, Medicare has the power to levy fines and penalities and exclude providers from the Medicare program. If improper coding patterns exist and are not corrected, then the provider of service will be penalized. Insurance carriers go by the rule "If it's not documented, then it was not performed," and they have the right to deny reimbursement.

Enforcement of Medical Record Keeping

Insurance carriers have become stricter in enforcing accurate coding substantiated by documentation. It is not uncommon for prepayment and postpayment random audits or reviews by Medicare carriers to occur that monitor accuracy of physicians' use of evaluation and management services and procedure codes. Medicare fiscal intermediaries have "walk-in rights" (access to a medical practice without an appointment or search warrant) that they may invoke to conduct documentation reviews, audits, and evaluations. Billing patterns that may draw attention to a medical practice for possible audit are:

- Bill intentionally for unnecessary services.
- Bill incorrectly for services of *physician extenders* (e.g., nurse practitioner, midwife, physician assistant).
- Bill for diagnostic tests without a separate report in the medical record.
- Change dates of service on insurance claims to comply with policy coverage dates.
- Waive copayments or deductibles or allow other illegal discounts.
- Order excessive diagnostic tests (e.g., laboratory tests, x-ray studies).
- Use two different provider numbers to bill the same services for the same patient.
- Misuse provider identification numbers, which results in incorrect billing.
- Use improper modifiers for financial gain.
- Fail to return overpayments made by Medicare program.

Documentation Guidelines for Evaluation and Management Services

The following is a brief overview of documentation guidelines regarding evaluation and management services.

1. The medical record should be accurate, complete (detailed), and legible.
2. The documentation of each patient encounter should include or provide reference to:
   a. Chief complaint and/or reason for the encounter
   b. Relevant history
   c. Examination
   d. Findings
   e. Prior diagnostic test results
   f. Assessment, clinical impression or diagnosis
   g. Plan for care
   h. Date and legible identity of the health care professional
3. The reason for the encounter and/or chief complaint should be stated, and the rationale should be documented or inferred for ordering diagnostic and other ancillary services.
4. Past and present diagnoses, including those in the prenatal and intrapartum period that affect the newborn, should be accessible to the treating and/or consulting physician.
5. Appropriate health risk factors should be identified.
6. The patient's progress, response to and changes in treatment, planned follow-up care and instructions, and diagnosis should be documented.
7. Patient refusal to follow medical advice should be documented and a letter sent to the patient about this noncompliance. Information on termination of a case is found at the end of this chapter.
8. Procedure and diagnostic codes reported on the health insurance claim form or billing statement should be supported by the documentation in the medical record and be at a level sufficient for a clinical peer to determine whether services have been accurately coded.
9. The confidentiality of the medical record should be fully maintained consistent with the requirements of medical ethics and the laws. An authorization form signed by the patient must be obtained to release information to the insurance carrier.
10. Each chart entry should be dated and signed, including the title or position of the person signing. If a signature log has been established, then initials are acceptable, because these would be defined in the log (Fig. 3–1). A *signature log* is a list of all staff members' names, job titles, signatures, and their initials. In regard to paperless documents, if passwords are used for restricted access, electronic signatures may be acceptable.
11. Charting procedures for progress notes should be standardized. Many physicians use a method called the SOAP style (Fig. 3–2). However, whatever method is used, make sure it is detailed enough to support current documentation requirements (Fig. 3–3).
12. Treatment plans should be written. Include patient/family education and specific instructions for follow-up. Treatment must be consistent with the working diagnosis.

SIGNATURE LOG

Name	Position	Signature or Initials	
Ann M. Arch	Receptionist	*Ann M. Arch*	*AMA*
John Bortolonni	Office manager	*John Bortolonni*	*JB*
Gerald Practon, MD	Provider	*Gerald Practon, MD*	*GP*
Rachel Vasquez, CPC	Insurance billing specialist	*Rachel Vasquez CPC*	*RV*
Mary Ann Worth	Clinical medical assistant	*Mary Ann Worth*	*MAW*

Figure 3–1. Example of a signature log.

13. Medications prescribed and taken should be listed, specifying frequency and dosage.

14. *Request* for a consultation from the attending/treating physician and the *need* for consultation must be documented. The consultant's opinion and any services ordered or performed must be documented and communicated to the requesting physician. Remember the three Rs: There must be a *requesting* physician, and the consultant must *render* an opinion and send a *report*.

15. Record a patient's failure to return for needed treatment by noting it in the medical record, in the appointment book, and on the financial record or ledger card. Follow up with a tele-

phone call or send a letter to the patient advising him or her that further treatment is indicated.

16. Use a permanent, not water-soluble, ink pen (legal copy pen) to cross out an incorrect entry on a patient's record. Mark it with a single line and write the correct information, and then date and initial the entry. Never erase, white out, or use self-adhesive paper over any information recorded on a patient record (see Example 3–1).

17. Document all laboratory tests ordered in the medical record. When the report is received, the physician should initial the report, indicating that it has been read. Each of these

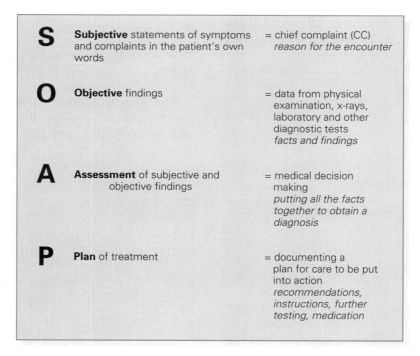

Figure 3–2. SOAP style progress note.

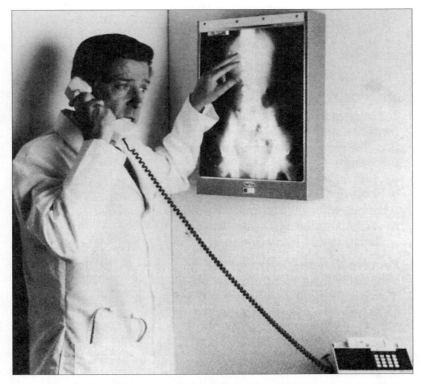

Figure 3–3. Physician dictating chart notes. (From Diehl, M.O, Fordney, MT: Medical Keyboarding, Typing, and Transcribing: Techniques and Procedures, 4th ed. Philadelphia, WB Saunders, 1997.)

documentations is considered an element and allows a point should the record undergo an external audit.

18. Ask the physician for approval for a different code(s) before submitting the claim to the insurance carrier if the insurance biller questions any procedure and/or diagnostic codes marked on the encounter form (Fig. 3–4).

19. Retain all records until you are positive they are no longer needed by conforming to federal and state laws as well as the physician's wishes. Retention of records is discussed at the end of the chapter and shown in Tables 3–4 and 3–5.

Contents of a Medical Report

The degree of documentation depends on the complexity of the service and the specialty of the physician. For example, a "normal chest examination" may have a different meaning to a cardiologist than it does to a family physician as far as the details of the examination and documentation.

The first time a new patient is seen, a family and social history is taken. When a new patient or an established patient comes to see the physician with a new injury or illness, the documentation should also include the patient's health history, the physical examination, results from any tests that are performed, the medical decision-making process, the diagnosis, and the treatment plan.

Documentation of History

The following documentation information for the history and physical examination are based on the 1997 Medicare guidelines.

The history includes the chief complaint (CC), the history of present illness (HPI), the review of systems (ROS), and past history, family, and/or

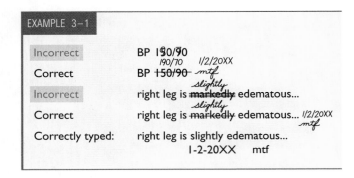

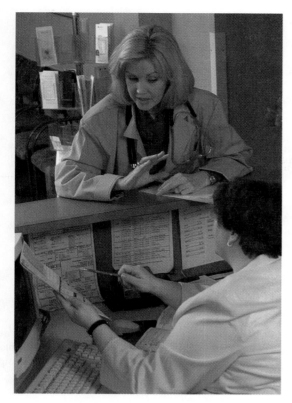

Figure 3–4. Insurance billing specialist checking information with physician before recording it on the insurance claim.

social history (PFSH).* The extent of the history is dependent on clinical judgment and on the nature of the presenting problem(s). Each history includes some or all of the following elements (Fig. 3–5).

Chief Complaint

The **chief complaint (CC)** is a concise statement describing the symptom, problem, condition, diagnosis, physician-recommended return, or other factor that is the *reason* for the encounter. *The chief complaint is a requirement for all levels of history*—problem focused, expanded problem focused, detailed, and comprehensive; these are described at the end of the section on history of present illness.

History of Present Illness

The **history of present illness (HPI)** is a chronologic description of the development of the pa-

tient's present illness from the first sign and/or symptom or from the previous encounter to the present. If the physician is unable to obtain a sufficient diagnosis for the patient's condition, the medical record documentation must reflect this. The history may include one or more of the eight following descriptive elements:

1. **Location**—area of the body where the symptom is occurring
2. **Quality**—character of the symptom/pain (burning, gnawing, stabbing, fullness)
3. **Severity**—degree of symptom and/or pain on a scale from 1–10. Severity can also be described with terms like severe, slight, persistent
4. **Duration**—how long the symptom/pain has been present and how long it lasts when the patient has it
5. **Timing**—when the pain/symptom occurs (e.g., morning, evening, after or before meals)
6. **Context**—situation associated with the pain/symptom (e.g., dairy products, big meals, activity)
7. **Modifying factors**—things done to make the symptom/pain worse or better (e.g., "If I eat spicy foods I get heartburn, but if I drink milk afterward the pain is not as bad.")
8. **Associated signs and symptoms**—symptom/pain and other things that happen when the symptom/pain occurs (e.g., chest pain leads to shortness of breath).

The documented elements are counted and totaled (Fig. 3–6*A*). The medical record should describe one to three elements of the present illness for a *brief level* of HPI. At least four elements of the HPI or the status of at least three chronic or inactive conditions is required for the *extended level* of HPI. Only two of three history elements are required for certain types of cases, such as newborns or subsequent hospital care. Figure 3–6*B* shows Section I of the review/audit sheet that depicts the history containing the HPI, ROS, and PFSH. The check marks and circled element in the HPI (Section I) of the figure relate to the case illustrated.

The types of evaluation and management services for the history are based on four levels of history. However, the review of systems (ROS) and past, family, and social histories (PFSH) must be totaled before the final decision on the level of service is assigned. The four levels of history may be defined as follows:

1. **Problem focused (PF):** chief complaint; brief history of present illness or problem
2. **Expanded problem focused (EPF):** chief complaint; brief history of present illness; problem-pertinent system review

---

*These abbreviations in the history portion of the report may vary depending on the physician who is dictating (i.e., PI for present illness, PH for past history, FH for family history, and SH for social history).

Hospital number: 00-83-06

Scott, Aimee

Rex Rumsey, MD

HISTORY

CHIEF COMPLAINT: Pain and bleeding after each bowel movement for the past 3-4 months.

PRESENT ILLNESS: This 68-year old white female says she usally has three bowel movements a day in small amounts, and there has been a change in the last 3 to 4 months in frequency, size and type of bowel movement. She has slight burning pain and irritation in the rectal area after bowel movements. The pain lasts for several minutes then decreases in intensity. She has had no previous anorectal surgery or rectal infection. She denies any blood in the stool itself or associated symptoms. Bright red blood occurs after stools have passed.

PAST HISTORY:
ILNESSES: The patient had polio at age 8 from which she has made a remarkable recovery. Apparently, she was paralyzed in both lower extremities and now has adequate use of these. She has no other serious illnesses.

ALLERGIES: ALLERGIC TO PENICILLIN. She denies any other drug or food allergies.

MEDICATIONS: None.

OPERATIONS: Right inguinal herniorrhaphy, 25 years ago.

SOCIAL HISTORY: She does not smoke or drink. She lives with her husband who is an invalid and for whom she cares. She is a retired former municipal court judge.

FAMILY HISTORY: One brother died of cancer of the throat (age 59), another has cancer of the kidney (age 63).

REVIEW OF SYSTEMS:
SKIN: No rashes or jaundice.

HEENT: Head normocephalic. Normal TMs. Normal hearing. Pupils equal, round, reactive to light. Deviated septum. Oropharynx clear.

CR: No history of chest pain, shortness of breath, or pedal edema. She has had some mild hypertension in the past but is not under any medical supervision nor is she taking any medication for this.

GI: Weight is stable. See present illness.

OB-GYN: Gravida II Para II. Climacteric at age 46, no sequelae.

EXTREMITIES: No edema.

NEUROLOGIC: Unremarkable.

mtf
D: 5-17-20XX
T: 5-20-20XX

_____
Rex Rumsey, MD

Figure 3–5. Example of a medical report done in modified block format showing the six components of a history.

3. **Detailed (D):** chief complaint; extended history of present illness; problem-pertinent system review extended to include a review of a limited number of additional systems; *pertinent* past, family, and/or social history directly related to the patient's problems

4. **Comprehensive (C):** chief complaint; extended history of present illness; review of systems that is directly related to the problem(s) identified in the history of the present illness plus a review of all additional body systems; *complete* past, family, and social history

Review of Systems

A **review of systems (ROS)** is an inventory of body systems obtained through a series of questions that is used to identify signs and/or symptoms that the patient might be experiencing or has experienced. Checklists are permitted, but if a body system is not considered then it should be crossed out. For an ROS, the following systems are recognized: constitutional symptoms (e.g., fever, weight loss), eyes, ears, nose, mouth, throat, cardiovascular, respiratory, gastrointestinal, genitourinary, musculoskeletal, integumentary (skin and/or breast), neurologic, psychiatric, endocrine, hematologic/lymphatic, and allergic/immunologic.

A

10-21-20XX

HISTORY OF PRESENT ILLNESS: This new patient is an 80-year-old white male who has had problems with voiding difficulty since 9-5 2000. During the night, the patient had only 50 cc output and was catheterized this morning because of his poor urinary output (200 cc). He was thought to have a distended bladder. He has not had any gross hematuria. He has voiding difficulty especially lying down and voiding in the supine position. His voiding pattern is improved while standing and sitting. However, the patient has developed a wound to his left lateral malleolus and is only able to ambulate with assistance.

— Location
— Duration
— Context
— Genitourinary (ROS)
— Modifying factor
— Integumentary (ROS)

Severity
Genitourinary (ROS)

Notice that there is no family or social history for this new patient.

PAST MEDICAL HISTORY: Unremarkable. He does have some slowing of his urinary stream and nocturia three to five times.

MEDICATIONS: He was on amitriptyline which may affect his bladder.

ALLERGIES: He has no known allergies.

PHYSICAL EXAMINATION: Shows the abdomen to be soft, nontender, and not distended. His bladder was nonpalpable and nondistended.

Notice that the examination of the wound is missing.

GENITOURINARY: Normal penis. Testes descended bilaterally. His prostate is 10 gm and benign in feeling.

IMPRESSION: Benign prostatic hypertrophy with some mild voiding difficulty exacerbated by the patient's poor ambulatory status.

I suspect that as his ambulatory status improves that his voiding pattern will improve. I will try him on Hytrin 5 mg by mouth q day. I will follow him as needed.

mtf   Gene Ulibarri, MD

B

SECTION I

CHIEF COMPLAINT:

HISTORY		Brief 1–3 elements	Brief	Extended	Extended
HPI (history of present illness) ☑ Location ☑ Severity ☐ Timing ☐ Modifying factors ☐ Quality ☑ Duration ☑ Context ☐ Associated signs and symptoms		Brief 1–3 elements		Extended	Extended ≥ 4 elements or status of ≥ 3 chronic or inactive conditions
ROS (review of systems) ☐ Constitutional (wt loss, etc) ☐ Eyes ☐ Ears, nose, mouth, throat ☐ Card/vasc ☐ Resp ☐ GI ☑ GU ☐ Musculo ☑ Integumentary (skin, breast) ☐ Neuro ☐ Psych ☐ Endo ☐ Hem/lymph ☐ All/imm ☐ "All others negative"	None	Pertinent to problem 1 system	Extended 2–9 systems	Complete ≥ 10 systems, or some systems with statement "all others negative"
PFSH (past family and social history) ☑ Past medical history ☐ Family history ☐ Social history Established/subsequent	None	None	One history area	Two or three history areas
No PFSH required: 99231–33, 99261–63, 99311–33 New/Initial	None	None	One or two history area(s)	Three history areas
Circle the entry farthest to the right for each history area. To determine history level, draw a line down the column with the circle farthest to the left.	PROBLEM FOCUSED	EXP. PROB. FOCUSED	DETAILED	COMPREHENSIVE

Descriptive elements of history

Systems of history

Review of history

Levels of history

Figure 3–6. *A,* Documentation from a medical record highlighting elements required for the history. *B,* Review/audit sheet Section I with check marks and circled elements to show how the history in the example is declared as detailed. This shows two of three history components *(arrow)* used for the purpose of determining the assignment of a procedure code at the appropriate level of service. (Reprinted with permission of the Iowa Medical Society, IMS Services, West Des Moines, IA, 1998.)

The body systems are counted and totaled. The medical record should describe 1 system of the ROS for a *pertinent to problem level*. For an *extended level*, 2 to 9 systems are required. For a *complete level*, at least 10 organ systems must be reviewed and documented. Refer to Figure 3–6*B* for a visual understanding of Section I of the review/audit sheet.

The check marks and circled element in the ROS (Section I) of the figure relate to the case illustrated.

Past, Family, and Social Histories

The past, family, and social histories (PFSH) consists of a review of three areas:

1. **Past history (PH)**—patient's past experiences with illnesses, operations, injuries, and treatments
2. **Family history (FH)**—review of medical events in the patient's family, including diseases that may be hereditary or place the patient at risk
3. **Social history (SH)**—age-appropriate review of past and current activities

The PFSH review areas are counted and totaled. The medical record must contain at least one history area for a *detailed extended level* and specific items from two of the three history areas for a *comprehensive level* of PFSH. Refer to Figure 3–6*B* for a visual guide of the PFSH in Section I of the review/audit sheet. Note the difference in the number of required elements for new versus established patients and the circled element for the case in question.

A vertical line is drawn down the right four columns that contain the most elements to determine whether the history is a PF, EPF, D, or C level.

Documentation of Examination

Physical Examination

The **physical examination** (PE or PX) is objective in nature; that is, it consists of the physician's findings by examination and/or test results. Figure 3–7 is an illustration of a single organ system examination that shows the details (elements) of examination for each body area within the genitourinary system. The three circled elements of the genitourinary system and one circled element of the gastrointestinal system relate to the case in question. For purposes of examination, the following body areas and organ systems are recognized.

Organ Systems/Body Areas—Elements of Examination

Constitutional (vital signs, general appearance)
Eyes
Ears, nose, mouth, and throat
Neck
Respiratory
Cardiovascular
Chest, including breasts and axillae
Gastrointestinal (abdomen)
Genitourinary (male)
Genitourinary (female)
Lymphatic
Musculoskeletal
Skin
Neurologic
Psychiatric

Note: In addition, any reasons for not examining a particular body area or system should be listed.

Types of Physical Examination

When performing an internal review of a patient's medical record, the number of elements identified by bullets are counted for each system and a total is obtained. The total is circled on Section II of the review/audit sheet as shown for the case illustrated (Fig. 3–8).

The levels of evaluation and management services are based on four types of physical examination (PE), as follows:

1. **Problem focused (PF)**: A limited examination of the affected body area or organ system. The medical record should describe 1 to 5 elements identified by a bullet for a *problem-focused level* of PE.
2. **Expanded problem focused (EPF)**: A limited examination of the affected body area or organ system and other symptomatic or related organ system(s). At least 6 elements identified by a bullet are required for an *expanded problem-focused level* of PE.
3. **Detailed (D)**: An extended examination of the affected body area(s) and other symptomatic or related organ system(s). At least 2 elements identified by a bullet from each of 6 areas/body systems OR at least 12 elements identified by a bullet in 2 or more areas/body systems are required for a *detailed level* of PE.
4. **Comprehensive (C)**: A general multisystem examination or complete examination of a single organ system. For a *comprehensive level* of PE, all elements must be identified by a bullet and documentation must be present for at least 2 elements identified by a bullet from each of 9 areas/body systems.

SINGLE ORGAN SYSTEM EXAMINATION REQUIREMENTS (SHADED)
CONTENT and DOCUMENTATION

Level of Exam	Perform and Document
(Problem focused)	**One to five** elements identified by a bullet.
Expanded Problem Focused	**At least six** elements identified by a bullet.
Detailed	**At least twelve** elements identified by a bullet.
Comprehensive	Perform all elements identified by a bullet; document every element in every shaded box and at least one element in every unshaded box.

Genitourinary

System/Body Area	Elements of Examination
Constitutional	• Measurement of **any three of the following seven** vital signs: 1) sitting or standing blood pressure, 2) supine blood pressure, 3) pulse rate and regularity, 4) respiration, 5) temperature, 6) height, 7) weight (may be measured and recorded by ancillary staff) • General appearance of patient *e.g. development, nutrition, body habitus, deformities, attention to grooming*
Neck	• Examination of neck *e.g. masses, overall appearance, symmetry, tracheal position, crepitus* • Examination of thyroid *e.g. enlargement, tenderness, mass*
Respiratory	• Assessment of respiratory effect *e.g. intercostal retractions, use of accessory muscles, diaphragmatic movement* • Auscultation of lungs *e.g. breath sounds, adventitious sounds, rubs*
Cardiovascular	• Auscultation of heart with notation of abnormal sounds and murmurs • Examination of peripheral vascular system by observation *e.g. swelling, varicosities* and palpation *e.g. pulses, temperature, edema, tenderness*
Chest (breasts)	See genitourinary (female)
Gastrointestinal (abdomen)	◉ Examination of abdomen with notation of presence of masses or tenderness • Examination for presence or absence of hernia • Examination of liver and spleen • Obtain stool sample for occult blood test when indicated
Genitourinary (male)	• Inspection of anus and perineum Examination (with or without specimen collection for smears and cultures) of genitalia including: • Scrotum *e.g. lesions, cysts, rashes* • Epididymides *e.g. size, symmetry, masses* ◉ Testes *e.g. size, symmetry, masses* • Urethral meatus *e.g. size, location, lesions, discharge* ◉ Penis *e.g. lesions, presence or absence of foreskin, foreskin retractability, plaque, masses, scarring, deformities* Digital rectal examination including: ◉ Prostate gland *e.g. size, symmetry, nodularity, tenderness* • Seminal vesicles *e.g. symmetry, tenderness, masses, enlargement* • Sphincter tone, presence of hemorrhoids, rectal masses
Genitourinary (female) Includes at least seven of the eleven elements to the right identified by bullets:	• Inspection and palpation of breasts *e.g. masses or lumps, tenderness, symmetry, nipple discharge* • Digital rectal examination including sphincter tone, presence of hemorrhoids, rectal masses Pelvic examination (with or without specimen collection for smears and cultures) including: • External genitalia *e.g. general appearance, hair distribution, lesions* • Urethral meatus *e.g. size, location, lesions, prolapse* • Urethra *e.g. masses, tenderness, scarring* • Bladder *e.g. fullness, masses, tenderness* • Vagina *e.g. general appearance, estrogen effect, discharge, lesions, pelvic support, cystocele, rectocele* • Cervix *e.g. general appearance, lesions, discharge* • Uterus *e.g. size, contour, position, mobility, tenderness, descent or support* • Adnexa/parametria *e.g. masses, tenderness, organomegaly, nodularity* • Anus and perineum

Genitourinary (continued)

System/Body Area	Elements of Examination
Lymphatic	• Palpation of lymph nodes in neck, axillae, groin and/or other location
Skin	• Inspection and/or palpation of skin and subcutaneous tissue *e.g. rashes, lesions, ulcers*
Neurological/ psychiatric	Brief assessment of mental status including: • Orientation to time, place and person • Mood and affect *e.g. depression, anxiety, agitation*

Skin

System/Body Area	Elements of Examination
Constitutional	• Measurement of **any three of the following seven** vital signs: 1) sitting or standing blood pressure, 2) supine blood pressure, 3) pulse rate and regularity, 4) respiration, 5) temperature, 6) height, 7) weight (may be measured and recorded by ancillary staff) • General appearance of patient *e.g. development, nutrition, body habitus, deformities, attention to grooming*
Eyes	• Inspection of conjuctivae and lids
Ears, nose, mouth and throat	• Inspection of lips, teeth and gums • Examination of oropharynx *e.g. oral mucosa, hard and soft palates, tongue, tonsils, and posterior pharynx*
Neck	• Examination of thyroid *e.g. enlargement, tenderness, mass*
Gastrointestinal (abdomen)	• Examination of liver and spleen • Examination of anus for condyloma and other lesions
Lymphatic	• Palpation of lymph nodes in neck, axillae, groin and/or other location
Extremities	• Inspection and palpation of digits and nails *e.g. clubbing, cyanosis, inflammation, petechiae, ischemia, infections, nodes*
Skin	• Palpation of scalp and inspection of hair of scalp, eyebrows, face, chest, pubic area (when indicated) and extremities • Inspection and/or palpation of skin and subcutaneous tissue *e.g. rashes, lesions, ulcers, susceptibility in and presence of photo damage* in **eight of the following ten areas:** 1) head including face, 2) neck, 3) chest including breasts and axilla, 4) abdomen, 5) genitalia, groin, buttocks, 6) back, 7) right upper extremity, 8) left upper extremity, 9) right lower extremity, 10) left lower extremity Note: For the comprehensive level, the examination of all eight anatomic areas must be performed and documented. For the three lower levels of examination, each body area is counted separately. For example, inspection and/or palpation of the skin and subcutaneous tissue of the head and neck extremities constitutes two areas. • Inspection of eccrine and apocrine glands of skin and subcutaneous tissue with identification and location of any hyperhidrosis, chromhidroses or bromhidrosis
Neurological/ psychiatric	Brief assessment of mental status including: • Orientation to time, place and person • Mood and affect *e.g. depression, anxiety, agitation*

Figure 3–7. Review/audit worksheet of a single organ system examination that shows the details (elements) of examination for each body area/system. Circled bullets relate to the example case shown in Figure 3–6A. (Reprinted with permission of the Iowa Medical Society, IMS Services, West Des Moines, IA, 1998.)

SECTION II

Four Elements identified

General Multi-system Exam		Single Organ System Exam
1-5 elements identified by •	PROBLEM FOCUSED	1-5 elements identified by •
≥6 elements identified by •	EXPANDED PROBLEM FOCUSED	≥6 elements identified by •
≥2 elements identified by • from 6 areas/ systems OR ≥12 elements identified by • from at least 2 areas/systems	DETAILED	≥12 elements identified by • EXCEPT ≥ 9 elements identified by • for eye and psychiatric exams
≥2 elements identified by • from 9 areas/ systems	COMPREHENSIVE	Perform all elements identified by • ; document all elements in shaded boxes; document ≥ 1 element in unshaded boxes.

Figure 3–8. Review/audit worksheet Section II for a general multisystem physical examination and single organ system examination. The circled item relates to a problem-focused examination for the example case (see Fig. 3–6A) for the purpose of coding. (Reprinted with permission of the Iowa Medical Society, IMS Services, West Des Moines, IA, 1998.)

The extent of the examination and what is documented depend on clinical judgment and the nature of the presenting problem(s). They range from limited examinations of single body areas to general multisystem or complete single-organ system examinations.

Documentation of Medical Decision-Making Complexity

In the medical decision-making process the physician must look at the number of diagnoses or treatment options, the amount and/or complexity of data to be reviewed, and the risk of complications and/or morbidity or mortality. *Morbidity* is a diseased condition or state whereas *mortality* has to do with the number of deaths in a given time or place.

▶ *Number of Diagnoses or Management Options.* This is based on the number and types of problems addressed during the visit, the complexity of establishing a diagnosis, and the number of management options that must be considered by the physician. For the case illustrated, the number of problems is 1, which equals 3 points (Fig. 3–9, top section).

▶ *Amount and/or Complexity of Data to be Reviewed.* This is based on the types of diagnostic tests ordered or reviewed. A decision to obtain and review old medical records and/or obtain history from sources other than the patient increases the amount and complexity of data to be analyzed. For the case illustrated, no points apply (see Fig. 3–9, middle section).

▶ *Risk of Complications, Morbidity, and/or Mortality.* This is based on other conditions associated with the presenting problem(s) known as the risk of complications, morbidity, and/or mortality, as well as comorbidities, the diagnostic procedure(s), and/or the possible management options (treatment rendered—surgery, therapy, drug management, services, and supplies). A **comorbidity** means underlying disease or other conditions present at the time of the visit.

To discover whether the *level of risk* is minimal, low, moderate, or high, bulleted elements are marked on the review/audit sheet (Fig. 3–10, Section III, Part C). For the case illustrated, the elements fall within the moderate level of risk category.

To conclude the internal review of a patient's medical record, a level from one of four types of medical decision making (straightforward (SF)*, **low complexity [LC], moderate complexity [MC], and high complexity [HC]**) must be determined.

---

*Straightforward medical decision making may be deleted when HCFA adopts guidelines in 2002.

SECTION III A AND B

A

NUMBER OF DIAGNOSES OR TREATMENT OPTIONS

Problems to exam physician	Number X points = Result		
Self-limited or minor (stable, improved or worsening)	Max = 2	1	
Est. problem (to examiner); stable, improved		1	
Est. problem (to examiner); worsening		2	
New problem (to examiner); no additional workup planned	Max = 1 1	3	3
New prob. (to examiner); add. workup planned		4	
		TOTAL	3

Bring total to line A in final result for complexity

B

AMOUNT AND/OR COMPLEXITY OF DATA TO BE REVIEWED

Data to be reviewed	Points
Review and/or order of clinical lab tests	1
Review and/or order of tests in the radiology section of CPT	1
Review and/or order of tests in the medicine section of CPT	1
Discussion of test results with performing physician	1
Decision to obtain old records and/or obtain history from someone other than patient	1
Review and summarization of old records and/or obtaining history from someone other than patient and/or discussion of case with another health care provider	2
Independent visualization of image, tracing or specimen itself (not simply review of report)	2
TOTAL	0

Bring total to line B in final result for complexity

Draw a line down the column with 2 or 3 circles and circle decision making level OR draw a line down the column with the center circle and circle the decision making level.

A	Number diagnoses or treatment options	≤ 1 Minimal	2 Limited	3 Multiple	≥ 4 Extensive
B	Amount and complexity of data	≤ 1 Minimal or low	2 Limited	3 Moderate	≥ 4 Extensive
C	Highest risk	Minimal	Low	Moderate	High
	Type of decision making	Straight-foward	Low complex	**Moderate complex**	High complex

Note: The wound was not a considering factor in the medical decision making.

Figure 3–9. Section III of the review/audit worksheet. Part A: Number of diagnoses or treatment options. Part B: Amount and/or complexity of data to be reviewed. Lower one third: Used to compile the results obtained from Parts A, B, and C (see Fig. 3–10) to determine the level of medical decision making. Circled points and words relate to a moderately complex level of decision making for the example case (see Fig. 3–6A) for the purpose of coding and billing. (Reprinted with permission of the Iowa Medical Society, IMS Services, West Des Moines, IA, 1998.)

SECTION III

C

RISK OF COMPLICATIONS AND/OR MORBIDITY OR MORTALITY

Level of risk	Presenting problem(s)	Diagnostic procedure(s) ordered	Management options selected
M I N I M A L	• One self-limited or minor problem, *e.g. cold, insect bite tinea corporis*	• Laboratory tests requiring venipuncture • Chest x-rays • KOH prep • EKG/EEG • Urinalysis • Ultrasound *e.g. echo*	• Rest • Gargles • Elastic bandages • Superficial dressings
L O W	• Two or more self-limited or minor problems • One stable chronic illness *e.g. well controlled hypertension, non-insulin dependent diabetes, cataract, BPH* • Acute uncomplicated illness or injury *e.g. cystitis, allergic rhinitis, simple sprain*	• Physiologic test not under stress *e.g. pulm. function tests* • Non-cardiovascular imaging studies with contrast *e.g. barium enema* • Superficial needle biopsies • Clinical laboratory tests requiring arterial puncture • Skin biopsies	• Over-the-counter drugs • Minor surgery with no identified risk factors • Physical therapy • Occupational therapy • IV fluids without additives
M O D E R A T E	• One or more chronic illnesses with mild exacerbation, progression or side effects of treatment • Two or more stable chronic illnesses • Undiagnosed new problem with uncertain prognosis *e.g. lump in breast* • Acute illness with systemic symptoms *e.g. pyelonephritis, pneumonitis, colitis* • Acute complicated injury *e.g. head injury with brief loss of consciousness*	• Physiologic test under stress *e.g. cardiac stress test, fetal contraction stress test* • Diagnostic endoscopies with no identified risk factors • Deep needle or incisional biopsy • Cardiovascular imaging studies with contrast and no identified risk factors *e.g. arteriogram, cardiac cath* • Obtain fluid from body cavity *e.g. lumbar puncture, thorocentesis culdocentesis*	• Minor surgery with identified risk factors • Elective major surgery (open percutaneous or endoscopic) with no identified risk factors • Prescription drug management • Therapeutic nuclear medicine • IV fluids with additives • Closed treatment of fracture or dislocation without manipulation
H I G H	• One or more chronic illnesses with severe exacerbation, progression or side effects of tx • Acute or chronic illnesses or injuries that may pose a threat to life or bodily function *e.g. multiple trauma, acute MI, pulmonary embolus, severe respiratory distress, progressive severe rheumatoid arthritis, psychiatric illness w/potential threat to self or others, peritonitis, acute renal failure* • An abrupt change in neurological status *e.g. seizure, TIA, weakness, sensory loss*	• Cardiovascular imaging studies with contrast with identified risk factors • Cardiac electrophysiological tests • Diagnostic endoscopies with identified risk factors • Discography	• Elective major surgery (open, percutaneous or endoscopic) with identified risk factor • Emergency major surgery (open, percutaneous or endoscopic) • Parenteral controlled substances • Drug therapy requiring intensive monitoring for toxicity • Decision not to resuscitate or de-escalate care because of poor prognosis

Figure 3–10. Section III, Part C of the review/audit worksheet used for determining the level of risk. The circled item and highlighted phrases relate to a moderate level of risk for the example case (see Fig. 3–6A) for the purpose of coding. (Reprinted with permission of the Iowa Medical Society, IMS Services, West Des Moines, Iowa, 1998.)

Now go to the bottom portion of Figure 3–9, Section III, and circle the results obtained from Parts A, B, and C. For the case illustrated, the number of diagnoses is declared *multiple*, there are *no data reviewed*, and the risk of complications is *moderate*; therefore, a *moderately complex* level of decision making has been assigned to be used for coding and billing purposes.

Documentation Terminology

Terminology for Evaluation and Management Services

While learning the complexities of medical documentation and how important it is as it relates to coding and billing, you have discovered that you must have a good foundation of medical terminology. To use the diagnostic and procedure code books efficiently, you must become familiar with their language, abbreviations, and symbols. The first terms introduced are most commonly used for evaluation and management services.

New versus Established Patient

In procedure coding, two categories of patients are considered: the new patient and the established patient. A **new patient** is one who *has not received* any professional services from the physician or another physician of the same specialty who belongs to the same group practice *within the past 3 years*. An **established patient** is one who *has received* professional services from the physician or another physician of the same specialty who belongs to the same group practice *within the past 3 years*.

There are several types of services that a physician may provide to evaluate and manage a patient who is seeking medical care (i.e., consultation, referral, concurrent care, continuity of care, critical care, emergency care, or counseling).

Consultation

A **consultation** includes services rendered by a physician whose opinion or advice is requested by another physician or agency in the evaluation or treatment of a patient's illness or a suspected problem. The request must be documented in the patient's medical record (e.g., "Patient is seen at the request of Dr. John Doe for a . . . reason."). Consultations may occur in a home, office, hospital, extended care facility, and other locations. A physician consultant recommends diagnostic or therapeutic services and may initiate these services if requested by the referring physician. The opinion must be in writing, documented in a consultation report, and communicated to the referring physician. The consultant may order a diagnostic and/or therapeutic service to formulate the opinion at an initial or subsequent visit. Reimbursement is significantly more than for an equivalent office visit.

Referral

A **referral** is the transfer of the total or specific care of a patient from one physician to another for known problems. It is *not* a consultation. For example, a patient is sent by a primary case physician to an orthopedist for care of a fracture.

However, when dealing with managed care plans, the term "referral" is also used when requesting an authorization for the patient to receive services elsewhere (e.g., referral for laboratory tests, radiology procedures, specialty care). As a courtesy, the physician may send a thank you note to the referring physician with comments about the patient's condition.

Concurrent Care

Concurrent care is the providing of similar services (e.g., hospital visits) to the same patient by more than one physician on the same day. Usually, such cases involve the presence of a physical disorder (e.g., diabetes) at the same time as the primary admitting diagnosis, and this may alter the course of treatment or lengthen recovery time for the primary condition. For example, two internists (a general internist and a cardiologist) see the same patient in the hospital on the same day. The general internist admitted the patient for diabetes and requested that the cardiologist also follow the patient's periodic chest pain and arrhythmia. If the second doctor is not identified in carrier records as a cardiologist, the claim may be denied. This is because the services appear to be duplicated by physicians of the same specialty. When billing insurance companies, physicians providing concurrent care may be cross referenced on the claim form. Medicare has a list that includes 62 specialties and subspecialties to help carriers more accurately judge whether concurrent care is necessary. Periodically, the physician should check with the carrier's provider service representative to see if the provider has updated its subspecialty status so claims for concurrent care are not denied.

Continuity of Care

If a case involves **continuity of care** (e.g., a patient who has received treatment for a condition and is then referred by the physician to a second physician for treatment for the same condition), both physicians are responsible to provide arrangements for the patient's continuing care. In such a case, records must be provided by the referring physician and the insurance billing specialist must obtain summaries or records of the patient's previous treatment. If the patient was seen in the hospital, emergency department, or outpatient department, obtain hospital reports before coding. Contact the hospital's medical record department for copies of reports after outpatient treatment or after a patient's discharge. In some cases, coding from hospital reports can increase reimbursement but can delay submission of claims because reports may not be available in a timely manner.

Critical Care

Critical care means the intensive care provided in a variety of acute life-threatening conditions requiring constant bedside "full attention" by a physician. A critical illness or injury acutely impairs one or more vital organ systems such that there is a high probability of imminent or life-threatening deterioration in the patient's condition. Examples of vital organ system failure include, but are not limited to, central nervous system failure, circulatory failure, shock, and renal, hepatic, metabolic, and/or respiratory failure. Critical care may sometimes, but not always, be rendered in a critical care area, such as a coronary care unit (CCU), intensive care unit (ICU), respiratory care unit (RCU), or emergency department (ED), also called the emergency room (ER).

Emergency Care

Emergency care differs from critical care in that it is given by the physician in a hospital emergency department. Advanced life support may be required and the physician may spend several hours attending to a patient. Office services may also be provided on an emergency basis.

In the Medicare program, an emergency medical condition is currently defined as a medical condition manifesting itself by acute symptoms of sufficient severity (including severe pain) such that the absence of immediate medical attention could reasonably be expected to result in placing the patient's health in serious jeopardy, serious impairment to body functions, or serious dysfunction of any body organ or part.

Counseling

Counseling is a discussion with a patient, family, or both concerning one or more of the following: diagnostic results, impressions, or recommended diagnostic studies; prognosis; risks and benefits of treatment options; instructions for treatment and/or follow-up; importance of compliance with chosen treatment options; risk factor reduction; and patient and family education.

Diagnostic Terminology and Abbreviations

When completing the medical record, some physicians write "imp" (impression) or "Dx" (diagnosis), which will usually serve as the diagnosis when completing the claim. If the diagnosis is not in the chart note and there is doubt about what the diagnosis is, always pull the chart and request that the physician review it. Attach a note to the insurance claim for the physician to read before signing the form. If the patient has been in the hospital, request a copy of the discharge summary, which contains the admitting and discharge diagnoses.

Official American Hospital Association policy states that "abbreviations should be totally eliminated from the more vital sections of the medical record, such as final diagnosis, operative notes, discharge summaries, and descriptions of special procedures." Many physicians are not aware of this policy, and the final diagnosis may appear as an abbreviation on the patient's record. Frequently, an abbreviation translates to several meanings. Use your medical dictionary (most list abbreviations alphabetically with the unabbreviated words) to interpret the abbreviation or ask the physician if clarification is needed. (If you are using the *Student Workbook for the Insurance Handbook for the Medical Office*, refer to the detailed list of common medical abbreviations in Appendix A.)

If a lay term appears on a patient record, the correct medical term should be substituted to locate the correct diagnostic code (e.g., "bruise" is known as "contusion").

An **eponym** (term including the name of a person) should not be used when a comparable anatomic term can be used in its place (see Example 3–2).

The word "**acute**" refers to a condition that runs a short but relatively severe course. The word "**chronic**" means a condition persisting over a long period of time. However, the word "recurrent" is preferable for certain conditions and should be used instead of "chronic." For example, if "chronic asthma" has been charted, it would be coded as "recurrent asthma."

Whenever the words "question of," "suspected," "rule out," or the abbreviation "R/O" are used in connection with a disease or illness, substitute the words "possible" or "probable" when trying to locate the appropriate diagnostic code number. These are only a few of the many terms used in documentation. For a comprehensive reference list of correct symptomatic and diagnostic terms with their lay equivalents, see Table 3–1.

EXAMPLE 3–2	
Eponym	**Comparable Medical Term**
Buerger's disease	thromboangiitis obliterans
Graves' disease	exophthalmic goiter
Wilks syndrome	myasthenia gravis

TABLE 3–1	Medical Terminology	
Lay Term	**Medical Term**	**Pronunciation**
Acute	Use "acute" when referring to a condition that runs a short but relatively severe course	ah-KŪT
Allergy	Allergic asthma	ah-LER-jik AZ-ma
	Allergic bronchitis	ah-LER-jik brong-KĪ-tis
	Bronchial asthma	BRONG-kē-al AZ-ma
Appetite loss (abnormal)	Anorexia nervosa	an"o-REK-sē-ah ner-VŌ-sa
Athlete's foot	Pedal epidermophytosis	PED-al ep"i-der"mō-fī-TŌ-sis
	Tinea pedis	TIN-e-ah PED-is
Bad breath	Halitosis	hal-i-TŌ-sis
Balance, sense of	Equilibrium	Ē-kwi-LIB-rē-um
Baldness	Alopecia	al" ō-PĒ-shē-ah
Bedsore	Decubitus ulcer	de-KŪ-bi-tus UL-ser
Bed-wetting	Enuresis	en"ū-RĒ-sis
Belching	Eructation	ē-ruk-TĀ-shun
Bleeder's disease	Hemophilia	hē"-mo-FIL-ē-ah
Bleeding	Hemorrhage	HEM-or-ij
Blood blister	Hematoma	hēm"ah-TŌ-mah
Blood clot	Thrombus	THROM-bus
Blood, in stools	Melena	MEL-e-nah or me-LĒ-nah
Blood, in urine	Hematuria	hēm"ah-TŪ-rē-ah
Blood poisoning	Septicemia	sep"ti-SĒ-mē-ah
Blood, spitting up of	Hemoptysis	hē-MOP-ti-sis
Bloody vomitus	Hematemesis	hēm"ah-TEM-ĕ-sis
Blue skin	Cyanosis	sī"ah-NŌ-sis
Boil	Furuncle	FU-rung-k'l
Bowel movement	Defecation	def"e-KĀ-shun
Bowleg	Genu varum	JE-nū VA-rum
Breathing, cessation of	Apnea	AP-nē-ah
Breathing, difficult	Dyspnea	DISP-nē-ah or disp-NĒ-ah
Breathing, normal	Eupnea	youp-NĒ-ah
Breathing, rapid	Tachypnea	tak"ip-NĒ-ah
Breathing, slow	Bradypnea	brad"ip-NĒ-ah or brad"IP-nē-ah
Breathing, upright position only	Orthopnea	or"thop-NĒ-ah
Bruise or injury not involving sutures	Contusion	kon-TOO-zhun
	Ecchymosis(ses)	ek"i-MO-sis(sēz)
	Hematoma	hēm"ah-TŌ-mah
	Extravasation	eks-trav"ah-SĀ-shun
Bulging of eyes	Exophthalmos	ek"-sof-THAL-mōs
Burning or cauterizing	Use "surgical removal of"	
Canker sore	Aphthous stomatitis	AF-thus stō-mah TĪ-tis
Cardiac arrest	Cardiac asystole	KAR-dē-ak ah-SIS-tō-le
	Cardiac standstill	KAR-dē-ak STAND-stil
Chafing	Intertrigo	in"ter-TRĪ-gō
Change of life	Menopause	MEN-ō-pawz
	Climacteric	kli"MAK-ter-ik
Chest pain with ECG but not cardiac case	Intercostal neuritis	in"ter-KOS-tal noo-RĪ-tis
	Neurasthenia	nūr"as-THĒ-nē-ah
Chickenpox	Varicella	var"i-SEL-ah
	Variola crystallina	vah-RĪ-ō-lah kris"tah-LĪ-nah
Chronic	Use "recurrent"	
Clubfoot	Talipes	TAL-i-pēz
Cold	Coryza	ko-RĪ-zah
Cold sore; fever blisters on lips	Herpes simplex	HER-pēz-SIM-plex
Cold with runny nose	Coryza with motor rhinitis	rī-NĪ-tis

continued

TABLE 3–1	**Medical Terminology** *Continued*	
Lay Term	**Medical Term**	**Pronunciation**
Collapsed lung	Pneumothorax	nū"mō-THOR-aks
Corn	Clavus	KLĀ-vus
	Heloma molle	he-LŌ-mah MŌL-le
Cross-eye	Convergent strabismus	kon-VER-jent strah BIZ-mus
	Esotropia	os"ō-TRŌ-pō-ah
Cut	Laceration (give location, length, depth)	las"er-Ā-shun
Cutting into	Incision of	in-SIZH-un
Cutting out	Excision of	ek-SIZH-un
Dandruff	Seborrhea capitis	seb"o-RĒ-ah CAP-i-tis
Degenerative joint disease	Osteoarthritis	os"tē-ō-ar-THRI-tis
Dim vision	Amblyopia	am"blē-Ō-pē-ah
Dizziness	Vertigo	VER-ti-go or ver-TI-go
Dog bite	Dog bite (one or more abrasions, give location and description)	
Double vision	Diplopia	di-PLŌ-pē-ah
Drooping eyelids	Ptosis	TŌ-sis
	Blepharoptosis	blef"ah-rō-TŌ-sis
Ear discharge	Otorrhea	o"to-RĒ-ah
Ear procedure involving opening of ear	Myringotomy	mir"in-GOT-ō-mē
Earache	Acute otitis	ah-KŪT-ō-TĪ-tis
	Otitis media	ō-TĪ-tis MĒ-dia
	Otalgia	ō-TAL-jē-ah
	Neuralgic pain in ear (left or right)	nū-RAL-jik
Eardrum	Tympanic membrane	tim-PAN-ik MEM-brān
Earwax removal	Cerumen syringed	see-ROO-men si-RINJD
Enlarged heart	Cardiomegaly	kar"dē-ō-MEG-ah-lē
Excessive eating	Polyphagia	pol"ē-FĀ-je-ah
Excessive thirst	Polydipsia	pol"ē DIP-sē-ah
Eye examination if more than just a check for eyeglasses	Refraction and eye examination	rē-FRAK-shun
Fainting	Syncope	SIN-ko-pē
Farsightedness	Hyperopia	hi"per-Ō-pe-ah
Fat	Obese	o-BĒS
	Exogenous obesity	eks-OJ-e-nus-ō-BĒS-i-tē
Felon	Paronychia	par"ō-NIK-ē-ah
Fever	Pyrexia	pi-REK-se-ah
Fever blister	Lesion of herpes simplex	HER-pēz SIM-plex
Fibroid of uterus	Leiomyoma	li"o-mī-Ō-mah
Fit	Convulsion	kon-VUL-shun
Flatfeet	Pes planus	pes PLA-nus
Flu	Influenza	in"floo-EN-zah
	La grippe	lah GRIP
Freckle	Lentigo	len-TĪ-go
	Ephelis	e-FĒ-lis
Gallstone	Cholelithiasis	kō"le-li-THĪ-ah-sis
Gas pain	Borborygmus	bor"bo-RIG-mus
Gas, passing	Flatulence	FLAT-ū-lens
Gastrointestinal case that is not a duodenal ulcer	Gastroenteritis	gas"trō-en-ter-Ī-tus
German measles	Rubella	roo-BEL-ah
Glands, swollen	Diffuse lymphadenitis	dif-FŪS lim-fad"e-NĪ-tis
Grippe; flu	Influenza	in"floo-EN-zah
	La grippe	lah GRIP
Hammer toe	Hallux malleus	HAL-uks MAL-lē-us
Hangnail	Agnail	AG-nāl

Lay Term	Medical Term	Pronunciation
Hardening of the arteries	Arteriosclerosis	ar-tē"-rē-ō-skle-RŌ-sis
Harelip	Cleft palate	kleft PAL-at
	Cleft lip	kleft lip
Hay fever	Allergic rhinitis	ah-LER-jik rī-NĪ-tis
	Rhinallergosis	rin"al-er-GŌ-sis
Headache	Acute cephalalgia	ah-KŪT sef"ah-LAL-jē-ah
	Cephalgia	se-FAL-jē-ah
Heart attack	Coronary thrombosis	KOR-ŏ-nā-rē throm-BŌ-sis
	Coronary occlusion	KOR-ŏ-na-re ŏ-KLOO-zhun
Heart wave (tracing)	Electrocardiogram (ECG), (EKG)	e-lek"tro-KAR-dē-o-gram
Heartbum	Pyrosis	pī-RŌ-sis
Hiccough; hiccup	Singultus	sing-GUL-tus
High blood pressure	Hypertension	hī"per-TEN-shun
Hives	Urticaria	ur"ti-KĀ-rē-ah
Hoarseness	Laryngitis	lar"in-JĪ-tis
	Dysphonia	dis-FŌ-nē-ah
Housemaid's knee	Prepatellar bursitis	prē"pah-TEL-ar bar-SĪ-tis
Humpback; hunchback	Kyphosis	ki-FŌ-sis
Incontinence of urine	Enuresis	en"ū-RĒ-sis
Indigestion	Dyspepsia	dis-PEP-sē-ah
Injury	Trauma	TRAW-mah
Itching	Pruritus	proo-RĪ-tus
Jaundice	Icterus	IK-ter-us
Kidney stone	Nephrolithiasis	ne-frō-li-THĪ-ah-sis
	Renal calculus	RĒ-nal KAL-kū-lus
Knock knees	Genu valgum	JE-nū VAL-gum
Lockjaw	Tetanus	TET-ah-nus
Loss of appetite	Anorexia	an"ō-REK-sē-ah
Loss of hearing	Deafness	DEF-nes
Loss of voice	Aphonia	ah-FŌ-nē-ah
Low blood pressure	Hypotension	hī"pō-TEN-shun
Malnutrition, general ill health	Cachexia	kah-KEK-sē-ah
Marble bones	Osteosclerosis	os"tē-ō-skle-RŌ-sis
Measles	Rubeola	roo-BĒ-ō-lah
Measles, German	Rubella	roo-BEL-ah
Milk leg	Phlebitis	fle-BĪ-tis
Miscarriage	Abortion (AB)	ah-BOR-shun
Mole(s)	Nevus(i)	NĒ-vus(Ī)
Mongolism	Down syndrome	down SIN-drōm
Monthly period	Menses	MEN-sēz
	Menstruation	men"stroo-Ā-shun
Mumps	Contagious parotitis	kon-TĀ-jus par"ō-TĪ-tis
Muscle wasting	Muscular atrophy	MUS-kū-lar AT-rō-fē
Muscular weakness	Atony	AT-ō-nē
Nearsightedness	Myopia	mī-Ō-pē-ah
Nosebleed	Epistaxis	ep"i-STAK-sis
	Rhinorrhagia	rī"no-RĀ-jē-ah
Overweight	Exogenous obesity	eks-OJ-e-nus ō-BĒS-i-tē
Painful periods	Dysmenorrhea	dis"men-o-RĒ-ah
Painful urination	Dysuria	dis-Ū-rē-ah
Pap smear	Papanicolaou smear	pap"ah-nik"-ō-LĀ-ōō-smēr
Piles	Hemorrhoids	HEM-o-roids
Pinkeye	Acute contagious conjunctivitis	ah-KŪT kon-TĀ-jus kon-junk"ti-VĪ-tis
Pneumonia	If both lungs are involved, use "bilateral pneumonitis"	bī-LAT-er-al nū"mō-NĪ-tis

continued

TABLE 3–1   **Medical Terminology** *Continued*

Lay Term	Medical Term	Pronunciation
Poison ivy; poison oak	*Rhus* 'oxicodendron sensitivity	rus tok"si-kō-DEN-dron sen"si-TIV-i-tē
	Rhus dermatitis	rus der"mah-TĪ-tis
Postnasal drip (PND)	Catarrh	kah-TAHR
Protrusion of eyeballs	Exophthalmos	ek"sof-THAL-mos
Pus, full of	Purulent	PŪ-roo-lent or PUR-ū-lent
Pus, in urine	Pyuria	pi-Ū-rē-ah
Question of	Use "possible" or "probable"	
Rabies	Hydrophobia	hi"drō-FŌ-bē-ah
Residual inquiry(ies)	Sequela(ae)	se-KWE-lah(ē)
Ringing in ears	Tinnitus	TIN-Ī-tus
Rule out (R/O)	Use "possible" or "probable"	
Ruptured spleen	Splenorrhexis	sple"no-REK-sis
St Vitus' dance	Chorea	kō-RĒ-ah
Scar	Cicatrix	sik-A-triks, SIK-ah-triks
Sciatica	Sciatic neuritis	sĪ-AT-ik nū-RĪ-tis
Scraping of uterus	Dilatation and curettage (D & C)	dil-ah-TĀ-shun and kū"rĕ-TAHZH
Sebaceous cyst	Steatoma	ste"ah-TŌ-mah
	Wen	wen
Shingles	Herpes zoster	HER-pēz-ZOS-ter
Sleeping sickness	Encephalitis	en"sef-ah-LĪ-tis
Slipped disk	Herniated intervertebral disk	HER-nē-āt"ed in"ter-VER-te-bral disc
Slow heart rate	Sinus bradycardia	SĪ-nus brad"ē-KAR-dē-ah
Smallpox	Variola	vah-RI-ō-lah
Sore throat	Laryngitis	lar"in-JĪ-tis
	Pharyngitis	far"in-JĪ-tis
	Tonsillitis	ton"si-LĪ-tis
	Alpha-hemolytic streptococcus (milder strep)	AL-fah hē"mō-LIT-ik strep"tō-KOK-us
	Beta-hemolytic streptococcus (real strep throat)	BĀ-tah hē"mō-LIT-ik strep"to-KOK-us
	Acute sore throat for any kind of sore throat unless it is strep	ah-KŪT sor thrōt
Speaking difficulty	Dysphonia	dis-FŌ-nē-ah
Spinal fusion	Arthrodesis	ar"thrō-DĒ-sis
Squint	Strabismus	strah-BIZ-mus
Stiff joint	Ankylosis	ang"ki-LŌ-sis
Stiff neck; wryneck	Torticollis	tor"ti-KOL-is
Stomach ache	Tonic abdominal spasm	TON-ik ab-DOM-i-nal spazm
	Gastritis	gas-TRĪ-tis
	Gastroenteritis	gas"trō-en-ter-Ī-tis
Stone(s)	Calculus(i)	KAL-kū-lus(Ī)
Stroke	Apoplexy	AP-ō-plek"se
	Cerebral hemorrhage	SER-e-bral HEM-or-ij
Stye	Hordeolum	hor-DĒ-o-lum
Swallowing difficulty	Dysphagia	dis-FĀ-je-ah
Swayback	Lordosis	lor-DŌ-sis
Tarry stool	Melena	me-LE-nah
Tennis elbow	Radiohumeral bursitis	ra"dē-ō-HŪ-mer-al ber-SĪ-tis
Tic douloureux	Trigeminal neuralgia	tri-JEM-i-nal nū-RAL-jē-ah
Tongue tie	Ankyloglossia	ang"ki-lo-GLOS-ē-ah
Trench mouth	Acute necrotizing ulcerative infection	ah-KŪT nek-ro-TĪ-zing UL-ser-ah-tiv in-FEK-shun

Lay Term	Medical Term	Pronunciation
	Vincent's angina	VIN-sents an-JĪ-nah
Undescended testicle	Cryptorchism	krip-TŌR-kizm
	Cryptorchidism	krip-TŌR-kĪ-dizm
Undulant fever	Brucellosis	broo"sel-LO-sis
Urination, excessive	Nocturia (nighttime)	nok-TŪ-rē-ah
	Polyuria	pol"ē-Ū-rē-ah
Urination, involuntary	Enuresis (bed-wetting)	en"ū-RĒ-sis
Urination, painful	Dysuria	dis-Ū-rē-ah
Urine, scanty	Oliguria	ol"i-GŪ-rē-ah
Urine, sugar in	Glycosuria	gli"kō-SŪ-rē-ah
Vomiting of blood	Hematemesis	hem"-ah-TEM-e-sis
Wall eye	Divergent strabismus	di-VER-jent strah-BIZ-mus
	Exotropia	ek"so-TRŌ-pē-ah
Wart(s)	Verruca(ae)	ve-ROO-kah(sē)
Water on the brain	Hydrocephalus	hĪ-drō-SEF-ah-lus
Water on the knee	Prepatellar bursitis	prē-pah-TEL-ar bur-SĪ-tis
Wen	Sebaceous cyst	sē-BĀ-shus sist
	Steatoma	stē"ah-TŌ-mah
Whooping cough	Pertussis	per-TUS-is
Womb	Uterus	Ū-ter-us
Wristdrop	Carpoptosis	kar"po-TŌ-sis
Writer's cramp	Graphospasm	GRAF-ō-spazm
Wryneck	Torticollis	tor"ti-KOL-is

A commonly seen phrase or abbreviation that may not support billing of services is "WNL" (within normal limits). For example, if used to document that "all extremities are within normal limits," this statement does not indicate how many extremities or which extremities were examined. Documentation must indicate exactly what limb was examined, and abbreviated wording would not pass an external audit.

Another phrase commonly used when examining a patient and the findings are within normal limits is the word, "negative" (e.g., "Ears, nose, and throat negative" or "chest x-rays negative"). The physician needs to document that there were no abnormalities in the system being examined. Detailed documentation justifies billed services by providing verification and allows points when an external audit is performed. Thus it should be dictated "Chest film (or report) was reviewed." or "Chest x-ray report was read."

Directional Terms

Some terms commonly used to describe location of pain and injuries to areas of the abdomen as shown in Figure 3–11*A* and *B* (*A,* Four quadrants and *B,* Nine regions) are:

Right upper quadrant (RUQ) or right hypochron-driac: liver (right lobe), gallbladder, part of the pancreas, parts of the small and large intestines

Epigastric: upper middle region above the stomach

Left upper quadrant (LUQ) or left hypochondriac: liver (left lobe), stomach, spleen, part of the pancreas, parts of the small and large intestines

Right and left lumbar: middle, right, and left regions of the waist

Umbilical: central region near the navel

Right lower quadrant (RLQ) or right inguinal: parts of the small and large intestines, right ovary, right uterine (fallopian) tube, appendix, right ureter.

Hypogastric: middle region below the umbilical region contains urinary bladder and female uterus.

Left lower quadrant (LLQ) or left inguinal: parts of the small and large intestines, left ovary, left uterine tube, left ureter.

Surgical Terminology

Surgical procedures of the integumentary system, such as repair of lacerations, are listed in the procedure code book as either *simple, intermediate,* or *complex* repairs. Simple lacerations are superficial requiring one-layer closure. Intermediate lacerations require layered closure of one or more of the deeper layers of the skin and tissues. Complex

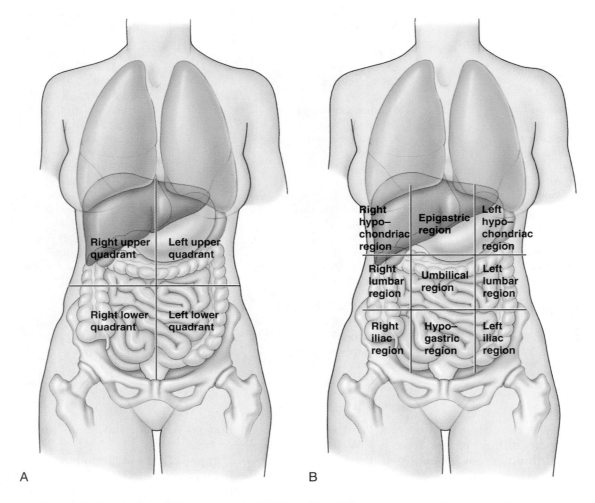

A

B

Figure 3–11. Regions of the abdomen. A, Four quadrants. B, Nine regions. (Reprinted with permission from Herlihy B, Maebius NK: The Human Body in Health and Illness. Philadelphia, WB Saunders, 2000.)

lacerations require more than layered closure and may require reconstructive surgery.

Documentation should list the length (in centimeters) of all incisions and layers of involved tissues (subcutaneous, fascia, muscle, grafts) so that correct procedure codes for excisions of lesions and type of repair can be determined.

Documentation should list the length of time spent on the procedure, especially if of unusual duration. This should be stated somewhere in the report.

If state of the art instruments or equipment are used, document the equipment as well as the time spent using it.

Therapeutic or cosmetic surgical procedures should be broken down into two categories—state how much of the procedure was functional and how much was cosmetic or therapeutic. Generally, the insurance carrier will pay for the functional portion of the procedure even if there is no coverage for cosmetic or therapeutic procedures.

If you type reports to be submitted with insurance claims to help justify the claim, you should also become familiar with the terms for various operational incisions (Fig. 3–12). Terms such as *undermining* (cut in a horizontal fashion), *take down* (to take apart), or *lysis of adhesions* (destruction of scar tissue) appear in many operations but should not be coded separately. Note the *position* (e.g., lithotomy, dorsal) of the patient during the operation and the *surgical approach* (e.g., vaginal, abdominal). These will help determine the proper code selection. Major errors can occur when an insurance biller is not familiar with the medical terms being used. Ask the physician to clarify the case if there is a question because medical terminology is very technical and can puzzle even the most knowledgeable of insurance billing specialists. Additional key words to look for that may affect code selection and reimbursement besides terminology shown in Table 3–2 are listed here along with brief definitions:

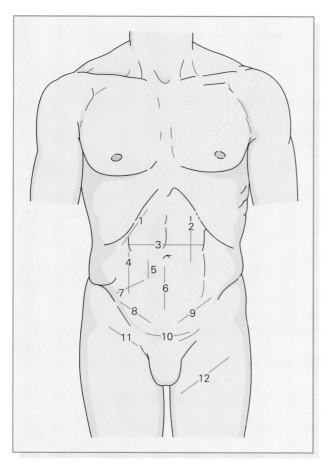

Figure 3–12. Operational incisions. Anterior (front) view: 1, subcostal incision; 2, paramedian incision; 3, transverse incision; 4, upper right rectus incision; 5, midrectus incision; 6, midline incision; 7, lower right rectus incision; 8, McBurney or right iliac incision; 9, left iliac incision; 10, suprapubic incision; 11, hernia incision; and 12, femoral incision.

bilateral: pertaining to both sides

blood loss of over 600 mL: severe bleeding

complete or total: entire or whole

complicated by: involved with other situations at the same time

hemorrhage: escape of blood from vessels; bleeding

initial: first procedure or service

multiple: affecting many parts of the body at the same time

partial: only a part, not complete

prolonged procedure due to: series of steps extended in time to get desired result

simple: single and not compound or complex

subsequent: second or more procedures or services

surgical: pertaining to surgery

uncomplicated: not intricately involved; straightforward (procedure)

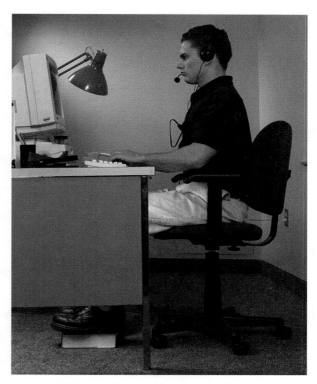

Figure 3–13. Medical transcriptionist typing a medical report.

unilateral: pertaining to one side

unusual findings or circumstances: rare or not usual conclusion

very difficult: hard to do, requiring extra effort and skill

Additional words used to detail accidents and injuries are shown in Chapter 14, Figures 14–5 through 14–9.

If you would like a more thorough discussion of medical terminology, many good books are available* (Fig. 3–13).

Review and Audit of Medical Records

Internal Reviews

Prospective Review

There are two types of **internal review.** The first type is **prospective review** which is done *before* billing is submitted. This may be done by some medical practices either daily, weekly, or monthly.

---

*Chabner DE: The Language of Medicine, 6th ed. Philadelphia, WB Saunders, 2001; Leonard PC: Building a Medical Vocabulary. Philadelphia, WB Saunders, 1997.

TABLE 3-2	Terminology Used in Coding Procedures

Medical Term	Definition
ablation	surgical removal of a body part, as by incision
acquired	condition or disorder contracted after birth; not hereditary or innate
amputation	removal of a body part, limb, or organ
anastomosis	surgical or pathologic connection of two tubular structures
anomaly	congenital or developmental defect; deviation from normal
arthrocentesis	surgical puncture of a joint to remove fluid
arthrodesis	to surgically immobilize a joint; fusion
aspiration	to draw in by inhaling or draw out by suction
biopsy	removal of living tissue for microscopic examination
cauterization	means of destroying tissue, treating infectious wounds, or stopping bleeding with use of chemicals (silver nitrate), heat, freezing, or electrical current
chemosurgery	use of chemicals to destroy tissue
chemotherapy	use of chemicals to treat disease
closed treatment	to treat a condition (such as a fracture) without surgically opening the location
closure	to bring together the edges of a wound
congenital	condition present from birth; believed to be inherited
curettage	scraping of a cavity to remove tissue, growths, or debris
débridement	excision of dead or damaged tissue and foreign matter from a wound
decompression	removal of pressure
decortication	removal of external layer (beneath the capsule) from any organ or structure
defect	imperfection, malformation, dysfunction, or absence
destructive	causing ruin; opposite of constructive
dialysis	to separate from the blood harmful waste products normally secreted in the urine
dilation	enlargement of a hollow structure or opening
discission	incision or cutting into
dissection	cutting of parts for the purpose of separation and study
drainage	continuous withdrawal of fluid from a wound, sore, or cavity
endoscopy	visual examination of the interior of a canal or hollow internal organ by means of a special instrument
evacuation	removal of waste material
excision	the act of cutting out
exploration	an active examination, usually involving endoscopy or a surgical procedure, to aid in diagnosis
fixation	the act of holding or fastening, immobilize; make rigid
foreign body	any substance or particle in the body that does not appear, form, or grow naturally
fulguration	destruction by means of high-frequency electric sparks
graft	any organ, tissue, or object used for implanting or transplanting to encourage healing, improve function, safeguard against infection, improve appearance, or replace a diseased body organ
immunoassay	any of several methods used for measuring chemical substances such as hormones, drugs, and specific proteins
implant	tissue or substance inserted or grafted into body
incision	to cut into
indwelling	located or implanted inside the body; such as a catheter or tube for drainage or administration of drugs
in situ	localized; in one specific location without disturbing or invading surrounding tissue
instrumentation	application or use of instruments or tools
internal	within the body
insertion	to place or implant; site of attachment
introduction	device for controlling and directing; to insert into the body via tube, needle, oral, or anal entrance
ligation	the process of binding or tying a body structure
lysis	destruction, decomposition, breakdown, or separation
manipulation	use of hands to produce a desired movement or effect in the body
marsupialization	surgical conversion of a closed cavity (abscess or cyst) into an open pouch to allow healing
obstruction	blockage of a structure that prevents it from functioning normally
occlusion	blockage of any passage, canal, opening, or vessel in the body; acquired or congenital
open treatment	to lay open internal parts to administer treatment

Medical Term	Definition
paring	surgical removal of foreign material or dead or damaged tissue by cutting or scraping
percutaneous	through the skin
qualitative	referring to the quality, value, or nature of something
quantitative	a measurable amount or portion
radical	extreme or drastic treatment or surgery aimed at eliminating a major disease by removing all affected tissue and any surrounding tissue that might be diseased
reconstitution	returning a substance that has been changed to its original state for preservation and storage
reconstruction	repair, mold, change, or alter to affect recovery
reduction	to restore to a normal position
repair	to remedy, replace, or heal; restore to a healthy state
replantation	surgical replacement of a body part
revision	to amend or alter to correct or improve
resection	partial excision of a body structure
shunt	an artificial passage constructed to divert flow from one route to another
suture	material (wire, thread, or staples) used in closing or attaching body tissue; to unite body tissue by stitching together; the seam formed by stitching body tissue together; line of union (border or joint) such as between the skull bones
therapy	treatment of disease or pathologic conditions
transection	a cross section; division by cutting transversely
transposition	displacement of an organ from one side of the body to the other; congenital anomaly in which a part of the body normally appearing on the right side is located on the left side of the body
traumatic	physical or psychological wound or injury

▶ Stage one of a prospective review is done to verify that completed encounter forms match patients seen according to the appointment schedule and have been posted on the daysheet. A prospective review is begun by obtaining the encounter form(s) and locating the dates in question for the review in the appointment schedule, printing the schedule as verification. The appointment schedule is then compared to the encounter forms to match patients for the date in question. Next check to see if all charges (procedures/services) have been posted on the daysheet or daily transaction register.

▶ Stage two of a prospective review is done to verify that all procedures/services and diagnoses listed on the encounter form match data on the insurance claim form. To perform this stage, use the completed claim form or print an insurance billing worksheet. Match the information on the claim/worksheet with the date of service, procedure/service, and diagnosis on the encounter form. It is possible that one or more diagnoses may not match. A common reason why this may occur is because an active diagnosis has not been entered into the computer system and the computer defaults to the last diagnosis given for an established patient. Another problem occurs when the diagnosis is not linked to the procedure. Such problems must be found prior to billing and corrected before claims are printed.

Retrospective Review

The second type of internal review is called **retrospective review,** which is done *after* billing insurance carriers. A coder or insurance biller may be asked to perform a retrospective review to determine whether there is a lack of documentation. To accomplish this, pull at random 15 to 20 medical records from the last 2 to 4 months. Recommended internal audit tools are:

pencil
internal record review worksheets
procedure code book
diagnostic code book
HCPCS code book
medical dictionary
abbreviation reference book
drug reference book (i.e., *Physicians' Desk Reference*)
laboratory reference book
provider's manual for insurance program or plan
insurance carrier's newsletters

Forms similar to the Internal Record Review Form shown in Figures 3–6 through 3–10 may be used as tools to gather information from the patient's record, laboratory reports, pathology reports, radiology reports, operative reports, and other diagnostic tests. If the physician's documentation is inadequate, errors or deficiencies will appear as the review is being conducted. You will discover that doing an internal review of this type is not an exact science and critical thinking skills are put into use. Because documentation guidelines and code policies are updated and refined periodically, it is extremely important to read and keep bulletins from all insurance carriers, especially from the local fiscal Medicare intermediary. Advise the physician of any new requirements. This resource may be the only notification of changes unless you routinely attend local or national workshops.

External Audit

An **external audit** is a retrospective review of medical and financial records by an insurance company or Medicare representative to investigate suspected fraud or abusive billing practices. Government officials discovered deficiencies in medical documentation as a result of external audits conducted by Medicare officials.

In 1984, Michigan signed into law the Health Care Claim Act with felony penalties ranging to 10 years in prison and fines of up to $50,000 per count for attempting to defraud an insurance company. Other states are following suit in establishing such laws.

Most insurance companies perform routine audits on unusual billing patterns. Insurance companies have computer software programs capable of editing and screening insurance claims to identify billing excesses or potential abuses before payment is rendered. Insurance carriers hire undercover agents who visit physicians' offices if overuse and abuse of procedure codes are suspected. Physicians who charge excessive fees are routinely audited by most carriers. Carriers spot check by sending questionnaires to patients and asking them if they received medical care from Dr. Doe to verify the services rendered. The answers are then compared with what the physician billed. Many insurance companies have installed anti-fraud telephone hotlines or billing question telephone lines for patients. Investigations can result from such calls, depending on the circumstances. Tips also come from peer review organizations, state licensing boards, whistle-blowing physicians, ex-staff members, and patients. If there is any suspicion of fraud, the insurance company will notify the medical practice, specify a date and time at which they will come to the office, and indicate which records they wish to audit (Fig. 3–14). Investiga-

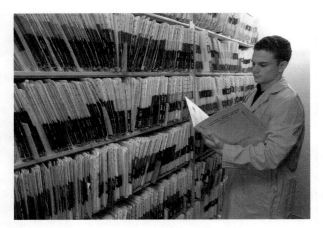

Figure 3–14. Insurance billing specialist searching for a patient's chart in the files to pull records for an external audit.

tors question the patient, look at the documentation in the medical record, and interview the staff and all physicians who have participated in the care of the patient. Points are awarded if documentation is present.

Audit Prevention

Compliance Program

In 1997 the Department of Health and Human Services (HHS) Office of the Inspector General (OIG) developed the concept of compliance planning as related to clinical documentation. OIG and HHS as well as the Health Care Compliance Association (HCCA) and many other health care agencies have asked physicians to voluntarily develop and implement compliance programs. OIG published guidelines to assist a physician and his or her staff in establishing a medical practice's compliance program to enhance documentation for Medicare cases as well as all patient's seen by the physician. Purposes of a compliance program are to reduce fraudulent insurance claims and to provide quality care to patients. A **compliance program** is composed of policies and procedures to accomplish uniformity, consistency, and conformity in medical record keeping that fulfills official requirements. If a medical practice experiences an external Medicare audit, HHS OIG and the Department of Justice considers that the medical practice made a reasonable effort to avoid and detect misbehavior if a compliance plan has been in place. When errors are found and a determination is made as to whether there was intent to commit health care fraud, a compliance plan provides evidence that any errors made were inadvertent. There is no single best compliance program because every medical practice is different. However, there are some elements that lead to a successful compliance program. These are

▶ written standards of conduct
▶ written policies and procedures
▶ compliance officer and/or committee to operate and monitor the program
▶ training program for all affected employees
▶ process to give complaints anonymously
▶ internal audit performed routinely
▶ investigation and remediation plan for problems that develop
▶ response plan for improper or illegal activities

A compliance program must be tailored to fit the needs of each medical practice depending on its corporate structure, mission, size, and employee composition. The statutes, regulations, and guidelines of the federal and state health insur-ance programs, as well as the policies and proce-dures of the private health plans should be inte-grated into every medical practice's compliance program. The ultimate goals are to improve quality of services and control of claims submission, and also to reduce fraud, waste, abuse, and the cost of health care to federal, state, and private health in-surers.

Edit Checks

An *edit check* is a good audit prevention measure to have in place because the software program au-tomatically screens transmitted insurance claims and electronically examines them for errors and/or conflicting code entries. Carriers accept a variety of levels of service; however, if only one or two levels are consistently listed, this is usually not

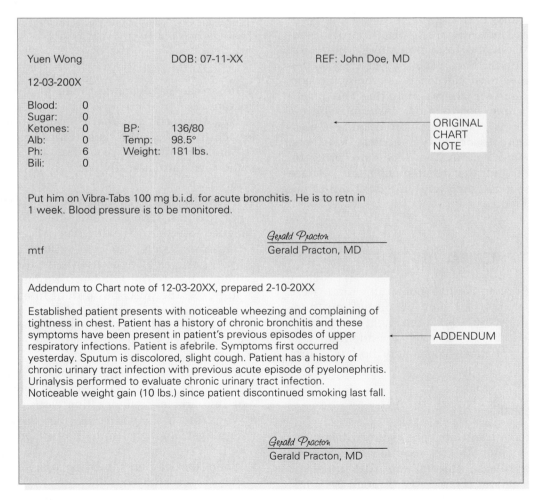

Figure 3–15. Example of an addendum to a patient's medical record to justify the level of service reported. The insurance carrier downcoded the services from level 99213 to 99212.

realistic and will attract attention and, possibly, an audit. If services are downcoded and the physician neglected to document the correct level of services performed, an addendum to a medical record must be made to justify the level of service reported (Fig. 3–15). Amended chart notes must be labeled "Addendum" or "Late entry," dated on the day of the amendment, and signed by the physician.

It is vital to be as correct as possible in your choice of diagnostic and procedural codes with modifiers. If the diagnosis does not match the service provided, the claim will be thrown out by the edit check of the computer program. It is equally important that everything involved in patient care be well documented and that records be complete (Fig. 3–16).

In subsequent chapters, you will obtain further knowledge on what needs to be documented in relationship to diagnostic and procedure codes. Information on the Civil Monetary Penalties Law to prosecute cases of Medicare and Medicaid fraud can be found in Chapter 12.

Once an individual has been found guilty of committing a Medicare or Medicaid program-related crime, exclusion from program participation is mandatory under Sec. 1128(a) of the Social Security Act. An individual can be anyone who participates in fraud or abuse, including the physician, nurse, home health aide, insurance billing specialist, claims assistance professional, electronic claims processor, and/or medical assistants. If ever suspended from the Medicare program, make sure to obtain a reinstatement letter because this will be needed when applying for a future position in the medical field.

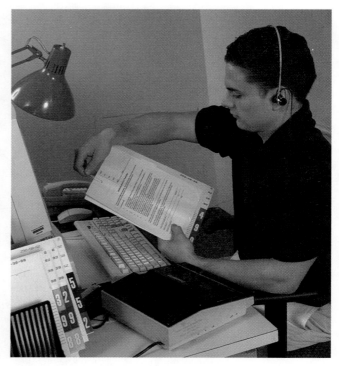

Figure 3–16. Medical transcriptionist inserting a transcribed chart note into a patient's medical record.

LEGALITIES OF MEDICAL RECORDS

The basics of confidential communication were provided in Chapter 1 where privileged and nonprivileged information and the right to privacy were discussed. In this chapter, confidentiality as it relates to the medical record and the law is presented.

Patient Confidentiality

The patient record and any photographs taken are confidential documents and require an authorization form to release information that must be signed by the patient (Figs. 3–17 through 3–19). If the form is a photocopy, it is necessary to state that the photocopy is approved by the patient or write to the patient and obtain an original signed document.

Unauthorized release of information is called **breach of confidential communication.**

Confidentiality between the physician and the patient is automatically waived in the following situations:

▶ When the patient is a member of a managed care organization (MCO) and the physician has signed a contract with the MCO that has a clause that says "for quality care purposes, the MCO has a right to access the medical records of their patients, and for utilization management purposes, the MCO has a right to audit those patients' financial records." Other managed care providers need to know about the patients if involved in the care and treatment of members of the MCO.

▶ When the physician examines a patient at the request of a third party who is paying the bill, as in workers' compensation cases.

▶ When the patient is suing someone, such as an employer, and wishes to protect herself or himself.

▶ When the patient's records are subpoenaed or there is a search warrant.

Other exceptions to the confidentiality requirement include when state law requires the release

Figure 3–17. Completed Authorization for Release of Information form for a patient relocating to another city. (From Federal Register, Vol. 64, No. 212, Appendix to Subpart E of Part 164—Model Authorization Form, November 3, 1999.)

AUTHORIZATION FOR RELEASE OF INFORMATION

Section A: Must be completed for all authorizations.

I hereby authorize the use or disclosure of my individually identifiable health information as described below.

I understand that this authorization is voluntary. I understand that if the organization authorized to receive the information is not a health plan or health care provider, the released information may no longer be protected by federal privacy regulations.

Patient name: _____Chloe E. Levy_____   **ID Number:** ____3075____

Persons/organizations providing information: **Persons/organizations receiving information:**
College Clinic, Gerald Practon, MD   Margaret L. Lee, MD
4567 Broad Avenue   328 Seward Street
Woodland Hills, XY 12345-0001   Anytown, XY 45601-0731

Specific description of information [including date(s)]: _Initial history and physical_ and complete medical records for last 3 years

Section B: Must be completed only if a health plan or a health care provider has requested the authorization.

1. The health plan or health care provider must complete the following:
   a. What is the purpose of the use or disclosure?__Patient relocating to another city__

   b. Will the health plan or health care provider requesting the authorization receive financial or in-kind compensation in exchange for using or disclosing the health information described above? Yes ____No X

2. The patient or the patient's representative must read and initial the following statements:
   a. I understand that my health care and the payment for my health care will not be affected if I do not sign this form.   Initials: _cel_
   b. I understand that I may see and copy the information described on this form if I ask for it, and that I get a copy of this form after I sign it.   Initials: _cel_

Section C: Must be completed for all authorizations.

The patient or the patient's representative must read and initial the following statements:

1. I understand that this form will expire on _09 / 01 /20XX_ (DD/MM/YR).
   Initials _cel_

2. I understand that I may revoke this authorization at any time by notifying the providing organization in writing , but if I do not it will not have any effect on any actions they took before they received the revocation.
   Initials: _cel_

Chloe E. Levy   June 1, 20XX
Signature of patient or patient's representative   **Date**
(Form MUST be completed before signing)

Printed name of patient's representative: _____

Relationship to the patient: _____

YOU MAY REFUSE TO SIGN THIS AUTHORIZATION
You may not use this form to release information for treatment or payment except when the information to be released is psychotherapy notes or certain research information.

NAME OF FACILITY
Consent for Release of Information

Date _May 16, 20XX_

1. I hereby authorize _College Hospital_ to release the following information from the
   health record(s) of _Martha T. Jacobson_
   _{Name of Institution}
   _{Patient name}

   52 East Rugby Street, Woodland Hills, XY 12345
   _{Address}

   covering the period(s) of hospitalization from:
   Date of Admission _January 3, 20XX_
   Date of Discharge _January 5, 20XX_
   Hospital # _278-1200_ Birthdate _June 27, 1960_

2. Information to be released:
   ☐ Copy of (complete) health record(s)   ☑ Discharge summary
   ☐ History and physical   ☐ Operative report
   ☐ Other _____

3. Information is to be released to: _Michael Hotta, MD_
   260 West Main Street, Woodland Hills, XY 12345

4. Purpose of disclosure _June 14, 20XX consultation_

5. I understand this consent can be revoked at any time except to the extent that disclosure
   made in good faith has already occurred in reliance to this consent.

6. Specification of the date, event, or condition upon which this consent expires:
   December 31, 20XX

7. The facility, its employees and officers, and attending physician are released from legal
   responsibility or liability for the release of the above information to the extent indicated and
   authorized herein.

Signed _Martha T. Jacobson_
            (Patient or Representative)

            _____
            (Relationship to Patient)

May 16, 20XX
            (Date of Signature)

Figure 3–18. Consent for Release of Information form. (Reprinted with permission from the American Health Information Management Association, Chicago, IL.)

of information that is for the good of society, such as cases of child or, in some states, elder abuse, certain highly contagious or infectious diseases, and gunshot wounds.

For information on confidentiality as it relates to computer use, refer to Chapter 7.

Principles for Release of Information

Some situations require the insurance billing specialist to release medical information to or for a patient, such as when a patient is seeking a second medical opinion, wishes to acquire insurance, needs it for personal record keeping or upcoming surgery, is transferring to another physician, or is relocating to another city. Some general guidelines are shown in Table 3–3.

To avoid misunderstanding of technical terms, it is preferable not to allow lay persons to examine records without the presence of the physician. If a

patient requests to view his or her medical record, inform the physician so that he or she can help interpret the language and abbreviations used in the record. When working in a hospital, the insurance billing specialist should check with the supervisor

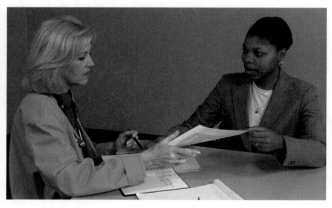

Figure 3–19. Patient signing a consent form.

TABLE 3–3   **Principles for Release of Information**

Request From or For	Policy
Physicians involved with patient care	Written consent of the patient
Physician referring a patient to another doctor for consultation	Referring physician sends summary of case or copies of patient's records without signed authorization
Patient moving to a new location or being released from medical care and transferred to another physician	Letter should be directed to the patient offering to transfer the patient's records with signed authorization to new physician
Managed care patient seen by different physicians at each office visit	Patient records may be read by all physicians involved with the case without a signed authorization.
Insurance companies and others concerned from a financial point of view	Written consent of the patient
Attorney in litigation case	Records may be released if subpoened; otherwise must have written consent of the patient
Any party in workers' compensation case	Insurance claims examiner can give patient copy of his or her records but physician cannot release record unless authorized by claims examiner. Authorization must be signed by employer and insurance company.
Any party via telephone	Either ask the caller to put the request in writing and to include the patient's signed authorization or obtain the name and telephone number of the caller and relationship to the patient and have the physician return the call.
Government and state agencies	Records may be reviewed without patient's consent to verify billing information and determine if services were medically necessary. Data in the records may be used only for audit and may not be released.
Employer	Written consent of patient. Special care should be exercised and the attending physician consulted before release of any information.
For psychiatric records	Consult psychiatrist or attending physician concerned with the case before records are released. If patient has threatened to harm himself or herself or someone else, the patient may lose the confidentiality privilege when he or she files litigation in which mental distress is claimed.
For publication	Written consent of patient. Care must be exercised in release of any information for publication because this constitutes an invasion of the patient's right to privacy and can result in legal action against the physician releasing such information.
For medical information in an acquired immunodeficiency syndrome (AIDS) or human immunodeficiency virus (HIV) infection case	Seek legal counsel and/or learn the state laws before releasing any information. Use the AHIMA consent form shown in Figure 3–18. Stamp all information released about a patient who has an HIV infection with a statement prohibiting redisclosure of the data to another party without prior consent of the patient. The party receiving the data should be requested to destroy the information after the stated need is fulfilled.
For medical information on a minor	If a minor patient is legally capable of consenting to medical treatment, only the minor patient may sign an authorization for disclosure. In all other cases, the authorization must be signed by the minor's parent, guardian, or other legal representative.
For medical information on a minor who has received alcohol and/or drug abuse treatment	Where state law permits the minor to apply for and obtain alcohol or drug abuse treatment, the minor may authorize disclosure.

at all times to make sure his or her actions conform with hospital policy. If employed by a health facility that has a policy manual, familiarize yourself with its rules regarding release of information. Regardless of the work setting, when in doubt about the release of any information, ask the physician or office manager for guidance and make sure you have obtained the patient's authorization in writing.

Faxing Documents

The common term *fax* is derived from the word **facsimile,** which means transmission of written and graphic matter by electronic means. Faxes have become an important communication tool. Fax transmission is a system of sending and receiving copies of information instantly over telephone lines. It is used to transmit insurance claims data directly to an electronic claims processor, resubmit an unpaid insurance claim, send further documentation on a claim to insurance carriers, obtain preauthorization for surgery on a patient, network with other insurance billers, and send medical reports between offices and to other medical facilities across the country. Documents to be faxed can be a graphic illustration, typewritten, or handwritten with pen. Pencil does not fax through as clear to the recipient. To prevent deterioration of documents faxed on thermal paper (when the machine is not a plain paper fax), photocopy the document onto regular paper before it is filed in medical records.

Sensitive Information

From the legal standpoint, protecting the patient's confidentiality in the fax process is critical. If, due to circumstances, medical records or a report must be faxed, you should have the patient sign an authorization to release information via facsimile equipment. The American Health Information Management Association (AHIMA) advises that fax machines should not be used for *routine* transmission of patient information. AHIMA recommends that documents should be faxed *only* when (1) hand or mail delivery will not meet the needs of immediate patient care or (2) required by a third party for ongoing certification of payment for a hospitalized patient.

Documents containing information on sexually transmitted diseases, drug or alcohol treatment, or human immunodeficiency virus (HIV) status should not be faxed. Psychiatric records should not be faxed except for emergency requests.

Fax machines should be located in secure or restricted access areas. Do not fax to machines in mail rooms, office lobbies, or other open areas unless they are secured with passwords. To ensure protection, a cover sheet should be used for all transmissions. This can be a half sheet, full sheet, or small self-adhesive form attached to the top of the first page. It should contain the following information:

- Name of recipient
- Name of sender
- Date
- Total number of pages including the cover sheet
- Fax and telephone numbers of recipient and sender in case of transmittal problems (e.g., lost page or dropped line)
- A statement that it is personal, privileged and confidential medical information intended for the named recipient only (Fig. 3–20).

Transmittal Destination

Noise or interference from telephone lines can be severe enough to distort a fax massage, so, when it is necessary, verify receipt. There are a number of ways to ensure that a faxed document has reached the correct destination.

- Place a telephone call to the requesting physician's office 10 to 15 minutes after faxing patient records to verify their receipt.
- Request that the authorized receiver sign and return an attached receipt form at the bottom of the cover sheet on receipt of the faxed information.
- Make arrangements with the recipient for a scheduled time for transmission.
- Send the fax to a coded mail box. Coded mail boxes require the sender to punch in a code indicating the individual to whom the fax is addressed and the receiver to then punch in his or her own code to activate the printer.
- Ask the receiving party for a patient reference number (e.g., the patient's Social Security number). Blank out the patient's name and write in the reference number on the document before faxing it. Also ask other providers to fax records by reference number rather than by patient name.

To safeguard against a fax sent to the wrong destination, telephone or fax a request to destroy misdirected information. Note the incident, along with the misdialed number, in the patient's medical record. Program frequently used numbers into the fax machine to avoid misdirecting faxed communications. Edit your release of records authorization form to allow for fax transmission because it is acceptable to honor an authorization sent via this method.

Medicare Guidelines

For Medicare patients, check with the Medicare fiscal intermediary to find out whether faxing of claims and documents is acceptable. The use of a fax transmittal system requires that the physician retain the original facsimile with the signature on it. Further information on digital fax may be found in Chapter 7, Electronic Data Interchange.

Financial Data

Never fax a patient's financial data. In court, faxing medical information can be justified on the basis of medical necessity, but faxing financial information cannot be justified.

Legal Documents

Consult an attorney to make sure that documents (e.g., contracts, proposals, insurance claims) requiring signatures are legally binding if faxed. To ensure legality do the following:

▶ Transmit the entire document, front and back, to be signed and not only the page to be signed so

Figure 3–20. Example of a fax cover sheet for medical document transmission.

FAX TRANSMITTAL SHEET

To: _____ University Hospital _____ Date __10-21-20XX__

Fax Number: ___013-273-0561___ Time __10:00 a.m.__

Number of pages (including this one): __3__

From: __Gerald Practon, MD__ Phone __013-486-9002__

Note: This transmittal is intended only for the use of the individual or entity to which it is addressed, and may contain information that is privileged, confidential, and exempt from disclosure under applicable law. If you are not the intended recipient, any dissemination, distribution, or photocopying of this communication is strictly prohibited. If you have received this communication in error, please notify this office immediately by telephone and return the original FAX to us at the address below by U.S. Postal Service. Thank you.

Remarks: ___Place laboratory reports done prior to patient's admission___ ___into the patient's hospital records.___

If you cannot read this FAX or if pages are missing, please contact:

PRACTON MEDICAL GROUP, INC.
4567 Broad Avenue
Woodland Hills, XY 12345-4700
Tel. 013/486-9002
Fax. No. 013/488-7815

INSTRUCTIONS TO THE AUTHORIZED RECEIVER: PLEASE COMPLETE THIS STATEMENT OF RECEIPT AND RETURN TO SENDER VIA THE ABOVE FAX NUMBER.

I, __Cheryl Watson, CMA__, verify that I have received __3__
                                                          (no. of pages including cover sheet)
from __Gerald Practon, MD__
        (sending facility's name)

the receiver has full disclosure of the agreement.

▶ Obtain confirmation that the receiver is in receipt of all pages sent, because an incomplete document may be invalid.

▶ Insert a clause in the contract stating that faxed signatures will be treated as originals.

▶ Follow up and obtain the original signature in hard copy form as soon as possible.

Subpoena

Subpoena literally means "under penalty." In legal language, it is a writ requiring the appearance of a witness at a trial or other proceeding. Strictly defined, a **subpoena duces tecum** requires the witness to appear and to bring and/or send certain records "in his possession." Frequently, however, only the records may be sent, and the physician is not required to appear in court.

A subpoena is a legal document signed by a judge or an attorney in the name of a judge. In cases in which a pretrial of evidence or deposition is set up, the subpoena may be issued by a notary public, in which event it is called a *notary subpoena.* If an attorney signs it, he or she must attest it in the name of a judge, the court clerk, or other proper officer.

It is possible for a state investigator to subpoena patient records and then file administrative charges against the physician, not because of the practice of shoddy medicine but rather because the case was inadequately documented for the treatment provided. Medical records may also be subpoenaed as proof in a medical malpractice case. Complete documentation and well-organized patient records help establish a strong defense in a medical professional liability claim.

The Subpoena Process

A subpoena must be personally served or handed to the prospective witness or the keeper of the medical records. Neither civil nor criminal subpoenas can be served via the telecopier (fax) machine. The acceptance of a document by someone authorized to accept it is the equivalent of personal service. The subpoena cannot be left on a counter or desk. In a state civil case, a "witness fee" and payment for travel to and from court are given, if demanded, at the time a subpoena is served. The fee is discretionary in criminal cases. In some states, provision is made for substitute service by mail or through newspaper advertisements. This is permitted only after all reasonable efforts to effect personal service have failed.

Never accept a subpoena or give records to anyone without the physician's prior authorization. The medical office should designate one person as keeper of the medical records. If the subpoena is only for medical records and/or financial data, the representative for the specific doctor can then usually accept it, and the physician will not be called to court.

If a physician is on vacation and there is no designated keeper of the records, tell the deputy that the physician is not in and cannot be served. Suggest the deputy contact the physician's attorney and relay this information.

When the "witness fee" has been received and the subpoena has been served, pull the chart and place it and the subpoena on the physician's desk for review. Willful disregard of a subpoena is punishable as contempt of court.

The medical office is given a prescribed time in which to produce the records. It is not necessary to show them at the time the subpoena is served unless the court order so states. The attorney usually employs a person or copy service to copy records that are under subpoena. At the time the subpoena is served, a date is usually agreed upon in which the representative will return and copy the portion of the record that is named in the subpoena. Often only the portion of the medical record requested is removed from the original chart and put in a copy folder. Items such as the patient registration information sheet, encounter form, and explanation of benefits should not be included. You may also telephone the attorney who sent the subpoena and ask if the records can be mailed. If so, mail them by registered mail with return receipt requested. Retain a copy of the records released. You will have to appear in court if specified in the subpoena. Verify with the court that the case is actually on the calendar. If you do not appear, you are in contempt of court and subject to a penalty, such as several days in jail.

If original records are requested, move them to a safe place, preferably under lock and key, so that they cannot be taken away or tampered with before the trial date. Make photocopies of the original records because this will prevent total loss of the records and facilitate discovery of any altering or tampering while they are out of your custody. Number the pages of the records so you will know if a page is missing.

On the day of your court appearance, comply with all instructions given by the court. *Do not*

TABLE 3-4	**Records Retention Schedule**

Temporary Record	Recommended Retention Period (Years)
Accounts receivable ledger cards	4
Appointment sheets	1
Balance sheets	5
Bank deposits and statements, reconciliations	6–8
Cash receipt records	10
Contracts and leases (expired)	7
Contracts with employees	6
Copies of estimated tax forms	6
Correspondence, general	1–5
Deceased patients' medical records	5
Depreciation schedules	3
Duplicate bank deposit slips	1
Employee time cards/sheets and schedules	5
Employment applications	3
Expense reports	7
Insurance claim forms (paid) in alpha files	3
Inventory records	3
Invoice and billing records	7
Medicare financial records	7
Payroll records	7
Petty cash vouchers	3
Postal and meter records	1

Permanent Record (Retained Indefinitely)

Accounts payable ledgers
Balance sheets
Bills of sale for important purchases
Canceled checks and check registers
Capital asset records
Cashbooks
Certified financial statements
Charts of accounts
Correspondence, legal
Credit history
Deeds, mortgages, contracts, leases, and property records
Equipment records
Inactive patient medical records purged from active files
Income tax returns and documents
Insurance policies and records
Journals
Patients' medical records, including x-ray films
Professional liability insurance policies
Property appraisals
Telephone records

Reproduced by permission from Fordney MT, Follis JJ: Administrative Medical Assisting. Albany, NY, Delmar Publishers, 1998.

give up possession of the records unless instructed to do so by the judge. *Do not* permit examination of the records by anyone before their identification in court. *Do not* leave the chart in the court unless it is in the possession of the judge or jury and a receipt for it has been obtained.

When you have questions, call the physician's attorney or the court's information and assistance staff.

Retention of Records

Today, most medical records are either stored in color-coded file folders containing a collection of paper documents or reside in multiple electronic databases displayed in a variety of formats via computer access. Regardless of the system used, there are general guidelines that must be followed to record information correctly, use it according to law, and retain it.

Medical Records

Preservation of medical records is governed by state and local laws. Individual states generally set a minimum of 7 to 10 years for keeping records, but it is the policy of most physicians to retain medical records of all living patients indefinitely. Proof materials for the establishment of evidence, such as x-ray films, laboratory reports, and pathologic specimens probably should be kept indefinitely. Calendars, appointment books, and telephone logs should also be filed and stored. Cases that involve radiologic injury claims (e.g., leukemia from radiation) may begin running the statute of limitations after discovery of the injury, which may occur 20 or 30 years after radiation exposure. Recommended retention periods for paper files are shown in Table 3–4. Electronic health records may have different retention periods depending on state law, as shown in Table 3–5.

A person's medical record may be of value not only to himself or herself in later years but also to the person's children. In some states a minor may file suit, after he or she has attained legal age, for any act performed during childhood that the person believes to be wrong or harmful. Sometimes a suit may be permitted even 2 to 3 years after the child has reached legal age. Thus, it is important to keep records until patients are 3 to 4 years beyond the age of majority.

Deceased patients' charts should be kept for at least 5 years. Shred documents that are no longer

| TABLE 3-5 | Electronic Health Records Retention Periods | | | | |

State	Routine Patients (Years)	X-Rays (Years)	Nursing Homes (Years)	Minors (Years)	Medicaid (Years)
Alabama	22	5	at least 5		
Alaska	7	5		at least 2	3
Arizona	10				
Arkansas	10			7	
California	7	7	1		
Colorado	10			majority +10	
Connecticut	25		10		
Delaware					
District of Columbia	10				
Florida	7	5	5		
Georgia	6			until 27th b-day	
Hawaii	7	7		majority +7	
Idaho	3	5	7	18th b-day +7	
Illinois	10–22		5		
Indiana	7	5			
Iowa	Statute of limitations		3		
Kansas	10			18th b-day +1	
Kentucky	5			majority +3	
Louisiana	10	3			
Maine	Statute of limitations				
Maryland	5			majority +3	
Massachusetts	5				
Michigan			6		
Minnesota	7				
Mississippi	7–10	4		majority +7	
Missouri	Statute of limitations		5		
Montana	10			majority +10	
Nebraska	10			majority +3	
Nevada	5		1		
New Hampshire	7	7	7	majority +7	
New Jersey	10	5		at least 23rd b-day	
New Mexico	10	4			
New York	6			majority +3	
North Carolina	Statute of limitations				
North Dakota	25		10	majority +3	
Ohio					
Oklahoma	5				6
Oregon		10	7	7	
Pennsylvania	7			majority +7	
Rhode Island	5			23rd b-day	
South Carolina	10		10		
South Dakota	Statute of limitations				
Tennessee	10	4	10	majority +1	
Texas	10			20th b-day	
Utah	10				
Vermont	10		6		
Virginia	5			23rd b-day	

State	Routine Patients (Years)	X-Rays (Years)	Nursing Homes (Years)	Minors (Years)	Medicaid (Years)
Washington	10			21st b-day	
West Virginia	NONE				
Wisconsin	5				
Wyoming	30	5			

From Amatayahul M, Brown L, Cavanaugh F, et al: Comprehensive Guide to Electronic Health Records. New York, Faulkner & Gray, 1997.

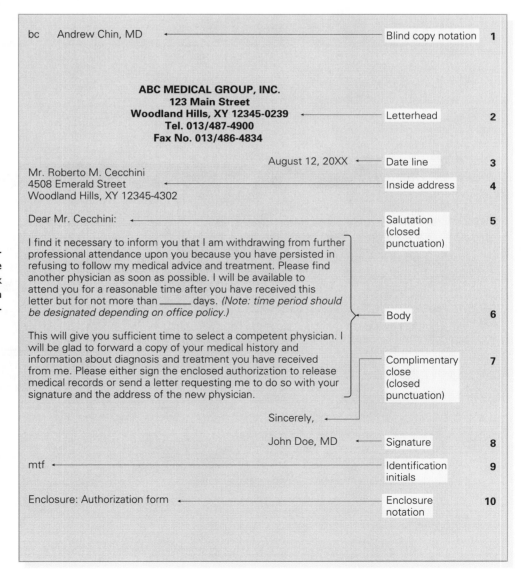

Figure 3–21. Example of letter of withdrawal from a case that is typed in modified-block style with closed punctuation and special notations (placement of parts of letter).

bc   Andrew Chin, MD ◄——————————————— Blind copy notation   **1**

ABC MEDICAL GROUP, INC.
123 Main Street
Woodland Hills, XY 12345-0239 ◄——— Letterhead   **2**
Tel. 013/487-4900
Fax No. 013/486-4834

August 12, 20XX ◄——— Date line   **3**

Mr. Roberto M. Cecchini
4508 Emerald Street ◄——————————————— Inside address   **4**
Woodland Hills, XY 12345-4302

Dear Mr. Cecchini: ◄——————————————— Salutation   **5**
(closed punctuation)

I find it necessary to inform you that I am withdrawing from further professional attendance upon you because you have persisted in refusing to follow my medical advice and treatment. Please find another physician as soon as possible. I will be available to attend you for a reasonable time after you have received this letter but for not more than _____ days. *(Note: time period should be designated depending on office policy.)* ——— Body   **6**

This will give you sufficient time to select a competent physician. I will be glad to forward a copy of your medical history and information about diagnosis and treatment you have received from me. Please either sign the enclosed authorization to release medical records or send a letter requesting me to do so with your signature and the address of the new physician. ——— Complimentary close (closed punctuation)   **7**

Sincerely, ◄—

John Doe, MD ◄——— Signature   **8**

mtf ◄——————————————— Identification initials   **9**

Enclosure: Authorization form ◄——————————————— Enclosure notation   **10**

A

UNITED STATES POSTAL SERVICE

‖‖‖

First-Class Mail
Postage & Fees Paid
USPS
Permit No. G-10

• Sender: Please print your name, address, and ZIP+4 in this box •

COLLEGE CLINIC
4567 BROAD AVENUE
WOODLAND HILLS, XY 12345 0001

B

SENDER: *COMPLETE THIS SECTION*	*COMPLETE THIS SECTION ON DELIVERY*	
■ Complete items 1, 2, and 3. Also complete item 4 if Restricted Delivery is desired. ■ Print your name and address on the reverse so that we can return the card to you. ■ Attach this card to the back of the mailpiece, or on the front if space permits.	A. Received by (*Please Print Clearly*)	B. Date of Delivery
	C. Signature X	☐ Agent ☐ Addressee
1. Article Addressed to: Mr. John Doe 2761 Fort Street Woodland Hills, XY 12345	D. Is delivery address different from item 1? ☐ Yes 　 If YES, enter delivery address below:　 ☐ No	
	3. Service Type ☒ Certified Mail　☐ Express Mail ☐ Registered　　☐ Return Receipt for Merchandise ☐ Insured Mail　　☐ C.O.D.	
	4. Restricted Delivery? (*Extra Fee*)	☐ Yes
2. Article Number (*Copy from service label*) 7000 0520 0020 3886 3129		

PS Form 3811, July 1999   Domestic Return Receipt   102595-00-M-0952

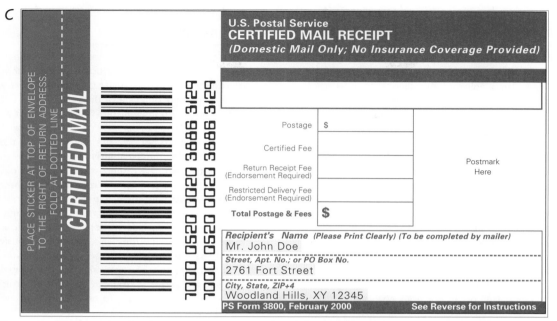

C

U.S. Postal Service
CERTIFIED MAIL RECEIPT
(Domestic Mail Only; No Insurance Coverage Provided)

Postage | $
Certified Fee |
Return Receipt Fee
(Endorsement Required) |
Restricted Delivery Fee
(Endorsement Required) |
Total Postage & Fees | **$**

Postmark
Here

CERTIFIED MAIL

PLACE STICKER AT TOP OF ENVELOPE
TO THE RIGHT OF RETURN ADDRESS.
FOLD AT DOTTED LINE

Recipient's Name *(Please Print Clearly) (To be completed by mailer)*
Mr. John Doe
Street, Apt. No.; or PO Box No.
2761 Fort Street
City, State, ZIP+4
Woodland Hills, XY 12345
PS Form 3800, February 2000   **See Reverse for Instructions**

Figure 3–22. Example of a domestic return receipt Postal Service Form 38-11 (*A* and *B*, front and back) and receipt (*C*) for certified mail Postal Service Form 3800 (U.S. Government Printing Office) shown completed.

Figure 3–23. Example of letter to confirm discharge by patient that is typed in modified-block style with open punctuation (no commas after salutation or complimentary close).

XYZ MEDICAL CLINIC
459 South Elm Street
Woodland Hills, XY 12345-4309
Tel. 013/487-9870
Fax No. 013/486-3400

September 3, 20XX

Mrs. Gregory Putnam
4309 North E Street
Woodland Hills, XY 12345-4398

Dear Mrs. Putnam

This will confirm our telephone conversation today during which you discharged me from attending you as your physician in your present illness. In my opinion, your medical condition requires continued treatment by a physician. If you have not already obtained the services of another physician, I suggest you do so without further delay.

You may be assured that, upon your written authorization, I will furnish your new physician with information regarding the diagnosis and treatment you have received from me.

Very truly yours

Mary Doe, MD

mtf

TABLE 3–6	Prevention of Lawsuits—Guidelines for Insurance Billing Specialists

1. Keep information about patients strictly confidential.
2. Obtain proper instruction and carry out responsibilities according to the employer's guidelines.
3. Keep abreast of general insurance program guidelines, annual coding changes, and medical and scientific progress to help when handling insurance matters.
4. Secure proper written consent in all cases before releasing a patient's medical record.
5. Do not refer to consent or acknowledgement forms as "releases." Use the word "authorization" forms because this has a better psychological understanding of the document to be signed.
6. Make sure documentation of patient care in the medical record corresponds with billing submitted on the insurance claim.
7. Exercise good judgment in what you write and how you word electronic mail because it does not give security against confidentiality.
8. Make every effort to reach an understanding with patients in the matter of fees by explaining what services will be received and what the "extras" may be. For hospital cases, it is advisable to explain that the fee the physician charges is for his or her services only and that charges for the bed or ward room, operating room, laboratory tests, and anesthesia will be billed separately in addition to the physician's charges.

9. Do not discuss other physicians with the patient. Patients sometimes invite criticism of the methods or results of former physicians. Remember that you are hearing only one side of the story.
10. Tell the physician immediately if you learn that a new patient is still under treatment by another physician and did not give this information to the physician during the initial interview.
11. Do not compare the respective merits of various forms of therapy and refrain from discussing patients' ailments with them. Patients come to talk to the physician about their symptoms, and you may give them incorrect information. Let the physician make the diagnosis. Otherwise, you may seriously embarrass the physician, yourself, or both of you.
12. Report a physician who is doing something illegal that you are aware of. You can be held responsible for being silent and failing to report an illegal action.
13. Say nothing to anyone except as required by the attorney of the physician or by the court if litigation is pending.
14. Be alert to hazards that may cause injury to anyone in the office and report such problems immediately.
15. Consult the physician before turning over a delinquent account to a collection agency.
16. Be courteous in dealing with patients and always act in a professional manner.

needed. Some practices prefer to use medical record storage companies, which may put records on microfilm before disposal. If records are disposed of by a professional company, be sure and obtain a document verifying method of disposal. Maintain a log of destroyed records showing the patient's name, Social Security number, date of last visit, and treatment.

Financial Documents

According to income tax regulations on record retention, accounting records should be kept a minimum of 4 years (following the due date for filing the tax return or the date the tax is paid, whichever is later). Always contact an accountant before discarding records that may determine tax liability. Suggested retention periods are shown in Table 3–4.

A federal regulation mandates that assigned claims for Medicaid and Medicare be kept for 7 years; the physician is subject to auditing during that period.

Termination of a Case

A physician may wish to withdraw formally from further care of a patient because the patient discharged the physician, did not follow instructions, did not take the recommended medication, failed to return for an appointment, or discontinues to pay on an overdue account. A physician may terminate a contract by

▶ Sending a letter of withdrawal (Fig. 3–21) to the patient by registered or certified mail with return of signature card (Fig. 3–22, Postal Service Form 3811) so that proof of termination is in the patient's medical record.

▶ Sending a letter of confirmation of discharge when the patient states that he or she no longer desires care. This should also be sent registered or certified mail with return receipt requested (Fig. 3–23).

▶ Sending a letter confirming that the patient left the hospital against medical advice or against the advice of the physician. If there is a signed statement in the patient's hospital records to this effect, it is not necessary to send a letter. If a letter is sent, a copy of the letter and return signature card from the post office must be filed with the patient's records.

Prevention of Legal Problems

After reading Chapters 1 through 3, you have discovered there are many instances in which an insurance biller must be careful in executing job duties to avoid the possibility of a lawsuit. A summary of guidelines for prevention of lawsuits is shown in Table 3–6.

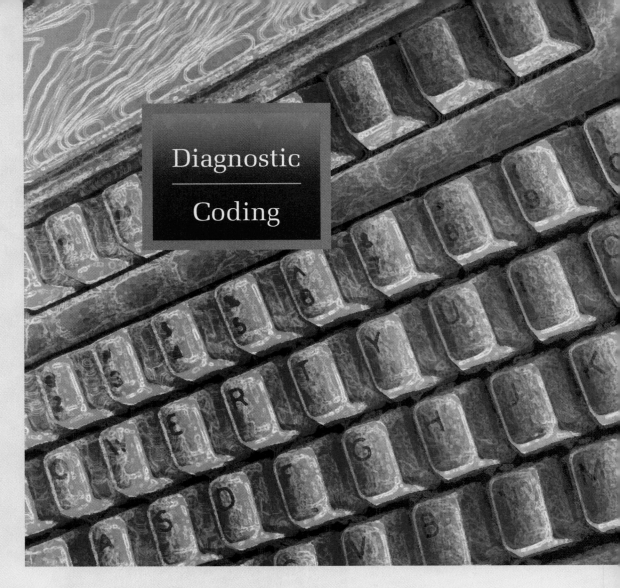

Diagnostic Coding

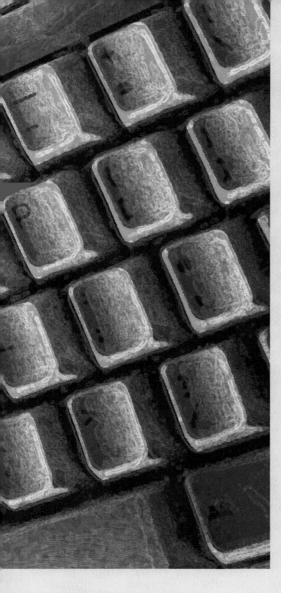

■ Perform diagnostic coding accurately after completing the problems in the *Workbook*.

OBJECTIVES*

After reading this chapter, you should be able to:

■ Give the history of diagnostic coding.
■ Explain the purpose and importance of coding diagnoses.
■ Use diagnostic code books properly and obtain accurate codes.
■ State the meaning of basic abbreviations and symbols in the code books.
■ Define diagnostic code terminology.

KEY TERMS

adverse effect

benign tumor

chief complaint (CC)

combination code

complication

E codes

etiology

in situ

International Classification of Diseases, Ninth Revision, Clinical Modification (ICD-9-CM)

intoxication

italicized code

late effect

malignant tumor

not elsewhere classifiable (NEC)

not otherwise specified (NOS)

physician's fee profile

poisoning

primary diagnosis

principal diagnosis

secondary diagnosis

slanted brackets

V codes

*Performance objectives and exercises for hands-on practical experience for this chapter appear in the *Workbook*.

The Diagnostic Coding System

This chapter deals with diagnostic coding for outpatient professional services, and the next chapter relates to coding of procedures. Proper coding can mean the financial success or failure of a medical practice. A working knowledge of medical terminology, including a basic course in anatomy and physiology, is essential to become a topnotch coder of diagnoses. The coding must be accurate because in many instances, such as with a patient under the Medicare program, payment for services may be based on the diagnosis. All diagnoses that affect the current status of the patient may be assigned a code. This includes conditions that exist at the time of the patient's initial contact with the physician as well as conditions that develop subsequently that affect the treatment received. Diagnoses that relate to a patient's previous medical problem that have no bearing on the patient's present condition are not coded. As presented by the American Health Information Management Association (AHIMA), diagnostic coding guidelines for outpatient services and diagnostic coding and reporting requirements for physician billing were shown in Chapter 1, Figure 1–3.

Types of Diagnostic Codes

Codes must be sequenced correctly on an insurance claim so that the chronology of patient care events and severity of disease can be understood. When submitting insurance claims for patients seen in a physician's office or in an outpatient hospital setting, the **primary diagnosis**, which is the main reason for the encounter, must be listed first. In an office setting, this is commonly called the **chief complaint (CC).** The **secondary diagnosis,** listed subsequently, is that which may contribute to the condition or defines the need for a higher level of care but is not the underlying cause. The underlying cause of a disease is referred to as the **etiology** and is sequenced in the first position. The **principal diagnosis,** used in hospital coding, is the diagnosis obtained after study that prompted the hospitalization. It is possible that the primary and principal diagnosis codes may be the same, but not in all cases. It is important to note that the concept of a "principal diagnosis" is only applicable to inpatient hospital orders.

Reasons for the Development and Use of Diagnostic Codes

Diagnostic coding was developed for the following reasons:

1. Tracking of disease processes
2. Classification of causes of mortality
3. Medical research
4. Evaluation of hospital service utilization

Medical practices use diagnostic codes on insurance claims instead of writing out the diagnostic description. The consequences of not using ICD-9-CM codes are many. For example, it affects the physician's level of reimbursement, claims can be denied, fines or penalties can be levied, and sanctions can be imposed. It is important to use diagnostic codes on all claims, and, if coding is correctly done, payments are accurate and prompt. When records are comprehensive, statistics can be gathered to make future payments more realistic for the physicians in private practice.

Occasionally an insurance company will reply to an insurance claim with an explanation of benefits or remittance advice stating "This procedure/item is not payable for the diagnosis as reported." For example, a patient has undergone magnetic resonance imaging of the brain. Medicare will not reimburse for magnetic resonance imaging for the diagnosis of transient ischemic attack or Alzheimer's disease but will pay for it with the diagnosis of cerebral insufficiency. The procedures that are diagnosis related include most imaging services (radiography, computed tomography, and magnetic resonance imaging), cardiovascular services (electrocardiograms, Holter monitors, echocardiography, Doppler and stress testing), neurologic services (electroencephalography and noninvasive ultrasonography), some laboratory services, and vitamin B12 injections. It is important to know the procedures that are diagnosis related and exactly which diagnosis relates to the procedure being billed. A reference book may be helpful in this situation, such as *St. Anthony's Medicare National Correct Coding Guide* or *St. Anthony's Medicare Correct Coding and Payment Manual for Procedures and Services.*

Physician's Fee Profile

A **physician's fee profile** is a compilation of each physician's charges and the payments made to him or her over a given period of time for each specific professional service rendered to a patient. Each insurance company keeps a profile on every provider for services that are processed for statistical purposes. As charges are increased, so are payments, and the profile is then updated through the use of statistical computer data. There are two types of profiles: *individual customary profile* and *prevailing profile*. Inquire from each insurance carrier whether the carrier will update the physician's fee profile on an annual basis. If so, send in an annual updated fee profile to those third party payers who implement this policy.

The use of nonspecific diagnostic codes may place the physician's practice at considerable risk regarding the development of his or her fee profile. Every claim form filed by a third party payer is entered into permanent computerized records. The compiled data (fees charged, procedure and diagnostic codes) may be used in the future as the basis for the physician's fee profile.

To ensure accuracy of future profiles, it is important that the insurance billing specialist use specific diagnostic codes on a routine basis. The coding must be accurate and precise if profiles are to be established for realistic payments.

History of Coding Diseases

From the beginnings of medicine, people have tried to name and classify diseases. Although many attempts have been made to systematize and clarify disease terminology, no one method has ever been accepted by the entire medical community.

About 1869, the American Medical Association prepared the *American Nomenclature of Diseases*. Then, in 1903, the *Bellevue Hospital Nomenclature of Diseases* was published. It was subsequently replaced by the *Standard Nomenclature of Diseases and Operations*. In the 1960s, the American Medical Association published *Current Medical Information and Terminology* (CMIT), which used a computer format to make frequent revisions easier. The medical terms were alphabetically arranged with detailed descriptions of the diseases and two- and four-digit code numbers. This book ceased publication in 1991.

Institutions (within a facility), pathologists, and those involved with generating medical reports and billing for laboratory medicine procedures use a system for retrieving types of diagnoses. These codes are found in a book entitled *Systematized Nomenclature of Human and Veterinary Medicine (SNOMED International)*, Volumes I through IV.* In addition, this system is used for managing patient records, teaching medical information science (informatics), and indexing and managing research data.

---

*Available from the College of American Pathologists, 325 Waukegan Road, Northfield, IL 60093-2750.

International Classification of Diseases

History

The *International Classification of Diseases* (ICD) had its beginnings in England during the 17th century. The United States began using the ICD toward the latter half of the 19th century to report causes of death and prepare mortality statistics. Hospitals began using the ICD in 1950 to classify and index diseases. The ninth revision of the *International Classification of Diseases* (ICD-9), published by the World Health Organization, is now being used by state health departments and the U.S. Public Health service for mortality reporting.

Organization and Format

In 1979, the *International Classification of Diseases, Ninth Revision, Clinical Modification* (**ICD-9-CM**) was published by the Department of Health Services in the United States. It is updated annually and has three volumes. Volume 1 is a Tabular List of Diseases, each having an assigned number. Volume 2 is an Alphabetic Index of Diseases. Volume 3 is a Tabular List and Alphabetic Index of Procedures used primarily in the hospital setting. The systematized arrangement in these books makes it possible to encode, computerize, store, and retrieve large volumes of information from the patient's medical record. ICD-9-CM is used by hospitals and other health care providers to code and report clinical information required for participation in various government programs, such as Medicare, Medicaid, and professional review organizations.

Volumes 1 and 2 are used in physicians' offices and other outpatient settings to complete insurance claims. These two volumes are almost completely compatible with the original international version (ICD-9). The code numbers have from three to five digits. Although abbreviated versions of the ICD-9-CM are available, it is preferable to obtain the complete ninth revision of Volumes 1 and 2.

The annual update of the ICD-9-CM occurs each October 1, and the changes are published in three publications—*Coding Clinic*, published by the American Hospital Association; the *American Health Information Management Association Journal*, published by the American Health Information Management Association; and the *Federal Register*, published by the U.S. Government Printing Office. Coding from an out-of-date manual can delay payment or cause costly mistakes that can lead to financial disaster. Many insurance carriers do not use the new codes until they have a chance to update their computer systems. It is important to verify with each carrier exactly when it plans to begin using the new codes. Refer to Appendix B to learn the names and addresses of several companies that publish the ICD-9-CM.

Psychiatric disorders are coded using the *Diagnostic and Statistical Manual of Mental Disorders*, Fourth Edition (DSM-IV). This code system is not discussed in this text. Refer to Appendix B to find out where to obtain this code book.

Contents

Table 4–1 is an outline of Volumes 1 and 2 of the ICD-9-CM. Volume 1 lists chapter headings with associated codes. The Supplementary Classification consists of V and E codes, which are discussed later in this chapter. Sections A, B, C, and D of the Appendices are not used in physician outpatient billing. Volume 2 contains three sections: an alphabetic index for diseases and injuries, a table of drugs and chemicals, and an alphabetic index to external causes of injuries and poisonings (E codes). In Chapter 16, Hospital Billing, an outline and information on how to find codes in Volume 3 are provided. This reference is used primarily in the hospital setting.

How To Use the Diagnostic Code Books Properly

To become a proficient coder, it is important to develop an understanding of the conventions and terminology of ICD-9-CM. Read all of the information at the beginning of Volumes 1 and 2 before coding. Volume 1, the Tabular List for the disease classifications, makes use of certain abbreviations, punctuation, symbols, and other conventions as shown in Table 4–2.

In Volume 2, the Alphabetic Index for the disease classification, the symbol of **slanted brackets** (*[ ]*) is used to indicate the need for another code. A code will be given after a listing followed by slanted brackets enclosing an additional code. Record both of these codes in the same sequence as indicated in the index.

An **italicized code** in the Tabular List may never be sequenced as principal or primary diagnoses.

Coding Instructions

Code only the conditions or problems that the physician is actively managing at the time of the visit. Some insurance carriers have restrictions

TABLE 4–1 Outline of Volumes 1 and 2 of ICD-9-CM	
Volume I Chapter Headings	**Codes**
1 Infectious and Parasitic Diseases	001–139
2 Neoplasms	140–239
3 Endocrine, Nutritional, and Metabolic Diseases and Immunity Disorders	240–279
4 Diseases of the Blood and Blood-Forming Organs	280–289
5 Mental Disorders	290–319
6 Diseases of the Nervous System and Sense Organs	320–389
7 Diseases of the Circulatory System	390–459
8 Diseases of the Respiratory System	460–519
9 Diseases of the Digestive System	520–579
10 Diseases of the Genitourinary System	580–629
11 Complications of Pregnancy, Childbirth, and the Puerperium	630–676
12 Diseases of the Skin and Subcutaneous Tissue	680–709
13 Diseases of the Musculoskeletal System and Connective Tissue	710–739
14 Congenital Anomalies	740–759
15 Certain Conditions Originating in the Perinatal Period	760–779
16 Symptoms, Signs, and Ill-Defined Conditions	780–799
17 Injury and Poisoning	800–999
Supplementary Classification	
Classification of Factors Influencing Health Status and Contact with Health Service	V01–V82
Classification of External Causes of Injury and Poisoning	E800–E999
Appendices	
A Morphology of neoplasms	
B Glossary of Mental Disorders	
C Classification of Drugs by American Hospital Formulary Service List Number and Their ICD-9-CM Equivalents	
D Classification of Industrial Accidents According to Agency	
E List of three-digit categories	
Volume 2	
Section 1: Index to Diseases and Injuries, alphabetic	
Section 2: Table of Drugs and Chemicals	
Section 3: Index to External Causes of Injuries and Poisonings	

on accepting codes, however, and may allow only one or two codes per claim. In those situations, it may not be possible to code all active problems. Always use both Volume 2, the Alpha-

TABLE 4–2	**ICD-9-CM Conventions**

Abbreviations

NEC	**Not Elsewhere Classifiable** (in the coding books). The category number for the term including NEC is to be used with ill-defined terms and only when the coder lacks the information necessary to code the term in a more specific category.

Example: Fibrosclerosis Familial multifocal NEC **710.8**

NOS	**Not Otherwise Specified** (by the physician). This abbreviation is the equivalent of "unspecified." It refers to a lack of sufficient detail in the diagnosis statement to be able to assign it to a more specific subdivision within the classification.

Example: 153.9 Colon, unspecified Large intestine NOS.

Punctuation

[ ]	Brackets are used to enclose synonyms, alternative wordings, or explanatory phrases.
( )	Parentheses are used to enclose supplementary words that may be present or absent in the statement of a disease or procedure without affecting the code number to which it is assigned.
:	Colons are used in the Tabular List after an incomplete term that needs one or more of the modifiers that follow to make it assignable to a given category.
{ }	Braces are used to enclose a series of terms, each of which is modified by the statement appearing at the right of the brace.

Symbols

□	The lozenge symbol printed in the left margin preceding the disease code indicates that the content of a four-digit category has been moved or modified.
§	The section mark symbol preceding a code denotes the placement of a footnote at the bottom of the page that is applicable to all subdivisions in that code.

The use of a medical dictionary will aid in accurate coding. Research any unfamiliar terminology, for example, amaurotic idiocy with severe mental retardation; impaludism.

Volume 2 elements are structured as follows:

▶ Main terms are classifications of diseases and injuries and appear as headings in **boldface** type.
▶ Subterms are listings under main terms and are indented two spaces to the right under main terms.
▶ Modifiers (often referred to as nonessential modifiers because their presence or absence does not affect the code assigned) provide additional description and are enclosed in parentheses.
▶ Carryover lines continue the text and are indented more than two spaces from the level of the preceding line.
▶ Subterms of subterms are additional listings and are indented two spaces to the right under the subterm (Table 4–3; see also Fig. 4–13).

Always code to the highest degree of specificity. The more digits a code has, the more specific the description. A three-digit code may be used only when the diagnostic statement cannot be further subdivided. When a three-digit code has subdivisions, the appropriate subdivision must be coded. Some insurance carrier computer systems kick out the lower-level codes (three-digit codes) and hold these claims for medical review, thereby delaying payment. *Do not* arbitrarily use a zero as a filler character when typing a diagnostic code number because this may be interpreted as indicating a different disease. The addition of a zero to a code number that does not require an additional digit can also cause a claim to be denied (see Example 4–1).

EXAMPLE 4–1	
Invalid code due to zero added	**Valid code**
373.20	373.2
496.0	496

Five-digit codes can appear:

1. At the beginning of a chapter
2. At the beginning of a section
3. At the beginning of a three-digit category
4. In a four-digit subcategory

The use of five digits is NOT optional; therefore, select a code book that has the categories marked and color coded so it will not be easy to overlook fifth digits. Near the end of this chapter (accompanying the section Rules for Coding, Diabetes Mellitus) is another example illustrating the use of five digits. Sometimes when the fourth or fifth digit is

betic Index, and Volume 1, the Tabular (numerical) List before assigning a code. Never use just one volume. Begin with the Alphabetic Index to locate the main term of the diagnosis. The main term is the condition. The primary arrangement of the Alphabetic Index, the disease index, is by *condition*. If you cannot find the condition listed, consider rearranging the word roots (e.g., crypt orchid/o or orchido crypt/o). Then substitute a similar suffix.

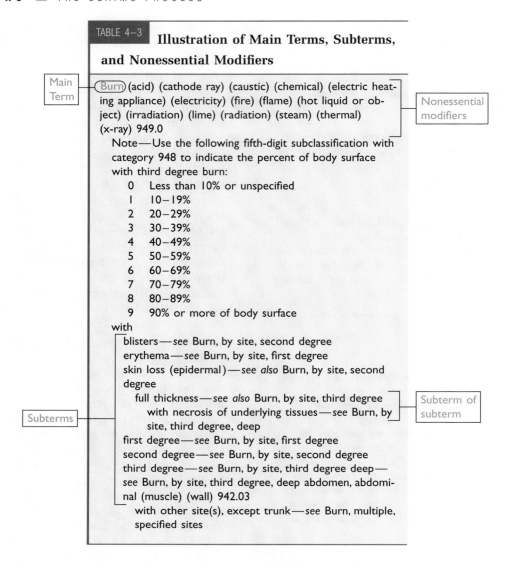

TABLE 4–3   **Illustration of Main Terms, Subterms, and Nonessential Modifiers**

Main Term

Burn (acid) (cathode ray) (caustic) (chemical) (electric heating appliance) (electricity) (fire) (flame) (hot liquid or object) (irradiation) (lime) (radiation) (steam) (thermal) (x-ray) 949.0

Nonessential modifiers

Note—Use the following fifth-digit subclassification with category 948 to indicate the percent of body surface with third degree burn:

0	Less than 10% or unspecified
1	10–19%
2	20–29%
3	30–39%
4	40–49%
5	50–59%
6	60–69%
7	70–79%
8	80–89%
9	90% or more of body surface

with

Subterms

blisters—see Burn, by site, second degree
erythema—see Burn, by site, first degree
skin loss (epidermal)—see also Burn, by site, second degree
    full thickness—see also Burn, by site, third degree
        with necrosis of underlying tissues—see Burn, by site, third degree, deep

Subterm of subterm

first degree—see Burn, by site, first degree
second degree—see Burn, by site, second degree
third degree—see Burn, by site, third degree deep—see Burn, by site, third degree, deep abdomen, abdominal (muscle) (wall) 942.03
    with other site(s), except trunk—see Burn, multiple, specified sites

---

EXAMPLE 4–2

§645   Prolonged pregnancy
[0, 1, 3]   Post-term pregnancy
            Pregnancy which has advanced beyond 42 weeks of gestation.
The section mark (§) requires a fifth digit; valid digits are in [brackets] under each code. Use 0 as the fourth digit for this category.

missing, the code is not complete and technically is not a code but rather a category (see Example 4–2).

When you are billing Medicare, you will find that some diagnostic codes are designated as invalid from year to year. If you work in a medical practice that sees Medicare patients, it is essential to read the regional Medicare bulletins and attend Medicare seminars periodically to keep abreast of these changes.

PROCEDURE: Basic Steps in Coding

Use a standard method and establish a routine for locating a code. Follow these recommended steps for coding the first diagnosis. There are no shortcuts. For each subsequent diagnosis in a patient's medical record, repeat these steps. Refer to Figure 4–1 as you go through Step 1.

1. Locate the main term in the Alphabetic Index, Volume 2. (anemia)
   - Refer to any notes under the main term. (none shown)
   - Read any terms enclosed in parentheses following the main term (nonessential modifiers). (none shown)
   - Look for appropriate subterm. (megaloblastic) *Do not* skip over any subterms indented under the main term.

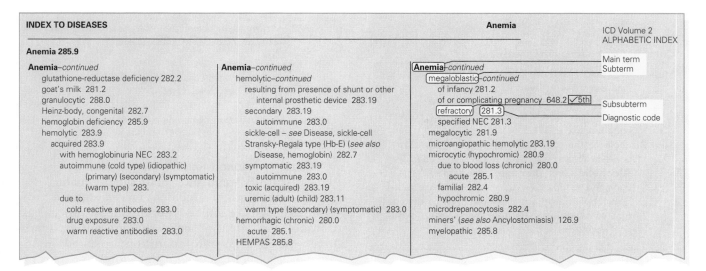

Figure 4–1. Excerpt from the Alphabetic Index of *International Classification of Diseases, 9th Revision, Clinical Modification* (ICD-9-CM), Volume 2.

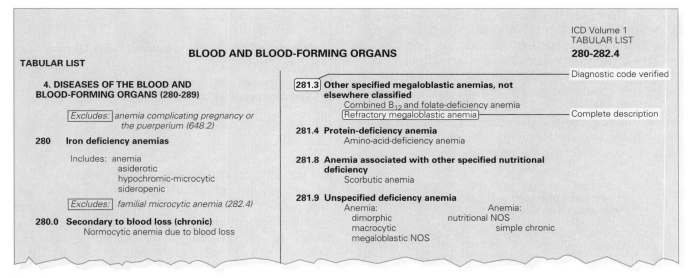

Figure 4–2. Excerpt from the Tabular List of *International Classification of Diseases, 9th Revision, Clinical Modification* (ICD-9-CM), Volume 1.

▶ Look for appropriate sub-subterm. (refractory)
▶ Follow any cross-reference instructions. (none given)
▶ Write down the code. (281.3)
2. Verify the code number in the Tabular List, Volume 1 (Fig. 4–2).
   ▶ Read and be guided by any instructional terms in the Tabular List. In this example, there are none given.
   ▶ Read complete description and assign the code to the highest specificity. (refractory megaloblastic anemia 281.3)

Now use a step-by-step approach to code chronic alcoholic liver disease and refer to each volume as shown in Example 4–3.

Code initially from the Alphabetic Index, Volume 2. Then go to the Tabular List, Volume 1, to *verify* that the code number selected is in accord with the desired classification of the diagnosis. Look for important instructions that often appear. Check for exclusion notes, which refer to terms or conditions that are not included within the code. These may further direct the coder to the correct ICD-9-CM code assignment (Fig. 4–3).

EXAMPLE 4–3

Chronic Alcoholic Liver Disease

Step 1. Look under **disease** (the condition) in Volume 2.
Find the subterm **liver.**
Locate the additional subterm **alcoholic.**
Look for the next subterm **chronic.** The correct code number is 571.3

Step 2. Look for the code number—*not* the page number—in Volume 1. Notice the wording **"571.3 Alcoholic Liver damage, unspecified."** The code and its title refer to any liver damage caused by alcoholism, without specification as to the nature of the disorder. Because there are no exclusion notes, this is the correct code.

An "excludes" box may appear listing diagnoses and additional codes to research to ensure that the correct code is assigned. As shown in Figure 4–3*B*, this example would appear on the insurance claim keyed without the decimal as: 5368

Note: Heartburn would not be coded because it is a symptom of dyspepsia and appears as an exclusion under dyspepsia in Volume 1.

Certain conditions are classified according to etiology (cause) of the disorder (Fig. 4–4). In these cases, you should follow the instructions "Code first underlying disease . . ." Code the etiology in the first position. Code the disorder in the second position. Words to look for in the diagnostic statement include "acquired," "congenital," "associated with,"

The Patient's Diagnosis is Dyspepsia and Heartburn, Code Number 536.8.

Step 1. Look for the code number—not the page number—in Volume 1.
Step 2. Notice that there is an exclusion note for heartburn indicating the code number 787.1
Step 3. Be sure to check code number 787.1 in the Tabular Listing.

536.8 Dyspepsia and other specified disorders of function of stomach

Achylia gastrica	Hyperchlorhydria
Hourglass contraction of stomach	Hypochlorhydria
Hyperacidity	Indigestion

Excludes:	achlorhydria (536.0)
	heartburn (787.1)

Figure 4–3. Example of a disease to look up in the Tabular List *(A)* and illustration of coding from the Tabular List *(B)* of *International Classification of Diseases, 9th Revision, Clinical Modification* (ICD-9-CM), Volume I showing an exclusion note.

713.1 Arthropathy associated with gastrointestinal conditions other than infections

Code first underlying disease as:
regional enteritis (555.0–555.9)
ulcerative colitis (556)

Figure 4–4. Illustration of coding by etiology.

"obstetric," "nonobstetric," "transmissible," "not transmissible," "traumatic," and "nontraumatic."

When the patient's medical record states a "versus" diagnosis, such as "peptic ulcer versus gastroesophageal reflux," code the presenting symptoms. When a specific condition is stated in the diagnosis as both acute (or subacute) and chronic and the Alphabetic Index provides separate codes at either the third-, fourth-, or fifth-digit level for acute and chronic, use both codes with the acute code given first (see Example 4–4).

EXAMPLE 4–4

Acute and Chronic Pelvic Inflammatory Disease

Condition:	Disease	
Subcategories:	Pelvis, Pelvic	
Subsubcategory:	Inflammatory	
	Acute	614.3
	Chronic	614.4

Four-digit subcategories .8 and .9 are usually, but not always, reserved for "other specified" and "unspecified" conditions, respectively. "Other specified" and "unspecified" subcategories are referred to as residual subcategories (Fig. 4–5). Residual subcategories are used for conditions that are specifically named in the medical record but not specifically listed under a code description. If there is a lack of details in the medical record and you cannot match to a specific subdivision, research the medical record for a qualifying statement in the physician's progress notes or history and physical examination report that will allow you to use a more specific diagnostic code (Fig. 4–6).

Diagnostic codes must match the age and gender of the patient. If an adult female patient with breast cancer is seen (excluding carcinoma in situ and skin cancer of breast), a code from 174.0 through 174.9 must be used. If a male with breast cancer is treated, a code from 175.0 through 175.9 must be chosen. Some codes apply only to newborns, such as code 775.10 for neonatal diabetes mellitus.

710.4 Polymyositis ◄

710.5 Eosinophilia myalgia syndrome ◄
  Toxic oil syndrome
  Use additional E code to identify drug if drug induced

[Specified]

710.8 Other specified diffuse diseases of connective tissue ◄——— Other specified
  Multifocal fibrosclerosis (idiopathic) NEC
  Systemic fibrosclerosing syndrome

710.9 Unspecified diffuse connective tissue disease ◄——— Unspecified
  Collagen disease NOS

Figure 4–5. Illustration of four-digit residual subcategories—specified, other specified, and unspecified disease conditions.

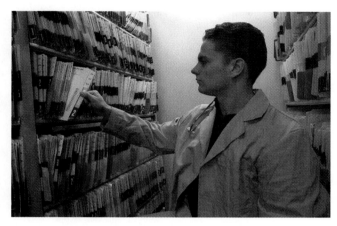

Figure 4–6. Insurance billing specialist looking up a diagnostic code.

Special Points to Remember in Volume 1

◗ Use two or more codes if necessary to completely describe a given diagnosis. *Example*: Arteriosclerotic cardiovascular *disease* (429.2) with congestive heart *failure* (428.0).

◗ Search for one code when two diagnoses or a diagnosis with an associated secondary process (manifestation) or complication is present. There are instances when two diagnoses are often classified with a single code number called a **combination code** (Fig. 4–7).

◗ Use category codes (three-digit codes) only if there are no subcategory codes (fourth-digit subdivisions) (Fig. 4–8).

Special Points to Remember in Volume 2

◗ Notice that appropriate sites and/or modifiers are listed in alphabetic order under the main terms, with further subterm listings as necessary.

◗ Examine all modifiers that appear in parentheses next to the main term.

◗ Check for nonessential modifiers that apply to any of the qualifying terms used in the state-

Figure 4–7. Illustration of combination coding.

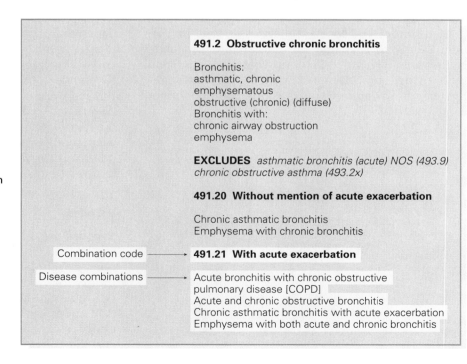

491.2 Obstructive chronic bronchitis

Bronchitis:
asthmatic, chronic
emphysematous
obstructive (chronic) (diffuse)
Bronchitis with:
chronic airway obstruction
emphysema

EXCLUDES *asthmatic bronchitis (acute) NOS (493.9)*
chronic obstructive asthma (493.2x)

491.20 Without mention of acute exacerbation

Chronic asthmatic bronchitis
Emphysema with chronic bronchitis

Combination code ———► **491.21 With acute exacerbation**

Disease combinations ———► Acute bronchitis with chronic obstructive
pulmonary disease [COPD]
Acute and chronic obstructive bronchitis
Chronic asthmatic bronchitis with acute exacerbation
Emphysema with both acute and chronic bronchitis

430 Subarachnoid hemorrhage

Meningeal hemorrhage
Ruptured:
berry aneurysm
(congenital) cerebral aneurysm NOS

Excludes: *syphilitic ruptured cerebral aneurysm (094.87)*

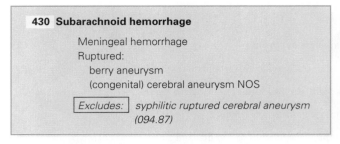

Figure 4–8. Illustration of three-digit coding.

ment of the diagnosis found in the patient's medical record (Fig. 4–9).

- Notice that eponyms appear as both main term entries and modifiers under main terms such as "disease" or "syndrome" and "operation." As mentioned in Chapter 3 and shown in Example 3–2, an *eponym* is the name of a disease, structure, operation, or procedure, usually derived from the name of a place or a person who discovered or described it first.
- Look for sublisted terms in parentheses that are associated with the eponym (Fig. 4–10).
- Locate closely related terms, code categories, and cross-referenced synonyms indicated by *see* and *see also* (Fig. 4–11).

Handy Hints in Diagnostic Coding

If your ICD-9-CM code books are not color-coded, mark manifestation (italicized) codes with a colored highlighter pen (i.e., 608.81 [italicized code]). This will remind you **to always code the underlying disease first.**

Many times you locate a diagnostic code in Volume 2 only to find that the cross-referenced code is the same when verified in Volume 1. Indicate these codes in Volume 2 with a colored highlighter pen to remind you that this code is correct

Obesity (constitutional) (exogenous) ← Nonessential modifiers
(familial) (nutritional) (simple) 278.0
adrenal 255.8
due to hyperalimentation 278.0
endocrine NEC 259.9
endogenous 259.9
Fröhlich's (adiposogenital dystrophy) 253.8
glandular NEC 259.9
hypothyroid (*see also* Hypothyroidism) 244.9
of pregnancy 646.1
pituitary 253.8
thyroid (*see also* Hypothyroidism) 244.9

Figure 4–9. Illustration of coding with modifiers in parentheses.

Eponym → **Cushing's**
basophilism, disease, or syndrome
(iatrogenic) (idiopathic) (pituitary basophilism) (pituitary dependent)
255.0 p. 154

Basophilism (corticoadrenal) (Cushing's)
(pituitary) (thymic) 255.0 p. 86

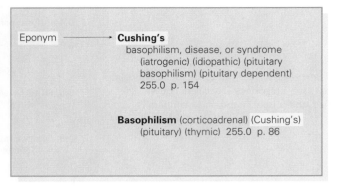

Figure 4–10. Illustration of coding diagnoses associated with an eponym.

Inflammation, inflamed, inflammatory
(with exudation)-*continued*

spinal
cord (*see also* Encephalitis) 323.9
late effect—*see* category 326
membrane—*see* Meningitis
nerve—*see* Disorder, nerve

Figure 4–11. Illustration of cross-referencing synonyms, closely related terms, and code categories from Volume 2 of *International Classification of Diseases, 9th Revision, Clinical Modification,* Alphabetic Index.

as described in Volume 2, saving the time you would use going to Volume 1.

Keep a list of diagnostic and CPT procedure codes that go well together. Some insurance companies publish lists of codes specifying diagnostic codes that are acceptable for specific procedures. Reference books are available that show codes that link between diagnostic and procedure codes. The American Medical Association publishes a list of the most common diagnostic codes at the end of each of their mini-specialty code books. See Appendix B for information on titles and how to obtain reference books that contain such data.

V Codes

V codes are a supplementary classification of coding located in a separate section at the end of Volume 1, Tabular List. In Volume 2, the Alphabetic Index, the V codes are included in the major section Index of Diseases.

V codes are used when a person who is not currently sick encounters health services for some specific purpose, such as to act as a donor of an

organ or tissue, to receive a vaccination, to discuss a problem that is not in itself a disease or an injury, to seek consultation regarding family planning, to request sterilization, or for the supervision of a normal pregnancy (see Example 4–5). These types of encounters are among the more common encounters for hospital outpatients and patients of private practitioners, health clinics, and others. In these situations, the V code would appear as a primary code and be placed first.

EXAMPLE 4–5

Supervision of First Pregnancy, Normal

Step 1. Find the heading **pregnancy** in Volume 2.
Step 2. Look for the subheading **supervision**.
Step 3. Look for the second subheading **normal** and a further subheading **first**, which gives you the code V22.0.
Step 4. Find **V22.0** in Volume 1, by where marked Tabular List, and you will see "**Supervision of normal first pregnancy.**"

V codes are also used when some circumstance or problem is present that influences the person's health status but is not in itself a current illness or injury, such as when the person is known to have an allergy to a specific drug. In this instance, the V code cannot be used as a stand-alone code and should be used only as a supplementary code.

Additional code numbers are given for occupational health examinations and routine annual physical examinations, so select specific codes depending on the circumstances (see Example 4–6).

EXAMPLE 4–6

Routine Annual Physical Examination

Step 1. Look up **examination**, and notice **annual** as a subterm and the code V70.0.
Step 2. Find **V70** in Volume 1, Tabular List, and the wording "**Routine general medical examination at a health facility.**"

Sometimes a patient receives a consultation for a preoperative medical evaluation as an inpatient or outpatient (see Example 4–7), and the majority of the results are negative for chronic or current illness. A good-health diagnosis code will trigger a rejection by the insurance carrier. Use an admission (encounter) code from the V72.X code series for "other specified examinations," instead of a treatment code. The term "admission (encounter)"

is equivalent to *encounter for* and does not refer to an admission to the hospital.

EXAMPLE 4–7

A patient to have surgery for gallstones is sent to a cardiologist for evaluation of suspected cardiovascular disease.
Step 1. In Volume 2, look up **admission (encounter) (for) examination, preoperative, cardiovascular V72.81.** Verify it in Volume 2.
Step 2. Code the reason for the surgery—574.xx, cholelithiasis.

When coding a healthy patient examination, V codes (V70.1 and V70.3 through V70.7) should be sequenced as primary diagnoses over all other diagnoses. Be cautious when using V codes as second or third diagnoses because Medicare will automatically reject the claim and insurance companies that adopt Medicare policies may possibly do so, too.

E Codes

E codes are also a supplementary classification of coding in which you look for external causes of injury rather than disease. E codes are given in a separate section of Volume 1, Tabular List, after V codes. In Volume 2, the E codes are also in a separate section, Index to External Causes of Injury and Poisoning, following the regular alphabetical index. E codes are also used in coding adverse reactions to medications (Fig. 4–12).

The use of an E code after the primary or other acute secondary diagnosis explains the mechanism

---

INDEX TO EXTERNAL CAUSES

Heat (apoplexy) (collapse) (cramps) (effects of) (excessive) (exhaustion) (fever) (prostration) (stroke)—*continued*
due to—*continued*
    weather (conditions) E900.0
from
    electric heating apparatus causing burning E924.8
    nuclear explosion in war operations E996
    generated in, boiler, engine, evaporator, fire room of boat, ship, watercraft E838
    inappropriate in local application or packing in medical or surgical procedure E873.5
    late effect of NEC E989

Figure 4–12. Illustration of E coding.

TABLE 4–4	Table of Drugs and Chemicals					
		External Cause (E Code)				
Substance	Poisoning	Accident	Therapeutic Use	Suicide Attempt	Assault	Undetermined
Acetylsalicylic acid....	965.1	E850.3	E935.3	E950.0	E962.0	E980.0

for the injury. Generally, E codes are not used for insurance claims submitted by physicians' offices, but some physicians may decide to use them for thoroughness when documenting a case. Instructions are included here for additional knowledge about the classification system.

The Table of Drugs and Chemicals found in Volume 2 (Table 4–4) contains a classification of drugs and other chemical substances for identifying poisoning states and external causes of adverse effects. Read the Foreword at the beginning of this table. Each of the substances listed in the table is assigned a code according to the poisoning classification (960 through 989). These codes are used when there is a state of poisoning, overdose, wrong substance given or taken, or intoxication.

Adverse effect is defined as an adverse or a pathologic reaction to a drug that occurs when appropriate doses are given to humans for prophylaxis (prevention of disease), diagnosis, and therapy (see Example 4–8). When an adverse effect occurs (e.g., drug reaction, hypersensitivity, drug intolerance, idiosyncratic reaction), a code is assigned to the diagnosis that classifies the specific reaction or symptom (e.g., dermatitis, syncope, tachycardia, urticaria). The E code identifying the agent involved is taken solely from the Therapeutic Use column. An E code may never be sequenced in the first position.

Poisoning is defined as a condition resulting from an intentional overdose of drugs or chemical substances or from the wrong drug or agent given or taken in error (see Example 4–9). **Intoxication** is defined as an adverse effect rather than a poisoning when drugs such as digitalis, steroid agents, and so on are involved. However, whenever the term *intoxication* is used, the biller should clarify with the physician the circumstances surrounding the administration of the drug or chemical before assigning the appropriate code.

EXAMPLE 4–8

Coding an Adverse Effect

The patient had an adverse effect (ventricular fibrillation) to the medication digoxin, which was prescribed by her physician and taken correctly.

Step 1. Refer to the Table of Drugs and Chemicals in Volume 2 and look up **digoxin**.
Step 2. Because this medication was for therapeutic use, locate the correct E code number under that column.
Step 3. The correct number is **E942.1.**
Step 4. Locate **fibrillation** in the index to diseases.
Step 5. Find the subheading **ventricular.**
Step 6. The correct code number is **427.41.**
Step 7. Be sure to check the code number 427.41 in Volume 1, the Tabular Listing.
Sequencing: 427.41   **Ventricular fibrillation**
           E942.1   **Therapeutic use, Digoxin**
Note: For outpatient billing, the E code would not be listed.

EXAMPLE 4–9

Coding a Poisoning

Baby Kathy got into the kitchen cabinet and ingested liquid household ammonia.
Step 1. Refer to the Table of Drugs and Chemicals in Volume 2 and locate **ammonia**.
Step 2. Find the subheading **liquid (household).**
Step 3. Locate the correct code number under the **Poisoning** column.
Step 4. The correct number is 983.2.
Step 5. Now look for the correct E code number by choosing the **Accident** column. (If the poisoning was a suicide attempt, the result of assault, or of undetermined nature, then you would choose a different column for the E code.) In this example, the correct E code number is **E861.4.**
Sequencing: The poisoning code should be sequenced in the first position:
        983.2   Poisoning, ammonia
        E861.4 Poisoning, accidental, ammonia
Note: Usually add the manifestation if it is documented in the medical record. For outpatient billing, the E code would not be listed.

Rules for Coding

Signs, Symptoms, and Ill-Defined Conditions

Chapter 16 of the ICD-9-CM—Symptoms, Signs, and Ill-Defined Conditions (codes 780.0–799.9)—contains many but not all codes for symptoms. If the final diagnosis at the end of the encounter or at the time of discharge is qualified by any of the following terms ("suspected," "suspicion of," "questionable," "likely," "probable," or "rule out"), *do not code* these conditions as if they existed or were established. Instead, code the chief complaint, sign, or symptom. Do not type "ruled out" on the insurance claim. This condition was suspected at one time but was ruled out after study and is no longer an active diagnosis. *Example*: Diabetes mellitus, ruled out. The condition(s) should be documented to the highest degree of certainty for each encounter or visit (e.g., signs, symptoms, abnormal test results, or other reason for the visit).

This is contrary to coding practices used by hospital medical record departments for coding the diagnoses of hospital inpatients. If one were to follow hospital coding guidelines and the patient was, for example, suspected of having a heart attack, this would be interpreted as a confirmed case of a myocardial infarction. The same would hold true for "possible epilepsy." If the patient had a convulsion and epilepsy was the probable cause but had not been proved, code the convulsion.

The following are instances in which sign and symptom codes can be used.

- No precise diagnosis can be made (see Examples 4–10 and 4–11).
- Signs or symptoms are transient, and a specific diagnosis was not made (see Example 4–12).
- Provisional diagnosis for a patient who does not return for further care (see Example 4–13).
- A patient is referred for treatment before a definite diagnosis is made (see Example 4–14).

EXAMPLE 4–10

The patient has an enlarged liver, and further diagnostic studies may or may not be done. Use code 789.10 for hepatomegaly.

EXAMPLE 4–11

The patient complains of painful urination, and urinalysis is negative. Use code 788.1 for dysuria.

EXAMPLE 4–12

The patient complains of **chest pain on deep inspiration**. On examination, the physician finds nothing abnormal and tells the patient to return in 1 week. When the patient returns, the pain has ceased. Use code **786.52 for painful respiration**.

EXAMPLE 4–13

On examination, the physician documents abnormal percussion of the chest. The patient is sent for a chest x-ray and asked to return for a recheck. The patient does not have the x-ray and fails to return. Use code **786.7 for abnormal chest sounds**.

EXAMPLE 4–14

A patient complains of nausea and vomiting and is referred to a gastroenterologist. Use code **787.01** for nausea with vomiting.

Sterilization

The code V25.2 is used only when the sterilization is performed for the major purpose of contraception rather than being an incidental result of the treatment of a disease. If the sterilization is purely elective, code V25.2 will suffice as a single code for the diagnosis. If the sterilization is performed for contraceptive purposes during a current admission for obstetric delivery, sequence code V25.2 in the second position. If the sterilization is the end result of a hysterectomy performed because of injury or damage to the uterus during delivery, do not use code V25.2 but instead code the condition and/or procedure.

Neoplasms

Neoplasms are new growths, and they may be benign or malignant tumors. A **benign tumor** is one that does not have the properties of invasion and metastasis (i.e., transfer of disease from one organ to another) and is usually surrounded by a fibrous capsule. Cysts and lesions are *not* neoplasms. A **malignant tumor** has the properties of invasion and metastasis. The term *carcinoma* refers to a cancerous or malignant tumor. Carcinoma **in situ** means cancer confined to the site of origin without invasion of neighboring tissues. A *primary* tumor means the original tumor site. A *secondary* tumor means a site of metastasis. If the diagnosis does not mention metastasis, then code the case as a primary tumor (see Example 4–15). Lymphomas and leukemias are not classified using the primary and secondary terminology.

The diagnostic statement "metastatic from" indicates primary stage carcinoma, whereas "metastatic to" indicates secondary stage carcinoma. If the diagnostic statement is "malignant neoplasm spread to," then code the primary site spread to

EXAMPLE 4–15

Primary cancerous tumor	189	**Malignant neoplasm of kidney and other and unspecified urinary organs**
		189.0 Kidney, except pelvis
		Kidney NOS
		Kidney parenchyma
Secondary cancerous tumor	198	**Secondary malignant neoplasm of other specified sites**
		Excludes *lymph node metastasis (196.0–196.9)*
		198.0 Kidney

the secondary site. The phrase "recurrent malignancy" is a new primary neoplasm.

The main entry "Neoplasm" contains a table with the column headings Malignant, Benign, Uncertain Behavior, and Unspecified. The table is found in the alphabetic index under "Neoplasm" in Volume 2 (Table 4–5). Code numbers for neoplasms are given by anatomic site. For each site, there are six possible code numbers, indicating whether the neoplasm in question is malignant (primary, secondary, or carcinoma in situ), benign, of uncertain behavior, or of unspecified nature. The description of the neoplasm often will indicate which of the six code numbers is appropriate (e.g., malignant melanoma of skin, benign fibroadenoma of breast, carcinoma in situ of cervix uteri, and so on) (see Example 4–16). For a tumor that has not been diagnosed as benign or malignant by the pathologist, use the codes in the column labeled

TABLE 4–5   Coding for Neoplasms

| | Malignant | | | | Uncertain | |
	Primary	Secondary	Ca in situ	Benign	Behavior	Unspecified
Neoplasm, neoplastic	199.1	199.1	234.9	229.9	238.9	239.9

Notes: 1. The list below gives the code numbers for neoplasms by anatomic site. For each site there are six possible code numbers according to whether the neoplasm in question is malignant, benign, in situ, of uncertain behavior, or of unspecified nature. The description of the neoplasm will often indicate which of the six columns is appropriate; e.g., malignant melanoma of skin, benign fibroadenoma of breast, carcinoma in situ of cervix uteri.

Where such descriptors are not present, the remainder of the Index should be consulted where guidance is given to the appropriate column for each morphologic (histologic) variety listed; e.g., Mesonephroma—*see* Neoplasm, malignant; Embryoma—*see also* Neoplasm, uncertain behavior; Disease, Bowen's—*see* Neoplasm, skin, in situ. However, the guidance in the Index can be overridden if one of the descriptors mentioned above is present, e.g., malignant adenoma of colon is coded to 153.9 and not to 211.3 because the adjective "malignant" overrides the Index entry "Adenoma—*see also* Neoplasm benign."

2. Sites marked with the sign * (e.g., face NEC*) should be classified to malignant neoplasm of skin of these sites if the variety of neoplasm is a squamous cell carcinoma or an epidermoid carcinoma and to benign neoplasm of skin of these sites if the variety of neoplasm is a papilloma (any type).

abdomen, abdominal	195.2	198.89	234.8	229.8	238.8	239.8
cavity	195.2	198.89	234.8	229.8	238.8	238.8
organ	195.2	198.89	234.8	229.8	238.8	238.8
viscera	195.2	198.89	234.8	229.8	238.8	239.8
wall	173.5	198.2	232.5	216.5	238.2	239.2
connective tissue	171.5	198.89	—	215.5	238.1	239.2
abdominopelvic	195.8	198.89	234.8	229.8	238.8	239.8
accessory sinus—*see* Neoplasm, sinus						
acoustic nerve	192.0	198.4	—	225.1	237.9	239.7
acromion (process)	170.4	198.5	—	213.4	238.0	239.2
adenoid (pharynx) (tissue)	147.1	198.89	230.0	210.7	235.1	239.0
adipose tissue (*see also* Neoplasm, connective tissue)	171.9	198.89	—	215.9	238.1	239.2
adnexa (uterine)	183.9	198.82	233.3	221.8	236.3	239.5
adrenal (cortex) (gland) (medulla)	194.0	198.7	234.8	227.0	237.2	239.7
ala nasi (external)	173.3	198.2	232.3	216.3	238.2	239.2
alimentary canal or tract NEC	159.9	197.8	230.9	211.9	235.5	239.0

EXAMPLE 4–16

Adenocarcinoma of the Breast with Metastases to the Pelvic Bone

Step 1. Look up **adenocarcinoma** in Volume 2. Do not use the morphology code, M8140/3. Notice it states "see also Neoplasm, by site, malignant."

Step 2. Locate **neoplasm** in the table in Volume 2. At the top of the page notice the Malignant heading with the subheadings **Primary, Secondary,** and **Ca In Situ. Primary** means the first site of development of the malignancy. **Secondary** means metastasis from the primary site to a second site. **Ca In Situ** means cancer confined to the epithelium of the site of origin without invasion of the basement membrane tissue of the site.

Step 3. Find the site of the adenocarcinoma (in this case the breast), and look under the Malignant and Primary headings. Note that the code given is **174.9.**

Step 4. Next, find **bone** as a subterm in the Neoplasm Table and look for the subterm **pelvic.** Now look at the three columns under Malignant and, using the Secondary column, find the **correct code number 198.5.** In listing these diagnoses on the insurance claim, you would give the following: **174.9 and 198.5.**

"Uncertain Behavior." If a tumor is suspected and not confirmed, use "mass." For example, a breast mass would be coded 611.72. When coding a neoplasm, ask yourself the following questions:

▶ What is it now?
▶ Where did it start?
▶ What happened to it?

Anatomic sites marked with an asterisk (*) are always considered to be neoplasms of the skin.

In Appendix A of the Tabular List of Volume 2, there is a section entitled Morphology of Neoplasms, which gives M codes. These codes are not used for billing insurance claims by physicians' offices.

Circulatory System Conditions

Diseases of the circulatory system are difficult to code because of the variety and lack of specific terminology used by physicians in stating the diagnoses. Carefully read all inclusion, exclusion, and "use additional code" notations contained in the Tabular List of Volume 1.

Hypertension

The lay term "high blood pressure" is medically termed *hypertension*. Hypertension can *cause* various forms of heart and vascular disease, or it can ac-

company some heart conditions. In fact, there is a syndrome called *malignant hypertension* that has nothing to do with tumor formation. A *syndrome* is another name for a *symptom complex* (a set or complex of signs, symptoms, or other manifestations resulting from a common cause or appearing in combination, presenting a distinct clinical picture of a disease or inherited abnormality). Malignant hypertension is a symptom complex of markedly elevated blood pressure (diastolic pressure of more than 140 mm Hg) associated with papilledema. The term *malignant* here means "life threatening." *Benign hypertension* refers to high blood pressure that runs a relatively long and symptomless course.

When the diagnostic statement indicates a cause by stating "heart condition *due* to hypertension" or "hypertensive heart disease," use codes 402.0X through 402.9X. If the diagnostic statement reads "*with* hypertension" or "cardiomegaly *and* hypertension," you will need two separate codes. Elevated blood pressure without mention of hypertension is coded 796.2. Secondary hypertension is coded 405.XX, and the cause of the hypertension should be coded when specified.

Myocardial Infarctions

A separate three-digit category (412) is provided for old myocardial infarction, healed myocardial infarction, or myocardial infarction diagnosed on electrocardiogram. Myocardial infarction of 8 weeks' duration or less is considered acute, if not specified otherwise. Symptoms of more than 8 weeks' duration are coded 414.8, Other Forms of Chronic Ischemic Heart Disease.

Chronic Rheumatic Heart Disease

The conditions presumed to be caused by rheumatic fever are as follows:

▶ Mitral valve of unspecified etiology 394
▶ Mitral valve insufficiency 394.1
▶ Mitral valve and aortic valve disorders of unspecified etiology 396
▶ Mitral stenosis 394.0

The following condition is *not* presumed to be caused by rheumatic fever:

▶ Aortic valve of unspecified etiology 424

Arteriosclerotic Cardiovascular Disease and Arteriosclerotic Heart Disease

In regard to a patient who has a diagnosis of arteriosclerotic cardiovascular disease (ASCVD), use code 429.2. If you refer to code 440.9, it excludes ASCVD because it is in conflict with the note given for 429.2. Code 429.2 is primary when the additional code 440.9 is needed. However, a patient with arteriosclerotic heart disease (ASHD) would be assigned code 414.0. In your copy of Volume 1, at code 429.2, write in "see code 440" after "use additional code to identify, if desired, the presence of arteriosclerosis." To distinguish between ASCVD and ASHD, cardiovascular means pertaining to heart and blood vessels throughout the body, whereas ASHD means acute or chronic heart disability resulting from an insufficient supply of oxygenated blood to the heart.

Diabetes Mellitus

There are two types of diabetes, type I and type II. The following are the clinical features important in the classification of diabetes.

Type I Diabetes	Type II Diabetes
Insulin dependency (IDDM)	Non-insulin dependency (NIDDM)
Patients *must* be treated with insulin	Patients *may* be treated with insulin
Insulin levels are very low	Insulin levels may be high, "normal," or low
Ketosis prone	Non-ketosis prone
Patients are usually lean	Patients are usually obese
Usually "juvenile onset" (peak onset at early puberty)	Usually "adult onset," although occasionally seen in children
Often little family history of diabetes mellitus	Often strong family history of diabetes mellitus

In type I diabetes (IDDM), the patient's pancreas does not function and produce the necessary insulin. Thus, this patient's body is dependent on insulin. In type II diabetes (NIDDM), the patient's pancreas produces some insulin, but the insulin is ineffective in doing its job, removing sugar from the bloodstream. This diabetic's problem may be controlled with diet, oral medication, or insulin.

Because of the types and complications that may accompany this disease, coding *always* requires five digits. Here is the way this classification appears in ICD-9-CM, Volume 2:

Fifth-digit subclassification with code 250 is not based on severity or age grouping of the case (Fig. 4–13). It is a *type grouping*; use the following:

250.00 for non-insulin-dependent diabetes (NIDDM)

Adult onset
Type two, Type II or unspecified
Stable or not stated as uncontrolled
Non-ketosis prone

250.01 for insulin-dependent diabetes (IDDM)

Juvenile onset
Type one, Type I
Stable or not stated as uncontrolled
Ketosis prone

250.02 for non-insulin-dependent diabetes (NIDDM)

Adult onset
Type two, Type II or unspecified
Uncontrolled

250.03 for insulin-dependent diabetes (IDDM)

Juvenile onset
Type one, Type I
Uncontrolled

When a medical record contains the statement "discharged on insulin" with no further explanation of the type of diabetes, always ask the physician for further clarification. Do not assume that a patient taking insulin has insulin-dependent diabetes.

Do not use code 250.0X if the diabetes is stated with delivery of a child or as a complication of pregnancy. Use code 648.01.

Pregnancy, Delivery, or Abortion

The following main sections are included:

630–633 Ectopic and Molar Pregnancy
634–639 Other Pregnancy with Abortive Outcome (*five-digit subclassifications must be used with categories 634–637*)
640–648 Complications Mainly Related to Pregnancy (*five-digit subclassifications must be used*)
650–659 Normal Delivery, and Other Indications for Care in Pregnancy, Labor, and Delivery (*five-digit subclassifications must be used in categories 651–659*)
660–669 Complications Occurring Mainly in the Course of Labor and Delivery (*five-digit subclassifications must be used*)
670–677 Complications of the Puerperium (*five-digit subclassifications must be used for categories 670–676*)

The following guidelines are used:

1. Code 650 is used for a completely *normal* delivery. This means normal spontaneous delivery, cephalic (vertex) presentation of one liveborn fetus, full-term gestation, with or without episiotomy, no manipulation required, and no laceration.

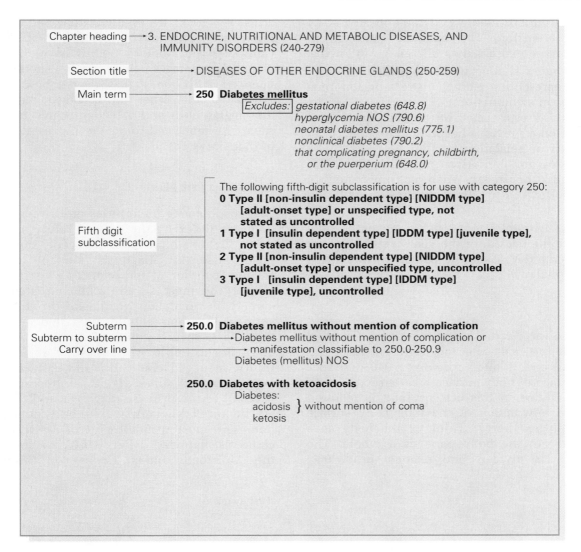

Chapter heading → 3. ENDOCRINE, NUTRITIONAL AND METABOLIC DISEASES, AND IMMUNITY DISORDERS (240-279)

Section title → DISEASES OF OTHER ENDOCRINE GLANDS (250-259)

Main term → **250 Diabetes mellitus**
Excludes: *gestational diabetes (648.8)*
hyperglycemia NOS (790.6)
neonatal diabetes mellitus (775.1)
nonclinical diabetes (790.2)
that complicating pregnancy, childbirth,
or the puerperium (648.0)

The following fifth-digit subclassification is for use with category 250:
0 Type II [non-insulin dependent type] [NIDDM type] [adult-onset type] or unspecified type, not stated as uncontrolled
1 Type I [insulin dependent type] [IDDM type] [juvenile type], not stated as uncontrolled
2 Type II [non-insulin dependent type] [NIDDM type] [adult-onset type] or unspecified type, uncontrolled
3 Type I [insulin dependent type] [IDDM type] [juvenile type], uncontrolled

Subterm → **250.0 Diabetes mellitus without mention of complication**
Subterm to subterm → Diabetes mellitus without mention of complication or
Carry over line → manifestation classifiable to 250.0-250.9
Diabetes (mellitus) NOS

250.0 Diabetes with ketoacidosis
Diabetes:
acidosis } without mention of coma
ketosis

Figure 4–13. Classification of diabetes mellitus showing fifth-digit subclassification from *International Classification of Diseases. Ninth Revision. Clinical Modification,* Volume II.

2. A code other than 650 should be used to provide greater detail about a **complication** of abortion, pregnancy, childbirth, or the puerperium when information is available, such as the presence of anemia, diabetes mellitus, or thyroid dysfunction (see Example 4–17). Complication of the puerperium is a complication within 6 weeks after labor.

EXAMPLE 4–17

| 648.01 | 250.00 | Pregnancy (delivered) with diabetes mellitus |
| 648.23 | 282.60 | Pregnancy (antepartum) with sickle cell anemia |

In most instances, an additional code is added to specify the patient's specific problem.

3. A multiple gestation (e.g., twins, triplets) is a complication of pregnancy and is considered high risk. When a patient delivers and experiences both antepartum and postpartum complications, different fifth digits may be applied on the codes to describe the episodes of care (see Example 4–18).

EXAMPLE 4–18

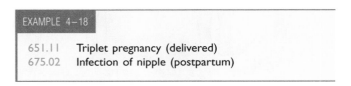

| 651.11 | Triplet pregnancy (delivered) |
| 675.02 | Infection of nipple (postpartum) |

Admitting Diagnoses

Some diagnosis codes are considered questionable when used as the first diagnosis on admittance of a patient to the hospital (e.g., 278.00 obesity, 401.1 benign hypertension). The inpatient admission diagnosis may be expressed as one of the following.

1. One or more significant findings (symptoms or signs) representing patient distress or abnormal findings on examination.
2. A diagnosis established on an ambulatory care basis or on a previous hospital admission.
3. An injury or poisoning.
4. A reason or condition not classifiable as an illness or injury, such as pregnancy in labor, follow-up inpatient diagnostic tests, and so on.

When your employer physician makes hospital visits, code the reason for the visit, which may *not* necessarily be the reason the patient was admitted to the hospital.

Burns

Burns are always coded using two codes. The first code is for the exact site and degree of the burn. The second code found in Category 948 describes the percentage of body surface area burned. A fifth digit is included in this category and is required to indicate how much of the total body surface had third-degree burns. Think of the body as a whole and not the body parts as a whole. The adult body is divided into regions: head, 9%;

arms, 9% each; trunk, 18% front and 18% back; legs, 18% each; and perineum, 1% (Fig. 4–14). Children's and infant's bodies have different regional percentages. Burn codes should be sequenced with the highest-degree burn first, followed by the other burn codes. But when a first-degree burn and a second-degree burn of the same site are listed, only the highest-degree burn of that site is coded.

Injuries and Late Effects

Diagnostic codes for injuries are listed in the Alphabetic Index by the type of injury and broken down by anatomic site. To code multiple injuries, list the diagnosis for the conditions treated in order of importance, with the diagnosis for the most severe problem listed first. If surgery is involved, the diagnostic code for the surgical problem should be listed first unless there is a severe injury of another part of the body. For example, in the case of an intracranial injury, managed medically, and a fractured phalanx, managed surgically, the intracranial injury is listed as the primary diagnosis and the diagnosis fractured phalanx would be sequenced second. The most difficult part of assigning injury codes is knowing what words to look for in the Alphabetic Index. Codes 800 through 959

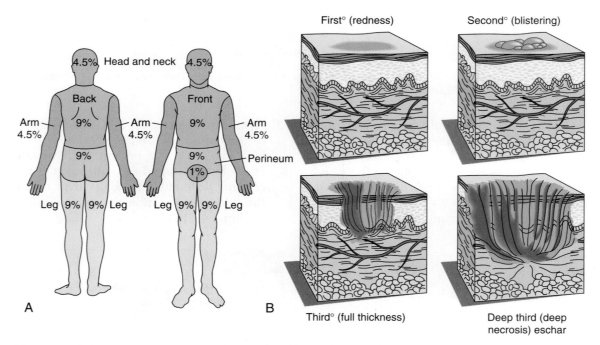

Figure 4–14. *A,* Illustration of the rules of nines for burn injury to the body. *B,* The degrees of burn involving the layers of the skin, i.e., first-degree includes the epidermis (redness), second-degree includes the epidermis and dermis (blistering), third-degree includes the first two layers and the subcutaneous tissues (full-thickness), and deep-third involves all layers of the skin with resulting eschar (deep necrosis).

include fractures, dislocations, sprains, and other types of injury. Injuries are coded according to the general type of injury and broken down within each type by anatomic site. A list of common injury medical terms and the types of injuries included for each is shown in Table 4–6. An injury may have a late effect, which must be coded in a different fashion.

A **late effect** means "the residual effect (condition produced) after the acute phase of an illness or injury has terminated." An effect is considered to be late if the diagnosis reads "due to an old injury," "late," "due to previous illness or injury," or "due to an injury or illness that occurred 1 year or more before the current admission of encounter." If time has passed between the occurrence of the acute illness or injury and the development of the residual effect, such as scarring, late effects may also be coded.

Example 4–19 illustrates late effects. Residuals are shown in italics, and the causes are shown in bold print. Code both the residual effect and the cause.

EXAMPLE 4–19
Malunion **fracture,** right tibia
Traumatic arthritis following **fracture** of right knee
Hemiplegia following **cerebrovascular thrombosis** 1 year ago
Scarring due to third-degree **burn** of right arm
Contracture of right heel tendons due to **poliomyelitis**

Use the following guides for coding injuries.

1. Decide whether a diagnosis represents a current injury or a late effect of an injury (see Example 4–20).
2. Fractures are coded as closed if there is no indication of whether the fracture is open or closed.
3. The word "with" indicates involvement of both sites, and the word "and" indicates involvement of either one or two sites when multiple injury sites are given (see Example 4–21).

TABLE 4–6	**Common Injury Medical Terms**
contusion	Bruise and hematoma without a fracture or open wound
crush	Crushing injury not complicated by concussion, fractures, injury to internal organs, or intracranial injury
dislocation	Displacement and subluxation. Dislocation may be open or closed. Closed dislocation may be either complete, partial, simple, or uncomplicated. Open dislocation may be either compound, infected, or with foreign body. A dislocation not indicated as closed or open is classified as closed.
fracture	Fractures may be open or closed. A fracture not indicated as open or closed is classified as closed. An injury described as fracture dislocation is coded as a fracture. Open fractures may be described as either compound, infected, missile, puncture, or with foreign body. Closed fractures may be described as either comminuted, depressed, elevated, fissured, greenstick, impacted, linear, march, simple, slipped, epiphyseal, or spiral.
injury, blood vessel	Described as either arterial hematoma, avulsion, laceration, rupture, traumatic aneurysm, or traumatic fistula
injury, internal	Includes all injuries to internal organs such as the heart, lung, liver, kidney, and pelvic organs. Types of injuries to internal organs include laceration, tear, traumatic rupture, penetrating wounds, blunt trauma, crushing, blast injuries, or open wounds to internal organs with or without fracture in the same region.
injury, intracranial	Includes concussion, cerebral laceration and contusion, or intracranial hemorrhage. These injuries may be open or closed. Intracranial injuries with skull fractures may be found under fracture.
injury, superficial	Includes abrasion, insect bite (nonvenomous), blister, or scratch
sprain/strain	Injury to the joint capsule, ligament, muscle, or tendon described by the following terms: avulsion, hemarthrosis, laceration (closed), rupture, or tear. Open laceration of these structures should be coded as open wounds.
wound, open	Includes open wounds not involving internal organs. Wounds may be to skin, muscle, or tendon, described as animal bite, avulsion, cut, laceration, puncture wound, or traumatic amputation. Open wounds may be complicated or uncomplicated. Complicated includes injuries with mention of delayed healing, delayed treatment, foreign body, or major infection.

EXAMPLE 4–20

824.8	**Current injury:** Fracture, left ankle
	OR
733.81 and 905.4	Late effect: Malunion fracture left ankle

EXAMPLE 4–21

| 806 | Fracture of the vertebral column **with** spinal cord injury |
| 813 | Fracture of radius **and** ulna |

Look up code 813 in your diagnostic code book and note that this code section relates to a fracture of the radius, the ulna, or both.

Now that you have learned the basics of ICD-9-CM coding, let's take the next step and begin to learn the new system based on ICD-10.

ICD-10-CM Diagnosis and Procedure Codes

For the past 20 years the ICD-9-CM diagnosis system has been used. Although it has been updated, the system has outlived its usefulness owing to advances in technology, discovery of new diseases, development of new procedures, and the need to report more details for statistical purposes. The time is fast approaching to adopt another system. Actually there are two systems, *International Classification of Diseases, 10th Revision, Clinical Modification* (ICD-10-CM—diagnostic codes) and *ICD-10 Procedure Coding System* (ICD-10-PCS—procedure codes). Both hospital and physician office insurance billers need to be concerned with the new diagnosis codes, but only hospital billers need to concern themselves with the procedure codes.

ICD-10 Volume 1: Tabular List was published by the World Health Organization in 1992. It is being clinically modified (CM) by the National Center for Health Statistics (NCHS) before code adoption. The CM provides the specifics that the United States needs for collecting data on our health status. Reasons for clinical modification are the removal of procedural codes, unique mortality codes, and "multiple" codes. ICD-10-PCS was developed in the mid 1990s by 3M Health Information Systems under contract with the Health Care Financing Administration (HCFA). This replaces Volume 3 of ICD-9-CM used in hospital billing but will not replace the *Current Procedural Terminology* (CPT) code book used in outpatient billing. Reasons for development of ICD-10-PCS are:

- ▶ ICD-10 did not have procedure classification.
- ▶ ICD-9-CM was not expandable, comprehensive, or multiaxial (broken down into many subdivisions).
- ▶ ICD-9-CM did not have standardized terminology and included diagnostic information.

As of the publication of this textbook, ICD-10-CM is to be implemented after October 1, 2001, and before 2003. ICD-10-PCS will follow after that and there are major organization changes. ICD-10-CM differs from ICD-9-CM in the following ways:

1. There are major changes in code book organization.
2. Many new categories and chapters have been added.
3. There is a replacement of the traditional numeric coding system with a six-digit alphanumeric scheme for ICD-10-CM (see Example 4–22).
4. Old injury (800–999) codes have been changed to S and T codes.
5. Explanatory notes and instructions for use have been greatly expanded.
6. The dagger-and-asterisk system of dual classification in ICD-10 has been considerably expanded for ICD-10-CM (see Example 4–23).
7. The E and V codes in ICD-9-CM are now Chapters XX and XXI.
8. The coding system allows for assignment of unique codes as new procedures are developed.

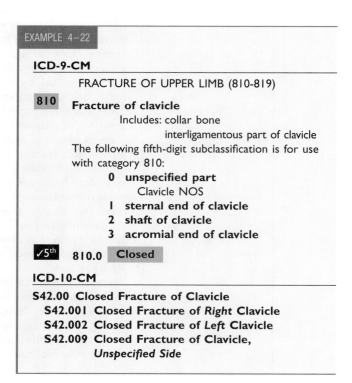

EXAMPLE 4–22

ICD-9-CM

FRACTURE OF UPPER LIMB (810-819)

810 **Fracture of clavicle**
      Includes: collar bone
               interligamentous part of clavicle
The following fifth-digit subclassification is for use with category 810:
      0 unspecified part
          Clavicle NOS
      1 sternal end of clavicle
      2 shaft of clavicle
      3 acromial end of clavicle

✓5th 810.0 **Closed**

ICD-10-CM

S42.00 Closed Fracture of Clavicle
  S42.001 Closed Fracture of *Right* Clavicle
  S42.002 Closed Fracture of *Left* Clavicle
  S42.009 Closed Fracture of Clavicle, *Unspecified Side*

EXAMPLE 4–23

ICD-10

A39.5†   **Meningococcal Heart Disease**
        Meningococcal:
            Carditis NOS (I52.0*)
            Endocarditis (I39.8*)

ICD-10-CM

A39.5   **Meningococcal Heart Disease**
       A39.50   Meningococcal Carditis . . .
       A39.51   Meningococcal Endocarditis

The second part, section, or volume of the ICD-10-CM is an instruction manual that provides definitions, standards, and rules for the tabular list. The last part or volume is an alphabetical index. These systems allow more code choices and require greater documentation in the medical record. An experienced coder will need to develop a proactive, positive attitude toward accepting and learning the ICD-10-CM. A coder must have a higher level of clinical knowledge. It would be wise to attend an anatomy and physiology course a year before the new system is adopted if you have not already done so. There has been a monumental change from ICD-9-CM to ICD-10-CM. After coding guidelines have been developed, training workshops will be offered. To gain knowledge and proficiency it may take about 80 hours of instruction to learn the new system. After learning how to code, it will take a longer time to code under the new system, especially if using ICD-10-PCS.

Publishers of ICD-10-CM may use different styles and format so it is important to study and compare the features of several books before making a decision to purchase. When choosing a book, the following questions should be asked: Is color coding being used for emphasis in locating items quickly? Are definitions or notes included to help one interpret and gain a better understanding of difficult medical terms and phrases? Are coding guidelines boxed for easy reference? All of these would benefit the coder.

Possible errors may occur when using the Tabular List and when coding diseases or conditions that begin with categories "O" and "I." These can also look like the numbers "zero" and "one" (e.g., I00 and O99 are correct and not 100 and 099). In these categories, special attention must be given.

As of the date of the printing of this textbook, guidelines have not been adopted, so training has not begun. The next edition of this textbook will feature how to code using ICD-10-CM.

STUDENT ASSIGNMENT LIST

✔ Study Chapter 4.
✔ Answer the review questions in the *Workbook* to reinforce theory learned in this chapter and to help prepare you for a future test.
✔ Complete the assignments in the *Workbook* to gain hands-on experience in diagnostic coding.
✔ Turn to the Glossary at the end of this textbook for a further understanding of the Key Terms used in this chapter.

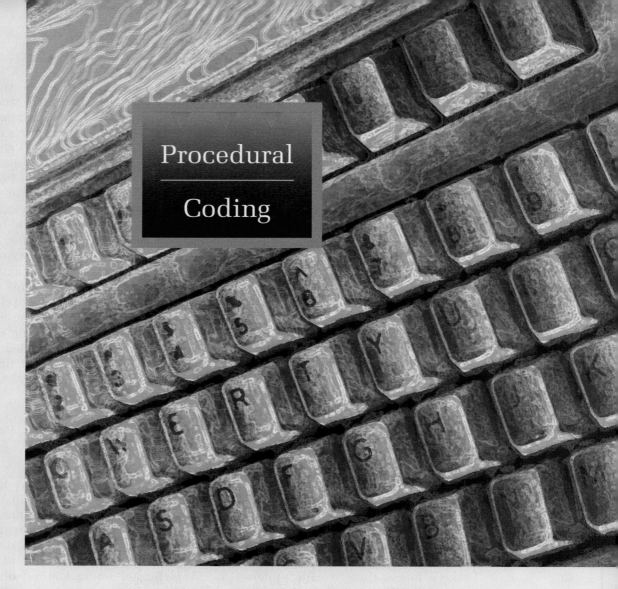

Procedural
Coding

5

CHAPTER OUTLINE

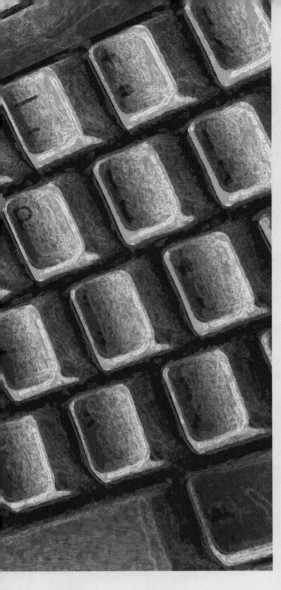

■ Code the *Workbook* problems using the CPT manual.
■ Describe the differences between CPT and RVS coding systems.
■ Describe various methods of payment by insurance companies and state and federal programs.

OBJECTIVES*

After reading this chapter you should be able to:

■ Explain the purpose of coding for professional services.
■ Use procedure code books properly.
■ Define procedure code terminology.
■ Explain the importance and usage of modifiers in procedure coding.

KEY TERMS

actual charge

bilateral

bundled codes

comprehensive code

conversion factor

customary fee

downcoding

fee schedule

global surgery policy

Health Care Financing Administration Common Procedure Coding System (HCPCS)

modifier

Current Procedural Terminology (CPT)

prevailing charge

procedure code numbers

professional component (PC)

reasonable fee

relative value studies (RVS)

star symbol

surgical package

technical component (TC)

unbundling

upcoding

usual, customary, and reasonable (UCR)

*Performance objectives and exercises for hands-on practical experience for this chapter appear in the *Workbook*.

Understanding the Importance of Procedural Coding Skills

Now that you have learned some terminology and the basics of diagnostic coding, the next step is to learn how to code procedures.

Procedure coding is the transformation of written descriptions of procedures and professional services into numeric designations (code numbers). The physician rendering medical care either writes or dictates this information into the patient's medical record. Then the insurance billing specialist abstracts pertinent information and assigns procedure codes. Routine office visits and procedures are usually listed with codes and brief descriptions on the encounter form. These are circled or checked off by the physician when they are performed on the patient.

With the use of the computer to produce insurance claims and the use of telecommunications, magnetic tape billing, or optical scanning equipment to process payment of these claims, more emphasis is being placed on procedure coding. Coding must be correct if claims are to be paid promptly. Every procedure or service must be assigned correct and complete code numbers. Because of the complexity of procedural coding, a working knowledge of medical terminology, including anatomy and physiology, is essential.

Procedure codes are a standardized method used to precisely describe the services provided by physicians and allied health care professionals. This then allows claim forms to be optically scanned by insurance companies. The general acceptance of the codes by insurance carriers and government agencies assures the physician who uses a standardized coding system that the services and procedures he or she performs can be objectively identified and priced. As presented by the American Health Information Management Association (AHIMA), diagnostic coding guidelines for outpatient services and procedure coding and reporting requirements for physician billing were shown in Chapter 1, Figure 1–3.

The primary coding system used in physicians' offices for professional services and procedures is *Current Procedural Terminology* (CPT), fourth edition,* published annually by the American Medical Association (AMA). Another rating scale, called relative value studies (RVS), is also used for

services and procedures (see later in this chapter).

Some managed care plans develop a few "plan codes" for use by the plan only. Sometimes, the codes are used for tracking; other times, they are used to provide reimbursement for a service not defined within CPT.

Various books are available for coding procedures for physicians. In some states, medical societies and medical specialty associations publish books for this purpose.

Current Procedural Terminology (CPT)

The first edition of ***Physicians' Current Procedural Terminology*** appeared in 1966, and the book was subsequently revised in 1970, 1973, and 1977. Since 1984, *Current Procedural Terminology (CPT),* fourth edition, has been updated and revised annually. Code numbers are added or deleted as new procedures are developed or existing procedures are modified. These changes are shown in each edition by the use of symbols as described and shown later in this chapter in Figure 5–2.

CPT uses a basic five-digit system for coding services rendered by physicians, plus two-digit add-on modifiers or separate five-digit numbers representing the modifiers to indicate complications or special circumstances. **Procedure code numbers** represent diagnostic and therapeutic services on medical billing statements and insurance forms (see Example 5–1).[†]

EXAMPLE 5–1

A 45-year-old woman is seen for an **initial office visit** for evaluation of recurrent right shoulder pain. The exam required a detailed history and physical examination (D HX & PX) with low complexity medical decision making (LCMDM) Patient complains of pain radiating down right arm. **Complete x-rays of the right shoulder** were taken in the office and read by the physician. A corticosteroid solution was **injected into the shoulder joint.**

CPT Code	Description of Services
99203	Office visit, new patient **(Evaluation and management [E/M] service)**
73030	Radiologic exam, shoulder, two views **(Diagnostic service)**
20610	Arthrocentesis inj.; major joint, shoulder **(Therapeutic service)**

---

[*]Available from Book and Pamphlet Fulfillment—OP-3416, American Medical Association, P.O. Box 10946, Chicago, IL 60610-0946 or visit CPT on the web at www.ama-assn.org/cpt.

[†]Examples shown in this chapter reflect wording pertinent to coding a specific procedure and may be missing complete chart entries; therefore, there may be a gap of information for the reader.

CPT codes, descriptions, and material are taken from *Current Procedural Terminology,* CPT 2001, Standard Edition, © 2001, American Medical Association. All Rights Reserved.

Almost all states use some method of procedural coding, and many states recommend CPT. CPT emerged as the procedural coding of choice when the federal government developed the **Health Care Financing Administration Common Procedure Coding System (HCPCS)** (pronounced "hick-picks") for the Medicare Program. The Medicare HCPCS consists of three levels of coding:

▶ Level I: the AMA CPT codes and modifiers (national codes)
▶ Level II: Health Care Financing Administration (HCFA) designated codes and alpha modifiers (national codes). Examples of this level may be found at the end of Appendix B of the *Workbook.*
▶ Level III: Codes specific to regional fiscal intermediary or individual insurance carrier (local codes) and not found in either levels I or II.

Level III, local codes, are used to identify new procedures or specific supplies for which there is no national code. These are five-digit alphanumeric codes and use the letters S, and W through Z. You may discover that one case can be coded in two or even three coding levels. When both a CPT and level II code have the same description, the CPT code should be used. If the descriptions are not identical (e.g., the CPT code narrative is generic and the HCPCS level II code is specific), the level II code should be used.

The formula for selecting a code that most accurately identifies the service reported is as follows:

Physician or provider service = CPT code
Supplies = HCPCS National code
Instructions to use from carrier = local code

Some private insurance companies have begun to accept level II HCPCS codes. It is always wise to check the carrier's provider manual or telephone the carrier before sending in claims for medications and durable medical equipment. The HCPCS is updated each spring. (See Chapter 11 for additional information on coding for Medicare cases.) In some states, the TRICARE and Medicaid programs accept HCPCS codes. In the majority of states, most private payers have adopted the HCPCS system.

Methods of Payment

Private insurance companies and federal and state programs adopt different methods for basing their payments on outpatient claims; they are (1) fee schedules; (2) usual, customary, and reasonable; and (3) relative value scales or schedules. Additional methods of payment for inpatient hospital claims are discussed in Chapter 16.

Fee Schedule

A **fee schedule** is simply a listing of accepted charges or established allowances for specific medical procedures. A medical practice can have more than one fee schedule unless specific state laws restrict this practice. The following situations can occur:

1. Providers *participating* in the Medicare program would typically have a fee schedule for Medicare patients and one for non-Medicare patients.
2. Providers *not participating* in the Medicare program would typically have two fee schedules: one based on limiting charges for each service set by the Medicare program and one used for non-Medicare patients.
3. Providers having a contractual arrangement with a managed care plan (e.g., health maintenance organization, individual practice association, or preferred provider organization) would probably have additional fee schedules in use.
4. Providers rendering services to those who have sustained industrial injuries would use a separate workers' compensation fee schedule (see Chapter 14).

Section 1128(b) of the Social Security Act says a physician may risk exclusion or suspension from the Medicare program if his or her Medicare charges are "substantially in excess of such individual's or entity's usual charges." Options are to either lower private rates to the Medicare fee schedule amount or use a separate Medicare fee schedule. An exception are charges negotiated for managed care contracts that are not considered the physician's usual charges. In those cases, it is possible that Medicare patients would be charged more than managed care patients.

The physician may want to evaluate one or all of the fee schedules in use to annually increase fees because of a rise in the cost of living. A process for accomplishing this is discussed and shown in the section of this chapter subtitled "Determining RVS Conversion Factors."

Usual, Customary, and Reasonable (UCR)

Usual, customary, and reasonable (UCR) is a complex system in which three fees are considered in calculating payment. UCR is used mostly in reference to fee-for-service reimbursement. Figure 5-1 illustrates how a surgeon's payment is determined under this method. The *usual fee* is the fee that a physician usually charges (submitted fee) for a given service to a private patient. A fee is **customary** if it is in the range of usual fees charged by providers of similar training and experience in a geographic area

PARTICIPATING SURGEON UCR CALCULATION

Four Example Cases

Surgeon's Bill	Usual fee	compared to	Customary fee		Payment
1) $400	$350	⟶	$350 ⟶	declared reasonable (extenuating circumstances)	$400
2) $400	$350	⟶	$350 ⟶	declared customary (no unusual circumstances)	$350
3) $375	$350	⟶	$400 ⟶	declared customary (does not exceed customary level)	$375
4) $350	$350	⟶	$400 ⟶	declared customary (falls within customary range)	$350

Usual Fee– usual submitted fee for a given service to patient.

Customary Fee– in the range of usual fees charged by providers of similar training and experience in a geographical area (i.e., the history of charges for a given service).

Reasonable fee– meets the aforementioned criteria or is, in the opinion of the medical review committee, justifiable considering the special circumstances of the case.

Payment– based on the lower of usual and customary fees.

Figure 5–1. UCR calculation for four participating surgeons' cases.

(i.e., the history of charges for a given service). The **reasonable fee** is the fee that meets the aforementioned criteria or is, in the opinion of the medical review committee, justifiable considering the special circumstances of the case. Reimbursement is based on the lower of the two fees (usual and customary) and determines the approved or allowed amount. In a UCR system, payment can be extremely low for a rarely performed but highly complex procedure because there may be no history of billed charges from other physicians on which to base payment. Many private health insurance plans use this method and will pay a physician's full charge if it does not exceed UCR charges. Depending on the insurance company policy, the UCR system is periodically updated. UCR is a method chosen by insurance carriers and not the provider. If the physician has a UCR that is significantly lower than those of other practices in his or her area, document this and ask the insurance carrier for a review and possible adjustment. Increasing numbers of plans are beginning to discontinue the UCR system and are adopting the Medicare Resource-Based Relative Value Scale (RBRVS) method for physician reimbursement. A description of this system is found under "Relative Value Studies," which follows, and additional information appears in Chapter 11.

Two other factors that Medicare takes into consideration while assigning UCR fees are actual charge and prevailing charge. The **actual charge** is the amount a physician actually bills a patient for a particular medical procedure or service. The **prevailing charge** is a charge that falls within the range of charges most frequently used in a locality for a particular medical service or procedure. Note that this is a general definition of UCR, and programs other than Medicare define it in a different way.

Relative Value Studies (RVS)

In 1956, the California Medical Association Committee on Fees published the first edition of the *California Relative Value Studies (CRVS).*

It was subsequently revised and published in 1957, 1960, 1964, 1969, and 1974. **RVS** is referred to as either **relative value studies** or scale. It is a coded listing of procedures with *unit values* that indicate the relative value of the various services performed, taking into account the time, skill, and overhead cost required for each service (see Example 5–2).

EXAMPLE 5–2

Procedure Code	Description	Units
10060	Incision & Drainage of cyst	0.8

Using a hypothetical figure of **$153/unit**, this procedure would be valued at $122.40.

Math: $153.00 × 0.8 = $122.40

The units in this scale are based on median charges of all physicians during the time period in which the RVS was published. A **conversion factor** is used to translate the abstract units in the scale to dollar fees for each service.

The RVS became a very sophisticated system for the coding and billing of professional services. After the successful use of the California RVS, many state and medical specialty associations adopted this method. In 1975, the Federal Trade Commission (FTC) challenged the legality of using the RVS as a fee schedule. Since that time, many medical societies and medical specialty associations have issued new publications that omit unit values for the procedures listed, retaining the procedure code portion of RVS.

Some states have passed legislation mandating the use of RVS codes for procedures and the unit values as the schedule of fees for workers' compensation claims. In these states, the conversion factor to be used in applying the units is also stated in the law. The insurance carrier pays a specific dollar amount for each unit listed for each procedure in the RVS code book.

An insurer or other third party could devise an RVS based on its own data. This RVS would not be created by physicians desiring to regulate their own fees and, therefore, would be acceptable to the FTC. One such book available is *St. Anthony's Relative Values for Physicians (RVP)* (refer to Appendix B, Relative Value Studies, for information on where to obtain this book). A national RVS developed under a government contract may be acceptable and would not be in violation of antitrust laws.

The *Resource-Based Relative Value Scale* (RBRVS) is an RVS developed for the HCFA by William Hsiao and associates of the Harvard School of Public Health. HCFA used it to devise the Medicare fee schedule that was phased in from 1992 through 1996. This approach to fees was developed to redistribute Medicare dollars more equitably among physicians. For further information, see Chapter 11, Medicare.

Determining Relative Value Studies Conversion Factors

If a physician's fees are too high or too low, they can be adjusted. But how to do this can present a problem. Determining the conversion factor can be of great assistance in realigning fees or setting a fee for a procedure for which the physician has not previously billed. Because there are six code sections in CPT, it is necessary to figure out the conversion factor for each section separately. Once the unit values are known and you discover the RVS being used by the insurance carriers that you bill, you can monitor the reimbursements to make sure the payments are correct. It is legal to use an RVS guide for setting, realigning, or evaluating fees as long as the physician does not enter into any price-fixing agreements. To set fees based on an RVS, obtain an RVS and make up a set of separate conversion factors for the Evaluation and Management (E/M), Anesthesia, Surgery, Radiology, Pathology, and Medicine sections. The workers' compensation board or the insurance commissioner in your state can supply you with an RVS.

Physicians who take x-ray films in their offices and bill for them will find an RVS radiology book to be of value. See Appendix B for information on how to obtain the code books mentioned in this chapter.

Use the following steps to determine conversion factors:

PROCEDURE: Determining Conversion Factors

1. Choose 10 or more procedures in the same section (Evaluation and Management [E/M], Anesthesia, Surgery, Radiology, Pathology, or Medicine) and put down the code numbers and fees you presently use.
2. Take each procedure and divide the fee you presently charge by the procedure's unit value. The unit value is listed next to the code number and procedure description in the RVS. Because some procedure descriptions change from year to year, be sure that the description of the service is the proper definition for the service you are giving for that particular fee.
3. Look at all the dollar figures in the section that you have determined. They should fall within the same general range. If they do not, then some of the fees that are too high or too low may have to be re-evaluated and readjusted depending on the service descriptions and competition.

4. Add all the conversion factors in the E/M section. Divide the sum by the total number of services in that sampling. Use this as the conversion factor for the Medicine section. Remember this is only a guideline, and the physician may elect to use the highest, lowest, or median figure depending on his or her own judgment and circumstances.

Repeat these steps with each of the sections to obtain at least five conversion factors. Once you have determined the conversion factors for each section, you can determine a dollar figure for a new procedure within the same general grouping by multiplying the unit value by the dollar conversion factor. This will give an approximate cost of each procedure's relative worth. After determining how to obtain a conversion factor, you may wish to evaluate the fee schedules annually to decide whether fees should be raised for certain procedures or services.

How To Use the CPT Code Book

The following are guidelines for the 2000 edition of the CPT. This code book is a systematic listing of five-digit code numbers with no decimals. It is divided into six code sections with categories and subcategories. The main code sections and appendices are as follows:

Evaluation and Management (E/M)	99201 to 99499
Anesthesia	00100 to 01999
Surgery	10040 to 69990
Radiology, Nuclear Medicine, and Diagnostic Ultrasound	70010 to 79999
Pathology and Laboratory	80048 to 89399
Medicine	90281 to 99199

Appendix A Modifiers
Appendix B Summary of Additions, Deletions, and Revisions
Appendix C Update to Short Descriptors
Appendix D Clinical Examples
Appendix E Summary of CPT Add-on Codes
Appendix F Summary of Codes Exempt from Modifier-51

Within each of the main sections are categories and subcategories divided according to anatomic body systems, procedure, condition, description, and specialties.

Read through the clinical examples presented in Appendix D. These will help familiarize you with some of the case scenarios that commonly occur for the codes that appear in the E/M section of the CPT.

When on the job, you might want to make your CPT into a reference manual by customizing it. This would help you find codes, modifiers, and rules, making your job easier. Break apart the manual into as many sections as required by the specialty where you work. Three-hole punch it, and place it into a binder. Add indexes with tabs to the frequently used sections. You can add coding edits, Medicare updates, and notes at any place in the binder. Color code any codes you usually have to add modifiers to or that should not be used until you have reviewed certain data. For example, use red to highlight codes, descriptions, or entire sections, to alert you or anyone using the reference to codes often denied. Use yellow highlight to indicate a code that needs to be checked before using it in combination with other codes. Use a symbol (e.g., * or ?) to identify services not covered under certain conditions. Since Appendix A is a comprehensive list of the modifiers, add any insurance plan bulletins pertinent to modifiers that affect the specialty you bill for in this section of the binder. Customizing the CPT with a reference like this can save you time and reduce errors made in coding claims.

Code Book Symbols

With each new issuance of CPT, new codes and description changes are added. It is important to become familiar with the new codes and any description changes for the specialized areas that will be used. Figure 5–2 shows you how to identify new codes and description changes by following the symbols that are used.

When using a new code, marked with a bullet (●), remember that it may take as long as 6 months before an insurance carrier has a mandatory value assignment; therefore, reimbursements will be received in varying amounts during that time. For revised codes or revised text, marked with a triangle (▲) or (► ◄), highlight what is new or what is deleted. This will save time in trying to figure out what was changed and will prevent using these codes incorrectly. Appendices B and C in the code book provide a summary of the additions, deletions, and revisions. Add-on codes, shown with a plus sign (+), and modifier -51 exempt, shown with a symbol (○) are explained at the end of this chapter. In the Surgery section, a **star symbol** (*) next to a procedure number, means all of the following:

Service includes surgical procedure only

10080* Incision and drainage of pilonidal cyst; simple

New code

● 57022 Incision and drainage of vaginal hematoma; post-obstetrical

Revised code (altered procedure descriptor)

▲ 82465 Cholesterol, serum or whole blood, total

New or revised text (other than the procedure descriptors)

▶◀ Critical care is the direct delivery by a physician(s) of medical care for a critically ill or ▶ critically ◀ injured patient.

Add-on code

+ 35400 Angioscopy (non-coronary vessels or grafts) during therapeutic intervention (List separately in addition to code for primary procedure)

Modifier –51 exempt

⊘ 20690 Application of a uniplane (pins or wires in one plane), unilateral, external fixation system

Figure 5–2. Symbols that appear in *Current Procedural Terminology* code book.

1. The listed service is for the surgical procedure only.
2. All postoperative care is added on a service-by-service basis (e.g., a return office visit, hospital visit, or suture removal).
3. Complications are added on a service-by-service basis.
4. Preoperative services are considered as one of the following:
   a. When the starred (*) procedure is carried out at the time of the initial (new patient) office visit and constitutes the major service provided at that visit, identify the procedure by listing the surgical procedure code and use code number 99025 instead of an E/M code for the new patient visit. This code may be found in the Medicine Section of the CPT code book (see correct method of listing codes in Example 5–3).
   b. When the starred (*) procedure is carried out at the time of the initial or other patient visit involving significant identifiable services (e.g., removal of a small skin lesion at the

EXAMPLE 5–3

This CPT coding shows that the starred surgical procedure performed on a new patient constitutes the major service. Two entries are required.

Medicine Section Code **99025**	**Initial new patient visit**	$00.00
Surgery Section Code **10060***	**Incision and drainage** of abscess	$00.00

time of a comprehensive history and physical examination), list the appropriate visit in addition to the starred (*) procedure and all follow-up care.

c. When the starred (*) procedure is carried out at the time of a follow-up (established patient) visit and this procedure constitutes the major service at that visit, the service visit is usually not added.

d. When the starred (*) procedure requires hospitalization, both the hospital visit and the starred (*) procedure should be listed, as well as all follow-up care.

Evaluation and Management Section

The insurance billing specialist must become familiar with the terminology in the procedure code book to use it efficiently. Basic procedural code terminology was reviewed in Chapter 3 to give you a good foundation to begin coding. By now you should know the differences between a new patient and an established patient, a consultation and a referral, and concurrent care versus continuity of care. This section will familiarize you with specific coding policies in relation to some of the terminology you have learned thus far.

Consultation

Some insurance policies will pay for only one consultation per patient per year and often require a written report to be generated.

A consulting physician must submit a written report to the requesting physician. Codes for consultations are as follows:

▶ Office or other outpatient consultations (new or established patient): 99241 through 99245

▶ Initial inpatient consultations (new or established patient): 99251 through 99255

▶ Follow-up inpatient consultations (established patient): 99261 through 99263

▶ Confirmatory consultations (new or established patient): 99271 through 99275. This type of consultation calls for an opinion only. If a second opinion is required by the insurance company, modifier -32 (mandated services) is added.

If after a consultation is completed the consulting physician assumes responsibility for management of a portion or all of the patient's condition(s), do not use the follow-up consultation codes. In the office setting, use the appropriate initial consultation code for the initial encounter, then the appropriate established patient code. In a hospital setting, use the appropriate inpatient hospital consultation code, and then subsequent hospital care codes.

Critical Care

You have learned that critical care can take place in a variety of departments, that is, the coronary care unit (CCU), intensive care unit (ICU), respiratory care unit (RCU), or emergency department (ED), also called the emergency room (ER). When a patient is seen in any one of these departments, codes 99291 or 99292 are used to report the total duration of time spent by the physician. The time spent on a given date does not have to be continuous and should be recorded in the patient's chart. Bedside care and related care spent in the hospital on the floor or unit may be used to calculate the total time spent. Activities that occur outside the hospital (e.g., telephone calls) may not be reported because the physician is not immediately available to the patient.

In the CPT, refer to the Critical Care Service guidelines preceding the critical care codes to determine what services are included in the critical care codes. All other services should be reported separately.

Critical care service definitions are the same for adult, child, and neonate. The neonate critical care codes are not reported as hourly services. They are 24-hour global codes. Critical care services provided to neonates (30 days or less at the time of admission to an ICU) are reported with codes 99295 through 99298. For critically ill infants older than 1 month of age at the time of admission to an ICU, report using codes 99291 and 99292.

In addition, miscellaneous service codes 99050 through 99054 may be used, depending on the hour at which the patient is seen in critical care. Other codes in the Medicine Section under Miscellaneous Services may be applicable for a patient receiving critical care, so be sure to scrutinize these carefully. The key to obtaining the highest level of reimbursement lies in selecting diagnostic codes that convey the critical nature of the patient's condition.

Emergency Care

Codes 99281 through 99285 describe various levels of emergency care. Code 99288 is used when advanced life support is required during emergency care. If office services are provided on an emergency basis, code 99058 found in the Medicine Section, may be used when billing private insurance cases in lieu of a code from the E/M Section. Medicare does not pay when code 99058 is used and other carriers may also deny this code. When a physician spends several hours attending to a patient, coding for prolonged services (modifier - 21), in addition to an E/M emergency department code, might be indicated. See section on modifiers for further explanation.

If a patient comes into the office requiring emergency care for a wound trauma, and you bill for the office visit, suturing of the laceration, and the surgical tray, most insurance carriers will pay only for the suturing. The physician will not get paid and the patient will have to pay for the office visit and tray since they are bundled (codes grouped together that are related to a procedure) with the surgical code. However, if you code the claim for office services provided on an emergency basis, most carriers will reimburse for the office visit (see Example 5–4).

Miscellaneous service codes 99050 through 99054 can be used depending on the hour at which the patient is seen as an emergency in the physician's office. Other codes under Miscellaneous Services in the Medicine Section may be applicable for a patient receiving emergency care, so be sure to scrutinize these carefully.

Counseling

Codes 99381–99397 include counseling that is provided at the time of the initial or periodic comprehensive preventive medicine examination. For reporting counseling given at an encounter separate from the preventive medicine examination, use codes 99401 through 99412.

Categories and Subcategories

The E/M section of CPT has categories and subcategories that have from three to five levels for reporting purposes. These levels are based on key compo-

---

EXAMPLE 5–4

Incorrect Coding

99212	Office visit, problem focused, est pt
12005	Suture of scalp 12.6 cm
99070	Surgical tray (itemized)

Correct Coding

99212	Office visit, problem focused, est pt
99058	Office services provided on an emergency basis
12005	Repair of 12.6 cm scalp laceration

---

nents, contributory factors, and face-to-face time with the patient and/or family. To begin the coding process, the insurance billing specialist must identify the category (e.g., office, hospital inpatient or outpatient, or consultation) and then select the subcategory (e.g., new patient or established patient). Read the description thoroughly to note the *key* components (e.g., history, examination, medical decision making) and the *contributory factors* (e.g., counseling, coordination of care, nature of the presenting problem), and also note the face-to-face time of the service. Review the sample in Figure 5–3 illustrating an E/M code for a new patient seen in the office or in an outpatient or ambulatory setting.

Because key components are clinical in nature, it is important that the physician give these factors and document them in the patient's record to assist in coding each case. In a case in which counseling and coordination of care dominate (more than 50%) the face-to-face physician/patient encounter, then *time* is considered the key component to qualify for a particular level of E/M services. Tables 5–1 and 5–2 give a concise view of the components for each code number.

Many physicians began ranking the E/M codes on a scale of from 1 to 5, with 5 as the highest, most complex level and 1 as the lowest, least complex level. These levels coincide with the last digit of the CPT code. It is common to hear a physician say, "Ted Brown was seen for a level 4 today." This terminology may appear on encounter forms with five-digit CPT code numbers and be referred to as levels 1 through 5 (see Example 5–5).

Alternatively, this terminology may be seen abbreviated as L-1, L-2, and so on, but this usage is not preferred because it can be confused with the nomenclature for the sections of the lumbar vertebrae. The level may also be written out as level one, level two, and so on, depending on the complexity of the case. A breakdown of the

---

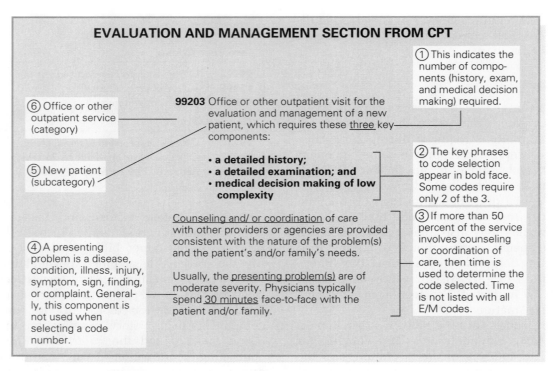

EVALUATION AND MANAGEMENT SECTION FROM CPT

① This indicates the number of components (history, exam, and medical decision making) required.

⑥ Office or other outpatient service (category)

99203 Office or other outpatient visit for the evaluation and management of a new patient, which requires these three key components:

⑤ New patient (subcategory)

- **a detailed history;**
- **a detailed examination; and**
- **medical decision making of low complexity**

② The key phrases to code selection appear in bold face. Some codes require only 2 of the 3.

Counseling and/ or coordination of care with other providers or agencies are provided consistent with the nature of the problem(s) and the patient's and/or family's needs.

④ A presenting problem is a disease, condition, illness, injury, symptom, sign, finding, or complaint. Generally, this component is not used when selecting a code number.

Usually, the presenting problem(s) are of moderate severity. Physicians typically spend 30 minutes face-to-face with the patient and/or family.

③ If more than 50 percent of the service involves counseling or coordination of care, then time is used to determine the code selected. Time is not listed with all E/M codes.

Figure 5–3. Evaluation and Management code 99203 defining the main words and phrases. This code is used for a new patient seen in the office or in an outpatient or ambulatory setting. (CPT codes, descriptions, and material are taken from *Current Procedural Terminology,* CPT 2001, Standard Edition, © 2001, American Medical Association. All Rights Reserved.)

E/M levels with code numbers is shown in Table 5–3.

In some billing cases, it is necessary to use a two-digit modifier or a separate five-digit code to give a more accurate description of the services rendered. This is used in addition to the procedure code. Refer to the comprehensive list of modifiers at the end of this chapter for more information.

Surgery Section

Coding from an Operative Report

When coding surgery, obtain a copy of the patient's operative report from the hospital. Make a photocopy that you can write on as you make notes. When scanning the report, use a ruler or highlighter pen. Use the ruler to read the report line by line. Highlight words that may indicate that the procedure performed may be altered by specific circumstances and when billing can remind you that a code modifier may be needed. Look up any unfamiliar terms and write the definition in the margin.

When coding a complex surgical procedure, either include an operative report or give a brief explanation in the proper block of the insurance claim

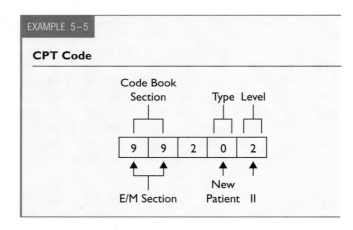

EXAMPLE 5–5

CPT Code

form so that the claims adjuster clearly understands the case and maximum payment is generated.

Use of code numbers that describe a part of the body treated may increase reimbursement (e.g., suturing of a facial laceration will pay a higher rate than suturing of laceration on the arm).

Code only the operations that were actually documented in the report. Do not code using only the name of the procedure given in the heading of the

---

TABLE 5-1	**Selection of Evaluation and Management Codes**

Code	History	Examination	Medical Decision Making	Problem Severity	Coordination of Care and Counseling	Time Spent (avg)
Office or Other Outpatient Services (Includes Hospital Observation Area)						
*New Patient**						
99201	Problem focused	Problem focused	Straightforward	Minor or self-limited	Consistent with problem(s) and patient's needs	10 min face to face
99202	Expanded problem focused	Expanded problem focused	Straightforward	Low to moderate	Consistent with problem(s) and patient's needs	20 min face to face
99203	Detailed	Detailed	Low complexity	Moderate	Consistent with problem(s) and patient's needs	30 min face to face
99204	Comprehensive	Comprehensive	Moderate complexity	Moderate to high	Consistent with problem(s) and patient's needs	45 min face to face
99205	Comprehensive	Comprehensive	High complexity	Moderate to high	Consistent with problem(s) and patient's needs	60 min face to face
*Established Patient**†						
99211	—	—	Physician supervision, but presence not required	Minimal	Consistent with problem(s) and patient's needs	5 min face to face
99212	Problem focused	Problem focused	Straightforward	Minor or self-limited	Consistent with problem(s) and patient's needs	10 min face to face
99213	Expanded problem focused	Expanded problem focused	Low complexity	Low to moderate	Consistent with problem(s) and patient's needs	15 min face to face
99214	Detailed	Detailed	Moderate complexity	Moderate to high	Consistent with problem(s) and patient's needs	25 min face to face
99215	Comprehensive	Comprehensive	High complexity	Moderate to high	Consistent with problem(s) and patient's needs	40 min face to face
Hospital Observation Services						
99217	—	—	—	—	—	—
99218	Detailed or comprehensive	Detailed or comprehensive	Straightforward or low complexity	Low	Consistent with problem(s) and patient's needs	—
99219	Comprehensive	Comprehensive	Moderate complexity	Moderate	Consistent with problem(s) and patient's needs	—
99220	Comprehensive	Comprehensive	High complexity	High	Consistent with problem(s) and patient's needs	—

| TABLE 5-1 | **Selection of Evaluation and Management Codes** *Continued* |

Code	History	Examination	Medical Decision Making	Problem Severity	Coordination of Care and Counseling	Time Spent (avg)
Hospital Inpatient Services						
Initial Care‡						
99221	Detailed or comprehen-sive	Detailed or comprehensive	Straightforward or low com-plexity	Low	Consistent with problem(s) and patient's needs	30 min unit/ floor
99222	Comprehensive	Comprehensive	Moderate complexity	Moderate	Consistent with problem(s) and patient's needs	50 min unit/ floor
99223	Comprehensive	Comprehensive	High complexity	High	Consistent with problem(s) and patient's needs	70 min unit/ floor
Hospital Inpatient Services						
Subsequent Care‡§						
99231	Problem focused interval	Problem focused	Straightforward or low complexity	Stable, recovering or improving	Consistent with problem(s) and patient's needs	15 min unit/ floor
99232	Expanded problem focused interval	Expanded problem focused	Moderate complexity	Inadequate response to treatment; minor complication	Consistent with problem(s) and patient's needs	25 min unit/ floor
99233	Detailed interval	Detailed	High complexity	Unstable; significant new problem or complication	Consistent with problem(s) and patient's needs	35 min unit/ floor
99238	Hospital discharge day management					

*Key component: For new patients for initial office and other outpatient services, all three components (history, physical examination, and medical decision making) are essential in selecting the correct code. For established patients, at least two of these three components are required.

†Includes follow-up, periodic reevaluation, and management of new problems.

‡Key components: For initial care, all three components (history, physical examination, and medical decision making) are essential in selecting the correct code. For subsequent care, at least two of these three components are required.

§All subsequent levels of service include a review of the medical record, diagnostic studies, and changes in the patient's status, such as history, physical condition, and response to treatment since the last assessment.

Reprinted with permission from St. Anthony's Coding for Physician Reimbursement, St. Anthony Publishing, Alexandria, Virginia, January 1992 and updated 2000.

CPT codes, descriptions, and material are taken from *Current Procedural Terminology,* CPT 2001, Standard Edition, © 2001, American Medical Association. All Rights Reserved.

operative report. Read the report thoroughly before coding to see whether additional procedures were performed and whether they were part of the main procedure, performed independently, or unrelated. Information on how to code multiple procedures that are not inherent in a major procedure may be found at the end of this chapter under modifier -51.

Reread the report to make certain that all procedural and diagnostic codes have been identified.

Compare the content with the codes you are using. You cannot code circumstances the physician relays to you verbally. If there were extensive complications, be sure the words "extensive complications" are in the report.

Surgical code descriptions may define a correct coding relationship where one code is part of another based on the language used in the description (see Example 5–6).

| TABLE 5–2 | Code Selection Criteria for Consultations |

E/M Code	History*	Examination	Medical Decision Making*	Problem Severity	Coordination of Care; Counseling	Time (avg)
			Office and Other Outpatient			
99241	Problem focused	Problem focused	Straightforward	Minor or self-limited	Consistent with problem(s) and patient's needs	15 min face to face
99242	Expanded problem focused	Expanded problem focused	Straightforward	Low	Consistent with problem(s) and patient's needs	30 min face to face
99243	Detailed	Detailed	Low complexity	Moderate	Consistent with problem(s) and patient's needs	40 min face to face
99244	Comprehensive	Comprehensive	Moderate complexity	Moderate to high	Consistent with problem(s) and patient's needs	60 min face to face
99245	Comprehensive	Comprehensive	High complexity	Moderate to high	Consistent with problem(s) and patient's needs	80 min face to face
			Initial Inpatient†			
99251	Problem focused	Problem focused	Straightforward	Minor or self-limited	Consistent with problem(s) and patient's needs	20 min unit/ floor
99252	Expanded problem focused	Expanded problem focused	Straightforward	Low	Consistent with problem(s) and patient's needs	40 min unit/ floor
99253	Detailed	Detailed	Low complexity	Moderate	Consistent with problem(s) and patient's needs	55 min unit/ floor
99254	Comprehensive	Comprehensive	Moderate complexity	Moderate to high	Consistent with problem(s) and patient's needs	80 min unit/ floor
99255	Comprehensive	Comprehensive	High complexity	Moderate to high	Consistent with problem(s) and patient's needs	110 min unit/ floor
			Follow-Up Inpatient†			
99261	Problem focused	Problem focused	Straightforward or low complexity	Stable, recovering or improving	Consistent with problem(s) and patient's needs	10 min unit/ floor
99262	Expanded problem focused interval	Expanded problem focused	Moderate complexity	Inadequate response to treatment; minor complication	Consistent with problem(s) and patient's needs	20 min unit/ floor
99263	Detailed interval	Detailed	High complexity	Unstable; significant new problem or complication	Consistent with problem(s) and patient's needs	30 min unit/ floor
			Confirmatory			
99271	Problem focused	Problem focused	Straightforward	Minor or self-limited	Consistent with problem(s) and patient's needs	—

CPT codes, descriptions, and material are taken from *Current Procedural Terminology*, CPT 2001, Standard Edition, © 2001, American Medical Association. All Rights Reserved.

TABLE 5-2 **Code Selection Criteria for Consultations** *Continued*

E/M Code	History*	Examination	Medical Decision Making*	Problem Severity	Coordination of Care; Counseling	Time (avg)
99272	Expanded problem focused	Expanded problem focused	Straightforward	Low	Consistent with problem(s) and patient's needs	—
99273	Detailed	Detailed	Low complexity	Moderate	Consistent with problem(s) and patient's needs	—
99274	Comprehensive	Comprehensive	Moderate	Moderate to high	Consistent with problem(s) and patient's needs	—
99275	Comprehensive	Comprehensive	High	Moderate to high	Consistent with problem(s) and patient's needs	—

*Key component: For office and initial inpatient consultations, all three components (history, physical examination, and medical decision making) are crucial for selecting the correct code. For follow-up consultations, two of these three components are required.
†These codes also are used for residents of nursing facilities.
Reprinted with permission from St. Anthony's Coding for Physician Reimbursement—Special Supplement, St. Anthony Publishing, Alexandria. Virginia, March 1992 and updated 1998.

Above all, be sure the report findings agree with the procedure codes on the claim.

Surgical Package

A phrase in the Surgery section commonly encountered when billing is **surgical package.** Procedures not followed by a star (*) include the "package" concept. Generally, a surgical procedure includes the operation, local infiltration, digital block or topical anesthesia, and normal, uncomplicated postoperative care (follow-up hospital visits, discharge, and/or follow-up office visits). This is referred to as a "package" for surgical procedures, and one fee covers the whole package (Fig. 5–4A). The majority of surgical procedures, including fracture care, are handled in this manner.

Preoperative services such as consultations, office visits, and initial hospital care are often billed separately. An appropriate five-digit E/M code

TABLE 5-3 **Levels with Code Numbers**

	Office Visits		Consultations	
	New	*Established*	*Office*	*Hospital*
Level 1	99201	99211	99241	99251
Level 2	99202	99212	99242	99252
Level 3	99203	99213	99243	99253
Level 4	99204	99214	99244	99254
Level 5	99205	99215	99245	99255

EXAMPLE 5-6

Partial and *complete,* which means the partial procedure is included in the complete procedure.
56620 Vulvectomy simple; partial
56625 complete
Partial and *total,* which means the partial procedure is included in the total procedure.
58940 Oophorectomy, partial or total, unilateral or bilateral
Unilateral and *bilateral,* which means the unilateral procedure is included in the bilateral procedure.
58900 Biopsy of ovary, unilateral or bilateral (separate procedure)
Single and *multiple,* which means the single procedure is included in the multiple procedure.
49320 Laparoscopy, abdomen, with or without collection of specimen(s) by brushing or washing (separate procedure)
49321 Laparoscopy, surgical; with biopsy (*single* or *multiple*)
49322 with aspiration of cavity or cyst (eg., ovarian cyst) (*single* or *multiple*)

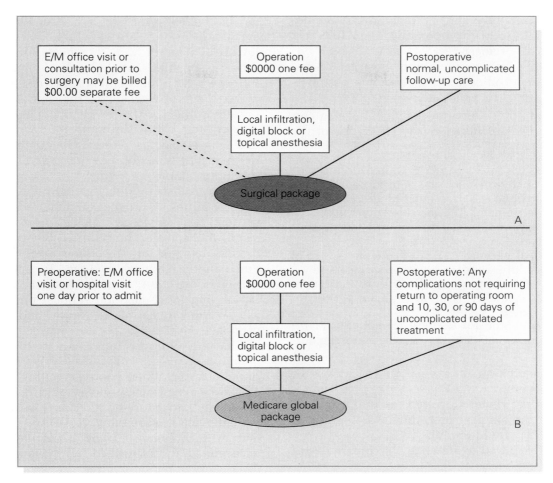

Figure 5–4. A, Surgical package concept. B, Medicare global package.

should be selected. Payment of these services depends on third party payment policy.

There are variations among insurance policies and managed care plans in regard to what is included in the package fee. Some follow Medicare guidelines, and some do not. Plans may include all visits several weeks before surgery, or they may include only visits that occur 1 day before the surgery. When a decision is made for surgery, a common question asked is whether a charge may be made for the consultation or office visit and admission if done on the same day. In most cases, the admission should be charged listing initial hospital care codes 99221–99223. However, for surgeons the guidelines are different. For example, if a surgeon sees a patient in consultation and recommends that the patient receive immediate trans-

fer of care to the surgeon and admission for surgery, then surgical package rules apply. The consultation that resulted in the decision for surgery may be billed, adding modifier -57 (decision for surgery) to the consultation procedure code number. The surgeon may not charge for an admission because all E/M services provided within 24 hours of surgery are bundled into the surgical fee.

Medicare Global Package

Medicare has a **global surgery policy** for major operations that is similar to the surgical package concept. The Medicare global fee is a single fee for all necessary services normally furnished by the surgeon before, during, and after the procedure. This became effective January 1, 1992 (see Fig. 5–4B). Included in the package are:

▶ Preoperative visits (1 day before or day of surgery)
▶ Intraoperative services that are a usual and necessary part of the surgical procedure

---

Remember the rule: Not documented, not done.

▸ Complications after surgery that do not require additional trips to the operating room (medical and surgical services)

▸ Postoperative visits including hospital visits, discharge, and office visits for variable postoperative period: 0, 10, or 90 days

In addition, procedures in the global period column of the *Federal Register* may show one of the following:

MMM A service furnished in uncomplicated maternity cases that include prenatal care, delivery, and postnatal care.

YYY Global period will be determined by the local Medicare carrier because the code is for an unlisted procedure.

XXX No global period. Visits, procedures, and follow-up services may be charged separately.

ZZZ The code is part of another service and falls within that service's global period.

Services provided for a Medicare patient *not included* in the global surgery package are the following:

▸ *Initial* consultation or evaluation (regardless of when it occurs)

▸ Postoperative visits unrelated to the diagnosis for which the surgical procedure was performed (modifier -24 would apply)

▸ Treatment required to stabilize a seriously ill patient before surgery

▸ Diagnostic tests and procedures

▸ Related procedure for postoperative complications that requires a return trip to the operating room (modifier -78 would apply)

▸ Immunosuppressive therapy after transplant surgery

If a Medicare patient is discharged from one hospital facility and admitted to a different hospital or facility on the same day, a provider may get paid for both, depending on the circumstances of the case. A low-level admission code, such as 99221, is used for the second hospital admit. A higher-level admission code may be used when the patient goes from a regular room to a specialized hospital of some type. Two separate claim forms, one for the discharge and another for the admission, must be used.

Follow-Up Days

The number of follow-up days that are allowed after surgery at no additional charge varies. The CPT code book does not specify how many days should be given, so an additional reference manual is needed. Most states use an RVS for workers' compensation cases, which will list the follow-up days allowed for most surgical procedures. Another source that lists surgical follow-up days for Medicare services is published in the *Federal Register* at the end of each year. Locate Appendix B (the Medicare Fee Schedule) and in the ninth column, follow-up days are listed as global fee period. Obtain the RVS used in your state or a copy of the *Federal Register* for this information.

Medicare lists a 90-day global period for all major procedures. A number of commercial insurance carriers have a 45-day global period for all or some of the major procedures. Some commercial carriers treat major procedures like minor procedures in the surgical package. To obtain specific carrier information, send the insurance company a list of your most common surgical procedures and ask for the surgical package rules and the number of global days that apply to each code. If you do not have this information, it is wise to bill the preoperative visit and all postoperative visits to the private carrier. When you receive this information, create a table showing global days on a payer-by-payer and procedure-by-procedure basis. On each patient's chart scheduled for surgery, show the date of the surgery and how many days the insurance policy allows. Bill for all visits after the surgical package period expires.

For office visits by the physician during the postoperative period, use CPT code number 99024 to indicate "No Charge." This code is located in the Medicine Section under Special Services and Reports; Miscellaneous Services. It has no value, is unbundled with other codes, and is used for tracking purposes. Always use 99024 for postoperative visits on itemized billing statements, because this lets the patient know how many office visits after surgery are being billed at no charge. There is no Medicare guideline for this code. Generally, it is not necessary to list this code when completing an insurance claim unless the insurance carrier has specific instructions requesting that it be shown. If the patient has to be seen beyond the normal postoperative time period, justify this by documenting the reason in the patient's medical record and submit an applicable procedure code and a fee for this on the claim form.

Repair of Lacerations

If multiple lacerations are repaired with the same technique and are in the same anatomic category,

EXAMPLE 5–7

Incorrect Coding

12011	Repair 2.5 cm laceration of face
12013	Repair 2.7 cm laceration of face
12013	Repair 3 cm laceration of face

Correct Coding

| 12015 | Repair 8.2 cm laceration of face |

EXAMPLE 5–8

Incorrect Coding

11055	Paring; single lesion
11056-51	two to four lesions
11057-51	more than four lesions
or	
11055 × 7	Paring; single lesion (× 7 corns)

Correct Coding

| 11057 | Paring; more than 4 lesions (7 corns) |

the insurance billing specialist should add up the total length of all the lacerations and report one code to obtain maximum reimbursement. Anatomic categories are the scalp, neck, axillae, external genitalia, trunk, extremities (hands or feet), face, ears, eyelids, nose, lips, and/or mucous membranes. If the patient had three repairs and each was listed with a different code, the second and third codes would be downcoded, so a smaller payment would be generated. If a patient has lacerations on both sides of the face, combine the lengths of all the lacerations since the anatomic region is the same and submit a claim for the total length. No modifier would be used, and the right and left side of the face would not be billed separately (see Example 5–7).

Multiple Lesions

The descriptions for the surgical codes that relate to accessory structures and lesions found in the integumentary system can cause confusion. Read code descriptions completely, including indentions, watching for terms such as complex, complicated, extensive, and multiple (lesions). See Example 5–8 as a guide to obtain maximum reimbursement for paring of seven corns.

Delay submission of the insurance claim for removal of a lesion or lesions until the pathology report is received. Usually, a malignant lesion is reimbursed at a higher rate because of the more detailed nature of the procedure.

Supplies

When billing for office surgery and supplies used, employ a checklist sheet for the items used on the sterile tray (Fig. 5–5A), as well as a checklist for determining complete and incomplete records (see Fig. 5–5B). These items can only be charged for if the surgery required the use of *additional* items not normally used for this type of surgery.

A **MINOR OPERATING ROOM INSTRUMENT TRAY SUPPLY CHECK LIST**

1 Adson Brown tissue forceps _____
1 Adson tissue forceps with teeth _____
1 long tissue forceps _____
2 mosquito clamps _____
1 Peck Joseph dissecting scissors _____
1 Kahn dissecting scissors _____
1 Reynolds dissecting scissors _____
1 Stratte needle holder _____
1 Webster needle holder _____
4 small piercing towel clips _____
2 double-skin hooks _____
2 single-skin hooks _____
1 knife handle _____
1 #15 blade _____
10 4 x 4s _____
2 cotton-tipped applicators _____
1 small basin _____
3 sterile towels (drapes) _____
1 Bovie pencil _____
Sutures: _____ _____ _____
Dressings: ½ inch Steri-strips _____

B **OFFICE SURGERY MEDICAL RECORD CHECK LIST**

Patient information sheet _____
H and P or progress note _____
Consent form _____
Diagnostic studies _____
Pathology report(s) _____
Anesthesia record _____
Circulating nurse's note _____
Doctor's orders _____
Discharge note _____
Operative report _____
Signature/operative report _____

Figure 5–5. *A,* Checklist to document supplies used when billing for office surgery. This list can be kept with the patient's medical record. *B,* Checklist for identifying complete and incomplete medical records used for a patient receiving office surgery. As each item or document is completed, it is checked off so that the person reviewing the chart can see at a glance what needs to be finalized.

Prolonged Services, Detention, or Standby

Code numbers 99354 through 99359 should be used to indicate prolonged services; for example, the physician has spent time beyond the usual amount allotted the service (i.e., 30 to 60 minutes). There are specific codes for face-to-face contact and without direct face-to-face contact. Prolonged service that is less than 30 minutes should not be billed using these codes because the time is included in the total work of the E/M codes. Time should be documented in the medical record to justify use of these codes. Reimbursement for prolonged detention in the hospital is higher than payment for many other types of care, and reimbursement for critical care is even higher.

Physician stand-by services are billed using code 99360. Some insurance programs or plans (e.g., Medicare) do not pay for operative standby, so be sure to check before billing to see whether the commercial carrier will pay. The charge is based on what the physician feels is the value of an hour of her or his time. An example is when a pediatrician is on standby during a high-risk cesarean section on a pregnant woman.

PROCEDURE: How to Code Effectively

To code effectively, follow these steps.

1. Always read the *Introduction* section at the beginning of the code book. This changes annually with each edition.
2. Read the *Guidelines* at the beginning of each of the six sections of the book. These define commonly used terms, explain classifications within each section, and give instructions specific to each section.
3. Read the *notes* and special subsection information throughout the Surgery, Radiology, Pathology, and Medicine sections. This information is listed throughout each section.
4. Use the index at the back of the book to locate a specific item by generalized code numbers, NOT by page numbers. Listings are given in four primary classes of main entries:
   a. Procedure or service
      Example: Anastomosis; Endoscopy; Splint
   b. Organ or other anatomic site
      Example: Salivary Gland; Tibia; Colon
   c. Condition
      Example: Abscess; Entropion; Tetralogy of Fallot
   d. Synonyms, eponyms, and abbreviations
      Example: EEG; Bricker operation; Clagett procedure

If the procedure performed is not listed, check for the organ involved. If the procedure or organ is difficult to find, look up the condition. Key words, such as synonyms or eponyms, and abbreviations will help you find the appropriate code.

5. Locate the code number in the code section and read through the narrative description to locate the most appropriate number to apply to the patient's procedure. Always start with the main term when reading the description. A semicolon (;) separates common portions from subordinate designations; subterms are indented (Fig. 5-6). Any terminology after the semicolon has a dependent status, as do the subsequent indented entries. In Figure 5-6 you see that procedure code number 11044 should read as follows: Debridement; skin, subcutaneous tissue, muscle, and bone. An example of how the billing should appear on an insurance claim for a patient who has had six corns pared is shown in Figure 5-7.
6. When trying to locate an E/M code, identify the place or type of service rendered. Then identify whether it is a new patient or established patient and locate the category or subcategory. Review any guidelines or instructions pertaining to the category or subcategory. Read the descriptors of the levels of E/M service. Identify the requirements necessary for code assignment. Make sure the components required were performed by the physician and documented in the chart, and then assign the E/M code.
7. Transfer the five-digit code number to the claim form exactly as given for each procedure. Be careful not to transpose code numbers. Also note the following:

11040	Debridement; skin, partial thickness
11041	skin, full thickness
11042	skin, and subcutaneous tissue
11043	skin, subcutaneous tissue, and muscle
11044	skin, subcutaneous tissue, muscle, and bone

Figure 5-6. Use of a semicolon. (CPT codes, descriptions, and material are taken from *Current Procedural Terminology,* CPT 2001, Standard Edition, © 2001, American Medical Association. All Rights Reserved.)

CODING FOR MULTIPLE LESIONS

Paring or Cutting

11055   Paring or cutting of benign hyperkeratotic lesion
(e.g. corn or callus); single lesion

11056   two to four lesions

11057   more than four lesions

A

24 A DATE(S) OF SERVICE						B Place of Service	C Type of Service	D PROCEDURES, SERVICES, OR SUPPLIES (Explain Unusual Circumstances) CPT/HCPCS | MODIFIER		E DIAGNOSIS CODE	F $ CHARGES		G DAYS OR UNITS	H EPSDT Family Plan	I EMG	J COB	K RESERVED FOR LOCAL USE
From MM	DD	YY	To MM	DD	YY												
1 05	11	2001				11		99203		1	00	00	1			46	27889700
2 05	11	2001				11		11057		1	00	00	1			46	27889700
3																	
4																	
5																	

B

Figure 5–7. *A,* Procedure codes from the Surgery Section of *Current Procedural Terminology. B,* Blocks 24A through 24K of the HCFA-1500 insurance claim form showing placement of the code on Line 2. (CPT codes, descriptions, and material are taken from *Current Procedural Terminology,* CPT 2001, Standard Edition, © 2001, American Medical Association. All Rights Reserved.)

▶ Parentheses ( ) further define the code and tell where other services are located (Fig. 5–8).

▶ Measurements throughout the code book are based on the metric system (Fig. 5–9).

▶ All anesthesia services are reported by use of the five-digit anesthesia code plus a physical status modifier. The use of other modifiers to explain a procedure further is optional. *Example:* Patient is a healthy 23-year-old white woman. Anesthesia given for a vaginal delivery. The procedure code would be 00946-P1.

▶ The Surgery section is the largest section in the code book. It has many subsections and subheadings. It is important to be able to break down a procedure and identify various terms that will direct you to the correct code (see Example 5–9*A*). Blocks 24A through 24K of the HCFA-1500 insurance claim form show

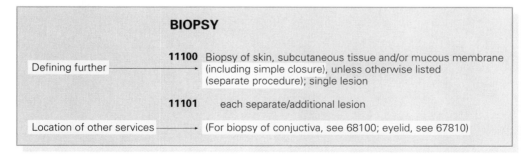

BIOPSY

Defining further ⟶ **11100**   Biopsy of skin, subcutaneous tissue and/or mucous membrane (including simple closure), unless otherwise listed (separate procedure); single lesion

11101   each separate/additional lesion

Location of other services ⟶   (For biopsy of conjunctiva, see 68100; eyelid, see 67810)

Figure 5–8. Use of parentheses in the Surgery Section of *Current Procedural Terminology.* (CPT codes, descriptions, and material are taken from *Current Procedural Terminology,* CPT 2001, Standard Edition, © 2001, American Medical Association. All Rights Reserved.)

CPT codes, descriptions, and material are taken from *Current Procedural Terminology,* CPT 2001, Standard Edition, © 2001, American Medical Association. All Rights Reserved.

Figure 5–9. Metric measurements from the Surgery Section of *Current Procedural Terminology*. (CPT codes, descriptions, and material are taken from *Current Procedural Terminology*, CPT 2001, Standard Edition, © 2001, American Medical Association. All Rights Reserved.)

13150	Repair, complex, eyelids, nose, ears and/or lips; 1.0 cm or less (See also 40650–40654, 67961–67975)
13151	1.1 cm to 2.5 cm
13152	2.6 cm to 7.5 cm

placement of the code on Line 2. (See Example 5–9, bottom.)

Unlisted Procedures

When a service is rendered that is not listed in the code book, use a code with a description stating "unlisted" (see Example 5–10). Unlisted codes end in -99 and are found at the end of each section or subsection. A comprehensive listing of unlisted codes is also found at the beginning of each section. Some Medicare fiscal agents will not pay for any of the special 99 adjunct codes.

When submitting a claim with an unlisted code, guidelines to follow to obtain maximum payment are:

▶ Always send supporting documentation with the claim that clearly identifies the procedure performed and the medical necessity for it. If detailed documentation cannot be electronically submitted or faxed to the carrier, then send a paper claim with supporting documentation in a large envelope so it is not folded. Do not use paper clips, staples, or tape to affix the attachments to the claim. Mark each attachment with the patient's name, insurance identification number, date of service, page number of the attachment, and total number of pages submitted (e.g., page 2 of 3). This helps the claim's processor match the documentation to the claim in the event they become separated.

▶ When unlisted procedures are performed frequently, ask the insurance carrier to assign a temporary local code so that it is not necessary to submit supporting documentation each time. This avoids manual processing and delays.

▶ File claims with unlisted procedure codes in a separate "tickler" file. Follow up about the status of the claim if there is no response within 1 month.

Coding Guidelines for Code Edits

In 1996 the Medicare program implemented a "Correct Coding Initiative" (CCI). This initiative

---

EXAMPLE 5–9

Closed manipulative treatment of a clavicular fracture.
Section: Surgery, Musculoskeletal System
Anatomic subheading: Shoulder
Condition: Fracture and/or Dislocation
Code: 23505

Thus, when completing an insurance claim form for closed manipulative tx, clavicular fracture, the billing portion would appear as follows:

24. A DATE(S) OF SERVICE From MM DD YYYY	To MM DD YYYY	B Place of Service	C Type of Service	D PROCEDURES, SERVICES, OR SUPPLIES (Explain Unusual Circumstances) CPT/HCPCS	MODIFIER	E DIAGNOSIS CODE	F $ CHARGES		G DAYS OR UNITS	H EPSDT Family Plan	I EMG	J COB	K RESERVED FOR LOCAL USE
010720XX		11		99203		1	00	00	1			46	27889700
010720XX		11		23505		1	00	00	1			46	27889700

CPT codes, descriptions, and material are taken from *Current Procedural Terminology,* CPT 2001, Standard Edition, © 2001, American Medical Association. All Rights Reserved.

99429	Unlisted preventive medicine service.

involves a code edit system consistent with Medicare policies to eliminate inappropriate reporting of CPT codes. *Code edit* is a function of computer software that performs online checking of codes on an insurance claim to detect unbundling, splitting of codes, and other types of improper code submissions. Such software is also used by private payers, other federal programs, and state Medicaid programs.

Because every medical practice has billing problems and questions unique to its specialty that arise due to denial or reduction in payment of claims, you must learn more about these edits. You must become a detective and discover how to obtain maximum reimbursements in the specialty in which you are working. The best way is to experiment and try out some new coding options and note how you are reimbursed. Coding takes expertise. It is an art, not an exact science. The following explanations of various ways of coding claims will help you obtain maximum reimbursement for each service rendered and avoid denials, lowered reimbursement, and possible audit.

Comprehensive/Component Edits

A **comprehensive code** means a single code that describes or covers two or more component codes that are bundled together as one unit. Each component code represents a portion of the service described in the comprehensive code and should be used only if a portion of the comprehensive service was performed (see Example 5–11).

Under the Medicare program, *component edits* are made involving procedures that meet any of the following criteria:

1. Code combinations that are specified as "separate procedures" by the CPT
2. Codes that are included as part of a more extensive procedure
3. Code combinations that are restricted by the guidelines outlined in the CPT
4. Component codes that are used incorrectly with the comprehensive code

If any one of these restricted code combinations is billed, Medicare allows payment for the procedure with the higher relative value (see Example 5–12).

comprehensive code	93015	Cardiovascular stress test
component codes	93016, 93017, 93018	

93015	Cardiovascular stress test using maximal or submaximal treadmill or bicycle exercise, continuous electrocardiographic monitoring, and/or pharmacological stress; with physician supervision, with interpretation and report
93016	physician supervision only, without interpretation and report
93017	tracing only, without interpretation and report
93018	interpretation and report only

Separate procedure example: Inguinal hernia repair with lesion excised from spermatic cord
Comprehensive code: 49505 Repair initial hernia age 5 years or older; reducible
Component code: 55520 Excision of lesion of spermatic cord (**separate procedure**)

When performing an inguinal hernia repair, the surgeon makes an incision in the groin and dissects tissue to expose the hernia sac, internal oblique muscle, and the spermatic cord. If a lesion is excised from the spermatic cord, it is considered a component of the comprehensive hernia repair procedure and not separately billable. Medicare will deny code 55520 as a component of procedure code 49505 when performed at the same operative session.

Mutually Exclusive Code Denials

Mutually exclusive edits relate to procedures that meet any of the following criteria:

1. Code combinations that are restricted by the guidelines outlined in the CPT
2. Procedures that represent two methods of performing the same service
3. Procedures that cannot reasonably be done during the same session
4. Procedures that represent medically impossible or improbable code combinations (see Example 5–13)

Because both of these procedures are different methods of accomplishing removal of the gallblad-

---

EXAMPLE 5–13

| 47605 | Excision, **cholecystectomy; with cholangiography** |
| 47563 | Laparoscopy, surgical; **cholecystectomy with cholangiography** |

---

der with cholangiography and represent duplication of efforts and overlapping of services, Medicare would deny code 47563 as mutually exclusive to code 47605.

Bundled Codes

When related to insurance claims, the phrase **bundled codes** means to group codes together that are related to a procedure. To completely understand bundled codes, one must have a thorough knowledge of the service or procedure that is being provided or use an unbundling book as a reference guide.

Example 5–14 illustrates one type of bundling found in the CPT code book. Because code 19271 does not include mediastinal lymphadenectomy and code 19272 does include it, reporting both codes together would be a contradiction in the actual performance of the services at the same session. Hence, when mediastinal lymphadenectomy is part of the procedure, submit code 19272 because code 19271 is bundled with it.

In the Medicare program, a number of services may be affected because HCFA considers the services bundled. Because many commercial carriers may follow Medicare guidelines, an understanding of this bundling concept is necessary. When dealing with private insurance, an Explanation of Benefits document may print out with a statement "Benefits have been combined," which means the same thing as bundling.

When listing, for example, a sterile tray for an in-office surgical procedure, the tray is bundled with the procedure unless additional supplies are needed over and above those usually used. CPT code 99070 (supplies and materials) is not recognized by Medicare for any supplies; however, level 2 alphanumeric codes may be used in such cases. The costs of some services and most supplies are bundled into E/M codes, for example, telephone services and reading of test results. However, Medicare will pay for slings, splints, rib belts, cast supplies, Hexcelite and light casts, pneumatic ankle-control splints, and prosthetics, but a supplier number is needed to bill for take-home surgical supplies and durable medical equipment (DME). Claims for supplies and DME go to one of four regional DME carriers whose addresses are listed in Appendix A. A reference book published by St. Anthony Publishing has comprehensive lists of the codes that HCFA considers bundled for the Medicare program (see Appendix B for further information).

Whenever appealing a claim, a great deal of time may be spent on paperwork only to discover that the code is bundled and denial is imminent. Whenever in doubt about whether services are combined or not, contact the insurance carrier and ask.

Unbundling

Unbundling is coding and billing numerous CPT codes to identify procedures that are usually described by a single code. It is also known as *exploding* or *à la carte* medicine.

Some practices do this unwittingly, but if it is done intentionally to gain increased reimbursement, it is considered fraud. Unbundling can lead to downward payment adjustments and possible audit of claims.

Types of unbundling are shown in Examples 5–15 through 5–18.

▶ Fragmenting one service into component parts and coding each component part as if it were a separate service (see Example 5–15).

EXAMPLE 5–14

| component code | 19271 | Excision of chest wall tumor involving ribs, with plastic reconstruction; without mediastinal lymphadenectomy |
| comprehensive code | 19272 | with mediastinal lymphadenectomy |

EXAMPLE 5–15

Incorrect Coding

| 43235 | Upper GI endoscopy |
| 43600 | Biopsy of stomach |

Correct Coding

| 43239 | Upper GI endoscopy with biopsy of stomach |

CPT codes, descriptions, and material are taken from *Current Procedural Terminology,* CPT 2001, Standard Edition, © 2001, American Medical Association. All Rights Reserved.

EXAMPLE 5–16

Unbundled Claim		Claim Coded Correctly	
58150	Total abdominal hysterectomy with removal of tubes and with removal of ovary ($1200)	**58150**	Comprehensive code for all three services ($1200)
58700	Salpingectomy ($650)		
58940	Oophorectomy ($685)		
Total charge: $2535		**Total charge: $1200**	

▶ Reporting separate codes for related services when one comprehensive code includes all related services (see Example 5–16).

▶ Coding **bilateral** (both sides of the body) procedures as two codes when one code is proper (see Example 5–17).

EXAMPLE 5–17

Incorrect Coding

76090-RT Right mammography
76090-LT Left mammography

Correct Coding

76091 Bilateral mammography

▶ Separating a surgical approach from a major surgical service that includes the same approach (see Example 5–18).

Insurers use special software that detects unbundling. To avoid this problem, always use up-to-date CPT and RVS code books. The use of outdated codes often inadvertently results in unbundling. Find out from insurers what edition they are using and always use the same edition as the insurer, especially during a transition period at the first of the year. When a new technology or technique is developed, it may have its own code, but as it becomes commonplace it may be bundled with another code. If the practice uses a billing service, request in writing that its computer system include no unbundling programming.

Downcoding

Approximately 35 different procedural coding systems are used in various regions across the United States. Generally, only three to five procedural coding systems are in use in any one given region at the same time. CPT and RVS codes have been emphasized in this chapter because they are the most commonly accepted, depending on what type of case you are billing—private, federal, state, or industrial. **Downcoding** occurs when the coding system used on a claim submitted to an insurance carrier does not match the coding system used by the company receiving the claim. The computer system converts the code submitted to the closest code in use, which is usually down one level from the submitted code. The payment that is generated is usually less than if the claim was not downcoded. To prevent downcoding, always monitor reimbursements and monitor downcodes to become knowledgeable about which codes are affected. Then call the insurance carrier and find out which code system is in use and obtain a reference list so you can code using the appropriate system (see Example 5–19).

Downcoding also occurs when the claims examiner must convert the CPT code submitted to a code in the RVS being used by the carrier. When

---

EXAMPLE 5–18

Incorrect Coding

49000	Exploratory laparotomy
44150	Total abdominal colectomy

Correct Coding

44150	Total abdominal colectomy (correct since it includes exploration of the surgical field)

EXAMPLE 5–19

Incorrect Coding

20010	Incision of abscess with suction irrigation (Note: 20010 has been deleted from CPT and would result in downcoding.)

Correct Coding

20005	Incision of abscess, complicated

CPT codes, descriptions, and material are taken from *Current Procedural Terminology,* CPT 2001, Standard Edition, © 2001, American Medical Association. All Rights Reserved.

there is a choice between two or three somewhat similar codes, the claims examiner will choose the lowest-paying code. Find out which RVS system is being used by the carrier before billing, and find the best match for the CPT code.

Downcoding may also occur when a claims examiner compares the code used with the written description of the procedure included in an attached document. If the two do not match, the carrier will reimburse according to the lowest-paying code that fits the description given (see Example 5–20). For additional information and solutions to downcoding, see Chapter 8.

EXAMPLE 5–20

Document states:	Excision of bone tumor from anterior tibial shaft.
Pathology report states:	Tibia bone tumor; benign

Incorrect Coding

11400	Excision of bone lesion, benign

Correct Coding

27635	Excision of bone tumor of tibia, benign

Upcoding

The term **upcoding** is used to describe deliberate manipulation of CPT codes for increased payment. This practice can be spotted by Medicare fiscal intermediaries and insurance carriers using prepayment and postpayment screens or "stop alerts," which are built into most coding computer software programs. An example of intentional upcoding would be when a physician selects one level

of service code for all visits with an attitude that the costs even out. This opens the door to audits and in the end may cost the practice money. Upcoding may also occur unintentionally if the coder is ill informed or does not keep current. Join a free list service (listserv) to keep current, to make coding contacts from all over the United States, and to post questions to someone who may know the answer to a current coding or billing dilemma; for example, go to the web site www.partbnews.com/enroll, fill out the enrollment form, and click "Done."

Code Monitoring

Monitoring of CPT codes is done to maximize reimbursement from all insurance carriers. First determine which codes are used most often in the physician's practice. Many computer programs can generate a list of codes, ranking them according to frequency of use. If the practice does not have a computer, take a sampling of the charge slips to find out the prevalent codes. Once the high-volume codes are known, focus on coding strategies for maximum reimbursement (see Figure 5–10).

Monitor every RA/EOB that comes to you directly or via the patients. Every private, Medicare, Medicaid, and TRICARE payment received should be checked for accuracy to see whether it is consistently the same or whether downcoding has occurred. Incorrect payments need to be investigated and possibly appealed. Examine all payments made for codes that do not match what you submitted. Be sure to appeal every payment that is less than half of what your physician bills. An example of a code and payment tracking log to help monitor payments received is shown in Figure 5–10.

Figure 5–10. Example of a code/payment tracking log.

CODE/PAYMENT TRACKING LOG					Date: 1-XX
CPT CODE	Practice Fee	Medicare date and amount paid	Medicaid date and amount paid	TRICARE date and amount paid	Blue Shield date and amount paid
99201	$00.00	11-XX $00.00	8-XX $00.00	7-XX $00.00	4-XX $00.00
99202	$00.00	12-XX $00.00	9-XX $00.00	10-XX $00.00	6-XX $00.00
99211	$00.00	12-XX $00.00			11-XX $00.00
99212	$00.00				12-XX $00.00
99221	$00.00				
99231	$00.00				
99232	$00.00				
99241	$00.00				

Helpful Hints in Coding

Office Visits

When an established patient is seen for an office visit and the medical assistant incidentally takes the patient's blood pressure per the physician's order, then the physician would include that service with the appropriate level of E/M code number (e.g., 99213, 99214). If the medical assistant takes the blood pressure and the patient is not seen by the physician but the physician reviews the results, then the appropriate code number is 99211 (presence of physician not required). If more than one office visit is required per day, read through the requirements for use of modifiers -25 and -59. One of them may be applicable before submitting a claim.

Some insurance policies allow only two moderate- or high-complexity office visits per patient per year. Therefore, it is important to contact the insurance company to learn whether there are any limitations. It is also important that a physician's practice has a system in place to track this.

Drugs and Injections

If the insurance claim has a description section (Block 19 on the HCFA-1500 claim form), give the name, amount, and strength of the medication as well as how it was administered. This information must also be documented in the patient's medical record. If a drug is experimental or expensive, it is good practice to include a copy of the invoice when sending in the insurance claim. Codes for injections are 90471 and 90472 and 90780 through 90799. Separate codes are used to identify the product being administered (see codes 90281 through 90399 and 90476 through 90749). Separate codes are available for combination vaccines. For allergy testing and immunotherapy, see codes 95004 through 95199. If an anesthetic agent is being used, determine whether it is diagnostic/therapeutic or prophylactic for pain. Medicare bills for immunosuppressive therapy are submitted to durable medical equipment carriers.

Adjunct Codes

Adjunct codes are referred to in the Medicine Section of the CPT as Special Services and Reports and fall under the category of Miscellaneous Services. They are important to consider when billing because these codes provide the reporting physician with a means of identifying special services and reports that are an adjunct to the basic services provided. The circumstances that are covered under these codes (99000 through 99090) include handling of laboratory specimens, telephone calls, seeing patients at odd hours, office emergency services, supplies and materials, special reports, travel, and educational services rendered to patients. If there is room on the insurance claim, explain the circumstances or include a report to justify the use of these codes. Some insurance companies will pay, but others will not.

Basic Life and/or Disability Evaluation Services

When reporting examinations done on patients for the purpose of trying to obtain life or disability insurance, use code 99450. For work-related or medical disability examinations, codes 99455 and 99456 may be used. Additional information about life or disability insurance examinations is given in Chapter 6.

Code Modifiers

The use of a CPT's two-digit add-on **modifier** or of separate five-digit numbers representing the modifiers permits the physician to indicate circumstances in which a procedure as performed differs in some way from that described by its usual five-digit code. A modifier can indicate:

▶ A service or procedure has either a professional or technical component.
▶ A service or procedure was performed by more than one physician and/or in more than one location.
▶ A service or procedure has been increased or reduced.
▶ A service or procedure was provided more than once.
▶ Only part of a service was performed.
▶ An adjunctive service was performed.
▶ A bilateral procedure was performed.
▶ Unusual events occurred.

In most cases, two-digit add-on modifiers are accepted. However, if an insurance company's input system accepts only five digits, such as with electronic claims, then it is always necessary to use five-digit modifiers. If in doubt, ask the insurance companies to express their desire of one form (two digits) over the other (five digits) (see Example 5−21).

EXAMPLE 5–21

2-digit	27590-**80** Amputation, thigh; **Assistant surgeon**
	or
	27590 Amputation, thigh
5-digit	**09980 Assistant surgeon**

When coding services or procedures, modifiers should be considered as an exception. The majority of professional services or procedures rendered are performed exactly as described by the CPT codes. Modifiers do not change the definition of a code but are used to describe modifying circumstances. It may be necessary when using a modifier to include an operative, pathology, x-ray, or special report to justify its use when submitting an insurance claim. A statement as to when a report is appropriate to include is noted for each modifier listed in Table 5–4.

Correct Use of Common CPT Modifiers

A choice of any modifier that fits the situation that is being coded may be used except when the modifier definition restricts the use of specific codes, for example, -51 Multiple procedures: "When multiple procedures, *other than Evaluation and Management Services . . .*" Some of the most commonly used modifiers will be discussed in detail here.

-21 Prolonged Evaluation and Management Services

This modifier is used to report a service longer than or greater than that described in the highest level evaluation and management service code (e.g., 99205, 99215, 99223). In addition, there are some five-digit codes for prolonged services involving *direct* (face-to-face) patient contact in either the inpatient or outpatient setting (99354 through 99357) and *without direct* (face-to-face) contact (99358 and 99359). Prolonged service of less than 30 minutes is not reported separately so these codes are used to report for time beyond that. Refer to the CPT for an illustration of correct reporting for these codes. Here is Example 5–22, showing use of this modifier.

-22 Unusual Procedural Service

Modifier -22 is used when the service(s) provided is greater than that usually required for the listed procedure. If you add the modifier -22 for unusual service, then the operative report must state that

EXAMPLE 5–22

An 80-year-old diabetic female is seen in a skilled nursing facility (SNF) by her internist for stage II decubitus ulcer with cellulitis. A revision in the treatment plan is indicated due to her condition. The physician performs a detailed interval history and a comprehensive physical examination, and the medical decision making is of moderate complexity. The physician meets with the patient's family to discuss treatment plans and future care (55 minutes).

99313-21   Subsequent nursing facility care—prolonged E/M service

unusual service was performed within the context of the normal procedure. Encourage your physician to use appropriate descriptions in the report, and call these words to his or her attention. Three guidelines are (1) the complications cannot be indicated by a separate code; (2) the procedure is lengthy and unusual; and (3) the services provided by the physician are increased because of unusual circumstances or complexities. This modifier may not be used with E/M services. Most insurance carriers send an insurance claim to medical review before payment is made if modifier -22, indicating unusual services, appears on the claim. Because payments may be delayed, it is important to be cautious when using this modifier. Comprehensive documentation will obtain 20% to 30% more reimbursement for the basic procedure. An operative report should be submitted with the claim. However, some Medicare carriers routinely deny any claim with modifier -22. An appeal for review can be made in such denials. See Chapter 8 for details on the Medicare review and appeal process.

-25 Significant, Separately Identifiable Evaluation and Management Service by the Same Physician on the Same Day of the Procedure or Other Service

For information on this modifier, see the explanation of modifier -57.

-26 Professional Component

Certain procedures are a combination of a **professional component (PC)** and a **technical component (TC).** These are usually seen in the radiology and pathology sections of CPT. The professional (physician) component refers to a portion of a test or pro-

(Text continued on page 147)

TABLE 5–4	Current Procedural Terminology Modifier Codes

Modifier Code	Explanation
-21	**_Prolonged Evaluation and Management Services:_** _When the face-to-face or floor/unit service(s) provided is prolonged or otherwise greater than that usually required for the highest level of evaluation and management service within a given category, it may be identified by adding modifier -21 to the evaluation and management code number or by use of the separate five-digit modifier code 09921. A report may also be appropriate._* **Example:** A physician spends an hour with a spouse and hospital inpatient, then an additional hour reviewing laboratory studies and x-ray films and reports, setting up a treatment plan with nurses, and coordinating care by two other specialists. **_Medicare Payment Rule:_** No effect on payment.
-22	**_Unusual Procedural Services:_** _When the services provided are greater than that usually required for the listed procedure, they may be identified by adding modifier-22 to the usual procedure number or by using the separate five-digit modifier code 09922. A report may also be appropriate._† **Example:** Removal of foreign body from stomach, which usually takes about 45 minutes, takes 2 hours on a particular patient; use modifier -22. A discharge summary or specially dictated statement should be attached to the claim form. This modifier increases the payment. **_Medicare Payment Rule:_** May result in increased payment based on supporting documentation of the unusual circumstances and complexity of the procedure performed.
-23	**_Unusual Anesthesia:_** _Occasionally, a procedure that usually requires either no anesthesia or local anesthesia must be done under general anesthesia because of unusual circumstances. This circumstance may be reported by adding the modifier -23 to the procedure code of the basic service or by using the separate five-digit modifier code 09923._† **Examples:** A proctoscopy might require no anesthesia. A skin biopsy or excision of a subcutaneous tumor might require local anesthesia. If general anesthesia is needed, append the procedure code with -23.
-24	**_Unrelated Evaluation and Management Service by the Same Physician During a Postoperative Period:_** _The physician may need to indicate that an evaluation and management service was performed during a postoperative period for a reason(s) unrelated to the original procedure. This circumstance may be reported by adding the modifier -24 to the appropriate level of E/M service, or the separate five-digit modifier 09924 may be used._† **Example:** A patient seen for a postoperative visit after an appendectomy complains of a lump on the leg. The physician takes a history and examines the site, and a biopsy is scheduled. The E/M code 99024 is used for the postsurgery examination and the modifier -24 is added for unrelated service rendered during a postoperative period. **_Medicare Payment Rule:_** No effect on payment: however, failure to use this modifier when appropriate may result in denial of the E/M service.
-25	**_Significant, Separately Identifiable Evaluation and Management Service by the Same Physician on the Day of a Procedure or Other Service:_** _The physician may need to indicate that on the day a procedure or service identified by a CPT code was performed, the patient's condition required a significant, separately identifiable E/M service above and beyond the other service provided or beyond the usual preoperative and postoperative care associated with the procedure that was performed. The E/M service may be prompted by the symptom or condition for which the procedure and/or service was provided. As such, different diagnoses are not required for reporting the E/M service on the same date._ **Example:** A patient is seen for a diabetic follow-up and the physician discovers a suspicious mole on the patient's neck (0.4 cm), which is removed. The physician makes a minor adjustment of the oral diabetes medication. This case illustrates a significant E/M service provided on the same day as a procedure, so -25 is added to the E/M code or a separate five-digit modifier 09925 may be used. Code 11420 is used for removal of the benign lesion. **Note:** _This modifier is not used to report an E/M service that resulted in a decision to perform surgery. See modifier -57._† **_Medicare Payment Rule:_** No effect on payment: however, failure to use this modifier when appropriate may result in denial of the E/M service.
-26	**_Professional Component:_** _Certain procedures are a combination of a professional physician component and a technical component. When the professional (physician) component is reported separately, the service may be identified by adding the modifier -26 to the usual procedure number or by using the five-digit modifier code 09926._* **Note:** The **professional component** comprises only the professional services performed by the physician during radiologic, laboratory, and other diagnostic procedures. These services include a portion of a test or procedure that the physician does, such as interpretation of the results. The **technical component** includes personnel, materials, including usual contrast media and drugs, film or xerograph, space, equipment, and other facilities but

CPT codes, descriptions, and material are taken from *Current Procedural Terminology,* CPT 2001, Standard Edition, © 2001, American Medical Association. All Rights Reserved.

Table continued on following page

TABLE 5-4	**Current Procedural Terminology Modifier Codes** *Continued*

Modifier Code	Explanation

excludes the cost of radioisotopes. When billing for the technical component, use the usual five-digit procedure number with modifier -TC.

Example:

70450-26 Computerized axial tomography, head or brain; without contrast material. *The modifier -26 indicates the physician interpreted this test only.*

70450-TC Computerized axial tomography, head or brain; without contrast material. *The modifier indicates the facility is billing only for the use of the equipment.*

-27 **Multiple Outpatient Hospital E/M Encounters on the Same Date:** For hospital outpatient reporting purposes, utilization of hospital resources related to separate and distinct E/M encounters performed in multiple outpatient hospital settings on the same date may be reported by adding the modifier -27 to each appropriate level outpatient and/or emergency department E/M code(s). This modifier provides a means of reporting circumstances involving E/M services provided by physician(s) in more than one (multiple) outpatient hospital setting(s) (e.g., hospital emergency department, clinic). Do not use this modifier for physician reporting of multiple E/M services performed by the same physician on the same date. See E/M, emergency department, or preventive medicine services codes.

Example: Patient is seen in a hospital outpatient clinic. The patient falls in the treatment room and receives a cut on the right arm. The patient is taken to the emergency department for two stitches and a dressing.

Medicare Payment Rule: Do not use modifier -27 for Medicare outpatients. Continue to use the -G0 (G-zero) modifier that HCFA established to cover multiple procedures, same patient, same day.

-32 ***Mandated Services:*** *Services related to mandated consultation and/or related services (e.g., PRO, third party payer, governmental, legislative or regulatory requirement), may be identified by adding the modifier -32 to the basic procedure, or the service may be reported by use of the five-digit modifier 09932.*‡

Example: A patient is referred to the physician by an insurance company for an unbiased opinion regarding permanent disability after a year of treatment following an accident. Add modifier -32 to the E/M code because the second opinion is mandated by the insurance company.

Medicare Payment Rule: No effect on payment

-47 ***Anesthesia by Surgeon:*** *Regional or general anesthesia provided by the surgeon may be reported by adding the modifier -47 to the basic service or by using the separate five-digit modifier code 09947 (this does not include local anesthesia).*†

Note: Modifier -47 or 09947 would not be used for anesthesia procedures 00100 through 01999.

Example: A gastroenterologist performs an endoscopy for removal of esophageal polyps using the snare technique. The physician sedates the patient with Versed to perform the procedure.

43217   Esophagoscopy with removal of polyps by snare technique

43217-47   Administered Versed

Medicare Payment Rule: Medicare will not reimburse the surgeon to administer anesthesia (any type).

-50 ***Bilateral Procedure:*** *Unless otherwise identified in the listings, bilateral procedures requiring a separate incision performed during the same operative session should be identified by the appropriate five-digit code describing the first procedure. The second (bilateral) procedure is identified either by adding modifier -50 to the procedure number or by using the separate five-digit modifier code 09950.*

Note: It is important to read each surgical description carefully to look for the word "bilateral."

Example A:

71060   Bronchography, bilateral (would be listed with no modifier)

Example B:

19200   mastectomy, radical

19200-50   mastectomy, radical; bilateral

Medicare Payment Rule: Payment is based on 150% (200% for x-rays) of the fee schedule amount.

-51 ***Multiple Procedures:*** *When multiple procedures, other than E/M services, are performed at the same session by the same provider, the primary procedure or service may be reported as listed. The additional procedure(s) or service(s) may be identified by adding the modifier -51 to the additional procedure or service code(s) or by using the separate five-digit modifier code 09551.*

Note: This modifier should not be appended to designated "add-on" codes (see Appendix E of CPT). Always list the procedure of highest dollar value first.

CPT codes, descriptions, and material are taken from *Current Procedural Terminology,* CPT 2001, Standard Edition, © 2001, American Medical Association. All Rights Reserved.

TABLE 5–4	Current Procedural Terminology Modifier Codes *Continued*

Modifier Code	Explanation
	Example: Patient had herniated disk in lower back with stabilization of the area where the disk was removed. 63030 Lumbar laminectomy with disk removal 22612-51 Arthrodesis (modifier used after the lesser of the two procedures) ***Medicare Payment Rules:*** Standard multiple surgery policy—100% of the fee schedule amount is allowed for the highest valued procedure, 50% for the second through fifth procedures, and "by report" for subsequent procedures.
-52	***Reduced Services:*** *Under certain circumstances a service or procedure is partially reduced or eliminated at the physician's election. Under these circumstances the service provided can be identified by its usual procedure number and the addition of the modifier -52 signifying that the service is reduced. This provides a means of reporting reduced services without disturbing the identification of the basic service. Modifier code 09952 may be used as an alternative to modifier -52.*§ **Note:** This means there will be no effect on the physician's fee profile in the computer data. It is not necessary to attach a report to the claim when using this modifier, because it indicates a reduced fee. When a physician performs a procedure but does not charge for the service, such as a postoperative follow-up visit that is included in a global service, remember to use code 99024. Some physicians prefer to bill the insurance carrier the full amount and accept what the carrier pays as payment in full. In such cases, a modifier would not be used. If only part of a procedure is performed and the physician feels a reduction in the service is warranted, to develop a reduced fee try calculating the reduced service by time. Calculate the amount (cost) per minute of the complete procedure by dividing the amount (cost) by the usual time it takes to complete the procedure. To determine how long the reduced procedure took, multiply the amount (cost) per minute by the time it took to do the reduced procedure. **Example:** A patient is not able to participate or cooperate in a minimal psychiatric interview (90801) and the physician decides to attempt this at a later date. Modify the code with -52. ***Medicare Payment Rule:*** Payment is based on the extent of the procedure or service performed. Submit documentation with the claim.
-53	***Discontinued Procedure:*** *Under certain circumstances, the physician may elect to terminate a surgical or diagnostic procedure. Due to extenuating circumstances or those that threaten the well-being of the patient, it may be necessary to indicate that a surgical or diagnostic procedure was started but discontinued. This circumstance may be reported by adding the modifier "-53" to the code for the discontinued procedure or by use of the separate five-digit modifier code 09953.* **Note:** This modifier is not used to report the elective cancellation of a procedure before the patient's anesthesia induction and/or surgical preparation in the operating suite. For outpatient hospital/ambulatory surgery center (ACS), see modifiers -73 and -74. **Example:** The physician is beginning a cholecystectomy on a patient. An earthquake of great magnitude occurs and the electricity is shut off. The backup generator comes on and electricity is restored; however, because of the disarray in the operative suite, the physician decides to discontinue the surgery. Code 47562 is used with -53 appended to it. ***Medicare Payment Rule:*** The carrier will determine the amount of payment "by report." Submit documentation with the claim identifying the extent of the procedure performed and the extenuating circumstances.
-54	***Surgical Care Only:*** *When one physician performs a surgical procedure and another provides preoperative and/or postoperative management, surgical services may be identified by adding the modifier -54 to the usual procedure number or by using the separate five-digit modifier code 09954.** **Note:** Because many surgical procedures encompass a "package" concept that includes normal uncomplicated follow-up care, the surgeon will be paid a reduced fee when using this modifier. **Example:** A patient presents in the emergency department with severe abdominal pain. Dr. A, the on-call surgeon, examines the patient and performs an emergency appendectomy. Dr. A is leaving on vacation the next morning so he calls his friend and colleague Dr. B. He asks him to visit the patient in the hospital the following day and take over the postoperative care. Dr. A bills using the appendectomy procedure code 44950 and modifies it with -54. ***Medicare Payment Rule:*** Payment is limited to the amount allotted for intraoperative services only.
-55	***Postoperative Management Only:*** *When one physician performs the postoperative management and another physician performs the surgical procedure, the postoperative component may be identified by adding the modifier -55 to the usual procedure number or by using the separate five-digit modifier code 09955.* **Note:** The fee to list would be approximately 30% of the surgeon's fee.

CPT codes, descriptions, and material are taken from *Current Procedural Terminology*, CPT 2001, Standard Edition, © 2001, American Medical Association. All Rights Reserved.

Table continued on following page

| TABLE 5–4 | **Current Procedural Terminology Modifier Codes** *Continued* |

Modifier Code	Explanation
	Example: The Dunmires are relocating to Memphis, Tennessee, when she discovers a lump on her arm. She visits her family physician, Dr. A, who tells her it needs to be excised. She wants her physician (Dr. A) to do the surgery and Dr. A agrees if she promises to arrange for a physician in Memphis to follow her postoperatively. She makes arrangements with Dr. B in Memphis. Dr. B bills using the correct excision code that he obtained from Dr. A and modifies it with -55.
	Medicare Payment Rule: Payment will be limited to the amount allotted for postoperative services only. Payment to more than one physician for split surgical care of a patient will not exceed the amount paid for the total global surgical package.
-56	**Preoperative Management Only:** *When one physician performs the preoperative care and evaluation and another physician performs the surgical procedure, the preoperative component may be identified by adding the modifier -56 to the usual procedure number or by using the separate five-digit modifier code 09956.*†
	Example: Dr. A sees Mrs. Jones and determines she needs to have a lung biopsy. He admits her to the hospital and Dr. A becomes ill. Dr. B is called in and performs the surgery. Dr. A bills for the preoperative care using the surgical code he obtained from Dr. B and modifies it with -56.
	Medicare Payment Rule: Payment for this component is included in the allowable for the surgery. If another physician performed the surgery, use an appropriate E/M code to bill for the preoperative service.
-57	**Decision for Surgery:** *An evaluation and management service that resulted in the initial decision to perform the surgery may be identified by adding the modifier -57 to the appropriate level of E/M service, or the separate five-digit modifier 09957 may be used.*‡
	Example: A patient is referred to a surgeon for a consultation to determine whether surgery is necessary. The patient consents to surgery. The surgeon bills the E/M consultation code and adds the -57 modifier. By adding this modifier, the third party payer is informed that the consultation is not part of the global surgical procedure. Medicare will pay if it is for major surgery that requires a 90-day postoperative follow-up but not for a minor surgical procedure (0- to 10-day postoperative follow-up).
	Medicare Payment Rule: Payment will be made for the E/M service in addition to the global surgery payment.
-58	**Staged or Related Procedure or Service by the Same Physician During the Postoperative Period:** *The physician may need to indicate that the performance of a procedure or service during the postoperative period was (a) planned prospectively at the time of the original procedure (staged); (b) more extensive than the original procedure; or (c) for therapy after a diagnostic surgical procedure. This circumstance may be reported by adding the modifier -58 to the staged or related procedure, or the separate five-digit modifier 09958 may be used.*‡
	Note: This modifier is not used to report the treatment of a problem that requires a return to the operating room. See modifier -78.
	Example: A patient has breast cancer, and a surgeon performs a mastectomy. During the postoperative global period, the surgeon inserts a permanent prosthesis. The -58 modifier is added to the code for inserting the prosthesis, indicating that this service was planned at the time of the initial operation. If the modifier is not used, the insurance carrier may reject the claim because surgery occurred during the surgery's global period.
-59	**Distinct Procedural Service:** *Under certain circumstances, the physician may need to indicate that a procedure or service was distinct or independent from other services performed on the same day. Modifier -59 is used to identify procedures/services that are not normally reported together but are appropriate under the circumstances. This may represent a different session or patient encounter, different procedure or surgery, different site or organ system, separate incision/excision, separate lesion, or separate injury (or area of injury in extensive injuries) not ordinarily encountered or performed on the same day by the same physician. However, when another already established modifier is appropriate it should be used rather than modifier -59. Only if no more descriptive modifier is available, and the use of modifier -59 best explains the circumstances, should modifier -59 be used. Modifier code 09959 may be used as an alternative to modifier -59.*
	Example: The patient is scheduled for a hysterectomy. She asks the physician if he will remove a lipoma (2.2 cm) from the right upper thigh area while she is under anesthesia. The surgeon bills for the hysterectomy, and bills for the lipoma removal (11403) modifying it with -59.
	Medicare Payment Rule: No effect on payment amount; however, failure to use modifier when appropriate may result in denial of payment for the services.
-60	**Altered Surgical Field:** Certain procedures involve significantly increased operative complexity and/or time in a significantly altered surgical field resulting from the effects of prior surgery, marked scarring, adhesions, inflamma-

TABLE 5–4	**Current Procedural Terminology Modifier Codes** *Continued*

Modifier Code	Explanation
	tion, or distorted anatomy, irradiation, infection, very low weight (i.e., neonates and small infants less than 10 kg), and/or trauma (as documented in the patient's medical record). These circumstances should be reported by adding modifier -60 to the procedure number or by using the separate five-digit modifier code 09960. **Note:** For unusual procedural services not involving an altered surgical field due to the late effects of previous surgery, irradiation, infection, very low weight and/or trauma, append modifier -22.
	Example: Ten years ago a patient had surgery for excision of a dermoid cyst, which required removal of the right ovary. Recently a hysterectomy is performed and the operative note clearly states the patient had "excessive adhesions in and surrounding the structures of the bowel, remaining ovary, and uterus, probably the etiology of the patient's progessive constipation." The procedure code should be appended with modifier -60 to alert the payer that this claim requires manual review due to the patient's scarring and adhesions for consideration of increased reimbursement.
	Medicare: Surgeons should continue to use modifier -22 instead of modifier -60 and only use modifier -60 for non-Medicare claims.
-62	**Two Surgeons:** *When two surgeons work together as primary surgeons performing distinct parts of a single reportable procedure, each surgeon should report his/her distinct operative work using the same procedure code and adding the modifier -62. If additional procedures (including add-on procedures) are performed during the same surgical session, separate codes may be reported without the modifier -62.*
	Note: If the co-surgeon acts as an assist in the performance of additional procedure(s) during the same surgical session, those services may be reported using separate procedure code(s) with modifier -80 or -81.
	Example: A procedure for scoliosis is performed by a thoracic surgeon who does the anterior approach and an orthopedic surgeon who does the posterior approach and repair.
	Medicare Payment Rule: Medicare allows 125% of the approved fee schedule amount for the -62 modifier if reported by both surgeons. That total fee is divided in half and dispersed to each surgeon at 62.5% of the approved amount.
-66	**Surgical Team:** *Under some circumstances, highly complex procedures (requiring the concomitant services of several physicians, often of different specialties, plus other highly skilled, specially trained personnel and various types of complex equipment) are carried out under the "surgical team" concept. Such circumstances may be identified by each participating physician with the addition of the modifier -66 to the basic procedure number used for reporting services. Modifier code 09966 may be used as an alternative to modifier -66.**
	Example: A kidney transplant, requiring use of a vascular surgeon, urologist and nephrologist, with the assistance of anesthesiologist, and pathologist, or open heart surgery using perfusion personnel, three cardiologists, and an anesthesiologist.
	Medicare Payment Rule: Carrier medical staff will determine the payment amounts for team surgeries on a report basis. Submit supporting documentation with the claim.
-76	**Repeat Procedure by Same Physician:** *The physician may need to indicate that a procedure or service was repeated subsequent to the original service. This circumstance may be reported by adding modifier -76 to the repeated service or by using the separate five-digit modifier code 09976.†*
	Example: A femoral-popliteal bypass graft (35556) is performed, the graft clots later that day, and the entire procedure is repeated. The original procedure is reported and the repeat procedure is reported using modifier -76. A report should be attached to the insurance claim when using this modifier.
	Medicare Payment Rule: Failure to use this modifier when appropriate (and to submit supporting documentation) may result in denial of the subsequent surgery.
-77	**Repeat Procedure by Another Physician:** *The physician may need to indicate that a basic procedure performed by another physician had to be repeated. This situation may be reported by adding modifier -77 to the repeated service or by using the separate five-digit modifier code 09977.†*
	Example: A femoral-popliteal bypass graft (35556) is performed in the morning and in the afternoon it becomes clotted. The original surgeon is not available and a different surgeon performs the repeat operation later in the day. The original surgeon reports 35556. The second surgeon reports 35556-77.
	Medicare Payment Rule: Failure to use this modifier when appropriate (and to submit supporting documentation) may result in denial of the subsequent surgery.
-78	**Return to the Operating Room for a Related Procedure During the Postoperative Period:** *The physician may*

Table continued on following page

| TABLE 5–4 | **Current Procedural Terminology Modifier Codes** *Continued* |

Modifier Code	Explanation
	need to indicate that another procedure was performed during the postoperative period of the initial procedure. When this subsequent procedure is related to the first, and requires the use of the operating room, it may be reported by adding the modifier -78 to the related procedure or by using the separate five-digit modifier 09978. (For repeat procedures on the same day, see -76.)†
	Example: A patient has an open reduction with fixation of a fracture of the elbow. While still hospitalized, the patient develops an infection and is returned to surgery for removal of the pin because it appears to be the cause of an allergic reaction. The original procedure would be billed for the open treatment of the fracture. The pin removal would be billed with modifier -78 because it is a related procedure.
	Medicare Payment Rule: Medicare will pay the full value of the intraoperative portion of a given procedure. Documentation should be submitted with the claim to describe the clinical circumstances.
-79	*Unrelated Procedure or Service by the Same Physician During the Postoperative Period*: The physician may need to indicate that the performance of a procedure or service during the postoperative period was unrelated to the original procedure. This circumstance may be reported by using the modifier -79 or by using the separate five-digit modifier 09979. (For repeat procedures on the same day, see -76).†
	Example: A patient in the hospital has colon resection surgery and is discharged home. After 7 days, the patient develops acute renal failure, is hospitalized, does not recover renal function, and hemodialysis is ordered. A nephrologist inserts a cannula for the dialysis. When billing for the nephrologist, the code for hemodialysis is shown with a -79 modifier indicating that this is unrelated to the initial surgery. If modifier -79 is not used, the insurance carrier may not realize the service is not related to the initial surgery and may reject the claim.
	Medicare Payment Rule: No effect on payment; however, failure to use this modifier when appropriate may result in denial of the subsequent surgery. Specific diagnostic codes will substantiate the medical necessity of the unrelated procedure. Documentation may be required to describe the clinical circumstances. A new global period begins for any procedure modified by -79.
-80	*Assistant Surgeon:* Surgical assistant services may be identified by adding the modifier -80 to the usual procedure number(s) or by using the separate five-digit modifier code 09980.*
	Note: Some insurance policies do not include payment for assistant surgeons, such as for 1-day surgery, but do pay for major or complex surgical assistance. In some instances, prior approval may be indicated owing to the patient's physiologic condition. Medicare will not pay assistant surgeons for operations that are not life threatening. Therefore, Medigap insurance will not pay on this service because the service is nonallowable. Assisting surgeons usually charge 16% to 30% of the primary surgeon's fee.
	Example: The primary surgeon performs a right ureterectomy submitting code 50650-RT. The assistant surgeon would bill using the primary surgeon's code with modifier -80 (50650-80).
	Medicare Payment Rule: Payment is based on the billed amount or 16% of the global surgical fee, whichever is lower, for procedures approved for assistant-at-surgery. Medicare will deny payment for an assistant-at-surgery for surgical procedures in which a physician is used as an assistant in less than 5% of the cases nationally.
-81	*Minimum Assistant Surgeon:* Minimum surgical assistant services are identified by adding the modifier -81 to the usual procedure number or by using the separate five-digit modifier code 09981.
	Note: Payment is made to physicians but not registered nurses or technicians who assist during surgery.*
	Example: A primary surgeon plans to perform a surgical procedure but during the operation circumstances arise that require the services of an assistant surgeon for a relatively short period of time. In this scenario, the second surgeon provides minimal assistance and may report using the procedure code with the -81 modifier appended.
-82	*Assistant Surgeon: (When qualified resident surgeon is not available.)* The unavailability of a qualified resident surgeon is a prerequisite for use of modifier -82 appended to the usual procedure code number(s) or the separate five-digit modifier code 09982.*
	Note: This modifier is usually used for services rendered at a teaching hospital.
	Example: A resident surgeon is scheduled to assist with an anorectal myomectomy (45108). Surgery is delayed due to the previous surgery, the shift rotation changes, and the resident is not available. A non-resident assists with the surgery and reports the procedure appending it with modifier -82 (45108-82).
-90	*Reference (Outside) Laboratory:* When laboratory procedures are performed by a party other than the treating or reporting physician, the procedure may be identified by adding the modifier -90 to the usual procedure number or by using the separate five-digit modifier code 09990.†

TABLE 5–4	Current Procedural Terminology Modifier Codes *Continued*

Modifier Code	Explanation
	Note: Use this modifier when the physician bills the patient for the laboratory work and the laboratory is not doing its own billing.
	Example: Dr. Input examines the patient, performs venipuncture, and sends the specimen to an outside laboratory for a liver panel. The physician has an arrangement with the laboratory to bill for the test, and, in turn, he bills the patient. Dr. Input bills for the examination (E/M code), venipuncture (36415 or for Medicare 0001), and liver panel (80058), using modifier -90 (80058–90) to append to the liver panel code.
-91	***Repeat Clinical Diagnostic Laboratory Test:*** *In the course of treatment of the patient, it may be necessary to repeat the same laboratory test on the same day to obtain subsequent (multiple) test results. Under these circumstances, the laboratory test performed can be identified by its usual procedure number and the addition of modifier -91.*
	Note: This modifier may not be used when tests are rerun to confirm initial results; due to testing problems with specimens or equipment; or for any other reason when a normal, one-time, reportable result is all that is required. This modifier may not be used when other code(s) describe a series of test results (e.g., glucose tolerance tests, evocative/suppression testing). This modifier may only be used for laboratory test(s) performed more than once on the same day on the same patient.
	Example: A patient is scheduled for a nonobstetrical dilation and curettage for dysfunctional uterine bleeding. When the patient arrives at the office, a routine hematocrit is obtained. During the procedure, the patient bleeds excessively. After the procedure, the physician orders a second hematocrit to check the patient for anemia due to blood loss. The first hematocrit is billed using CPT code 85013. The second hematocrit is billed using the same code appended with modifier -91 (85013-91).
-99	***Multiple Modifiers:*** *Under certain circumstances, two or more modifiers may be necessary to delineate a service completely. In such situations modifier -99 should be added to the basic procedure, and other applicable modifiers may be listed as part of the description of the service. Modifier code 09999 may be used as an alternative to modifier -99.‡*
	Example: An assistant surgeon helps repair an enterocele where unusual circumstances appear because of extensive hemorrhaging.
	57270-99 Repair of enterocele 　　　-22 Extensive hemorrhaging (unusual service) 　　　-80 Assistant surgeon
	Medicare Payment Rule: No effect on payment; however, the individual modifier payment policies apply, including any inherent effect they may have on payment.

*This modifier may have an effect on reimbursement.
†This modifier may affect reimbursement, depending on the payer.
‡Modifier is informational in nature. Do not ask for an adjustment in reimbursement. Monitor reimbursement when using this modifier.
§This modifier affects reimbursement but not the physician's fee profile.
Modified with permission from the American Medical Association, Chicago, Illinois.s

cedure that the physician does, such as interpreting an electrocardiogram (ECG), reading an x-ray film, or making an observation and determination using a microscope. The technical component refers to the use of the equipment and its operator that performs the test or procedure, such as ECG machine and technician, radiography machine and technician, and a microscope and technician. Do not modify procedures that are either 100% technical or 100% professional or when the physician performs both the professional and technical components. Modifier -26 represents the professional component only. Use of this modifier alerts the insurance company to expect a separate claim from another provider or facility for the technical component.

In Example 5–23, the physician is performing only one of two services—he or she is interpreting the results of bilateral hip x-ray films.

The facility where the patient went to have the x-ray would bill only for the technical component by modifying the same code with a -TC (73520-TC). If the physician owned the equipment and read the x-ray film, there would be no need to modify the x-ray code (73520).

-51 Multiple Procedures

There are many occasions when multiple procedures are performed at the same session by the same provider. In such cases, report the primary service or procedure, which can easily be deter-

EXAMPLE 5–23

73520-**26** or 73520 and 09926	Professional component *only* for an x-ray of both hips. *Use to bill physician's fee for interpretation of x-ray film.*	$
73520-**TC**	Technical component *only* for an x-ray of both hips. *Use to bill facility fee that owns equipment and employs technician.*	$
		=
73520	Radiologic examination (x-ray), hips, bilateral. *Use to bill complete fee when physician owns equipment, employs technician, and interprets x-ray film.*	$$

mined by highest dollar value, as listed. Identify all additional services or procedures by appending code(s) with modifier -51 or use separate five-digit modifier 09951 (see Example 5–24).

EXAMPLE 5–24

Excision of 2.0-cm benign lesion on the nose and at the same session a biopsy of the skin and subcutaneous tissue of the forearm.

| 11442 | $$ | Excision, benign lesion |
| 11100-**51** | $ | Biopsy of skin |

The operative report should clearly state which procedures were done through separate incisions and which were done through the same incision. There are many circumstances when multiple procedures are performed. Modifier -51 may be used to identify:

▶ Multiple medical procedures performed at the same session by the same provider
▶ Multiple, related surgical procedures performed at the same session by the same provider
▶ Surgical procedures performed in combination at the same session, whether through the same or another incision or involving the same or different anatomy
▶ A combination of medical and surgical procedures performed at the same session by the same provider

Usually payment for the primary code is 100% of the allowable charge, second code 50%, third code 25%, fourth and remaining codes 10%. However, Medicare pays 50% of the allowable for two

to five secondary procedures and does not require the assignment of modifier -51. The computer system can determine code order and automatically make the code adjustment. Always bill the full amount and let the insurance carrier make the payment adjustments for percentage considerations. For all insurance carriers, it is recommended to monitor the Remittance Advice/Explanation of Benefits to ensure correct payment. A decision flow chart is provided for reference to simplify applying modifiers to multiple surgical procedures. As you read through the remainder of this chapter, follow the steps by answering the questions in Figure 5–11*A* as they apply to your billing scenario and refer to Figure 5–11*B* for key information and descriptions.

Do not use this modifier with Evaluation and Management services, add-on codes designated with a " + " (see Appendix E in CPT), or codes listed as exempt to modifier -51 (see Appendix F in CPT). Add-on codes are codes that cannot stand alone. When billing with add-on codes, you *always* have to list another code referred to as the "parent code" to give full description for service billed (see Example 5–25).

When making a decision about when to use an add-on code, look for a clue phrase that indicates additional procedures, such as "each additional," "list in addition to," and "second lesion."

EXAMPLE 5–25

| **parent code** | 11000 | Biopsy of skin . . . single lesion |
| **add-on code** | 11101 | each separate/additional lesion (list separately in addition to code for primary procedure) |

-52 Reduced Services

Use of this modifier indicates that under certain circumstances a service or procedure is partially reduced or eliminated at the physician's discretion. It would be wise to provide an explanation of why the service was reduced. A cover letter or a copy of the operative report does not need to accompany these claims because usually they are not sent to medical review and such documents may impede processing. Never use this modifier if the fee is reduced due to a patient's inability to pay.

-57 Decision for Surgery

This modifier is used strictly to report an E/M service that resulted in the initial decision to perform

---

CPT codes, descriptions, and material are taken from *Current Procedural Terminology,* CPT 2001, Standard Edition, © 2001, American Medical Association. All Rights Reserved.

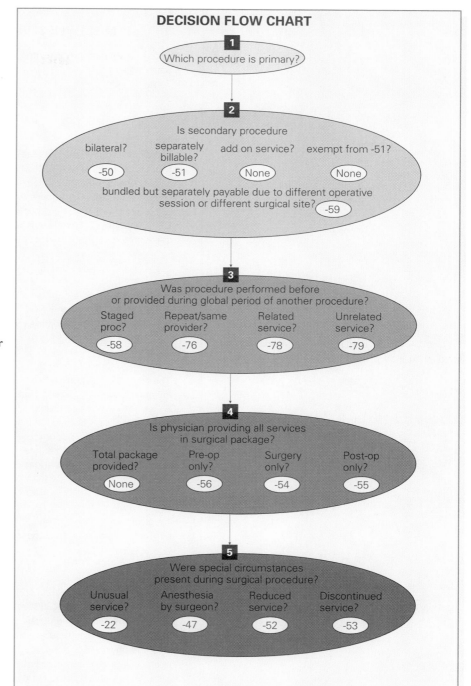

Figure 5–11. *A*, Decision flow chart for surgical procedures.

a major surgical procedure within 24 hours of the office visit (e.g., those with a 90-day follow-up period); see Examples 5–26 and 5–27. A -57 modifier may be used for inpatient or outpatient consultations, inpatient hospital visits, and new or established patient visits that occur the day of or the day before surgery. Do not attach modifier -57 to a hospital visit code for the day before surgery or the day of surgery when a decision for a major surgical procedure was made a week before surgery. Think of -57 as telling the insurance company that the office visit *is not* part of the global fee.

MULTIPLE SURGICAL PROCEDURES

Multiple services must be related to:
- Same patient
- Same provider
- Same date of service

- List all procedures in order of reimbursement, highest to lowest
- Most comprehensive service brings greatest reimbursement and is considered primary
- Check all procedures to make sure there is no unbundling, i.e., using two codes when one code describes procedure
- Decision making expands at this point. Follow numbered question to determine correct modifier usage

-50 bilateral procedure, not described by code
-51 not bundled, separately billable
-59 ordinarily bundled, separately payable due to special circumstance

Figure 5–11. *B*, Description of modifiers for multiple surgical procedure flow chart.

- The term "primary procedure" can also refer to the first procedure initiating a global surgical period
-58 Current service was planned prospectively at time of first service
-76 Physician repeats procedure subsequent to original procedure
-78 Return to operating room for subsequent procedure, complication relating to original procedure
-79 Unrelated procedure performed during global period of previous surgery

- Surgical package means one fee covers the whole package, surgical procedure and postoperative care

5

-22 An extremely difficult procedure due to altered anatomy or unusual circumstances (add 10–30% to reimbursement)
-47 When the surgeon administers regional or general anesthesia
-52 Procedure/service reduced or eliminated at the discretion of the physician
-53 Procedure is discontinued due to extenuating circumstances or because of threat to the patient

B

-25 Significantly Separately Identifiable E/M Service

In some cases, you may be confused whether to assign modifier -25 or -57. Modifier -25 is defined as "Significant, separately identifiable evaluation and management service by same physician on the same day of the procedure or other service." The industry standard is to use -25 when a diagnostic procedure or minor *non-starred procedure* is involved (e.g., those with 0- to 10-day follow-up period). Typically, E/M services that would be modi-

A new patient is seen in the office complaining of a great deal of pain. Cholangiography is done and reveals blocked bile ducts. The patient is scheduled for surgery the next day.

| 8-1-20XX | 99204-**57** | New patient office visit | $00.00 |
| 8-2-20XX | 47600 | Cholecystectomy | $000.00 |

fied with -25 are office visits performed on the day of a minor (non-starred) procedure for an established patient. However, the confusion results because the CPT code book states, "This modifier is

A new patient comes to the office after sustaining a fall while in-line skating. She is in distress, complaining of right wrist pain and swelling of the joint. The injury is evaluated **(1)** with an x-ray film **(2)**. It is determined that the patient has a Smith fracture and manipulation is performed. A long-arm cast is applied **(3)** using fiberglass (Hexcelite) material **(4)**.

(1)	99203-**57**	Initial office evaluation (detailed) **with decision for surgery**
(2)	73100-RT	Radiologic examination, right wrist, AP and lat views
(3)	25605	Closed treatment of distal radial fracture (e.g., Colles or Smith type), with manipulation
(4)	99070	Supplies: Casting material (private carrier) Medicine Section code
	or	
		Supplies: Hexcelite material (Medicare carrier)
	A4590	HCPCS Level II code

The patient returns in 4 weeks for follow-up care **(1)**. The wrist is x-rayed again **(2)**, the long-arm cast is removed **(3)**, and a short-arm cast is applied **(4)** using plaster material **(5)**.

(1)	No code	Follow-up care included in global fee
(2)	73100-RT	Radiologic examination, right wrist, AP and lat views
(3)	No code	Cast removal included in original fracture care (25605)
(4)	29075-**58**	Application, plaster, elbow to finger (short arm) **staged procedure**
(5)	99070	Supplies: Casting material (private carrier) Medicine Section code
	or	
		Supplies: Plaster material (Medicare carrier)
	A4580	HCPCS Level II code

not used to report an E/M service that resulted in a decision to perform surgery. See modifier -57."

Another consideration when a decision to perform surgery takes place on the same day as the procedure is code 99025 from the Medicine Section of CPT, Special Services and Reports, Miscellaneous Services. Code 99025, however, can only be used in lieu of an E/M code for an initial (new patient) visit, when a starred (*) surgical procedure constitutes major services at that visit (see Example 5–3).

When making the decision regarding which code/modifier to use for a surgical procedure performed within 24 hours of an office visit, consult Figure 5–12.

In Medicare cases, the HCFA has published in the *Correct Coding Initiative* the specific codes for modifier -25 use after October 2000. Refer to the bulletin or newsletter pertinent to this update.

-58 Staged or Related Procedure

This modifier is used to indicate that the performance of a procedure or service during the postoperative period was

◗ Planned (staged) at the time of the original procedure.
◗ More extensive than the original procedure.
◗ For therapy after a diagnostic surgical procedure.

Such circumstances should be reported by adding modifier -58 to the staged or related procedure, or the separate five-digit modifier may be used (09958). The use of this modifier requires accurate documentation of events leading up to surgeries and any subsequent surgeries. It is only possible to modify procedures if the coder has all of the relevant facts and circumstances. In Example 5–27, the fracture is considered surgery because it is in the surgery section of the CPT book. All fracture codes have 90-day postoperative periods.

-62, -66, -80, -81, -82 More Than One Surgeon

If more than one surgeon is involved, clarify for whom you are billing by using two-digit modifiers (-62, co-surgeon; -66, team surgery; -80, assistant at surgery; -81, minimum assistant surgeon, or -82, assistant surgeon when a qualified resident surgeon is not available) (see Examples 5–21 and 5–28).

Modifier -80 (assistant at surgery) is commonly used when billing for a physician who assists another (primary) physician in performing a surgical procedure (see Example 5–28).

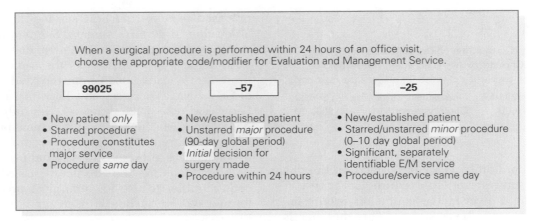

When a surgical procedure is performed within 24 hours of an office visit, choose the appropriate code/modifier for Evaluation and Management Service.

99025	–57	–25
• New patient *only*	• New/established patient	• New/established patient
• Starred procedure	• Unstarred *major* procedure	• Starred/unstarred *minor* procedure
• Procedure constitutes major service	(90-day global period)	(0–10 day global period)
• Procedure *same* day	• *Initial* decision for surgery made	• Significant, separately identifiable E/M service
	• Procedure within 24 hours	• Procedure/service same day

Figure 5–12. Reference chart for making a decision when to select code 99025 or modifiers -57 or -25.

EXAMPLE 5–28

Closure of intestinal cutaneous fistula
Operating surgeon reports   44640   **No modifier**
Assistant surgeon reports   44640-80   **With modifier**

The assisting doctor is usually paid a fee of 16% to 30% of the allowed fee the primary surgeon receives for performing the surgery. The assisting physician uses the same surgical code as the primary surgeon and adds the -80 modifier to it. The fee indicating a reduced percentage is typically listed as the fee on the claim form. However, some insurance carriers may prefer having the full fee listed and making the reduction on their end. Under Medicare guidelines, there may be some surgical procedures that restrict payment for an assistant surgeon, so refer to the provider manual or contact the fiscal intermediary for information.

-99 Multiple Modifiers

If a procedure requires more than one modifier code, use the two-digit modifier -99 after the usual five-digit code number, all typed on one line, or a separate five-digit code (09999) in addition to the basic five-digit procedure code number, each typed on separate lines. Some insurance companies require -99 with a separate note in Block 19 of the HCFA-1500 claim form or in the freeform area of electronic submissions, indicating which two or more modifiers are being used. Remember to ask the insurance company which format is preferred when submitting claims that reflect modifier -99 (see Example 5–29).

EXAMPLE 5–29

A physician sees a patient who is grossly obese. The operative report documents that a bilateral sliding-type inguinal herniorrhaphy was performed, and the procedure took 2 hours 15 minutes.

49525-99	Bilateral repair sliding inguinal hernia re-
-50	quiring 2 hours 15 minutes
-22	

OR

49525	Repair sliding inguinal hernia
09999	Multiple modifiers
09950	Bilateral procedure
09922	Unusual services requiring increased time (2 hours 15 minutes)

HCPCS Modifiers

Besides CPT and RVS modifiers, HCPCS level II and III modifiers are used by Medicare and level II may be used by some commercial carriers. HCPCS level II modifiers may be two alpha digits (see Example 5–30), two alphanumeric characters (Fig. 5–13), or a single alpha digit used for reporting ambulance services or results of PET scans. A brief list of these modifiers may be found in Appendix A of the CPT code book. A comprehensive list may be found in an HCPCS national level II code book. HCPCS reference books may be obtained from resources listed in Appendix B.

Use the two-digit HCPCS modifiers whenever they are required. HCPCS modifiers further describe the services provided and can either *increase* or *decrease* the physician's fee. If not used properly, they

---

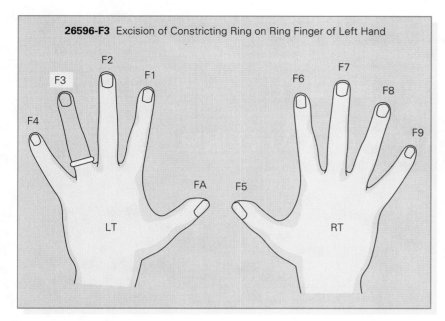

26596-F3 Excision of Constricting Ring on Ring Finger of Left Hand

Figure 5–13. HCPCS digital alphanumeric modifiers FA through F9 used to identify fingers of right and left hands.

EXAMPLE 5–30

When taking x-ray films of both feet, the billing portion of the insurance claim would appear as follows:

| 05/06/XX | 73620 **RT** | $00.00 Radiologic examination, foot—right |
| 05/06/XX | 73620 **LT** | $00.00 Radiologic examination, foot—left |

Table 5–4 to gain information on additional modifiers and their use illustrated by clinical examples.

STUDENT ASSIGNMENT LIST

✔ Study Chapter 5.
✔ Answer the review questions in the *Workbook* to reinforce the theory learned in this chapter and to help prepare you for a future test.
✔ Complete the assignments in the *Workbook* to assist you in hands-on practical experience in procedural coding as well as learning medical abbreviations.
✔ Turn to the Glossary at the end of this textbook for a further understanding of the Key Terms used in this chapter.

can drastically affect the physician's fee profile by reducing future payments to the physician.

Comprehensive List of Modifier Codes

Now that you have learned about some basic modifiers, read through the comprehensive list shown in

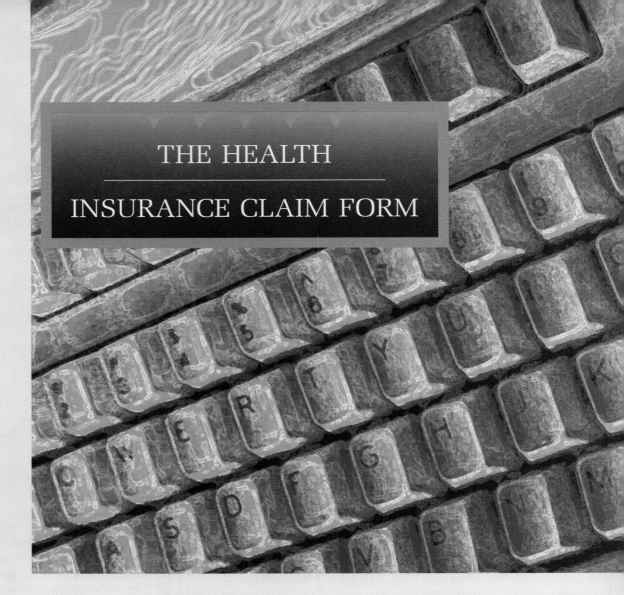

THE HEALTH
INSURANCE CLAIM FORM

6

CHAPTER OUTLINE

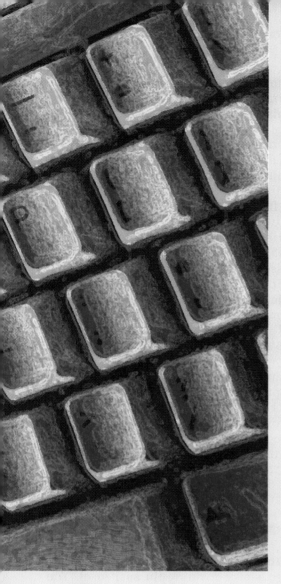

- Explain the difference between clean, pending, rejected, incomplete, and invalid claims.
- Abstract from the patient record relevant information for completing the HCFA-1500 insurance claim form.
- Describe reasons why claims are rejected.
- Minimize the number of insurance forms returned because of improper completion.
- Identify techniques required for optically scanned insurance claims.
- Execute general guidelines for completing the HCFA-1500 claim form for federal, state, and private payer insurance contracts.

OBJECTIVES*

After reading this chapter, you should be able to:

- Give the history of the Health Insurance Claim Form (HCFA-1500).
- State when the HCFA-1500 claim form may or may not be used.
- Expedite the handling and processing of the HCFA-1500 insurance claim form.
- Define two types of claims submission.

KEY TERMS

clean claim

digital fax claim

dingy claim

dirty claim

durable medical equipment (DME) number

electronic claim

employer identification number (EIN)

facility provider number

group provider number

Health Insurance Claim Form (HCFA-1500)

incomplete claim

intelligent character recognition (ICR)

invalid claim

national provider identifier (NPI)

optical character recognition (OCR)

"other" claims

paper claim

pending claim

physically clean claim

provider identification number (PIN)

rejected claim

Social Security number (SSN)

state license number

unique provider identification number (UPIN)

---

*Performance objectives and exercises for hands-on practical experience for this chapter appear in the *Workbook*.

History

In 1958, the Health Insurance Association of America (HIAA) and the American Medical Association (AMA) attempted to standardize the insurance claim form by jointly developing the Standard Form. It was not universally accepted by all third party payers, and as the types of coverage became more variable, new claim forms were instituted that required more information than the original Standard Form. The form eventually became known as COMB-1, or Attending Physician's Statement. In 1968, the HIAA decided to revamp the form so that it would be more adaptable to electronic data processing.

In April 1975, the AMA approved a "universal claim form," called the **Health Insurance Claim Form (HCFA-1500)**, that could be used for both group and individual claims. The HCFA-1500 claim form answered the needs of many health insurers processing claims manually. The National Association of Blue Shield Plans Board of Directors adopted a motion supporting the concept of a uniform national claim form.

Then, in 1990, the HCFA-1500 was revised and printed in red ink, which would allow claims to be optically scanned by the insurance carriers. Beginning on May 1, 1992, all services for Medicare patients from physicians and suppliers except for ambulance services had to be billed on the scannable HCFA-1500 form.

The revised form was adopted by TRICARE Management Activity (TMA) formerly known as the Office of Civilian Health and Medical Programs of the Uniformed Services (OCHAMPUS). It also received the approval of the AMA Council on Medical Services. The HIAA endorses and recommends that their members, who are private insurance companies, accept the form. In some states, the Medicaid program, as well as industrial (workers' compensation) cases, use this form to process claims.

Widespread use of this form will save time and simplify processing of claims for both physicians and carriers, because it eliminates having to complete many various insurance forms brought into the office by patients. Another way of billing that may be accepted by insurance companies is to complete the HCFA-1500 and attach it to the patient's form. Make sure the patient's and employer's portions of the private insurance form are complete and accurate and that the patient has signed the release of information box and the assignment of benefits, if applicable. Both forms are sent directly to the insurance carrier. If the patient is insured with two companies, obtain release of information and assignment for both insurance carriers. Determine which carrier is primary and submit the claim to that carrier first. After the primary insurance carrier has paid, submit a claim to the secondary carrier.

Insurance carriers with various computer programs and equipment that optically scan claims may have instructions on completion of the form that will vary from locality to locality and program to program. Always contact local representatives of insurance carriers to find out whether the form is acceptable before submitting any claims. If the form is processed by the insurance carrier through scanning equipment, a photocopy is not acceptable. Quantities of the HCFA-1500 can be purchased from many medical office supply companies as well as from the American Medical Association, 515 North State Street, Chicago, IL 60610.

In this chapter, instructions for completing a claim using optical character recognition format is emphasized. However, the federal government prefers electronic claims submission to reduce costs and expedite reimbursement. Chapter 7 takes you through the intricacies of transmitting electronic claims as well as the do's and don'ts of transmitting a digital fax claim.

Types of Claims

Claims are either paper or electronic and can be designated as clean or pending (in suspense). You may come across the term "encounter record." This is a buzz term for a claim.

A **paper claim** is one that is submitted on paper, including optically scanned claims that are converted to electronic form by insurance companies. Paper claims may be typed or generated via computer.

An **electronic claim** is one that is submitted to the insurance carrier via a central processing unit (CPU), tape diskette, direct data entry, direct wire, dial-in telephone, or personal computer via modem. Electronic claims are never printed on paper.

A **digital fax claim** is sent to the insurance carrier as a paper claim via fax but never printed to paper at the receiving end. The fax is encoded by an optical code reader and is transmitted into the claims processing system. It is not considered an electronic claim.

Claim Status

A **clean claim** means that the claim was submitted within the program or policy time limit and contains all necessary information so it can be processed and paid promptly. A **physically clean claim** is one that has no staples or highlighted areas and on which the bar code area has not been deformed.

A **pending claim** is an insurance claim that is held in suspense due to review or other reason. These claims may be cleared for payment or denied.

Medicare Claim Status

In the Medicare program, besides the phrase "clean claims," specific terms, such as *incomplete, rejected, invalid, dirty,* and *dingy,* are used to describe various claim processing situations. These terms may or may not be used by other insurance programs.

A *clean claim* means the following:

1. The claim has no deficiencies and passes all electronic edits.
2. The carrier does not need to investigate outside of the carrier's operation before paying the claim.
3. The claim is investigated on a postpayment basis, meaning a claim is not delayed before payment and may be paid.
4. The claim is subject to medical review with attached information or forwarded simultaneously with electronic medical claim (EMC) records.

Medicare claims not considered "clean" claims, which require investigation or development on a prepayment basis (developed for Medicare Secondary Payer information), are known as **"other" claims.**

Participating provider electronic submissions are processed within approximately 14 days of receipt. Participating provider paper submissions and nonparticipating provider claims are not processed until at least 27 days after receipt.

An **incomplete claim** is any Medicare claim missing required information. It is identified to the provider so it can be resubmitted.

A **rejected claim** is one that requires investigation and needs further clarification and possibly answers to some questions. Such a claim may need to be resubmitted.

An **invalid claim** is any Medicare claim that contains complete, necessary information but is illogical or incorrect (e.g., listing an incorrect provider number for a referring physician). An invalid claim is identified to the provider and may be resubmitted.

A **dirty claim** is a claim submitted with errors, one requiring manual processing for resolving problems, or one rejected for payment. Pending or suspense claims are placed in this category be-

cause something is holding the claim back from payment, perhaps review or some other problem.

A **dingy claim** happens when the Medicare contractor cannot process a claim for a particular service or bill type. These claims are held until the necessary systems changes are implemented to pay the claim correctly.

Abstracting from Medical Records

You may be asked to abstract technical information from patient records in either of three situations: (1) to complete insurance claim forms; (2) when sending a letter to justify a health insurance claim after professional services are rendered; or (3) when a patient applies for life, mortgage, or health insurance. Abstracting to complete insurance claims is discussed later in this chapter.

Cover Letter Accompanying Insurance Claims

A letter accompanying insurance claims should include the patient's name, subscriber identification number, date and type of service, a short history, and a clear but concise explanation of the medical necessity, difficulty or complexity, or unusual circumstance (i.e., emergency). Send the letter and insurance claim to the attention of the claims supervisor so it may be directed to the appropriate person for processing.

Life or Health Insurance Applications

When a patient applies for insurance, the insurance company may request information from the patient's private physician and/or may require a physical examination.

On some application forms (Fig. 6–1), the release of medical information signed by the patient may appear as a separate sheet or as a perforated attachment to a multiple-paged form. In the latter, page 1 is completed by the insurance agent when interviewing the client, page 2 is filled in by the prospective insured, and page 3 is completed by the physician at the time of the physical examination of the prospective insured. Sometimes a form is sent to the client's attending physician along with a check requesting medical information (Fig. 6–2). The amount of the check may vary, depending on how much information is requested. If the check is not included, the physician should request a fee based on the length of the report before sending in the completed report form. You must have the fee before completion of the form, or you may not receive payment.

PART II of Application to the MASSACHUSETTS INDEMNITY AND LIFE INSURANCE COMPANY

PROPOSED
INSURED
OR ANNUITANT: _Jason F. Reed_

Date of Birth _March 10, 1972_
Mo.   Day   Year

1. a. Name and address of your personal physician? _Gerald Practon, MD 4567 Broad Ave.,_
(If none, so state)
   b. Date and reason last consulted? _November 4, 1999_   _Woodland Hills, XY 12345_
   c. What treatment was given or medication prescribed? _Rx flumadine_

	Yes	No
2. Have you ever been treated for or ever had any known indication of:		
a. Disorder of eyes, ears, nose, or throat?	☐	☑
b. Dizziness, fainting, convulsions, recurrent headache, speech defect, paralysis or stroke, mental or nervous disorder?	☐	☑
c. Shortness of breath, persistent hoarseness or cough, blood spitting, bronchitis, pleurisy, asthma, emphysema, tuberculosis or chronic respiratory disorder?	☐	☑
d. Chest pain, palpitation, high blood pressure, rheumatic fever, heart murmur, heart attack or other disorder of the heart or blood vessels?	☐	☑
e. Jaundice, intestinal bleeding, ulcer, hernia, appendicitis, colitis, diverticulitis, hemorrhoids, recurrent indigestion, or other disorder of the stomach, intestines, liver or gallbladder?	☐	☑
f. Sugar, albumin, blood or pus in urine, venereal disease, stone or other disorder of kidney, bladder, prostate or reproductive organs?		
g. Diabetes, thyroid or other endocrine disorders?	☐	☑
h. Neuritis, sciatica, rheumatism, arthritis, gout or disorder of the muscles or bones, including the spine, back, or joints?	☐	☑
i. Deformity, lameness or amputation?	☐	☑
j. Disorder of skin, lymph glands, cyst, tumor or cancer?	☐	☑
k. Allergies, anemia or other disorder of the blood?	☐	☑
l. Excessive use of alcohol, tobacco, sedatives, or any habit-forming drugs?	☐	☑
3. Are you now under observation or taking treatment?	☐	☑
4. Have you had any change in weight in the past year?	☐	☑
5. Other than above, have you within the past 5 years:	☐	☑
a. Had any mental or physical disorder not listed above?	☑	☐
b. Had a checkup consultation, illness, injury, surgery?	☐	☑
c. Been a patient in a hospital, clinic, sanatorium, or other medical facility?	☐	☑
d. Had electrocardiogram, X-ray, blood sugar, basal metabolism, other diagnostic test?	☑	☐
e. Been advised to have any diagnostic test, hospitalization, or surgery which was not completed?	☐	☑
6. Have you ever had military service deferment, rejection or discharge because of a physical or mental condition?	☐	☑
7. Have you ever requested or received a pension, benefits, or payment because of an injury, sickness or disability?	☐	☑
8. Family History: Tuberculosis, diabetes cancer, high blood pressure, heart or kidney disease, mental illness or suicide?	☑	☐

DETAILS of "Yes" answers. (IDENTIFY QUESTION NUMBER, CIRCLE APPLICABLE ITEMS: Include diagnoses, dates, duration and names and addresses of all attending physicians and medical facilities.)

5b. Last checkup 1997
(G. Procton MD)

5d. Blood serology

8. Father is diabetic

	Age if Living	Cause of Death?	Age at Death?
Father	55		
Mother	54		
Brothers and Sisters	2		
No. Living			
No. Dead			

(For non-medical cases only)
Height _ _ _ _ _ _ _ Weight _ _ _ _ _ _ _

9. Females only:	Yes	No
a. Have you ever had any disorder of menstruation, pregnancy or of the female organs or breasts?	☐	☐
b. To the best of your knowledge and belief are you now pregnant?	☐	☐

I HEREBY DECLARE that, to the best of my knowledge and belief, the statements and answers in Part II of this Application are full, complete, and true. These statements and answers are to be considered as the basis for any insurance written hereon.

Signed at: (City & State) _Woodland Hills, XY_   Dated: _January 25, 20XX_

X _Jason F. Reed_

_ _
Signature of witness   Signature of PROPOSED INSURED

Form MD (70)a

Figure 6–1. The prospective insured completes this side of the insurance application form.

PART III—PHYSICIAN'S EXAMINATION REPORT

Acct. No. _145_ District or Agency _____ Name of Agent _James Santor_

Date _Jan. 25, 20xx_ Name of Insuring Company _Hartman Insurance Company_

PROPOSED INSURED: _Reed_ (Last Name) _Jason_ (First Name) _F._ (Middle Initial) Date of Birth _3_ Mo. _10_ Day _1972_ Year

10a.	Height (In Shoes)	Weight (Clothed)	Chest (Full Inspiration)	Chest (Forced Expiration)	Abdomen, at Umbilicus	Details of "Yes" answers. (Identify item.)
	_5_ ft. _11_ in.	_180_ lbs.	_43_ in.	_42_ in.	_38_ in.	

b. Did you weigh?...... ☒ Yes ☐ No Did you measure?.......... ☒ Yes ☐ No

c. Is appearance unhealthy or older than stated age?............... ☐ Yes ☒ No

11. Blood Pressure (Record ALL readings)

Systolic	120		
Diastolic { 4th phase	80		
{ 5th phase			

12. Pulse:

Rate	At Rest	After Exercise	3 minutes later
	60	86	66
Irregularities per min.			

13. Heart: Is there any:

Enlargement............... ☐ Yes ☒ No   Dyspnea.............. ☐ Yes ☒ No

Murmur(s).................. ☐ Yes ☒ No   Edema.............. ☐ Yes ☒ No

(describe below—if more than one, describe separately)

Location [   ] [   ]

MCL

			Indicate:
Constant	☐	☐	Apex by X
Inconstant	☐	☐	Murmur area by ↻
Transmitted	☐	☐	
Localized	☐	☐	Point of greatest intensity by O
Systolic	☐	☐	
Presystolic	☐	☐	Transmission by ▶
Diastolic	☐	☐	
Soft (Gr. 1–2)	☐	☐	
Mod. (Gr. 3–4)	☐	☐	
Loud (Gr. 5–6)	☐	☐	For comments and your impression?

After Exercise:

Increased	☐	☐
Absent	☐	☐
Unchanged	☐	☐
Decreased	☐	☐

14. Is there on examination any abnormality of the following: Yes No
(Circle applicable items and give details.)

(a) Eyes, ears, nose, mouth, pharynx? ☐ ☒
(If vision or hearing markedly impaired, indicate degree and correction)

(b) Skin (incl. scars); lymph nodes; varicose veins or peripheral arteries?.................... ☐ ☒

(c) Nervous system (include reflexes, gait, paralysis)?......... ☐ ☒

(d) Respiratory system? .... ☐ ☒

(e) Abdomen (include scars)? .... ☐ ☒

(f) Genitourinary system (include prostate)?.............. ☐ ☒

(g) Endocrine system (include thyroid and breasts)? .... ☐ ☒

(h) Musculoskeletal system (include spine, joints, amputations, deformities)?....................... ☐ ☒
(A confidential report may be sent to the Medical Director)

15. (a) Are there any hernias? .... ☐ ☒
   (b) Any hemorrhoids?........................ ☐ ☒

16. Are you aware of any additional medical history?............... ☐ ☒

17. Was the examination conducted in the English language?.... ☒ ☐
If No, complete the following:
   a. Was an interpreter used?................. ☐ ☒
   b. What language was used? _____
   c. Relationship of interpreter to proposed insured?_____

Urinalysis: Specific Gravity   Albumin _0_   Sugar _trace_

Is specimen being sent?.............. ☒ Yes ☐ No
If Yes, where? _ABC laboratory_

Send Specimen: (Details according to Company) _____

Date: _1-25-20xx_   Time: _10_ ⓐ.M./P.M.   City: _Woodland Hills_   State: _XY_

Signature of Medical Examiner: _Gerald Practon_   M.D.   Physical Measurements Information_____

PMI-188R—1-88

Figure 6–2. Sample of a life insurance application form with the check to the physician omitted. The physician completes this side of the form at the time of the examination of the patient, the prospective insured.

A

Block 24A
Dates of
Service

Block 24D
Documentation
of professional
services
rendered

Block 14
Date of last
menstrual
period

Block 21
Primary and
secondary
diagnoses

DATE	PROGRESS
2-10-2000	This 35-year-old Hispanic female recently moved to this city. She is employed as a legal secretary. She began having labor pains and was admitted to College Hospital on 2/10/2000. LMP 5-5-99. Primiparous. Healthy 6 lb 4 oz baby girl was delivered vaginally.
	mtf Bertha Caesar, MD
2-11-2000	Hospital visit. Normal postpartum. Patient resting comfortably.
	mtf Bertha Caesar, MD
2-12-2000	Hospital visit.
	mtf Bertha Caesar, MD
2-13-200	Discharged from hospital. Patient has been off work since Jan. 25, 2 weeks before delivery and will return to work March 29, six weeks after delivery. Patient to be seen in the office for two week check up.
	mtf Bertha Caesar, MD

Block 18
Dates of
hospitalization

Block 16
Dates of
disability

B

14. DATE OF CURRENT: MM DD YYYY 05 5 1999 ◄ ILLNESS (First symptom) OR INJURY (Accident) OR PREGNANCY (LMP)

15. IF PATIENT HAS HAD SAME OR SIMILAR ILLNESS GIVE FIRST DATE MM DD YY

16. DATES PATIENT UNABLE TO WORK IN CURRENT OCCUPATION FROM MM DD YYYY 01 25 20XX TO MM DD YYYY 03 28 20XX

17. NAME OF REFERRING PHYSICIAN OR OTHER SOURCE

17a. I.D. NUMBER OF REFERRING PHYSICIAN

18. HOSPITALIZATION DATES RELATED TO CURRENT SERVICES FROM MM DD YYYY 02 10 20XX TO MM DD YYYY 02 13 20XX

19. RESERVED FOR LOCAL USE

20. OUTSIDE LAB? ☐ YES ☒ NO $ CHARGES

21. DIAGNOSIS OR NATURE OF ILLNESS OR INJURY. (RELATE ITEMS 1,2,3 OR 4 TO ITEM 24E BY LINE)

1. 650
2. V27 0
3.
4.

22. MEDICAID RESUBMISSION CODE ORIGINAL REF. NO.

23. PRIOR AUTHORIZATION NUMBER

24. A DATE(S) OF SERVICE From MM DD YYYY	To MM DD YYYY	B Place of Service	C Type of Service	D PROCEDURES, SERVICES, OR SUPPLIES (Explain Unusual Circumstances) CPT/HCPCS MODIFIER	E DIAGNOSIS CODE	F $ CHARGES	G DAYS OR UNITS	H EPSDT Family Plan	I EMG	J COB	K RESERVED FOR LOCAL USE
1 0210 20XX		21		59410	1 2	1600 00	1			43	05675700
2											
3											
4											
5											
6											

25. FEDERAL TAX I.D. NUMBER 725713051 SSN ☐ EIN ☒

26. PATIENT'S ACCOUNT NO.

27. ACCEPT ASSIGNMENT? (For govt. claims, see back) ☒ YES ☐ NO

28. TOTAL CHARGE $ 1600 00

29. AMOUNT PAID $

30. BALANCE DUE $ 1600 00

31. SIGNATURE OF PHYSICIAN OR SUPPLIER INCLUDING DEGREES OR CREDENTIALS (I certify that the statements on the reverse apply to this bill and are made a part thereof.)
BERTHA CAESAR MD
SIGNED 021520XX DATE

32. NAME AND ADDRESS OF FACILITY WHERE SERVICES WERE RENDERED (if other than home or office)
COLLEGE HOSPITAL
4500 BROAD AVENUE
WOODLAND HILLS XY 12345 0001
95 0731067

33. PHYSICIAN'S, SUPPLIER'S BILLING NAME, ADDRESS, ZIP CODE AND PHONE #
COLLEGE CLINIC
4567 BROAD AVENUE
WOODLAND HILLS XY 12345 0001
013 486 9002
PIN# GRP# 3664021CC

reference initials

FORM RRB-1500

ICD-9-CM
650 Normal delivery
V27.0 Single liveborn

CPT
59410 Vaginal delivery only (with or without episiotomy and/or forceps); including postpartum care

Figure 6–3. *A,* Example of a chart note illustrating important information to read through and abstract for insurance claim completion. *B,* The location of the abstracted information placed in the blocks on an HCFA-1500 insurance claim form in OCR format.

If you are asked to abstract medical information from the patient's record, be extremely accurate. Figure 6–3 is a chart note identifying important abstracting components. Be certain that you understand abbreviations on the chart. Give only the information requested. If the form has questions about high blood pressure, kidney infection, or heart problems, you could prohibit a patient from obtaining life, health, or mortgage insurance if your answers are derogatory. If the urine sample shows albumin or sugar, a person could also be denied insurance. If a patient has had a chronic illness, ask the physician if a euphemism can be substituted. A *euphemism* is a word or phrase substituted for one considered offensively explicit, such as "remains" for "corpse."

If a patient tests positive for human immunodeficiency virus (HIV), legal counsel may be necessary, because some state laws allow information on HIV infection and the acquired immunodeficiency syndrome (AIDS) to be given only to the patient or to the patient's spouse. In some states, it is illegal to require a blood test for HIV antibodies, a urinalysis for HIV, or an HIV antigen test as a condition of coverage. It may also be illegal to question applicants about HIV status or prior symptoms of and treatment for AIDS or other forms of immune deficiency. Sometimes, private group plans allow medical coverage for people testing positive for HIV or an AIDS-related illness through a state major risk medical insurance program. However, if the maximum enrollment number is reached, the waiting period may exceed 1 year.

Sometimes a narrative report dictated by the physician is preferable to filling in the form, especially if there are long columns to check and no space for comments. It may even be necessary to attach a copy of an operative, pathology, laboratory, or radiology report and an electrocardiogram (ECG) tracing. ECG tracings mounted upside-down have resulted in rejections of insurance applications.

Place a "Please Read" note on the insurance questionnaire to have the physician check it over thoroughly before signing it and to make sure that the information is accurate and properly stated.

An insurance company may ask a copy service to come to your office to photocopy the patient's record. This is usually done at the office's convenience, and an appointment should be made. Remind the insurance company that you must have an authorization form signed by the patient to release medical information. Charge accordingly and quote the fee at the time of the telephone request. The physician should review the records in advance to see that they are in proper order.

Health Insurance Claim Form (HCFA-1500)

Basic Guidelines for Submitting a Claim

Use the HCFA-1500 insurance claim form as often as possible. It is accepted by nearly all private insurance carriers as well as Medicaid, Medicare, TRICARE, and workers' compensation.

Complete and submit a claim form whenever you are asked to do so by the patient, even though you think there is no coverage, unless the patient accepts your tactful suggestion that he or she is not covered. If in question, check with the insurance carrier for eligibility status. An official rejection from the insurance company is the best answer to present to the patient in this situation. The patient may be unaware of major medical credits accrued because of nonpayment of benefits from a basic plan. It is feasible to bill and get paid for services rendered even though the patient may not think that he or she is covered.

Individual Insurance

When a patient brings in a form from a private insurance plan that is not like the HCFA-1500 claim form, have him or her sign it. In addition, have the patient sign the HCFA-1500 claim form in two places (the Assignment of Benefits and Release of Information, Blocks 12 and 13). Make sure the patient's portion of the private insurance form is complete and accurate. Mail the forms together to the insurance carrier. Some companies allow staples and some do not. It is not recommended to let patients direct their own forms to insurance companies or employers. Patients have been known to lose forms or alter data on documents before mailing, forget to send them, or mail them to an incorrect address.

Group Insurance

When a patient has group insurance through an employer, look for an employer's section and make sure this part of the private insurance form has been completed. If it is not completed, send the form to the employer before completing the physician's section of the HCFA-1500 claim form. If the employer's section is complete, send both forms directly to the insurance carrier after the physician's portion is completed.

Secondary Insurance

When two insurance policies are involved (sometimes called dual coverage), one is considered pri-

A husband and wife have insurance through their employers and each has added the spouse to their plans for secondary coverage. If the wife is seen for treatment, then the insurance plan sponsored by her employer would be primary and her husband's plan would be secondary.

mary and the other secondary (see Example 6–1). The primary policy is the policy held by the patient when the patient and his or her spouse are both insured. Always obtain the patient's signature for release of information and assignment of benefits for both insurance companies.

After payment is made by the primary plan, then a claim is submitted with a copy of the explanation of benefits from the primary carrier to the secondary carrier.

Completion of Insurance Claim Forms

Check with private insurance carriers to see if they optically scan insurance claim forms. If a claim is optically scanned by the insurance company, do NOT put any comments in blocks that are unanswerable or do not apply. Leave them blank. The computer scanner will kick out the claim if any marks are entered into nonapplicable blocks. If a form is not optically scanned by the insurance carrier, then it may be a good idea to answer all questions on the form. If any are unanswerable, type DNA (Does Not Apply) or NA or N/A (Not Applicable) or simply put a dashed line.

Diagnosis

In Block 21, diagnosis field, insert all accurate diagnostic codes that affect the patient's condition, listing the primary diagnosis code first followed by any secondary diagnosis codes. Never submit a diagnosis without supporting documentation in the medical record. Be certain the diagnosis agrees with the treatment. If there is no formal diagnosis at the conclusion of an encounter, submit the code(s) for the patient's symptom(s).

To avoid confusion, it is best to list only one illness or injury and its treatment per form, unless there are concurrent conditions.

Service Dates

Do not ditto dates for services performed. Do not submit charges for services rendered in different years on the same claim form. Sometimes such practices can be affected by deductible and eligibility factors, thereby delaying reimbursement.

Consecutive Dates

Some carriers allow hospital and/or office visits to be grouped if each visit is consecutive, occurs in the same month, uses the same procedure code, and results in the same fee. The fee for a single procedure should be listed in Block 24F, and the number of times the procedure was performed should be listed in Block 24G as illustrated in the graphic at the bottom of this page. However, check with private insurance carriers because some carriers require a total fee listed in Block 24F rather than the fee for a single procedure. If there is a difference in the procedure code or fee for several visits listed on the claim, each hospital/office visit must be itemized and each procedure code and charge entered on separate lines.

No Charge

Do not submit a claim for services that have no charge unless the patient requests that you send it in. These services should appear documented in the patient's medical and financial records.

Physicians' Identification Numbers

Insurance companies and federal and state programs require certain identification numbers on claim forms submitted from individuals and facilities who provide and bill for services to patients. Because there are so many different numbers, this can be confusing to the beginner as well as someone experienced in insurance billing procedures. Therefore, an explanation will be given.

24.	A				B	C	D		E		F		G	H	I	J	K
	DATE(S) OF SERVICE				Place of Service	Type of Service	PROCEDURES, SERVICES, OR SUPPLIES (Explain Unusual Circumstances)		DIAGNOSIS CODE		$ CHARGES		DAYS OR UNITS	EPSDT Family Plan	EMG	COB	RESERVED FOR LOCAL USE
	From MM DD YY		To MM DD YY				CPT/HCPCS	MODIFIER									
1	10 04 2000		10 08 2000		21		99232		1		55	56	5				
2																	

▶ **State License Number:** To practice within a state, each physician must obtain a physician's **state license number**. Sometimes this number is requested on forms and used as a provider number.

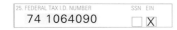

▶ **Employer Identification Number:** In a medical group or solo practice, each physician must have his or her own federal tax identification number, known as an **employer identification number (EIN)**. This is issued by the Internal Revenue Service for income tax purposes.

25. FEDERAL TAX I.D. NUMBER		SSN	EIN
74 1064090		☐	X

▶ **Social Security Number:** In addition, each physician has a **Social Security number (SSN)** for other personal use and may have one or more *tax identification numbers (TIN)* for financial reasons. These are not typically used on the claim form unless the provider does not have an EIN.

25. FEDERAL TAX I.D. NUMBER		SSN	EIN
082 19 1707		X	☐

Provider Numbers

Claims may require three provider identification numbers, one for the referring physician, one for the ordering physician, and one for the performing physician (billing entity). It is possible that the ordering physician and the performing physician are the same. On rare occasions, the number may be the same for all three, but more frequently three different numbers are required depending on the circumstances of the case. For placement of the provider number on the HCFA-1500 claim form, refer to the block-by-block instructions for Blocks 17a and 24j–k. Keep in mind what role the physician(s) and their numbers represent in relationship to the provider listed in Block 33. The following examples of blocks from the HCFA-1500 insurance claim form show where these numbers are commonly placed.

To assist you with claims completion, compile a reference list of provider numbers for all ordering physicians and physicians who frequently refer patients. To obtain the physicians' provider numbers, call their offices or obtain them through your Medicare carrier. When completing Workbook assignments, refer to Appendix A for all physician provider numbers.

▶ **Provider Identification Number:** Every physician who renders services to patients may be issued a carrier-assigned **provider identification number (PIN)** by the insurance company.

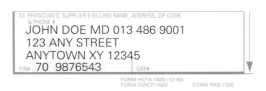

▶ **Unique Provider Identification Number:** The Medicare program issues each physician a **unique provider identification number (UPIN)**.

17a. I.D. NUMBER OF REFERRING PHYSICIAN
4627889700

▶ **Performing Provider Identification Number:** Each physician has a separate PPIN for each group office/clinic in which he or she practices. If a doctor practices in two of the group's four offices, he or she will have two PPINs. In the Medicare program, in addition to a group number, each member of a group is issued an 8-character *performing provider identification number (PPIN)*, which correlates to that particular group's location. (see Example 6–2).

EXAMPLE 6–2

College Clinic
4567 Broad Avenue
Woodland Hills, XY
12345-0001   **Group PIN: 3664021CC**
Cosmo Graff, MD   **PPIN: WA 24516B**

College Clinic
20 South Main Street
Louisville, XY 12670-0341   **Group PIN: 3664021CC**
Cosmo Graff, MD   **PPIN: WA 01021A**

▶ **Group Provider Number:** The **group provider number** is used instead of the individual physician's number (PIN) for the performing provider who is a member of a group practice that submits claims to insurance companies under the group name.

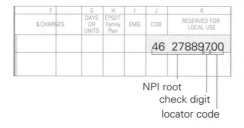

33. PHYSICIAN'S, SUPPLIER'S BILLING NAME, ADDRESS, ZIP CODE & PHONE #
COLLEGE CLINIC 013 486 9002
4567 BROAD AVENUE
WOODLAND HILLS XY 12345 0001
PIN#   GRP#   3664021CC

FORM HCFA-1500 (12-90)
FORM OWCP-1500   FORM RRB-1500

▶ **National Provider Identifier:** In 1997 the Health Care Financing Administration (HCFA) began issuing each provider a Medicare lifetime 10-digit **national provider identifier (NPI)** but as of this printing an implementation date has not been released. When adopted, it will be recognized by Medicaid, Medicare, TRICARE, and CHAMPVA programs and may eventually be used by private insurance carriers. It is possible it may replace some of the existing identification numbers.

F	G	H	I	J	K
$ CHARGES	DAYS OR UNITS	EPSDT Family Plan	EMG	COB	RESERVED FOR LOCAL USE
					46 27889700

NPI root
check digit
locator code

▶ **Durable Medical Equipment Number:** Medicare providers who charge patients a fee for supplies and equipment, such as crutches, urinary catheters, ostomy supplies, surgical dressings, and so forth must bill Medicare using a **durable medical equipment (DME) number**.

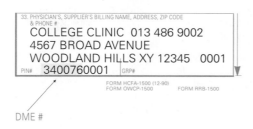

33. PHYSICIAN'S, SUPPLIER'S BILLING NAME, ADDRESS, ZIP CODE & PHONE #
COLLEGE CLINIC 013 486 9002
4567 BROAD AVENUE
WOODLAND HILLS XY 12345 0001
PIN#   3400760001   GRP#

FORM HCFA-1500 (12-90)
FORM OWCP-1500   FORM RRB-1500

DME #

▶ **Facility Provider Number:** Each facility (e.g., hospital, laboratory, radiology office, skilled nursing facility) is issued a **facility provider number** to be used by the performing physician to report services done at the location.

32. NAME AND ADDRESS OF FACILITY WHERE SERVICES WERE RENDERED (If other than home or office)
COLLEGE HOSPITAL
4500 BROAD AVENUE
WOODLAND HILLS XY 12345
95 0731067

A final note: **A PIN number pays!**

Physician's Signature

Have the physician sign the insurance claim form above or under the typed or preprinted physician's name. A stamped signature is allowed in some instances and discussed later in this chapter. To help the physician locate where to sign the claim, use a removable indicator "Sign Here" tag.

Insurance Biller's Initials

The insurance billing specialist should place his or her initials in the bottom left or top right corner of the claim form. Be consistent in placing this reference. Three good reasons to adopt this habit are:

▶ To identify who in the office is responsible for the insurance form
▶ To decrease errors
▶ To avoid being accused of someone else's error, especially if the previous biller submitted a fraudulent claim

Proofread

Proofread every claim. Be aware of larger, more complex claims, because they involve greater sums of money and may be more difficult to complete. Proofread for transposition of numbers (group, policy, physician's I.D., procedure and diagnostic codes), misspelled name, missing date of birth, blanks, and attachments.

Supporting Documentation

Occasionally claims need supporting documents to further explain services billed and to obtain maximum reimbursement.

On any submitted report, include the patient's name, subscriber's name (if different from that of the patient), and insurance identification number in case the document becomes separated from the claim during processing.

If a medication is expensive or experimental, send a copy of the invoice received from the supply house or pharmacy.

When a procedure is complicated, include a copy of all pertinent reports (operative, radiology, laboratory, pathology, discharge summary).

For a treatment not listed in the procedure code book, send in a detailed report, giving the nature, extent, and need for the services. If the claim is submitted electronically, this description should be typed in the narrative field. Use the correct code number for unlisted services or procedures, which usually end in "99" (see Example 6–3).

EXAMPLE 6–3

Unlisted Allergy Testing Procedure 95199

Office Pending File

As mentioned in Chapter 2, file the office copy of the insurance form in a separate alpha (tickler) file for insurance claim copies (which is preferred) or in the back of the patient's medical chart.

Common Reasons Why Claim Forms Are Delayed or Rejected

For quicker claim settlements and to reduce the number of appeals, it is wise to be aware of common billing errors and how to correct them. This may help avoid additional administrative burdens, such as telephone calls, resubmission of claims, appeal letters, and so on. Also see Chapter 8 for information on solutions to denied or delayed claims as well as prevention measures. The following is a list of some reasons why claims are rejected or delayed and suggested solutions when completing the HCFA-1500 insurance claim form blocks.

Problem: Block 1. The claim was submitted to the secondary insurer instead of the primary insurer.

Solution: Obtain data from the patient during the first office visit as to which company is the primary insurer, depending on illness, injury, or accident. Submit the claim to the primary carrier and then send in a claim with the explanation of benefits (EOB) to the secondary carrier.

Problem: Blocks 1–13. Information missing on patient portion of the claim form.

Solution: Obtain a complete patient registration form from which information can be extracted. Educate patients on data requirements at the time of the first visit to the physician's office if patients are filling out their portion.

Problem: Block 1a. The patient's insurance number is incorrect or transposed (especially in Medicare and Medicaid cases).

Solution: Proofread numbers carefully from source documents. Always photocopy front and back sides of insurance identification cards.

Problem: Block 2. Patient's name and insured's name are entered as the same when the patient is a dependent.

Solution: Verify the insured party and check for Sr., Jr., and correct birth date.

Problem: Block 3. Incorrect gender identification, resulting in a diagnosis or procedure code that is inconsistent with patient's gender.

Solution: Proofread claim before mailing and review patient's medical record to locate gender, especially if the patient's first name could be male or female.

Problem: Blocks 9a–d. Incomplete entry for other insurance coverage.

Solution: Accurately abstract data from the patient's registration form. Telephone the patient if information is incomplete.

Problem: Block 10. Failure to indicate whether patient's condition is related to employment or an "other" type of accident.

Solution: Review patient's medical history to find out details of injury or illness and proofread claim before mailing. Telephone the employer to see if permission was given to treat the patient as a workers' compensation case.

Problem: Blocks 12 and 13. Patient's signature is missing.

Solution: Always check the form after the patient signs this block or check the patient's medical record to see if the patient's signature is on file.

Problem: **Block 14**. Date of injury is missing, date of last menstrual period (LMP), or dates of onset of illness are omitted. This information is important for determining whether accident benefits apply, whether patient is eligible for maternity benefits, and whether there was a preexisting condition.

Solution: Do not list unless dates are clearly documented in the patient's medical record. Read the patient's medical history and call patient to obtain date of accident or LMP. Compose an addendum to the record, if necessary. Always proofread claim before mailing so no data are missing.

Problem: **Block 17–17a**. Incorrect or missing name and/or UPIN/NPI of referring physician on claim for consultation or other services requiring this information.

Solution: Check the patient registration form and the chart note for reference to the referring physician. Obtain a list of UPIN/NPI numbers for all physicians in the area.

Problem: **Block 19**. Attachments (e.g., prescription, operative report, manufacturer's invoice) or Medicaid verification (e.g., labels, identification numbers) is missing.

Solution: Submit all information required for pricing or coverage on 8.5- × 11-inch paper with the patient's name, subscriber name (if other than patient), and insurance identification number on each attachment (enclosure). Type the word "AT-TACHMENT" in Block 19 or 10d. Never staple or clip documentation to a claim.

Problem: **Block 21**. Diagnostic code is missing, incomplete, invalid, not in standard nomenclature (e.g., missing fourth or fifth digit), includes a written description, or does not correspond to the treatment (procedure code) rendered by the physician.

Solution: Update encounter forms annually. Verify and submit correct diagnostic codes by referring to an updated diagnostic code book and reviewing the patient record. Check with the physician if diagnosis code listed does not go with the procedure code shown.

Problem: **Block 24A**. Omitted, incorrect, overlapping, or duplicate dates of service.

Solution: Verify against the encounter form or medical record that all dates of service are listed and accurate and appear on individual lines. Date spans for multiple services must be adequate for the number and types of services provided. Each month should be on a separate line and year should be on a separate claim.

Problem: **Block 24B**. Missing or incorrect place of service code.

Solution: Verify the place of service from the encounter form or medical record and list the correct code for place of service and submitted procedure.

Problem: **Block 24C**. Missing or incorrect type of service code for Medicaid, TRICARE, or workers' compensation claims.

Solution: Verify and list the type of service code and confirm that it is correct for the submitted procedure code(s).

Problem: **Block 24D**. Procedure codes are incorrect, invalid, or missing.

Solution: Verify the coding system used by the insurance company and submit correct procedure code(s) by referring to a current procedure code book. For Medicare patients and certain private insurance plans, check the HCPCS manual for HCFA national and local procedure codes.

Problem: **Block 24D**. Incorrect or missing modifier(s).

Solution: Verify usage of modifiers by referring to a current procedure code book and HCPCS manual. Submit valid modifiers with the correct procedure codes (see Chapter 5).

Problem: **Block 24F**. Omitted or incorrect amount billed.

Solution: Be certain the fee column is filled in. Check the amounts charged with the appropriate fee schedule.

Problem: **Block 24G**. Reasons for multiple visits made in 1 day are not stated on an attachment sheet.

Solution: Depending on insurance guidelines, submit documentation explaining reason for multiple visits. Use appropriate modifiers or upcode evaluation and management services to include all visits.

Problem: **Block 24G**. Incorrect quantity billed.

Solution: Verify charge amounts. Make sure that the number of units listed is equal to the date span when more than one date of service is billed (e.g., hospital visits).

Problem: Block 24J–K. Provider's identification number is missing.

Solution: Verify and insert the required provider's number in these blocks.

Problem: Block 24A–K, Line 6. Squeeze in more than six lines per claim form.

Solution: Insert service date and corresponding procedure on lines 1–6 only. If more services need to be billed, complete an additional claim form.

Problem: Block 28. Total amounts do not equal itemized charges.

Solution: Total charges for each claim and verify amounts with patient account. If number of units listed in 24G is more than 1, multiply the units by the fee listed in 24F and add to all other charges listed.

Problem: Block 31. Physician's signature is missing.

Solution: Have the physician or physician's representative sign the claim using a removable indicator "Sign Here" tag to indicate the correct location.

Problem: Block 32. Information is not centered in block as required.

Solution: Enter data centered in block.

Problem: Block 33. Provider's address or PIN or Group number is missing.

Solution: Obtain provider's data from a list that contains all physicians' professional information.

Additional Reasons Why Claim Forms Are Delayed

Problem: No record of the claim at the insurance company.

Solution: Always keep copies of paper claims or electronic transmission receipts. Send claims with large dollar amounts by certified mail, return receipt requested.

Problem: Claim form submitted is illegible.

Solution: Never hand-write a claim form. Check printer ink, toner, or typewriter ribbon and replace when necessary.

Problem: Untimely or lack of response to claim development letters.

Solution: Pay close attention to the due date shown in the letter, and reply to development letters (insurance company's request for additional information) as soon as possible. Send a copy of the claim with the letter and appropriate medical documentation listing the claim control number, if assigned.

Optical Scanned Format Guidelines

Optical Character Recognition

Optical character recognition (OCR) or **intelligent character recognition (ICR)** devices (scanners) are being used more frequently across the nation in processing insurance claims because of their speed and efficiency. A scanner can transfer printed or typed text and bar codes to the insurance company's computer memory. Scanners read at such a fast speed that they reduce data entry cost and decrease processing time.

By using OCR, more control is gained over data input. It improves accuracy, thus reducing coding errors because the claim is entered exactly as coded by the insurance biller.

Do's and Don'ts for Optical Character Recognition

The HCFA-1500 form was developed so insurance carriers could process claims efficiently by OCR or ICR. Typing or keying a form for OCR scanning requires different techniques than preparing one for standard claims submission. Because the majority of insurance carriers accept the OCR format, it is suggested that it be routinely used. Basic do's and don'ts for completing claims using OCR format are given.

DO: use original claim forms printed in red ink; photocopies cannot be scanned.

DON'T: hand-write information on the document. Handwriting is only accepted for signatures. Handwritten claims require manual processing.

Incorrect

APPROVED OMB-0938-008

2 nd request

HEALTH INSURANCE CLAIM FORM   PICA

FECA BLK LUNG (SSN)	OTHER (ID)	1a. INSURED'S I.D. NUMBER	(FOR PROGRAM IN ITEM 1)
		111704521	A482

DO: align the typewriter or printer correctly so characters appear in the proper fields. Enter all information within designated fields.

Correct

DON'T: allow characters to touch lines.

Correct

HEALTH INSURANCE CLAIM FORM

Incorrect

HEALTH INSURANCE CLAIM FORM

DON'T: use script, slant, minifont, or italicized fonts or expanded, compressed, bold, or proportional print. If typing on a typewriter, use an OCR or Manifold typing element in pica Courier 10 or 12 font so that shifting for capitals is unnecessary. Use fonts that have the same width for each character.

DO: use black typewriter ink, high carbon content one-time Mylar or OCR printer ribbons. Change ribbons and/or cartridges frequently for clear print quality.

DO: enter all information in upper case (CAPITAL) letters. Keep characters within the borders of each field.

Correct

DOE JANE E

Incorrect

Doe, Jane E.

DON'T: strike over any errors when correcting or crowd preprinted numbers; OCR equipment does not read corrected characters on top of correction tape or correction fluid.

Correct

Incorrect

DO: indicate a deletion for a delete field and go to the next line to insert the data if an optically scanned form has a delete field. Lines, marks, or characters entered in a delete field will cause deletion of the entire line.

DO: complete a new form for additional services if the case has more than six lines of service.

Correct

Incorrect

DON'T: use highlighter pens or colored ink on claims because OCR equipment will not pick these up.

DO: use alpha or numeric symbols.

DON'T: use symbols (#, −, /), periods (.), ditto marks, parentheses, or commas (,).

Correct

123 45 6789

Incorrect

123-45-6789

DON'T: use decimals in Block 21 or dollar ($) signs in the money column.

Correct

F
$ CHARGES
10000

Incorrect

F
$ CHARGES
$10000

DON'T: use narrative descriptions of procedures, modifiers, or diagnoses; code numbers are sufficient.

Correct

D
PROCEDURES, SERVICES, OR SUPPLIES (Explain Unusual Circumstances)
CPT/HCPCS | MODIFIER
42820 |

Incorrect

D
PROCEDURES, SERVICES, OR SUPPLIES (Explain Unusual Circumstances)
CPT/HCPCS | MODIFIER
42820 | tonsill- ectomy

DON'T: use N/A or DNA when information is not applicable. Leave the space blank.

Correct

17. NAME OF REFERRING PHYSICIAN OR OTHER SOURCE

Incorrect

17. NAME OF REFERRING PHYSICIAN OR OTHER SOURCE
DNA

DO: enter comments in Block 19 (e.g., ATTACH-MENT) for primary EOB submitted with claim to secondary insurance company.

Correct

19. RESERVED FOR LOCAL USE
ATTACHMENT

Incorrect

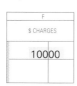

1. MEDICARE	MEDICAID	CHAMPUS	CHAMPVA
☐ (Medicare #)	☐ (Medicaid #)	☐ (Sponsor's SSN)	☐ (VA File #)

2. PATIENT'S NAME (Last Name, First Name, Middle Initial)
FOREHAND HARRY N
5. PATIENT'S ADDRESS
1456 MAIN STREET

CITY	STATE
WOODLAND HILLS	XY

ZIP CODE	TELEPHONE (Include Area Code)
12345 0000	(013) 490 9876

DON'T: use paper clips, cellophane tape, or staples.

DON'T: staple over the bar code area of the claim form.

DO: enter eight-digit date formats: 06012000 or 06 01 2000, depending on the block instructions.

Correct

24. A					
DATE(S) OF SERVICE					
From			To		
MM	DD	YY	MM	DD	YY
03	03	20XX			

Incorrect

24. A					
DATE(S) OF SERVICE					
From			To		
MM	DD	YY	MM	DD	YY
03	03	XX			

DO: keep signature within signature block. Rubber stamps may be used if they are accepted by insurance carrier and produce complete, clean images, without smudges or missing letters.

Correct

| 31. SIGNATURE OF PHYSICIAN OR SUPPLIER INCLUDING DEGREES OR CREDENTIALS (I certify that the statements on the reverse apply to this bill and are made a part thereof.) |
| CONCHA ANTRUM MD |
| 030320XX |
| SIGNED *Concha Antrum MD* DATE |

reference initials

Incorrect

| 31. SIGNATURE OF PHYSICIAN OR SUPPLIER INCLUDING DEGREES OR CREDENTIALS (I certify that the statements on the reverse apply to this bill and are made a part thereof.) |
| CONCHA ANTRUM MD |
| 030320XX |
| SIGNED   DATE |

Concha Antrum MD
reference initials

DON'T: overtrim or undertrim forms when bursting. Use care in separating forms and discard any form with tears or holes.

DON'T: fold or spindle forms when mailing because they will not feed into OCR equipment properly if creased or torn.

DO: enter information via machine printing (e.g., typewriter, word processor, or computer keyboard). Use clean equipment and quality ink jet, laser, or letter-quality matrix printers, if possible, not dot matrix. Clean line printers frequently. Adjust hammer density to prevent shadows and satellites. Monitor phase adjustment to ensure character clarity side to side and top to bottom.

PROCEDURE: Instructions for the Health Insurance Claim Form (HCFA-1500)

The Health Insurance Claim Form is divided into two major sections: patient information and physician information. The Patient and Insured (Subscriber) Information section is the upper portion of the claim form and contains 13 blocks numbered 1 through 13 (11 data elements and two signature blocks). The Physician or Supplier Information section is the lower portion of the claim form and consists of 20 blocks numbered 14 through 33 (19 data elements and 1 signature block). Some of the blocks are subdivided with subdivisions labeled a, b, c, d, and so forth. There is a total of over 100 places to enter specific information.

The instructions are straightforward and contain all pertinent information needed to complete a claim (see Figs. 6–6 through 6–15). However,

much information on specific coverage guidelines, program policies, and practice specialties could not be included here.

A brief description of each block and of its applicability to the requirements of private insurance payers, Medicaid, Medicare, TRICARE, CHAMPVA, and workers' compensation is presented. Because guidelines vary at the state and local levels for completing the HCFA-1500 claim form for the aforementioned insurance plans, consult your local intermediary or private carriers. For completing Medi-Cal claims in California, refer to Appendix C.

When generating paper claims via computer, many software programs insert the insurance carrier's name and address in the top right corner of the HCFA-1500 claim form. When typing a claim form, it is suggested that this same procedure be followed.

Block numbers match those on the Health Insurance Claim Form. Italicized sections refer students to guidelines in completing the *Workbook* assignments when there are optional ways of completing a block. Icon meanings are as follows:

 All payers: All payer guidelines including all private insurance companies and all federal and state programs.

 All private payers: All private insurance companies.

 Medicaid: State Medicaid programs.

 Medicare: Federal Medicare programs, Medicare/Medicaid, Medicare/Medigap, and Medicare Secondary Payer (MSP).

 TRICARE: TRICARE Standard (formerly CHAMPUS), TRICARE Prime, TRICARE Extra.

 CHAMPVA: Civilian Health and Medical Program of the Department of Veterans' Affairs.

 Workers' Compensation: State workers' compensation programs.

TOP OF FORM

Enter name and address of insurance company in the top right corner of the insurance form using all capital letters and no punctuation.

PLEASE
DO NOT
STAPLE
IN THIS
AREA

PRUDENTIAL INSURANCE COMPANY
5450 WILSHIRE BOULEVARD
WOODLAND HILLS XY 12345 0000

APPROVED OMB-0938-008

CARRIER

PICA   **HEALTH INSURANCE CLAIM FORM**   PICA

1. MEDICARE	MEDICAID	CHAMPUS	CHAMPVA	GROUP HEALTH PLAN	FECA BLK LUNG	OTHER	1a. INSURED'S I.D. NUMBER	(FOR PROGRAM IN ITEM 1)
(Medicare #)	(Medicaid #)	(Sponsor's SSN)	(VA File #)	X (SSN or ID)	(SSN)	(ID)	111704521	A482

2. PATIENT'S NAME (Last Name, First Name, Middle Initial)	3. PATIENT'S BIRTH DATE MM DD YY	SEX	4. INSURED'S NAME (Last Name, First Name, Middle Initial)
FOREHAND HARRY N	01 06 1946	M X F☐	SAME

BLOCK 1

PLEASE
DO NOT
STAPLE
IN THIS
AREA

PRUDENTIAL INSURANCE COMPANY
5450 WILSHIRE BOULEVARD
WOODLAND HILLS XY 12345 0000

APPROVED OMB-0938-008

CARRIER

PICA   HEALTH INSURANCE CLAIM FORM   PICA

1. MEDICARE	MEDICAID	CHAMPUS	CHAMPVA	GROUP HEALTH PLAN	FECA BLK LUNG	OTHER	1a. INSURED'S I.D. NUMBER	(FOR PROGRAM IN ITEM 1)
(Medicare #)	(Medicaid #)	(Sponsor's SSN)	(VA File #)	X (SSN or ID)	(SSN)	(ID)	111704521	A482

2. PATIENT'S NAME (Last Name, First Name, Middle Initial)	3. PATIENT'S BIRTH DATE MM DD YY	SEX	4. INSURED'S NAME (Last Name, First Name, Middle Initial)
FOREHAND HARRY N	01 06 1946	M X F☐	SAME

All Private Payers:
Individual Health Plan: Check "Other" for an individual who is covered under an individual policy.
Group Health Plan: Check this box for those covered under any group contract insurance (e.g., insurance obtained through employment); also for patients who receive services paid by managed care programs (e.g., HMOs, PPOs, IPAs).
▶ *When completing the* Workbook *assignments, if the insured is employed, assume the insurance is through the employer and is "group" insurance; otherwise, assume it is an individual policy and enter "other."*

Medicaid: Check for person receiving Medicaid benefits.

Medicare: Check for patient who receives Medicare benefits.
Medicare/Medicaid: Check "Medicare" and "Medicaid" if the patient is covered under Medicare and Medicaid programs.
Medicare/Medigap: Check "Medicare" and, if the patient has group or individual or Medigap coverage, check "Group" or "Other," depending on health plan.

▶ *When completing the* Workbook *assignments, if the insured is employed, assume the insurance is through the employer and is "group" insurance; otherwise, assume it is an individual policy and enter "other."*

MSP: Check "Group" or "Other" (depending on health plan) and "Medicare" when a Medicare patient has insurance primary to Medicare coverage.

TRICARE: Check "CHAMPUS" for individual receiving TRICARE benefits.

CHAMPVA: Check "CHAMPVA" for individual receiving CHAMPVA benefits.

Workers' Compensation: Check "Other" for all workers' compensation claims except FECA Black Lung. Check "FECA Black Lung" for patients who receive black lung benefits under the Federal Employee Compensation Act.

BLOCK 1a

PLEASE
DO NOT
STAPLE
IN THIS
AREA

APPROVED OMB-0938-008

PRUDENTIAL INSURANCE COMPANY
5450 WILSHIRE BOULEVARD
WOODLAND HILLS XY 12345 0000

CARRIER

	PICA		HEALTH INSURANCE CLAIM FORM	PICA	

1. MEDICARE	MEDICAID	CHAMPUS	CHAMPVA	GROUP HEALTH PLAN	FECA BLK LUNG	OTHER	1a. INSURED'S I.D. NUMBER	(FOR PROGRAM IN ITEM 1)
☐ (Medicare #)	☐ (Medicaid #)	☐ (Sponsor's SSN)	☐ (VA File #)	☒ (SSN or ID)	☐ (SSN)	☐ (ID)	111704521	A482

2. PATIENT'S NAME (Last Name, First Name, Middle Initial)	3. PATIENT'S BIRTH DATE MM DD YY	SEX	4. INSURED'S NAME (Last Name, First Name, Middle Initial)
FOREHAND HARRY N	01 06 1946	M ☒ F ☐	SAME

All Private Payers: Enter the patient's policy (identification or certificate) number in the left portion of the block and the group number, if applicable, in the right portion of the block as it appears on the insurance card, without punctuation.

Medicaid: Enter the Medicaid number in the left portion of the block. Do not enter dashes or other special characters in this block.

Medicare: Enter the patient's Medicare Health Insurance Claim (HIC) number from the patient's Medicare card in the left portion of this block, regardless of whether Medicare is the primary or secondary payer.

Medicare/Medicaid: Enter the patient's Medicare number in the left portion of this block.

Medicare/Medigap: Enter the patient's Medicare number in the left portion of this block.

MSP: Enter the patient's Medicare number in the left portion of this block. Refer to Block 11 for primary insurance.

TRICARE: First enter sponsor's Social Security number (SSN) in the left portion of this block. Then, if the patient is a NATO beneficiary, add "NATO" or, if sponsor is a security agent, add "SECURITY." Do not provide the patient's SSN unless the patient and sponsor are the same.

CHAMPVA: Enter the Veterans Affairs file number (omit prefix or suffix) or sponsor's Social Security number in the left portion of this block. Do not use any other former service numbers.

Workers' Compensation: Enter the claim number. If none is assigned, enter the employer's policy number or patient's Social Security number.

BLOCK 2

PLEASE
DO NOT
STAPLE
IN THIS
AREA

APPROVED OMB-0938-008

PRUDENTIAL INSURANCE COMPANY
5450 WILSHIRE BOULEVARD
WOODLAND HILLS XY 12345 0000

← CARRIER →

HEALTH INSURANCE CLAIM FORM

| PICA | | | | | | | PICA |

1. MEDICARE	MEDICAID	CHAMPUS	CHAMPVA	GROUP HEALTH PLAN	FECA BLK LUNG	OTHER	1a. INSURED'S I.D. NUMBER	(FOR PROGRAM IN ITEM 1)
(Medicare #)	(Medicaid #)	(Sponsor's SSN)	(VA File #)	X (SSN or ID)	(SSN)	(ID)	111704521	A482

2. PATIENT'S NAME (Last Name, First Name, Middle Initial)	3. PATIENT'S BIRTH DATE MM DD YY	SEX	4. INSURED'S NAME (Last Name, First Name, Middle Initial)
FOREHAND HARRY N	01 06 1946	M X F	SAME

All Payers: Enter the last name, first name, and middle initial of the patient—in that order—as shown on the patient's identification card, even if it is misspelled. Do not use nicknames or abbreviations. Do not use commas. If a name is hyphenated, a hyphen may be used (see Example 6–4).

EXAMPLE 6–4

Hyphenated name: Smith-White = SMITH-WHITE
Prefixed name: MacIverson = MACIVERSON
Seniority name with numeric suffix: John R. Ellis, III = ELLIS III JOHN R

BLOCK 3

PLEASE
DO NOT
STAPLE
IN THIS
AREA

APPROVED OMB-0938-008

PRUDENTIAL INSURANCE COMPANY
5450 WILSHIRE BOULEVARD
WOODLAND HILLS XY 12345 0000

CARRIER

| | | PICA | | HEALTH INSURANCE CLAIM FORM | | PICA | | |

1. MEDICARE	MEDICAID	CHAMPUS	CHAMPVA	GROUP HEALTH PLAN	FECA BLK LUNG	OTHER	1a. INSURED'S I.D. NUMBER	(FOR PROGRAM IN ITEM 1)
(Medicare #)	(Medicaid #)	(Sponsor's SSN)	(VA File #)	X (SSN or ID)	(SSN)	(ID)	111704521	A482

2. PATIENT'S NAME (Last Name, First Name, Middle Initial)	3. PATIENT'S BIRTH DATE			4. INSURED'S NAME (Last Name, First Name, Middle Initial)
	MM	DD	YY	SEX	
FOREHAND HARRY N	01	06	1946 M X F ☐	SAME

All Payers: Enter the patient's birth date using eight digits (01272000). The patient's age must be as follows to correlate with the diagnosis in Block 21:

▶ Birth: Newborn diagnosis
▶ Birth to 17 years: Pediatric diagnosis
▶ 12 to 55 years: Maternity diagnosis
▶ 15 to 124 years: Adult diagnosis

Check the appropriate box for the patient's sex. If left blank, gender block defaults to "female."

BLOCK 4

PLEASE
DO NOT
STAPLE
IN THIS
AREA

APPROVED OMB-0938-008

PRUDENTIAL INSURANCE COMPANY
5450 WILSHIRE BOULEVARD
WOODLAND HILLS XY 12345 0000

CARRIER

| | | PICA | | HEALTH INSURANCE CLAIM FORM | | PICA | | |

1. MEDICARE	MEDICAID	CHAMPUS	CHAMPVA	GROUP HEALTH PLAN	FECA BLK LUNG	OTHER	1a. INSURED'S I.D. NUMBER	(FOR PROGRAM IN ITEM 1)
(Medicare #)	(Medicaid #)	(Sponsor's SSN)	(VA File #)	X (SSN or ID)	(SSN)	(ID)	111704521	A482

2. PATIENT'S NAME (Last Name, First Name, Middle Initial)	3. PATIENT'S BIRTH DATE			4. INSURED'S NAME (Last Name, First Name, Middle Initial)
	MM	DD	YY	SEX	
FOREHAND HARRY N	01	06	1946 M X F ☐	SAME

All Private Payers: Enter "SAME" when the insured is also the patient. If the insured is not the patient, enter the name of the insured (last name first).

Medicaid: Refer to Medicare guidelines.

Medicare: Leave blank if the insured is also the patient. Enter the insured's name, if different from the patient's.
Medicare/Medicaid: Refer to Medicare guidelines.
Medicare/Medigap: Refer to Medicare guidelines.
MSP: Enter the name of the insured (last name first).

TRICARE: Enter the sponsor's last name, first name, and middle initial, not a nickname or abbreviation. Enter "SAME" if the sponsor and patient are the same.

CHAMPVA: Enter the veteran's name, last name first.

Workers' Compensation: Enter the employer's name. If the employer is a large corporation, enter the name of the insured corporation in Block 4 and the local employer in Block 11b (e.g., Harcourt General is the insured corporation [4] and W. B. Saunders is the employer and would be typed in Block 11b).

BLOCK 5

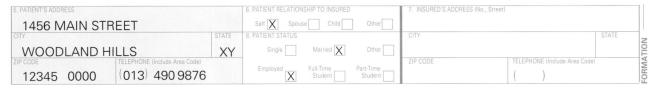

All Private Payers: Enter the patient's mailing address and residential telephone number.

Medicaid: Enter the patient's mailing address and residential telephone number.

Medicare: Enter the patient's mailing address and residential telephone number. On the first line, enter the street address; on the second line, the city and two-character state code (e.g., AZ = Arizona); on the third line, enter the ZIP code and residential telephone number. Punctuation is not necessary (e.g., ST LOUIS, no period after ST).

Medicare/Medicaid: Enter the patient's mailing address and residential telephone number.

Medicare/Medigap: Enter the patient's mailing address and residential telephone number.

MSP: Enter the patient's mailing address and residential telephone number.

TRICARE: Enter the patient's mailing address and residential telephone number. Do not enter a post office box number; provide the actual place of residence. If a rural address, the address must contain the route and box number. An APO/FPO address should not be used unless that person is residing overseas.

CHAMPVA: Enter the patient's mailing address and residential telephone number. Do not enter a post office box number; provide the actual place of residence. If a rural address, the address must contain the route and box number. An APO/FPO address should not be used unless that person is residing overseas.

Workers' Compensation: Enter the patient's mailing address and residential telephone number.

BLOCK 6

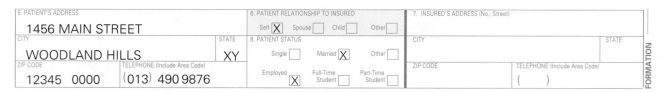

5. PATIENT'S ADDRESS		6. PATIENT RELATIONSHIP TO INSURED	7. INSURED'S ADDRESS (No., Street)	
1456 MAIN STREET		Self [X] Spouse [ ] Child [ ] Other [ ]		
CITY WOODLAND HILLS	STATE XY	8. PATIENT STATUS Single [ ] Married [X] Other [ ]	CITY	STATE
ZIP CODE 12345 0000	TELEPHONE (Include Area Code) (013) 490 9876	Employed [X] Full-Time Student [ ] Part-Time Student [ ]	ZIP CODE TELEPHONE (Include Area Code) ( )	

All Private Payers: Check the patient's relationship to the insured. If the patient is an unmarried "domestic partner," check "Other."

Medicaid: Leave blank. Check appropriate box only if there is third party coverage.

Medicare: Indicate relationship to insured when Block 4 is completed; otherwise, leave blank.
Medicare/Medicaid: Refer to Medicare guidelines.
Medicare/Medigap: Refer to Medicare guidelines.
MSP: Indicate relationship to insured.

TRICARE: Check the patient's relationship to the sponsor. If patient is the sponsor, check "self" (e.g., retiree). If the patient is a child or stepchild, check the box for child. If "other" is checked, indicate how the patient is related to the sponsor in Block 19 or on an attachment (e.g., former spouse).

CHAMPVA: Indicate the patient's relationship to the sponsor. If patient is the sponsor, check "self." If the patient is a child or stepchild, check the box for child. If "other" is checked, indicate how the patient is related to the sponsor (e.g., former spouse).

Workers' Compensation: Check "Other."

BLOCK 7

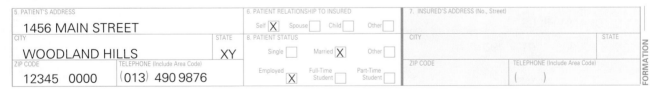

All Private Payers: Leave blank if Block 4 indicates "same." Enter "SAME" if Block 4 is completed and the address is identical to that listed in Block 5. Enter address if different from that listed in Block 5.

Medicaid: Refer to Medicare guidelines.

Medicare: Leave blank if Block 4 is blank. Enter "SAME" if Block 4 is completed and the address is identical to that listed in Block 5. Enter address if different from that listed in Block 5.
Medicare/Medicaid: Refer to Medicare guidelines.
Medicare/Medigap: Refer to Medicare guidelines.
MSP: Complete only when Block 4 is completed. If insured is other than the patient, list insured's address and if the address is the same as in Block 5, enter "SAME."

TRICARE: Enter "SAME" if address is the same as that of the patient listed in Block 5. Enter the sponsor's address (e.g., an APO/FPO address or active duty sponsor's duty station or the retiree's mailing address) if different from the patient's address.

CHAMPVA: Enter "SAME" if address is the same as that of the patient. Enter the sponsor's address if different from the patient's address.

Workers' Compensation: Enter the employer's address.

BLOCK 8

5. PATIENT'S ADDRESS			6. PATIENT RELATIONSHIP TO INSURED	7. INSURED'S ADDRESS (No., Street)		
1456 MAIN STREET			Self [X] Spouse [ ] Child [ ] Other [ ]			
CITY		STATE	8. PATIENT STATUS	CITY		STATE
WOODLAND HILLS		XY	Single [ ] Married [X] Other [ ]			
ZIP CODE	TELEPHONE (Include Area Code)		Employed [X] Full-Time Student [ ] Part-Time Student [ ]	ZIP CODE	TELEPHONE (Include Area Code)	
12345 0000	(013) 490 9876				( )	

All Private Payers: Check the appropriate box for the patient's marital status and whether employed or a student. The "other" box should be checked when a patient is covered under his or her children's health insurance plan or for a domestic partner. For individuals between the ages of 19 and 23, some insurance carriers require documentation from the school verifying full-time student status. This may be obtained as a signed letter from the school or by using a special form supplied by the insurance company.

Medicaid: Leave blank.

Medicare: Check the appropriate box or boxes for the patient's marital status and whether employed or a student (e.g., a beneficiary may be employed, a student, and married). Check "single" if widowed or divorced. In some locales, this block is not required by Medicare.

Medicare/Medicaid: Check appropriate box for the patient's marital status and whether employed or a student. Check "single" if widowed or divorced.

Medicare/Medigap: Check appropriate box for the patient's marital status and whether employed or a student. Check "single" if widowed or divorced.

MSP: Check appropriate box for the patient's marital status and whether employed or a student. Check "single" if widowed or divorced.

TRICARE: Check the appropriate box for the patient's marital status and whether employed or a student.

CHAMPVA: Check the appropriate box for the patient's marital status and whether employed or a student.

Workers' Compensation: Check "Employed." Some workers' compensation carriers may have requirements for marital status; otherwise, leave blank.

▶ *When completing the* Workbook *assignments, leave marital status blank.*

BLOCK 9

9. OTHER INSURED'S NAME (Last Name, First Name, Middle Initial)	10. IS PATIENT'S CONDITION RELATED TO:	11. INSURED'S POLICY GROUP OR FECA NUMBER	
a. OTHER INSURED'S POLICY OR GROUP NUMBER	a. EMPLOYMENT? (CURRENT OR PREVIOUS) ☐ YES ☒ NO	a. INSURED'S DATE OF BIRTH MM DD YY SEX M ☐ F ☐	PATIENT AND INSURED IN
b. OTHER INSURED'S DATE OF BIRTH MM DD YY SEX M ☐ F ☐	b. AUTO ACCIDENT? PLACE (State) ☐ YES ☒ NO	b. EMPLOYER'S NAME OR SCHOOL NAME	
c. EMPLOYER'S NAME OR SCHOOL NAME	c. OTHER ACCIDENT? ☐ YES ☒ NO	c. INSURANCE PLAN NAME OR PROGRAM NAME	
d. INSURANCE PLAN NAME OR PROGRAM NAME	10d. RESERVED FOR LOCAL USE	d. IS THERE ANOTHER HEALTH BENEFIT PLAN? ☐ YES ☒ NO *If yes*, return to and complete item 9 a-d.	

All Private Payers: For submission to primary insurance, leave blank. If patient has secondary insurance, enter patient's full name in last name, first name, and middle initial order.

Medicaid: For primary insurance, leave blank. For secondary insurance, enter patient's full name in last name, first name, and middle initial order.

Medicare: For primary insurance, leave blank. Do not list Medicare supplemental coverage (private, not Medigap) on the primary Medicare claim. Beneficiaries are responsible for filing a supplemental claim if the private insurer does not contract with Medicare to send claim information electronically.
Medicare/Medicaid: Enter Medicaid patient's full name in last name, first name, and middle initial order.
Medicare/Medigap: Enter the last name, first name, and middle initial of the Medigap enrollee if it differs from that in Block 2; otherwise, enter "SAME." Only Medicare participating physicians and suppliers should complete Block 9 and its subdivisions, and only when the beneficiary wishes to assign his/her benefits under a Medigap policy to the participating physician or supplier. If no Medigap benefits are assigned, leave blank.
MSP: Leave blank.

TRICARE: For primary insurance, leave blank. For secondary insurance held by someone other than the patient, enter the name of the insured. Blocks 11a–d should be used to report *other health insurance held by the patient.*

CHAMPVA: For primary insurance, leave blank. For secondary insurance held by someone other than the patient, enter the name of the insured. Blocks 11a–d should be used to report *other health insurance held by the patient.*

Workers' Compensation: Leave blank. If case is pending and not yet declared workers' compensation, insert other insurance.

BLOCK 9a

All Private Payers: Enter the policy and/or group number of the other (secondary) insured's insurance coverage.

Medicaid: Leave blank.

Medicare: Refer to appropriate secondary coverage guidelines.

Medicare/Medicaid: Enter Medicaid policy number here or in Block 10d. However, some states may have different guidelines; so, if in doubt, check with your local fiscal intermediary.

▶ *When completing the* Workbook *assignments, enter the Medicaid policy number in Block 10d.*

Medicare/Medigap: Enter the policy and/or group number of the Medigap enrollee preceded by the word "MEDIGAP," "MG," or "MGAP." In addition to Medicare/Medigap, if a patient has a third insurance (i.e., employer-supplemental), all information for the third insurance should be submitted on an attachment.

▶ *When completing the* Workbook *assignments, enter the word "MEDIGAP."*

MSP: Leave blank.

TRICARE: Enter the policy or group number of the other (secondary) insured's insurance policy.

CHAMPVA: Enter the policy or group number of the other (secondary) insured's insurance policy.

Workers' Compensation: Leave blank.

BLOCK 9b

All Private Payers: Enter the other insured's date of birth and gender.

Medicaid: Leave blank.

Medicare: Refer to appropriate secondary coverage guidelines.

Medicare/Medicaid: Enter the Medicaid enrollee's birth date, using eight digits (e.g., 03062000), and gender. If same as patient's, leave blank.

Medicare/Medigap: Enter the Medigap enrollee's birth date, using eight digits (e.g., 03062000), and gender. If same as patient's, leave blank.

MSP: Leave blank.

TRICARE: For secondary coverage held by someone other than the patient, enter the other insured's date of birth and check the appropriate box for gender.

CHAMPVA: For secondary coverage held by someone other than the patient, enter the other insured's date of birth and check the appropriate box for gender.

Workers' Compensation: Leave blank.

BLOCK 9c

All Private Payers: For secondary coverage, enter employer's name, if applicable.

Medicaid: Leave blank.

Medicare: Refer to appropriate secondary coverage guidelines.
Medicare/Medicaid: Leave blank.
Medicare/Medigap: Enter the Medigap insurer's claims processing address. Ignore "employer's name or school name." Abbreviate the street address to fit in this block by deleting the city, and using the two-letter state postal code and ZIP code. For example, 1234 Wren Drive, Any City, Pennsylvania 19106 would be typed "1234 WREN DR PA 19106." *Note: If a carrier-assigned unique identifier (sometimes called "Other Carrier Name and Address," or OCNA) for a Medigap insurer appears in Block 9d, then Block 9c may be left blank.*
MSP: Leave blank.

TRICARE: For secondary coverage held by someone other than the patient, enter the name of the other insured's employer or name of school.

CHAMPVA: For secondary coverage held by someone other than the patient, enter the name of the other insured's employer or name of school.

Workers' Compensation: Leave blank.

BLOCK 9d

All Private Payers: Enter name of secondary insurance plan or program.

Medicaid: Leave blank.

Medicare: Refer to appropriate secondary coverage guidelines.
Medicare/Medicaid: Leave blank.
Medicare/Medigap: Enter the Medigap insurer's nine-digit alphanumeric PAYERID number if known (often called the OCNA key), and Block 9c may be left blank. If not known, enter the name of the Medigap enrollee's insurance company. If you are a participating provider, all of the information in Blocks 9 through 9d must be complete and correct or the Medicare carrier cannot electronically forward the claim information to the Medigap insurer. For multiple insurance information, enter "ATTACHMENT" in Block 10d and provide information on an attached sheet.
MSP: Leave blank.

TRICARE: For secondary coverage held by someone other than the patient, insert name of insured's other health insurance program. On an attached sheet, provide a complete mailing address for all other insurance information and enter the word "ATTACHMENT" in Block 10d. If the patient is covered by a Health Maintenance Organization, attach a copy of the brochure showing that the service is not covered by the HMO.

CHAMPVA: For secondary coverage held by someone other than the patient, insert name of insured's other health insurance program. On an attached sheet, provide a complete mailing address for all other insurance information and enter the word "ATTACHMENT" in Block 10d. If the patient is covered by a Health Maintenance Organization, attach a copy of the brochure showing that the service is not covered by the HMO.

Workers' Compensation: Leave blank.

BLOCK 10a

9. OTHER INSURED'S NAME (Last Name, First Name, Middle Initial)	10. IS PATIENT'S CONDITION RELATED TO:	11. INSURED'S POLICY GROUP OR FECA NUMBER	PATIENT AND INSURED IN
a. OTHER INSURED'S POLICY OR GROUP NUMBER	a. EMPLOYMENT? (CURRENT OR PREVIOUS) ☐ YES ☒ NO	a. INSURED'S DATE OF BIRTH MM DD YY M ☐ SEX F ☐	
b. OTHER INSURED'S DATE OF BIRTH MM DD YY M ☐ SEX F ☐	b. AUTO ACCIDENT? PLACE (State) ☐ YES ☒ NO	b. EMPLOYER'S NAME OR SCHOOL NAME	
c. EMPLOYER'S NAME OR SCHOOL NAME	c. OTHER ACCIDENT? ☐ YES ☒ NO	c. INSURANCE PLAN NAME OR PROGRAM NAME	
d. INSURANCE PLAN NAME OR PROGRAM NAME	10d. RESERVED FOR LOCAL USE	d. IS THERE ANOTHER HEALTH BENEFIT PLAN? ☐ YES ☒ NO *If yes*, return to and complete item 9 a-d.	

All Payers: Check "yes" or "no" to indicate whether patient's diagnosis described in Block 21 is the result of an accident or injury that occurred on the job or an industrial illness.

BLOCK 10b

All Private Payers: A "yes" checked in Block 10b indicates a third party liability case; file the claim with the other liability insurance or automobile insurance company. List the abbreviation of the state in which the accident took place (e.g., CA for California).

Medicaid: Check appropriate box.

Medicare: Check "no." If "yes," bill the liability insurance as primary insurance and Medicare as secondary insurance.
Medicare/Medicaid: Refer to Medicare guidelines.
Medicare/Medigap: Refer to Medicare guidelines.
MSP: Refer to Medicare guidelines.

TRICARE: Check "yes" or "no" to indicate whether automobile liability applies to one or more of the services described in Block 24. If "yes," provide information concerning potential third party liability. If a third party is involved in the accident, the beneficiary must complete Form DD 2527 (Statement of Personal Injury—Possible Third-Party Liability) and attach it to the claim.

CHAMPVA: Check "yes" or "no" to indicate whether automobile liability applies to one or more of the services described in Block 24. If "yes," provide information concerning potential third party liability.

Workers' Compensation: Check "yes" to indicate an automobile accident that occurred while the patient was on the job.

BLOCK 10c

All Private Payers: Check "yes" or "no" to indicate whether the patient's condition is related to an accident other than automobile or employment. Verify primary insurance.

Medicaid: Check if applicable.

Medicare: Check "yes" or "no" to indicate whether the patient's condition is related to an accident other than automobile or employment. Verify primary insurance.
Medicare/Medicaid: Refer to Medicare guidelines.
Medicare/Medigap: Refer to Medicare guidelines.
MSP: Refer to Medicare guidelines.

TRICARE: Check "yes" or "no" to indicate whether another accident (not work related or automobile) applies to one or more of the services described in Block 24. If so, provide information concerning potential third party liability. If third party is involved in the accident, the beneficiary must complete Form DD 2527 (Statement of Personal Injury—Possible Third-Party Liability) and attach it to the claim.

CHAMPVA: Refer to TRICARE guidelines.

Workers' Compensation: Check "no."

BLOCK 10d

All Private Payers: Leave blank.

Medicaid: Generally, this block is used exclusively for Medicaid as a secondary payer. Enter the patient's Medicaid (MCD) number preceded by "MCD." Note, however, that this guideline is under discussion, so carriers may not yet notify providers of a usage change for this block. Some carriers state that if more than one type of other insurance applies to the claim, the identifiers for each type should be shown, for example:

Medicare/Medigap and Medicaid coverage = MG/MCD
Medicare/Medigap and Employer-Supp coverage = MG/SP
Medicaid and Employer-Supp coverage = MCD/SP
Primary (MSP) and Medicaid Secondary coverage = MSP/MCD
Two primary insurance plans = 2MSP

▶ *When completing the* Workbook *assignments, enter the patient's Medicaid number preceded by "MCD."*

Medicare: Leave blank.
Medicare/Medicaid: Enter the patient's Medicaid (MCD) number preceded by "MCD."
Medicare/Medigap: Leave blank.
MSP: Leave blank.

TRICARE: Generally, leave blank unless regional fiscal intermediary gives special guidelines. However, if Block 11d is checked "yes," the mailing address of the insurance carrier must be attached to the claim form, and in this block enter "ATTACHMENT."
▶ *When completing the* Workbook *assignments, leave blank.*

CHAMPVA: Generally, leave blank unless regional fiscal intermediary gives special guidelines. If Block 11d is checked "yes," the mailing address of the insurance carrier must be attached to the claim form, and in this block enter "ATTACHMENT."
▶ *When completing the* Workbook *assignments, leave blank.*

Workers' Compensation: Leave blank.

BLOCK 11

9. OTHER INSURED'S NAME (Last Name, First Name, Middle Initial)	10. IS PATIENT'S CONDITION RELATED TO:	11. INSURED'S POLICY GROUP OR FECA NUMBER
a. OTHER INSURED'S POLICY OR GROUP NUMBER	a. EMPLOYMENT? (CURRENT OR PREVIOUS) ☐ YES ☒ NO	a. INSURED'S DATE OF BIRTH MM ┊ DD ┊ YY SEX M ☐ F ☐
b. OTHER INSURED'S DATE OF BIRTH MM ┊ DD ┊ YY SEX M ☐ F ☐	b. AUTO ACCIDENT? PLACE (State) ☐ YES ☒ NO	b. EMPLOYER'S NAME OR SCHOOL NAME
c. EMPLOYER'S NAME OR SCHOOL NAME	c. OTHER ACCIDENT? ☐ YES ☒ NO	c. INSURANCE PLAN NAME OR PROGRAM NAME
d. INSURANCE PLAN NAME OR PROGRAM NAME	10d. RESERVED FOR LOCAL USE	d. IS THERE ANOTHER HEALTH BENEFIT PLAN? ☐ YES ☒ NO *If yes*, return to and complete item 9 a-d.

(right margin: PATIENT AND INSURED IN)

All Private Payers: Leave Blocks 11 through 11c blank if no private secondary coverage. If (private) secondary insurance, see Blocks 9–9d.

Medicaid: Generally, leave blank. Enter a rejection code if the patient has other third party insurance coverage and the claim was rejected.

Medicare: If other insurance is not primary to Medicare, enter "NONE" and go to Block 12. Block 11 must be completed. By completing this block, the physician/supplier acknowledges having made a good faith effort to determine whether Medicare is the primary or secondary payer.
Medicare/Medicaid: Refer to Medicare guidelines.
Medicare/Medigap: Refer to Medicare guidelines.
MSP: When insurance is primary to Medicare, enter the insured's policy and/or group number and complete Blocks 11a through 11c.

TRICARE: Leave blank.

CHAMPVA: Enter the three-digit number of the VA station that issued the identification card.

Workers' Compensation: Leave blank.

BLOCK 11a

All Private Payers: Leave blank.

Medicaid: Leave blank.

Medicare: Leave blank.
Medicare/Medicaid: Leave blank.
Medicare/Medigap: Leave blank.
MSP: Enter the insured's eight-digit date of birth (06122000) and gender if different from that listed in Block 3.

TRICARE: Enter sponsor's date of birth and gender, if different from that listed in Block 3.

CHAMPVA: Enter sponsor's date of birth and gender, if different from that listed in Block 3.

Workers' Compensation: Leave blank.

BLOCK 11b

All Private Payers: When submitting to secondary insurance, enter the name of the employer, school, or organization if primary policy is a group plan; otherwise, leave blank.

Medicaid: Leave blank.

Medicare: Leave blank.
Medicare/Medicaid: Leave blank.
Medicare/Medigap: Leave blank.
MSP: Enter the employer's name of primary insurance. Also use this block to indicate a change in the insured's insurance status (e.g., "RETIRED" and the eight-digit retirement date). Submit paper claims with a copy of the primary payer's Remittance Advice (RA) document to be considered for Medicare Secondary Payer benefits. Instances when Medicare may be secondary include the following:

1. Group health plan coverage
   a. Working aged
   b. Disability (large group health plan)
   c. End-stage renal disease
2. No fault and/or other liability
   a. Automobile
   b. Homeowner
   c. Commercial
3. Work-related illness/injury
   a. Workers' compensation
   b. Black lung
   c. Veterans' benefits

TRICARE: Indicate sponsor's branch of service, using abbreviations (e.g., United States Navy = USN).

CHAMPVA: Indicate sponsor's branch of service, using abbreviations (e.g., United States Army = USA).

Workers' Compensation: If a large corporation's name is listed in Block 4, enter the name of the patient's local employer; otherwise, leave this block blank.

BLOCK 11c

All Private Payers: When submitting to secondary insurance, enter the name of the primary insurance plan; otherwise, leave this block blank.

Medicaid: Leave blank.

Medicare: Leave blank.
Medicare/Medicaid: Leave blank.
Medicare/Medigap: Leave blank.
MSP: Enter the complete name of the insurance plan or program that is primary to Medicare. Include the primary payer's claim processing address directly on the EOB.

TRICARE: Leave blank.

CHAMPVA: Indicate name of the secondary coverage held by the patient, if applicable; otherwise, leave this block blank.

Workers' Compensation: Leave blank.

BLOCK 11d

All Private Payers: Check "yes" or "no" to indicate if there is another health plan. If "yes," Blocks 9a through 9d must be completed.

Medicaid: Leave blank.

Medicare: Generally, leave blank; some regions require "yes" or "no" checked, so verify this requirement with your local fiscal intermediary.
▶ *When completing the* Workbook *assignments, leave blank.*
Medicare/Medicaid: Refer to guidelines for Medicare.
Medicare/Medigap: Refer to guidelines for Medicare.
MSP: Leave blank.

TRICARE: Check "yes" or "no" to indicate if there is another health plan. If "yes," Blocks 9a through 9d must be completed.

CHAMPVA: Check "yes" or "no" to indicate if there is another health plan. If "yes," Blocks 9a through 9d must be completed.

Workers' Compensation: Leave blank.

BLOCK 12

READ BACK OF FORM BEFORE COMPLETING & SIGNING THIS FORM.	13. INSURED'S OR AUTHORIZED PERSON'S SIGNATURE I authorize
12. PATIENT'S OR AUTHORIZED PERSON'S SIGNATURE I authorize the release of any medical or other information necessary to process this claim. I also request payment of government benefits either to myself or to the party who accepts assignment below.	payment of medical benefits to the undersigned physician or supplier for services described below.
SIGNED _Harry N. Forehand_ DATE _March 3, 20XX_	SIGNED _Harry N. Forehand_

or

READ BACK OF FORM BEFORE COMPLETING & SIGNING THIS FORM.	13. INSURED'S OR AUTHORIZED PERSON'S SIGNATURE I authorize
12. PATIENT'S OR AUTHORIZED PERSON'S SIGNATURE I authorize the release of any medical or other information necessary to process this claim. I also request payment of government benefits either to myself or to the party who accepts assignment below.	payment of medical benefits to the undersigned physician or supplier for services described below.
SIGNED _____ SOF _____ DATE _____	SIGNED _____ SOF _____

All Private Payers: A signature here authorizes the release of medical information for claims processing. Have the patient or the authorized representative sign and date this block. If the patient has signed an authorization form, "Signature on File" or "SOF" can be entered here. The authorization form must be current, may be lifetime, and must be in the physician's file. When the patient's representative signs, the relationship to the patient **must** be indicated. If the signature is indicated by a mark (X), a witness must sign his or her name and enter the address next to the mark.
▶ *When completing the* Workbook *assignments, enter "SOF" in this block.*

Medicaid: Leave blank.

Medicare: A signature here authorizes payment of benefits to the physician (if the physician accepts assignment) *and* release of medical information for claims processing. Have the patient or the authorized representative sign and date this block. If the patient has signed an authorization form, "Signature on File" or "SOF" can be typed here. Be sure the form includes both authorizations just mentioned. The form must be current, may be lifetime, and must be in the physician's file. When the patient's representative signs, the relationship to the patient **must** be indicated. If the signature is by mark (X), a witness must sign his or her name and enter the address next to the mark.
▶ *When completing the* Workbook *assignments, enter "SOF" in this block.*
Medicare/Medicaid: Refer to Medicare guidelines.
Medicare/Medigap: Refer to Medicare guidelines.
MSP: Guidelines for this block are the same as for Medicare.

TRICARE: A signature here authorizes payment of benefits to the physician (if the physician accepts assignment) and release of medical information for claims processing. Have the patient or the authorized representative sign and date this block. If the patient has signed an authorization form, "Signature on File" or "SOF" can be typed here. Be sure the form includes both authorizations mentioned above. The form must be current, may be lifetime, and must be in the physician's file. When the patient's representative signs, the relationship to the patient **must** be indicated. If the signature is by mark (X), a witness must sign his or her name and enter the address next to the mark.
▶ *When completing the* Workbook *assignments, enter "SOF" in this block.*

CHAMPVA: Refer to TRICARE guidelines.

Workers' Compensation: No signature is required.

BLOCK 13

| READ BACK OF FORM BEFORE COMPLETING & SIGNING THIS FORM.
12. PATIENT'S OR AUTHORIZED PERSON'S SIGNATURE I authorize the release of any medical or other information necessary to process this claim. I also request payment of government benefits either to myself or to the party who accepts assignment below.

SIGNED *Harry N. Forehand*   DATE *March 3, 20XX* | 13. INSURED'S OR AUTHORIZED PERSON'S SIGNATURE I authorize payment of medical benefits to the undersigned physician or supplier for services described below.

SIGNED *Harry N. Forehand* |

or

| READ BACK OF FORM BEFORE COMPLETING & SIGNING THIS FORM.
12. PATIENT'S OR AUTHORIZED PERSON'S SIGNATURE I authorize the release of any medical or other information necessary to process this claim. I also request payment of government benefits either to myself or to the party who accepts assignment below.

SIGNED   SOF   DATE | 13. INSURED'S OR AUTHORIZED PERSON'S SIGNATURE I authorize payment of medical benefits to the undersigned physician or supplier for services described below.

SIGNED   SOF |

All Private Payers: Patient's signature is required when benefits are assigned. "SOF" may be listed if the patient's signature is on file.
▶ *When completing the* Workbook *assignments, enter "SOF" in this block.*

Medicaid: Leave blank.

Medicare: Leave blank.

Medicare/Medicaid: Leave blank.

Medicare/Medigap: For participating provider, a signature here authorizes payment of "mandated" Medigap benefits when required Medigap information is included in Blocks 9 through 9d. List the signature of the patient or authorized representative, or list "SOF" if the signature is on file as a separate Medigap authorization.

▶ *When completing the* Workbook *assignments, enter "SOF" in this block.*

MSP: The signature of the patient or authorized representative should appear in this block or list "SOF" if the signature is on file for benefits assigned from the primary carrier.

▶ *When completing the* Workbook *assignments, enter "SOF" in this block.*

TRICARE: Leave blank.

CHAMPVA: Leave blank.

Workers' Compensation: Leave blank. All payment goes directly to the physician.

BLOCK 14

14. DATE OF CURRENT: ◀ ILLNESS (First symptom) OR INJURY (Accident) OR PREGNANCY (LMP)	15. IF PATIENT HAS HAD SAME OR SIMILAR ILLNESS. GIVE FIRST DATE	16. DATES PATIENT UNABLE TO WORK IN CURRENT OCCUPATION
MM 03 DD 01 YY 2000	MM DD YY	MM DD YY FROM — MM DD YY TO
17. NAME OF REFERRING PHYSICIAN OR OTHER SOURCE PERRY CARDI MD	17a. I.D. NUMBER OF REFERRING PHYSICIAN 6780502700	18. HOSPITALIZATION DATES RELATED TO CURRENT SERVICES MM DD YY FROM — MM DD YY TO
19. RESERVED FOR LOCAL USE		20. OUTSIDE LAB? ☐ YES ☒ NO $ CHARGES

All Private Payers: Enter the eight-digit date the patient's first symptoms occurred from the current illness, if stated in the medical record; date of injury or accident; or for pregnancy, first day of last menstrual period. For chiropractic treatment, enter the eight-digit date that treatment began.

Medicaid: Leave blank.

Medicare: Enter the eight-digit date the patient's first symptoms occurred from the current illness, if stated in the medical record; date of injury or accident; or for pregnancy, first day of last menstrual period. For chiropractic treatment, enter the eight-digit date that treatment began.
Medicare/Medicaid: Refer to Medicare guidelines.
Medicare/Medigap: Refer to Medicare guidelines.
MSP: Refer to Medicare guidelines.

TRICARE: Enter the eight-digit date the patient's first symptoms occurred from the current illness, if stated in the medical record; date of injury or accident; or for pregnancy, first day of last menstrual period. For chiropractic treatment, enter the eight-digit date that treatment began.

CHAMPVA: Refer to TRICARE guidelines.

Workers' Compensation: Enter first date of injury, accident, or industrial illness; it should coincide with the date specified in the Doctor's First Report of Injury.

BLOCK 15

14. DATE OF CURRENT: ILLNESS (First symptom) OR INJURY (Accident) OR PREGNANCY (LMP)	15. IF PATIENT HAS HAD SAME OR SIMILAR ILLNESS. GIVE FIRST DATE MM DD YY	16. DATES PATIENT UNABLE TO WORK IN CURRENT OCCUPATION
MM DD YY 03 01 2000		FROM MM DD YY TO MM DD YY
17. NAME OF REFERRING PHYSICIAN OR OTHER SOURCE PERRY CARDI MD	17a. I.D. NUMBER OF REFERRING PHYSICIAN 6780502700	18. HOSPITALIZATION DATES RELATED TO CURRENT SERVICES FROM MM DD YY TO MM DD YY
19. RESERVED FOR LOCAL USE		20. OUTSIDE LAB? ☐ YES ☒ NO $ CHARGES

All Private Payers: Enter date when patient had same or similar illness, if applicable, and documented in the medical record.

Medicaid: Leave blank.

Medicare: Leave blank.
Medicare/Medicaid: Leave blank.
Medicare/Medigap: Leave blank.
MSP: Leave blank.

TRICARE: Enter date when patient had same or similar illness, if applicable and documented in the medical record.

CHAMPVA: Refer to TRICARE guidelines.

Workers' Compensation: Enter date if appropriate and documented in the medical record.

BLOCK 16

14. DATE OF CURRENT:	15. IF PATIENT HAS HAD SAME OR SIMILAR ILLNESS.	16. DATES PATIENT UNABLE TO WORK IN CURRENT OCCUPATION
MM | DD | YY ◄ ILLNESS (First symptom) OR / INJURY (Accident) OR / PREGNANCY (LMP) 03 | 01 | 2000	GIVE FIRST DATE MM | DD | YY	MM | DD | YY MM | DD | YY FROM TO
17. NAME OF REFERRING PHYSICIAN OR OTHER SOURCE PERRY CARDI MD	17a. I.D. NUMBER OF REFERRING PHYSICIAN 6780502700	18. HOSPITALIZATION DATES RELATED TO CURRENT SERVICES MM | DD | YY MM | DD | YY FROM TO
19. RESERVED FOR LOCAL USE		20. OUTSIDE LAB? $ CHARGES ☐ YES ☒ NO

All Private Payers: Enter dates patient is employed but cannot work in current occupation. *From*: Enter first *full* day patient was unable to perform job duties. *To*: Enter last day patient was disabled before returning to work.

Medicaid: Leave blank.

Medicare: Enter eight-digit dates patient is employed but cannot work in current occupation. *From*: Enter first *full* day patient was unable to perform job duties. *To*: Enter last day patient was disabled before returning to work.
Medicare/Medicaid: Refer to Medicare guidelines.
Medicare/Medigap: Refer to Medicare guidelines.
MSP: Refer to Medicare guidelines.

TRICARE: Refer to Medicare guidelines.

CHAMPVA: Refer to Medicare guidelines.

Workers' Compensation: May be completed but is not mandatory and must be verified with documentation in Doctor's First Report of Injury. *From*: Enter first *full* day patient was unable to perform job duties. *To*: Enter last day patient was disabled before returning to work.

▶ *When completing the* Workbook *assignments, enter information when documented in the medical record.*

BLOCK 17

14. DATE OF CURRENT: MM | DD | YY ◀ILLNESS (First symptom) OR INJURY (Accident) OR PREGNANCY (LMP) 03 | 01 | 2000	15. IF PATIENT HAS HAD SAME OR SIMILAR ILLNESS. GIVE FIRST DATE MM | DD | YY	16. DATES PATIENT UNABLE TO WORK IN CURRENT OCCUPATION MM | DD | YY MM | DD | YY FROM TO
17. NAME OF REFERRING PHYSICIAN OR OTHER SOURCE PERRY CARDI MD	17a. I.D. NUMBER OF REFERRING PHYSICIAN 6780502700	18. HOSPITALIZATION DATES RELATED TO CURRENT SERVICES MM | DD | YY MM | DD | YY FROM TO
19. RESERVED FOR LOCAL USE		20. OUTSIDE LAB? $ CHARGES ☐ YES ☒ NO

All Private Payers: Enter complete name and degree of referring physician, when applicable. Do not list other referrals (i.e., family or friends).

Medicaid: Enter complete name and degree of referring physician, when applicable. Do not list other referrals (i.e., family or friends).

Medicare: Enter the name and degree of the referring or ordering physician on all claims for Medicare-covered services and items resulting from a physician's order or referral. Use a separate claim form for each referring and/or ordering physician.

Surgeon: A surgeon must complete this block. When the patient has not been referred, enter the surgeon's name. On an assistant surgeon's claim, enter the primary surgeon's name.

Referring physician: A physician who requests a service for the beneficiary for which payment may be made under the Medicare program. When a physician extender (e.g., nurse practitioner) refers a patient for a consultative service, enter the name of the physician supervising the physician extender.

Ordering physician: A physician who orders nonphysician services for the patient, such as diagnostic radiology/laboratory/pathology tests, pharmaceutical services, durable medical equipment (DME), parenteral and enteral nutrition, or immunosuppressive drugs, and consultations.

When the ordering physician is also the performing physician (e.g., the physician who actually performs the in-office laboratory tests), the performing physician's name and assigned UPIN/NPI number must appear in Blocks 17 and 17a.

When a patient is referred to a physician who also orders and performs a diagnostic service, *a separate claim form* is required for the diagnostic service.

▶ Enter the original referring physician's name and NPI in Blocks 17 and 17a of the first claim form.

▶ Enter the ordering (performing) physician's name and NPI in Blocks 17 and 17a of the second claim form.

Medicare/Medicaid: Refer to Medicare guidelines.

Medicare/Medigap: Refer to Medicare guidelines.

MSP: Refer to Medicare guidelines.

TRICARE: Enter name, degree, and address of referring provider. This is required for all consultation claims. If the patient was referred from a Military Treatment Facility (MTF), enter the name of the MTF and attach DD Form 2161 or SF 513, "Referral for Civilian Medical Care."

CHAMPVA: Refer to TRICARE guidelines.

Workers' Compensation: Indicate name and degree of referring provider.

BLOCK 17a

14. DATE OF CURRENT: ◀ ILLNESS (First symptom) OR INJURY (Accident) OR PREGNANCY (LMP)	15. IF PATIENT HAS HAD SAME OR SIMILAR ILLNESS. GIVE FIRST DATE MM	DD	YY	16. DATES PATIENT UNABLE TO WORK IN CURRENT OCCUPATION
MM	DD	YY 03	01	2000		FROM MM	DD	YY TO MM	DD	YY
17. NAME OF REFERRING PHYSICIAN OR OTHER SOURCE PERRY CARDI MD	17a. I.D. NUMBER OF REFERRING PHYSICIAN 6780502700	18. HOSPITALIZATION DATES RELATED TO CURRENT SERVICES FROM MM	DD	YY TO MM	DD	YY
19. RESERVED FOR LOCAL USE		20. OUTSIDE LAB? ☐ YES ☒ NO $ CHARGES

All Private Payers: Enter the referring physician's UPIN/NPI number.

Medicaid: Enter the referring physician's UPIN/NPI number.

Medicare: Enter the HCFA-assigned UPIN/NPI of the referring or ordering physician (or the supervising physician for a physician extender) as detailed in Medicare Block 17. Temporary "surrogate" NPIs are issued until permanent ones are assigned for physicians in the following categories: residents and interns, retired physicians, nonphysicians (nurse practitioners, clinical nurse specialists, other state licensed nonphysicians), Veterans Affairs/US Armed Services, Public Health/Indian Health Services, and any physician not meeting the just described criteria for a surrogate that has not been issued an NPI.

Medicare/Medicaid: Refer to Medicare guidelines.

Medicare/Medigap: Refer to Medicare guidelines.

MSP: Refer to Medicare guidelines.

TRICARE: Enter the referring physician's federal tax identification number or Social Security number.

▶ *When completing the* Workbook *assignments, enter the physician's federal tax identification number.*

CHAMPVA: Refer to TRICARE guidelines.

Workers' Compensation: Leave blank.

BLOCK 18

14. DATE OF CURRENT: ILLNESS (First symptom) OR INJURY (Accident) OR PREGNANCY (LMP)	15. IF PATIENT HAS HAD SAME OR SIMILAR ILLNESS. GIVE FIRST DATE MM | DD | YY	16. DATES PATIENT UNABLE TO WORK IN CURRENT OCCUPATION MM | DD | YY MM | DD | YY FROM TO
MM | DD | YY 03 | 01 | 2000		
17. NAME OF REFERRING PHYSICIAN OR OTHER SOURCE PERRY CARDI MD	17a. I.D. NUMBER OF REFERRING PHYSICIAN 6780502700	18. HOSPITALIZATION DATES RELATED TO CURRENT SERVICES MM | DD | YY MM | DD | YY FROM TO
19. RESERVED FOR LOCAL USE		20. OUTSIDE LAB? $ CHARGES ☐ YES X NO

All Payers: Complete this block when a medical service is furnished as a result of, or subsequent to, a related (inpatient) hospitalization, skilled nursing facility, or nursing home visit. Do not complete for outpatient hospital services, ambulatory surgery, or emergency department services. Enter eight-digit admitting and discharge dates. If the patient is still hospitalized at the time of the billing, enter 8 zeros in the "TO" field.

BLOCK 19

14. DATE OF CURRENT:			ILLNESS (First symptom) OR INJURY (Accident) OR PREGNANCY (LMP)	15. IF PATIENT HAS HAD SAME OR SIMILAR ILLNESS. GIVE FIRST DATE MM	DD	YY	16. DATES PATIENT UNABLE TO WORK IN CURRENT OCCUPATION MM	DD	YY MM	DD	YY FROM TO
MM	DD	YY					
03	01	2000					
17. NAME OF REFERRING PHYSICIAN OR OTHER SOURCE				17a. I.D. NUMBER OF REFERRING PHYSICIAN			18. HOSPITALIZATION DATES RELATED TO CURRENT SERVICES MM	DD	YY MM	DD	YY FROM TO
PERRY CARDI MD				6780502700			
19. RESERVED FOR LOCAL USE							20. OUTSIDE LAB? $ CHARGES ☐ YES ☒ NO

All Private Payers: This block may be completed in a number of different ways depending on commercial carrier guidelines. Some common uses are:

▶ Enter the word "ATTACHMENT" when an operative report, discharge summary, invoice, or other attachment is included.

▶ Enter an explanation regarding unusual services or unlisted services.

▶ Enter all applicable modifiers when modifier -99 is used in Block 24D (e.g., 99–80 51). If -99 appears with more than one procedure code, list the line number (24–1, 2, 3, and so on) for each -99 listed (see Example 6–5).

EXAMPLE 6–5

2–80 51   3–80 51

▶ Enter the drug name and dosage when submitting a claim for Not Otherwise Classified (NOC) drugs. Enter the word "ATTACHMENT" and attach the invoice.

▶ Describe the supply when the code 99070 is used.

▶ Enter the x-ray date for chiropractic treatment.

Medicaid: Check with the regional fiscal intermediary who may have special guidelines for entries in this block.

▶ *When completing the* Workbook *assignments, refer to private payer guidelines.*

Medicare: Although the block is labeled "Reserved for Local Use," HCFA guidelines state it may be completed in a number of different ways depending on the circumstances of the services provided to the patient. This block can only contain up to three conditions per claim. Some common uses are:

▶ Enter the attending physician's NPI and the eight-digit date of the patient's latest visit for claims submitted by a physical or occupational therapist, psychotherapist, chiropractor, or podiatrist.

▶ Enter the drug's name and dosage when submitting a claim for Not Otherwise Classified (NOC) drugs. Enter the word "ATTACHMENT" and include a copy of the invoice.

▶ Describe the procedure for *unlisted procedures.* If there is not sufficient room in this block, send an attachment.

▶ Enter all applicable modifiers when modifier -99 is used in Block 24D (e.g., 99-80 51). If -99 appears with more than one procedure code, list the line number (1, 2, 3, and so on) for each -99 listed (see Example 6–5).

▶ Enter "Homebound" when an independent laboratory renders an electrocardiogram or collects a specimen from a patient who is homebound or institutionalized.

▶ Enter the statement "Patient refuses to assign benefits" when a Medicare beneficiary refuses to assign benefits to a participating provider. No payment to the physician will be made on the claim in this case.

▶ Enter "Testing for hearing aid" when submitting a claim to obtain an intentional denial from Medicare as the primary payer for hearing aid testing and a secondary payer is involved.

▶ Enter the specific dental surgery for which a dental examination is being performed.

▶ Enter the name and dosage when billing for low osmolar contrast material for which there is no Level 2 HCPCS code.

▶ Enter "Pump" or "Reservoir" to indicate which is used when codes 63750 and/or 63780 are used.

▶ Enter the eight-digit assumed and relinquished dates of care for each provider when providers share postoperative care for global surgery claims.

▶ Enter the statement "Attending physician, not hospice employee" when a physician gives service to a hospice patient but the hospice in which the patient resides does not employ the physician.

Medicare/Medicaid: Refer to Medicare guidelines.

Medicare/Medigap: Refer to Medicare guidelines.

MSP: Refer to Medicare guidelines.

TRICARE: Generally this block is reserved for local use (e.g., to indicate referral number or enter x-ray date for chiropractic treatment).

CHAMPVA: Refer to TRICARE guidelines.

Workers' Compensation: Leave blank.

BLOCK 20

14. DATE OF CURRENT: ◀ ILLNESS (First symptom) OR INJURY (Accident) OR PREGNANCY (LMP)	15. IF PATIENT HAS HAD SAME OR SIMILAR ILLNESS. GIVE FIRST DATE	16. DATES PATIENT UNABLE TO WORK IN CURRENT OCCUPATION
MM DD YY 03 01 2000	MM DD YY	FROM MM DD YY TO MM DD YY
17. NAME OF REFERRING PHYSICIAN OR OTHER SOURCE PERRY CARDI MD	17a. I.D. NUMBER OF REFERRING PHYSICIAN 6780502700	18. HOSPITALIZATION DATES RELATED TO CURRENT SERVICES FROM MM DD YY TO MM DD YY
19. RESERVED FOR LOCAL USE		20. OUTSIDE LAB? ☐ YES ☒ NO $ CHARGES

All Private Payers: Enter "yes" or "no" when billing diagnostic laboratory tests. *NO* means the tests were performed by the billing physician/laboratory. *YES* means that the laboratory test was performed *outside* of the physician's office and that the physician is billing for the laboratory services. If "yes", enter purchase price of the test in the Charges portion of this block and complete Block 32.

Medicaid: Check "no"; outside laboratories must bill direct.

Medicare: Enter "yes" or "no" when billing diagnostic laboratory tests. *NO* means the tests were performed by the billing physician/laboratory. *YES* means that the laboratory test was performed *outside* of the physician's office and that the physician is billing for the laboratory services. If "yes", enter purchase price of the test in the Charges portion of this block and complete Block 32. *Clinical laboratory services must be billed to Medicare on an assigned basis.*
Medicare/Medicaid: Refer to Medicare guidelines.
Medicare/Medigap: Refer to Medicare guidelines.
MSP: Refer to Medicare guidelines.

TRICARE: Refer to Medicare guidelines.

CHAMPVA: Refer to Medicare guidelines.

Workers' Compensation: Refer to Medicare guidelines.

BLOCK 21

21. DIAGNOSIS OR NATURE OF ILLNESS OR INJURY. (RELATE ITEMS 1,2,3 OR 4 TO ITEM 24E BY LINE)						22. MEDICAID RESUBMISSION CODE	ORIGINAL REF. NO.
1. 382 00			3.				
2.			4.			23. PRIOR AUTHORIZATION NUMBER	

24.	A			B	C	D	E	F	G	H	I	J	K	
	DATE(S) OF SERVICE			Place of Service	Type of Service	PROCEDURES, SERVICES, OR SUPPLIES (Explain Unusual Circumstances) CPT/HCPCS | MODIFIER	DIAGNOSIS CODE	$ CHARGES	DAYS OR UNITS	EPSDT Family Plan	EMG	COB	RESERVED FOR LOCAL USE	INFORMATION
	From MM DD YY	To MM DD YY												
1														

ICD-9-CM
    382.00 Acute suppurative otitis media without
          spontaneous rupture of ear drum

All Payers: Enter up to four diagnostic codes in priority order, with the primary diagnosis in the first position. Codes must be carried out to their highest degree of specificity. Do not use decimal points or add any code narratives unless required in your locale. Code only the conditions or problems that the physician is actively treating and that relate directly to the services billed.

BLOCK 22

21. DIAGNOSIS OR NATURE OF ILLNESS OR INJURY. (RELATE ITEMS 1,2,3 OR 4 TO ITEM 24E BY LINE)							22. MEDICAID RESUBMISSION CODE	ORIGINAL REF. NO.			

1. 382 00   3. |___.___

                                             4. |___.___

                                  23. PRIOR AUTHORIZATION NUMBER

2. |___.___

24. A						B	C	D		E		F	G	H	I	J	K	
	DATE(S) OF SERVICE					Place of Service	Type of Service	PROCEDURES, SERVICES, OR SUPPLIES (Explain Unusual Circumstances)		DIAGNOSIS CODE		$ CHARGES	DAYS OR UNITS	EPSDT Family Plan	EMG	COB	RESERVED FOR LOCAL USE	INFORMATION
	From			To				CPT/HCPCS	MODIFIER									
MM	DD	YY	MM	DD	YY													
1										1								

All Private Payers: Leave blank.

Medicaid: Complete for resubmission.

Medicare: Leave blank.
Medicare/Medicaid: Refer to Medicaid guidelines.
Medicare/Medigap: Leave blank.
MSP: Leave blank.

TRICARE: Leave blank.

CHAMPVA: Leave blank.

Workers' Compensation: Leave blank.

BLOCK 23

21. DIAGNOSIS OR NATURE OF ILLNESS OR INJURY. (RELATE ITEMS 1,2,3 OR 4 TO ITEM 24E BY LINE)						22. MEDICAID RESUBMISSION CODE / ORIGINAL REF. NO.					
1. ⌐382 ⌐00	3. ⌐___⌐___					23. PRIOR AUTHORIZATION NUMBER					
2. ⌐___⌐___	4. ⌐___⌐___										

24. A DATE(S) OF SERVICE						B Place of Service	C Type of Service	D PROCEDURES, SERVICES, OR SUPPLIES (Explain Unusual Circumstances) CPT/HCPCS | MODIFIER	E DIAGNOSIS CODE	F $ CHARGES	G DAYS OR UNITS	H EPSDT Family Plan	I EMG	J COB	K RESERVED FOR LOCAL USE
From MM	DD	YY	To MM	DD	YY				1						

All Private Payers: Enter the professional or peer review organization (PRO) 10-digit prior authorization number.

Medicaid: Enter the Professional (Peer) Review Organization (PRO) 10-digit prior authorization or precertification number for procedures requiring PRO prior approval. If billing for an investigational device, enter the Investigational Device Exemption (IDE) number.

Medicare: Although this block is labeled "Prior Authorization Number," HCFA guidelines state it may be completed in a number of different ways depending on the circumstances of the services provided to the patient. Some common uses are:

▶ Enter the Professional (Peer) Review Organization (PRO) 10-digit prior authorization or precertification number for procedures requiring PRO prior approval.
▶ Enter the Investigational Device Exemption (IDE) number if billing for an investigational device.
▶ Enter the 10-digit CLIA (Clinical Laboratory Improvement Amendments) federal certification number when billing for laboratory services billed by a physician office laboratory.
▶ Enter the 6-digit Medicare provider number of the hospice or home health agency (HHA) when billing for care plan oversight services.

Medicare/Medicaid: Refer to Medicare guidelines.
Medicare/Medigap: Refer to Medicare guidelines.
MSP: Refer to Medicare guidelines.

TRICARE: Enter the Professional (Peer) Review Organization (PRO) 10-digit prior authorization or precertification number for procedures requiring PRO prior approval. If billing for an investigational device, enter the Investigational Device Exemption (IDE) number. Attach a copy of the authorization.

CHAMPVA: Refer to TRICARE guidelines.

Workers' Compensation: Leave blank.

Blocks 24A through 24K may not contain more than six detail lines. If the case requires more than six detail lines, put the additional information on a separate claim form and treat it as an independent claim totalling all charges on each claim. Claims cannot be "continued" from one to another. Do not list a procedure on the claim form for which there is no charge.

BLOCK 24A

24. A DATE(S) OF SERVICE From MM DD YY — To MM DD YY	B Place of Service	C Type of Service	D PROCEDURES, SERVICES, OR SUPPLIES (Explain Unusual Circumstances) CPT/HCPCS | MODIFIER	E DIAGNOSIS CODE	F $ CHARGES	G DAYS OR UNITS	H EPSDT Family Plan	I EMG	J COB	K RESERVED FOR LOCAL USE
1 030320XX	11		99203	1	70 92	1			12	45897700
2										
3										
4										
5										
6										

25. FEDERAL TAX I.D. NUMBER SSN EIN	26. PATIENT'S ACCOUNT NO.	27. ACCEPT ASSIGNMENT? (For govt. claims, see back)	28. TOTAL CHARGE	29. AMOUNT PAID	30. BALANCE DUE
74 1064090 ☐ ☒	010	☒ YES ☐ NO	$ 70 92	$	$ 70 92

24. A DATE(S) OF SERVICE From MM DD YY — To MM DD YY	B Place of Service	C Type of Service	D PROCEDURES, SERVICES, OR SUPPLIES (Explain Unusual Circumstances) CPT/HCPCS | MODIFIER	E DIAGNOSIS CODE	F $ CHARGES	G DAYS OR UNITS	H EPSDT Family Plan	I EMG	Initials	Date COB	RESERVED FOR LOCAL USE
1 113020XX	21		99231	1	37 74	1				32	78312700
2 120120XX 120320XX	21		99231	1	37 74	3				32	78312700
3											
4											
5											
6											

25. FEDERAL TAX I.D. NUMBER SSN EIN	26. PATIENT'S ACCOUNT NO.	27. ACCEPT ASSIGNMENT? (For govt. claims, see back)	28. TOTAL CHARGE	29. AMOUNT PAID	30. BALANCE DUE
75 6721022 ☐ ☒	102	☒ YES ☐ NO	$ 150 96	$	$ 150 96

All Private Payers: Enter the month, day, and year (eight digits with no spaces) for each procedure, service, or supply reported in Block 24D. Make sure the dates shown are no earlier than the date of the current illness if listed in Block 14. If the "from" and "to" dates are the same, enter only the "from" date. Enter the "to" date when reporting a consecutive range of dates for the same procedure code. Use a separate line for each month. Some third party payers may use different date formats (e.g., December 4, 20XX = 20001204).

Medicaid: Enter an eight-digit "from" date (month, day, and year with no spaces) for each service or supply. Leave "to" date blank. No date ranging is allowed for consecutive dates.

Medicare: Enter the month, day, and year (eight digits with no spaces) for each procedure, service, or supply reported in Block 24D. Make sure the dates shown are no earlier than the date of the current illness if listed in Block 14. If the "from" and "to" dates are the same, enter only the "from" date. Enter the "to" date when reporting a consecutive range of dates for the same procedure code. Use a separate line for each month except when reporting weekly radiation therapy, durable medical equipment, or oxygen rental.

Medicare/Medicaid: Refer to Medicare guidelines.
Medicare/Medigap: Refer to Medicare guidelines.
MSP: Refer to Medicare guidelines.

TRICARE: Enter the month, day, and year (eight digits with no spaces) for each procedure, service, or supply reported in Block 24D. Make sure the dates shown are no earlier than the date of the current illness if listed in Block 14. If the "from" and "to" dates are the same, enter only the "from" date. Enter the "to" date when reporting a consecutive range of dates for the same procedure code. Use a separate line for each month.

CHAMPVA: Refer to TRICARE guidelines.

Workers' Compensation: Enter the month, day, and year (eight digits with no spaces) for each procedure, service, or supply reported in Block 24D. Date ranging is not the preferred format for consecutive dates.

BLOCK 24B

24. A DATE(S) OF SERVICE		B Place of Service	C Type of Service	D PROCEDURES, SERVICES, OR SUPPLIES (Explain Unusual Circumstances) CPT/HCPCS | MODIFIER	E DIAGNOSIS CODE	F $ CHARGES	G DAYS OR UNITS	H EPSDT Family Plan	I EMG	J COB	K RESERVED FOR LOCAL USE
From MM DD YY	To MM DD YY										
1	030320XX	11		99203	1	70 92	1			12	45897700
2											
3											
4											
5											
6											

25. FEDERAL TAX I.D. NUMBER	SSN EIN	26. PATIENT'S ACCOUNT NO.	27. ACCEPT ASSIGNMENT? (For govt. claims, see back)	28. TOTAL CHARGE	29. AMOUNT PAID	30. BALANCE DUE
74 1064090	☐ ☒	010	☒ YES ☐ NO	$ 70 92	$	$ 70 92

All Payers: Enter the appropriate "Place of Service" code shown in Figure 6–4. Identify by location where the service was performed or an item was used. Use the inpatient hospital code only when a service is provided to a patient admitted to the hospital for an overnight stay. Enter the name, address, and provider number of the hospital in Block 32.

PLACE OF SERVICE CODES   (24B)

11 Doctor's office
12 Patient's home
21 Inpatient hospital
22 Outpatient hospital
23 Emergency department—hospital
24 Ambulatory surgical center
25 Birthing center
26 Military treatment facility/ uniformed service
    treatment facility
31 Skilled nursing facility (swing bed visits)
32 Nursing facility (intermediate/long-term care facilities)
33 Custodial care facility (domiciliary or rest home
    services)
34 Hospice (domiciliary or rest home services)
35 Adult living care facilities (residential care facility)
41 Ambulance–land
42 Ambulance–air or water
50 Federally qualified health center
51 Inpatient psychiatric facility
52 Psychiatric facility–partial hospitalization
53 Community mental health care (outpatient, twenty-
    four-hours-a-day services, admission screening,
    consultation, and educational services)
54 Intermediate care facility/mentally retarded
55 Residential substance abuse treatment facility
56 Psychiatric residential treatment center
60 Mass immunization center
61 Comprehensive inpatient rehabilitation facility
62 Comprehensive outpatient rehabilitation facility
65 End-stage renal disease treatment facility
71 State or local public health clinic
72 Rural health clinic
81 Independent laboratory
99 Other unlisted facility

Figure 6–4.

BLOCK 24C

24. A DATE(S) OF SERVICE						B Place of Service	C Type of Service	D PROCEDURES, SERVICES, OR SUPPLIES (Explain Unusual Circumstances) CPT/HCPCS | MODIFIER		E DIAGNOSIS CODE	F $ CHARGES		G DAYS OR UNITS	H EPSDT Family Plan	I EMG	J COB	K RESERVED FOR LOCAL USE
	From			To													
MM	DD	YY	MM	DD	YY												
030320XX						11		99203		1	70	92	1			12	45897700

25. FEDERAL TAX I.D. NUMBER	SSN EIN	26. PATIENT'S ACCOUNT NO.	27. ACCEPT ASSIGNMENT? (For govt. claims, see back)	28. TOTAL CHARGE	29. AMOUNT PAID	30. BALANCE DUE
74 1064090	☐ ☒	010	☒ YES ☐ NO	$ 70 92	$	$ 70 92

All Private Payers: Leave blank.

Medicaid: Enter the appropriate "Type of Service" code from Figure 6–5.

Medicare: Leave blank. "Type of Service" codes are used on Medicare Remittance Advice (RA) documents and electronic claims.
Medicare/Medicaid: Refer to Medicare guidelines.
Medicare/Medigap: Refer to Medicare guidelines.
MSP: Refer to Medicare guidelines.

TRICARE: Enter the appropriate "Type of Service" code from Figure 6–5. Codes may vary according to regions and claim administrators.
▶ *When completing the* Workbook *assignments, use the codes shown in Figure 6–5.*

CHAMPVA: Refer to guidelines for TRICARE.

Workers' Compensation: Enter the appropriate "Type of Service" code shown in Figure 6–5. These codes may not be used or may vary according to regions and claim administrators.
▶ *When completing the* Workbook *assignments, use the codes shown in Figure 6–5.*

BLOCK 24C TYPE OF SERVICE CODES FOR MEDICAID, TRICARE, AND WORKERS' COMPENSATION

These codes should be selected depending on the procedure code used on each line. Codes may vary according to regions and claim administrators.

1 Medical care (e.g., evaluation and management services)
2 Surgery
3 Consultation
4 Diagnostic x-ray (e.g., ultrasound and nuclear testing)
5 Diagnostic laboratory
6 Radiation therapy
7 Anesthesia
8 Assistant at surgery
9 Other medical service (e.g., laboratory, venipuncture, handling of specimen)
0 Blood or packed red cells
A DME rental/purchase
B Drugs
C Ambulatory surgery
D Hospice
E Second opinion on elective surgery
F Maternity
G Dental
H Mental health care
I Ambulance
J Program for persons with disabilities
L Renal supply in home
M Alternate payment for maintenance
N Kidney donor
V Pneumococcal vaccine
Z Third opinion on elective surgery

Figure 6–5.

BLOCK 24D

24. A DATE(S) OF SERVICE							B Place of Service	C Type of Service	D PROCEDURES, SERVICES, OR SUPPLIES (Explain Unusual Circumstances) CPT/HCPCS | MODIFIER		E DIAGNOSIS CODE	F $ CHARGES		G DAYS OR UNITS	H EPSDT Family Plan	I EMG	J COB	K RESERVED FOR LOCAL USE
MM	From DD	YY	MM	To DD	YY													
1	03 03 20 XX						11		99203			1	70	92	1			12	45897700
2																		
3																		
4																		
5																		
6																		

25. FEDERAL TAX I.D. NUMBER	SSN EIN	26. PATIENT'S ACCOUNT NO.	27. ACCEPT ASSIGNMENT? (For govt. claims, see back)	28. TOTAL CHARGE	29. AMOUNT PAID	30. BALANCE DUE
74 1064090	☐ ☒	010	☒ YES ☐ NO	$ 70 92	$	$ 70 92

CPT   99203   Office visit, new patient

All Private Payers: Enter the appropriate CPT/HCPCS code for each procedure, service, or supply and applicable modifier without a hyphen. If it is necessary to use more than two modifiers with a procedure code, enter modifier -99 in Block 24D and list applicable modifiers in Block 19.

Medicaid: Enter the appropriate CPT/HCPCS code for each procedure, service, or supply and applicable modifier without a hyphen.

Medicare: Enter CPT/HCPCS code and applicable modifiers without a hyphen for procedures, services, and supplies without a narrative description. When procedure codes do not require modifiers, leave modifier area blank—do not enter 00 or any other combination. For multiple surgical procedures, list the procedure with the highest fee first. For unlisted procedure codes, include a narrative description in Block 19 (e.g., 99499, "Unlisted Evaluation and Management Service"). If information does not fit in Block 19, include an attachment. When entering an unlisted surgery code, submit the operative notes with the claim as an attachment.
Medicare/Medicaid: Refer to Medicare guidelines.
Medicare/Medigap: Refer to Medicare guidelines.
MSP: Refer to Medicare guidelines.

TRICARE: Enter the appropriate CPT/HCPCS code for each procedure, service, or supply and applicable modifier without a hyphen. If it is necessary to use more than two modifiers with a procedure code, enter modifier -99 in Block 24D and list applicable modifiers in Block 19. When Not Otherwise Classified (NOC) codes are submitted (e.g., supplies and injections), provide a narrative of the service in Block 19 or on an attachment.

CHAMPVA: Refer to TRICARE guidelines.

Workers' Compensation: Enter appropriate RVS codes and applicable modifiers (without a hyphen) used in your state or region.
▶ *When completing the* Workbook *assignments, use appropriate CPT codes.*

BLOCK 24E

21. DIAGNOSIS OR NATURE OF ILLNESS OR INJURY (RELATE ITEMS 1,2,3 OR 4 TO ITEM 24E BY LINE)		22. MEDICAID RESUBMISSION CODE	ORIGINAL REF. NO.
1. 382 00	3.	23. PRIOR AUTHORIZATION NUMBER	
2.	4.		

24. A DATE(S) OF SERVICE		B Place of Service	C Type of Service	D PROCEDURES, SERVICES, OR SUPPLIES (Explain Unusual Circumstances) CPT/HCPCS | MODIFIER	E DIAGNOSIS CODE	F $ CHARGES	G DAYS OR UNITS	H EPSDT Family Plan	I EMG	J COB	K RESERVED FOR LOCAL USE
From MM DD YY	To MM DD YY										
1 030320XX		11		99203	1	70 92	1			12	45897700
2											
3											
4											
5											
6											

25. FEDERAL TAX I.D. NUMBER	SSN EIN	26. PATIENT'S ACCOUNT NO.	27. ACCEPT ASSIGNMENT? (For govt. claims, see back)	28. TOTAL CHARGE	29. AMOUNT PAID	30. BALANCE DUE
74 1064090	☐ ☒	010	☒ YES ☐ NO	$ 70 92	$	$ 70 92

All Private Payers: Enter only one diagnosis code reference "pointer" number per line item (unless you have verified that independent carriers allow more than one) linking the diagnostic code listed in Block 21. When multiple services are performed, enter the corresponding diagnostic reference number for each service (e.g., 1, 2, 3, or 4). DO NOT USE ACTUAL ICD-9-CM CODES IN THIS BLOCK.

▶ *When completing* Workbook *assignments, more than one diagnosis reference "pointer" number per line item is allowed.*

Medicaid: Refer to Medicare guidelines. In some states, completion may not be required.

Medicare: Enter only one diagnosis code reference "pointer" number per line item linking the diagnostic codes listed in Block 21. When multiple services are performed, enter the corresponding diagnostic reference number for each service (e.g., 1, 2, 3, or 4). DO NOT USE ACTUAL ICD-9-CM CODES IN THIS BLOCK.

Medicare/Medicaid: Refer to Medicare guidelines.

Medicare/Medigap: Refer to Medicare guidelines.

MSP: Refer to Medicare guidelines.

TRICARE: Enter the diagnosis reference number (i.e., indicating up to four ICD-9-CM codes) as shown in Block 21 to relate the date of service and the procedures performed to the appropriate diagnosis. If multiple procedures are performed, enter the diagnosis code reference number for each service.

CHAMPVA: Refer to TRICARE guidelines.

Workers' Compensation: Enter all appropriate diagnosis code reference "pointer" numbers from Block 21 to relate appropriate diagnosis to date of service and procedures performed. A maximum of four diagnosis pointers may be referenced. Place commas between multiple diagnosis reference pointers on the same line.

BLOCK 24F

24. A DATE(S) OF SERVICE		B Place of Service	C Type of Service	D PROCEDURES, SERVICES, OR SUPPLIES (Explain Unusual Circumstances) CPT/HCPCS | MODIFIER	E DIAGNOSIS CODE	F $ CHARGES	G DAYS OR UNITS	H EPSDT Family Plan	I EMG	J COB	K RESERVED FOR LOCAL USE
From MM DD YY	To MM DD YY										
030320XX		11		99203	1	70 92	1			12	45897700

25. FEDERAL TAX I.D. NUMBER	SSN EIN	26. PATIENT'S ACCOUNT NO.	27. ACCEPT ASSIGNMENT? (For govt. claims, see back)	28. TOTAL CHARGE	29. AMOUNT PAID	30. BALANCE DUE
74 1064090	☐ ☒	010	☒ YES ☐ NO	$ 70 92	$	$ 70 92

All Payers: Enter the fee for each listed service from the appropriate fee schedule. DO NOT ENTER DOLLAR SIGNS OR DECIMAL POINTS. ALWAYS INCLUDE CENTS. If the same service is performed on consecutive days, list the fee for one service in this block and the number of units (times it was performed) in Block 24G (see bottom graphic on page 204). The total for consecutive services should be computed and added into the claim total shown in Block 28.

▶ *When completing the* Workbook *assignments for private, Medicaid, TRICARE, and workers' compensation cases, use the **Mock Fee**. For Medicare participating provider cases, use the **Participating Provider Fee**. For nonparticipating provider cases, use the **Limiting Charge**.*

BLOCK 24G

24. A DATE(S) OF SERVICE						B Place of Service	C Type of Service	D PROCEDURES, SERVICES, OR SUPPLIES (Explain Unusual Circumstances) CPT/HCPCS | MODIFIER		E DIAGNOSIS CODE	F $ CHARGES		G DAYS OR UNITS	H EPSDT Family Plan	I EMG	J COB	K RESERVED FOR LOCAL USE
From MM	DD	YY	MM	To DD	YY												
1	03 03 20 XX						11		99203		1	70	92	1			12	45897700
2																	
3																	
4																	
5																	
6																	

25. FEDERAL TAX I.D. NUMBER	SSN EIN	26. PATIENT'S ACCOUNT NO.	27. ACCEPT ASSIGNMENT? (For govt. claims, see back)	28. TOTAL CHARGE	29. AMOUNT PAID	30. BALANCE DUE
74 1064090	☐ ☒	010	☒ YES ☐ NO	$ 70 92	$	$ 70 92

All Private Payers: Enter the number of days or units that apply to each line of service. This block is important for calculating multiple visits, anesthesia minutes, or oxygen volume (see bottom graphic on page 204).

Medicaid: Each service must be listed on separate lines (no date ranging). Indicate that each service was performed one time by listing "1" in this block. List number of visits in 1 day.

Medicare: Enter the number of days or units that apply to each line of service. This block is important for calculating multiple visits, number of miles, units of supplies including drugs, anesthesia minutes, or oxygen volume. For example, when a physician reports consecutive hospital care services using CPT code number 99231, on May 6, 7, 8, and 9, it would be totalled and shown as on page 204. See the Medicare Manual for reporting anesthesia time/units and for rounding out figures when billing gas and liquid oxygen units.
Medicare/Medicaid: Refer to Medicare guidelines.
Medicare/Medigap: Refer to Medicare guidelines.
MSP: Refer to Medicare guidelines.

TRICARE: Refer to guidelines for Medicare.

CHAMPVA: Refer to Medicare guidelines.

Workers' Compensation: Refer to Medicare guidelines.

BLOCK 24H

24. A DATE(S) OF SERVICE		B Place of Service	C Type of Service	D PROCEDURES, SERVICES, OR SUPPLIES (Explain Unusual Circumstances) CPT/HCPCS | MODIFIER	E DIAGNOSIS CODE	F $ CHARGES	G DAYS OR UNITS	H EPSDT Family Plan	I EMG	J COB	K RESERVED FOR LOCAL USE
From MM DD YY	To MM DD YY										
1 030320XX		11		99203	1	70 92	1			12	45897700
2											
3											
4											
5											
6											

25. FEDERAL TAX I.D. NUMBER	SSN EIN	26. PATIENT'S ACCOUNT NO.	27. ACCEPT ASSIGNMENT? (For govt. claims, see back)	28. TOTAL CHARGE	29. AMOUNT PAID	30. BALANCE DUE
74 1064090	☐ ☒	010	☒ YES ☐ NO	$ 70 92	$	$ 70 92

All Private Payers: Leave blank.

Medicaid: EPSDT means early, periodic, screening, diagnosis, and treatment and this refers to a Medicaid service program for children 12 years of age or younger. Enter "E" for EPSDT services or "F" for family planning services, if applicable.

Medicare: Leave blank.
Medicare/Medicaid: Leave blank.
Medicare/Medigap: Leave blank.
MSP: Leave blank.

TRICARE: Leave blank.

CHAMPVA: Leave blank.

Workers' Compensation: Leave blank.

BLOCK 24I

24. A DATE(S) OF SERVICE						B Place of Service	C Type of Service	D PROCEDURES, SERVICES, OR SUPPLIES (Explain Unusual Circumstances) CPT/HCPCS | MODIFIER	E DIAGNOSIS CODE	F $ CHARGES		G DAYS OR UNITS	H EPSDT Family Plan	I EMG	J COB	K RESERVED FOR LOCAL USE
From MM	DD	YY	To MM	DD	YY											
1	03	03	20XX				11		99203	1	70	92	1			12	45897700
2																
3																
4																
5																
6																

25. FEDERAL TAX I.D. NUMBER SSN EIN	26. PATIENT'S ACCOUNT NO.	27. ACCEPT ASSIGNMENT? (For govt. claims, see back) YES NO	28. TOTAL CHARGE	29. AMOUNT PAID	30. BALANCE DUE
74 1064090 ☐ ☒	010	☒ YES ☐ NO	$ 70 92	$	$ 70 92

All Private Payers: Leave blank.

Medicaid: EMG stands for the word "emergency" and means that the service was rendered in a *hospital emergency department*. Enter "X" if emergency care is provided in an emergency department.

Medicare: Leave blank.
Medicare/Medicaid: Leave blank.
Medicare/Medigap: Leave blank.
MSP: Leave blank.

TRICARE: Enter "X" in this block to indicate that the service was provided in a hospital emergency department.

CHAMPVA: Enter "X" in this block to indicate that the service was provided in a hospital emergency department.

Workers' Compensation: Leave blank.

BLOCK 24J

24. A DATE(S) OF SERVICE						B Place of Service	C Type of Service	D PROCEDURES, SERVICES, OR SUPPLIES (Explain Unusual Circumstances) CPT/HCPCS | MODIFIER	E DIAGNOSIS CODE	F $ CHARGES		G DAYS OR UNITS	H EPSDT Family Plan	I EMG	J COB	K RESERVED FOR LOCAL USE
	From MM	DD	YY	To MM	DD	YY											
1	03	03	20XX				11		99203	1	70	92	1			12	45897700
2																	
3																	
4																	
5																	
6																	

25. FEDERAL TAX I.D. NUMBER	SSN EIN	26. PATIENT'S ACCOUNT NO.	27. ACCEPT ASSIGNMENT? (For govt. claims, see back)	28. TOTAL CHARGE	29. AMOUNT PAID	30. BALANCE DUE
74 1064090	☐ ☒	010	☒ YES ☐ NO	$ 70 92	$	$ 70 92

All Private Payers: Refer to the note under Block 24K.

Medicaid: COB means coordination of benefits. Check, if applicable, when the patient has other insurance.

Medicare: Refer to the note for Block 24K.
Medicare/Medicaid: Refer to the note for Block 24K.
Medicare/Medigap: Refer to the note for Block 24K.
MSP: Refer to the note for Block 24K.

TRICARE: Leave blank.

CHAMPVA: Leave blank.

Workers' Compensation: Leave blank.

BLOCK 24K

| 24. A DATE(S) OF SERVICE | | | | | | B Place of Service | C Type of Service | D PROCEDURES, SERVICES, OR SUPPLIES (Explain Unusual Circumstances) CPT/HCPCS \| MODIFIER | E DIAGNOSIS CODE | F $ CHARGES | | G DAYS OR UNITS | H EPSDT Family Plan | I EMG | J COB | K RESERVED FOR LOCAL USE |
From MM	DD	YY	To MM	DD	YY											
1 030320XX						11		99203	1	70	92	1			12	45897700
2																
3																
4																
5																
6																

25. FEDERAL TAX I.D. NUMBER	SSN	EIN	26. PATIENT'S ACCOUNT NO.	27. ACCEPT ASSIGNMENT? (For govt. claims, see back)	28. TOTAL CHARGE	29. AMOUNT PAID	30. BALANCE DUE
74 1064090	☐	☒	010	☒ YES ☐ NO	$ 70 92	$	$ 70 92

All Private Payers: Enter the HCFA-assigned Provider Identification Number (PIN) or National Provider Identifier (NPI) for each line of service when the performing physician/supplier is in a *group practice* and billing under a group I.D. number. An individual physician's PIN/NPI is not required if he or she is in solo practice or when billing under his or her individual I.D. number. **Note:** *Enter the first two digits of the NPI in Block 24J. Enter the remaining eight digits of the NPI in Block 24K, including the two-digit location identifier.*

Medicaid: Leave blank.

Medicare: Enter the HCFA-assigned Provider Identification Number (PIN) or National Provider Identifier (NPI) for each line of service when the performing physician/supplier is in a *group practice* and billing under a group I.D. number. An individual physician's PIN/NPI is not required if he or she is in solo practice or when billing under his or her individual I.D. number. **Note:** *Enter the first two digits of the NPI in Block 24J. Enter the remaining eight digits of the NPI in Block 24K, including the two-digit location identifier.*
Medicare/Medicaid: Refer to Medicare guidelines.
Medicare/Medigap: Refer to Medicare guidelines.
MSP: Refer to Medicare guidelines.

TRICARE: Enter the physician's state license number when billing for a group practice using one group I.D. number. The state license number is an alpha character followed by six numeric digits. If there are not six digits, enter appropriate number of zero(s) after the alpha character (i.e., A1234 would be A001234).

CHAMPVA: Refer to TRICARE guidelines.

Workers' Compensation: Leave blank.

BLOCK 25

25. FEDERAL TAX I.D. NUMBER	SSN EIN	26. PATIENT'S ACCOUNT NO.	27. ACCEPT ASSIGNMENT? (For govt. claims, see back)	28. TOTAL CHARGE	29. AMOUNT PAID	30. BALANCE DUE
74 1064090	☐ ☒	010	☒ YES ☐ NO	$ 70 92	$	$ 70 92

31. SIGNATURE OF PHYSICIAN OR SUPPLIER INCLUDING DEGREES OR CREDENTIALS (I certify that the statements on the reverse apply to this bill and are made a part thereof.)	32. NAME AND ADDRESS OF FACILITY WHERE SERVICES WERE RENDERED (If other than home or office)	33. PHYSICIAN'S, SUPPLIER'S BILLING NAME, ADDRESS, ZIP CODE & PHONE #
CONCHA ANTRUM MD 030320XX SIGNED *Concha Antrum MD* DATE	SAME	COLLEGE CLINIC 4567 BROAD AVENUE WOODLAND HILLS XY 12345 0001 013 486 9002 PIN# GRP# 3664021CC

reference initials

All Payers: Enter the physician/supplier's federal tax I.D. This number may be the Employer Identification Number (EIN) or Social Security Number (SSN). Check the corresponding box.
▶ A Medicaid case may or may not require a physician's tax I.D. number, depending on individual state guidelines.
▶ In a Medicare/Medigap case, the physician's federal tax I.D. number is required for Medigap transfer.
▶ *When completing the* Workbook *assignments, enter the physician's EIN number and check the appropriate box.*

BLOCK 26

25. FEDERAL TAX I.D. NUMBER	SSN EIN	26. PATIENT'S ACCOUNT NO.	27. ACCEPT ASSIGNMENT? (For govt. claims, see back)	28. TOTAL CHARGE	29. AMOUNT PAID	30. BALANCE DUE
74 1064090	☐ ☒	010	☒ YES ☐ NO	$ 70 92	$	$ 70 92

31. SIGNATURE OF PHYSICIAN OR SUPPLIER INCLUDING DEGREES OR CREDENTIALS (I certify that the statements on the reverse apply to this bill and are made a part thereof.)	32. NAME AND ADDRESS OF FACILITY WHERE SERVICES WERE RENDERED (If other than home or office)	33. PHYSICIAN'S, SUPPLIER'S BILLING NAME, ADDRESS, ZIP CODE & PHONE #
CONCHA ANTRUM MD 030320XX SIGNED *Concha Antrum MD* DATE	SAME	COLLEGE CLINIC 4567 BROAD AVENUE WOODLAND HILLS XY 12345 0001 013 486 9002 PIN# GRP# 3664021CC

reference initials

All Payers: Enter the patient's account number assigned by the physician's accounting system. Do not use dashes or slashes. When Medicare is billed electronically, this block *must be completed.*
▶ *When completing the* Workbook *assignments, list the patient account number when provided.*

BLOCK 27

25. FEDERAL TAX I.D. NUMBER SSN EIN	26. PATIENT'S ACCOUNT NO.	27. ACCEPT ASSIGNMENT? (For govt. claims, see back)	28. TOTAL CHARGE	29. AMOUNT PAID	30. BALANCE DUE
74 1064090 ☐ ☒	010	☒ YES ☐ NO	$ 70│92	$	$ 70│92

31. SIGNATURE OF PHYSICIAN OR SUPPLIER INCLUDING DEGREES OR CREDENTIALS (I certify that the statements on the reverse apply to this bill and are made a part thereof.)	32. NAME AND ADDRESS OF FACILITY WHERE SERVICES WERE RENDERED (If other than home or office)	33. PHYSICIAN'S, SUPPLIER'S BILLING NAME, ADDRESS, ZIP CODE & PHONE #
CONCHA ANTRUM MD 030320XX SIGNED *Concha Antrum MD* DATE	SAME	COLLEGE CLINIC 4567 BROAD AVENUE WOODLAND HILLS XY 12345 0001 013 486 9002 PIN# GRP# 3664021CC

reference initials

All Private Payers: Check "yes" or "no" to indicate whether the physician accepts assignment of benefits. If yes, then the physician agrees to accept the allowed amount paid by the third party plus any copayment and/or deductible as payment in full.

▶ *When completing the* Workbook *assignments, check "yes."*

Medicaid: Check "yes."

Medicare: Check "yes" or "no" to indicate whether the physician accepts assignment of benefits. If yes, then the physician agrees to accept the allowed amount paid by the third party plus any copayment or deductible as payment in full. If this field is left blank, "no" is assumed, and a participating physician's claim will be denied. The following provider/supplier must file claims on an assignment basis:

◗ Clinical diagnostic laboratory services performed in physician's office

   Physicians wishing to accept assignment on clinical laboratory services but not other services should submit two separate claims, one "assigned" for laboratory and one "nonassigned" for other services. Submit all charges on a nonassigned claim, as indicated in Block 27, and write "I accept assignment for the clinical laboratory tests" at the bottom of Block 24.

◗ Participating physician/supplier services
◗ Physician's services to Medicare/Medicaid patients
◗ Services of: physician assistants, nurse practitioners, clinical nurse specialists, nurse midwives, certified registered nurse anesthetists, clinical psychologists, clinical social workers
◗ Ambulatory surgical center services
◗ Home dialysis supplies and equipment paid under Method II (monthly capitation payment)

▶ *When completing the* Workbook *assignments, check "yes."*

Medicare/Medicaid: Check "yes."
Medicare/Medigap: Check "yes."
MSP: Check "yes" or "no" to indicate whether the physician accepts assignment of benefits for primary insurance and Medicare.

▶ *When completing the* Workbook *assignments, check "yes."*

TRICARE: Refer to Medicare guidelines. However, participation in TRICARE may be made on a case-by-case basis.

CHAMPVA: Refer to Medicare guidelines.

Workers' Compensation: Leave blank.

BLOCK 28

25. FEDERAL TAX I.D. NUMBER SSN EIN	26. PATIENT'S ACCOUNT NO.	27. ACCEPT ASSIGNMENT? (For govt. claims, see back)	28. TOTAL CHARGE	29. AMOUNT PAID	30. BALANCE DUE
74 1064090 ☐ ☒	010	☒ YES ☐ NO	$ 70	92	$	$ 70	92

| 31. SIGNATURE OF PHYSICIAN OR SUPPLIER INCLUDING DEGREES OR CREDENTIALS (I certify that the statements on the reverse apply to this bill and are made a part thereof.)

CONCHA ANTRUM MD 030320XX

SIGNED *Concha Antrum MD* DATE | 32. NAME AND ADDRESS OF FACILITY WHERE SERVICES WERE RENDERED (If other than home or office)

SAME | 33. PHYSICIAN'S, SUPPLIER'S BILLING NAME, ADDRESS, ZIP CODE & PHONE #

COLLEGE CLINIC
4567 BROAD AVENUE
WOODLAND HILLS XY 12345 0001
013 486 9002
PIN#   GRP#   3664021CC |

reference initials

All Payers: Enter total charges for services listed in Block(s) 24F. If more than one unit is listed in Block 24G, multiply the number of units by the charge and add the amount into the total charge (see page 204, bottom). Do not enter dollar signs or decimal points. Always include cents.

BLOCK 29

25. FEDERAL TAX I.D. NUMBER SSN EIN	26. PATIENT'S ACCOUNT NO.	27. ACCEPT ASSIGNMENT? (For govt. claims, see back)	28. TOTAL CHARGE	29. AMOUNT PAID	30. BALANCE DUE
74 1064090 ☐ ☒	010	☒ YES ☐ NO	$ 70	92	$	$ 70	92

| 31. SIGNATURE OF PHYSICIAN OR SUPPLIER INCLUDING DEGREES OR CREDENTIALS (I certify that the statements on the reverse apply to this bill and are made a part thereof.)

CONCHA ANTRUM MD 030320XX

SIGNED *Concha Antrum MD* DATE | 32. NAME AND ADDRESS OF FACILITY WHERE SERVICES WERE RENDERED (If other than home or office)

SAME | 33. PHYSICIAN'S, SUPPLIER'S BILLING NAME, ADDRESS, ZIP CODE & PHONE #

COLLEGE CLINIC
4567 BROAD AVENUE
WOODLAND HILLS XY 12345 0001
013 486 9002
PIN#   GRP#   3664021CC |

reference initials

All Private Payers: Enter only the amount paid for the charges listed on the claim.

Medicaid: Enter only the payment on claim by a third party payer, excluding Medicare.

Medicare: Enter only the amount paid for the charges listed on the claim.
Medicare/Medicaid: Refer to Medicare guidelines.
Medicare/Medigap: Enter only the amount paid for charges listed on the claim.
MSP: Enter only the amount paid for charges listed on the claim. It is mandatory to enter amount paid by primary carrier and attach an explanation of benefits document when billing Medicare.

TRICARE: Enter only amount paid by *other carrier* for the charges listed on the claim. If the amount includes payment by any other health insurances, the other health insurance explanation of benefits, work sheet, or denial showing the amounts paid must be attached to the claim. Payment from the beneficiary should not be included.

CHAMPVA: Refer to TRICARE guidelines.

Workers' Compensation: Leave blank.

BLOCK 30

25. FEDERAL TAX I.D. NUMBER	SSN EIN	26. PATIENT'S ACCOUNT NO.	27. ACCEPT ASSIGNMENT? (For govt. claims, see back)	28. TOTAL CHARGE	29. AMOUNT PAID	30. BALANCE DUE
74 1064090	☐ ☒	010	☒ YES ☐ NO	$ 70 | 92	$	$ 70 | 92

31. SIGNATURE OF PHYSICIAN OR SUPPLIER INCLUDING DEGREES OR CREDENTIALS (I certify that the statements on the reverse apply to this bill and are made a part thereof.)	32. NAME AND ADDRESS OF FACILITY WHERE SERVICES WERE RENDERED (If other than home or office)	33. PHYSICIAN'S, SUPPLIER'S BILLING NAME, ADDRESS, ZIP CODE & PHONE #
CONCHA ANTRUM MD 030320XX SIGNED *Concha Antrum MD* DATE	SAME	COLLEGE CLINIC 4567 BROAD AVENUE WOODLAND HILLS XY 12345 0001 013 486 9002 PIN# GRP# 3664021CC

reference initials

All Private Payers: Enter balance due on claim (Block 28 less Block 29).

Medicaid: Leave blank or enter balance due on claim depending on individual state guidelines.
► *When completing the* Workbook *assignments, enter the balance due.*

Medicare: Leave blank.
Medicare/Medicaid: Leave blank.
Medicare/Medigap: Leave blank.
MSP: Leave blank.

TRICARE: Enter balance due on claim (Block 28 less Block 29).

CHAMPVA: Enter balance due on claim (Block 28 less Block 29).

Workers' Compensation: Enter balance due on claim (Block 28 less Block 29).

BLOCK 31

25. FEDERAL TAX I.D. NUMBER SSN EIN	26. PATIENT'S ACCOUNT NO.	27. ACCEPT ASSIGNMENT? (For govt. claims, see back)	28. TOTAL CHARGE	29. AMOUNT PAID	30. BALANCE DUE
74 1064090 ☐ ☒	010	☒ YES ☐ NO	$ 70 | 92	$	$ 70 | 92
31. SIGNATURE OF PHYSICIAN OR SUPPLIER INCLUDING DEGREES OR CREDENTIALS (I certify that the statements on the reverse apply to this bill and are made a part thereof.) CONCHA ANTRUM MD 030320XX SIGNED *Concha Antrum MD* DATE	32. NAME AND ADDRESS OF FACILITY WHERE SERVICES WERE RENDERED (If other than home or office) SAME		33. PHYSICIAN'S, SUPPLIER'S BILLING NAME, ADDRESS, ZIP CODE & PHONE # COLLEGE CLINIC 4567 BROAD AVENUE WOODLAND HILLS XY 12345 0001 013 486 9002 PIN# GRP# 3664021CC		

reference initials

All Payers: Type the provider's name and show the signature of the physician or the physician's representative above or below the name. Enter the eight-digit date the form was prepared. Most insurance carriers will accept a stamped signature, but the stamp must be completely inside the block. *Do not* type the name of the association or corporation.

BLOCK 32

25. FEDERAL TAX I.D. NUMBER	SSN EIN	26. PATIENT'S ACCOUNT NO.	27. ACCEPT ASSIGNMENT? (For govt. claims, see back)	28. TOTAL CHARGE	29. AMOUNT PAID	30. BALANCE DUE
74 1064090	☐ ☒	010	☒ YES ☐ NO	$ 70 92	$	$ 70 92

31. SIGNATURE OF PHYSICIAN OR SUPPLIER INCLUDING DEGREES OR CREDENTIALS (I certify that the statements on the reverse apply to this bill and are made a part thereof.)	32. NAME AND ADDRESS OF FACILITY WHERE SERVICES WERE RENDERED (If other than home or office)	33. PHYSICIAN'S, SUPPLIER'S BILLING NAME, ADDRESS, ZIP CODE & PHONE #
CONCHA ANTRUM MD 030320XX SIGNED *Concha Antrum MD* DATE	SAME	COLLEGE CLINIC 4567 BROAD AVENUE WOODLAND HILLS XY 12345 0001 013 486 9002 PIN# GRP# 3664021CC

reference initials

All Private Payers: Enter the word "SAME" in the center of the block if the facility furnishing services is the same as that of the biller listed in Block 33. *If other* than home, office, nursing facility, or community mental health center, enter the name, address, and provider number of the facility (e.g., hospital name for physician's hospital services). For durable medical equipment, enter the *location* where the *order is taken*. If a test is performed by a mammography screening center, enter the six-digit certification number approved by the Food and Drug Administration (FDA). When billing for purchased diagnostic tests performed outside the physician's office but billed by the physician, enter the facility's name, address, and HCFA-assigned NPI where the test was performed.

Medicaid: Refer to Medicare guidelines when completing this block; however, use Medicaid facility provider number.

Medicare: Enter "SAME" in the center of the block if the facility furnishing services is the same as that of the biller listed in Block 33. *If other* than home, office, nursing facility, or community mental health center, enter the name, address, and provider number of the facility (e.g., hospital name for physician's hospital services). For hospital services performed by a physician, the Medicare provider number must be preceded by "HSP." For durable medical equipment, enter the *location* where the *order is taken*. If the test is performed by a mammography screening center, enter the six-digit FDA-approved certification number. When billing for purchased diagnostic tests performed outside the physician's office but billed by the physician, enter the facility's name, address, and HCFA-assigned NPI where the test was performed.

Medicare/Medicaid: Refer to Medicare guidelines.

Medicare/Medigap: Refer to Medicare guidelines.

MSP: Refer to Medicare guidelines.

TRICARE: Refer to private payer guidelines. For partnership providers, indicate the name of the Military Treatment Facility.

CHAMPVA: Refer to private payer guidelines.

Workers' Compensation: Refer to private payer guidelines.

BLOCK 33

25. FEDERAL TAX I.D. NUMBER SSN EIN	26. PATIENT'S ACCOUNT NO.	27. ACCEPT ASSIGNMENT? (For govt. claims, see back)	28. TOTAL CHARGE	29. AMOUNT PAID	30. BALANCE DUE
74 1064090 ☐ ☒	010	☒ YES ☐ NO	$ 70 | 92	$	$ 70 | 92

| 31. SIGNATURE OF PHYSICIAN OR SUPPLIER INCLUDING DEGREES OR CREDENTIALS (I certify that the statements on the reverse apply to this bill and are made a part thereof.)

CONCHA ANTRUM MD 030320XX

SIGNED *Concha Antrum MD* DATE | 32. NAME AND ADDRESS OF FACILITY WHERE SERVICES WERE RENDERED (If other than home or office)

SAME | 33. PHYSICIAN'S, SUPPLIER'S BILLING NAME, ADDRESS, ZIP CODE & PHONE #
COLLEGE CLINIC
4567 BROAD AVENUE
WOODLAND HILLS XY 12345 0001
013 486 9002
PIN#   GRP# 3664021CC |

reference initials

All Private Payers: Refer to Medicare guidelines.

Medicaid: Refer to Medicare guidelines except use Medicaid's facility provider number.

Medicare: Enter the name, address, and telephone number for the physician, clinic, or supplier billing for services. Either enter the PIN/NPI for a performing physician or supplier who is *not* a member of a group practice in the lower left section of the block or enter the *group number* for a performing physician or supplier who belongs to a group practice and is billing under the group I.D. number in the right lower section of the block.
Medicare/Medicaid: Refer to Medicare guidelines.
Medicare/Medigap: Refer to Medicare guidelines.
MSP: Refer to Medicare guidelines.

TRICARE: Enter the name, address, and telephone number for the physician, clinic, or supplier billing for services. Radiologists, pathologists, and anesthesiologists may use their billing address if they have no *physical address*. Enter the NPI or TRICARE assigned PIN for a performing physician or supplier in the lower left section of the block; *the group number is not required.*
▶ *When completing the* Workbook *assignments, enter the performing physician's NPI in the lower left section of the block.*

CHAMPVA: Refer to TRICARE guidelines.

Workers' Compensation: Enter the name, address, and telephone number of the physician. Individual or group provider numbers or state license number are generally required depending on the insurance carrier's requirements.
▶ *When completing* Workbook *assignments, follow Medicare guidelines.*

BOTTOM OF FORM

Enter insurance billing specialist's initials in lower left corner of the insurance claim form.

Insurance Program Templates

The following pages show completed HCFA-1500 insurance claim forms and templates for the most common insurance programs encountered in a medical practice. Screened areas on each form do not apply to the insurance program example shown and should be left blank. Add a tab at the page margin for ease in flipping to this reference section when completing *Workbook* assignments. Examples illustrating entries for basic cases are:

Figure 6−6   Private payer

Figure 6−7   Back of HCFA-1500 insurance claim form

Figure 6−8   Medicaid

Figure 6−9   Medicare

Figure 6−10   Medicare/Medicaid—a crossover claim

Figure 6−11   Medicare/Medigap—a crossover claim

Figure 6−12   MSP—other insurance primary and Medicare secondary

Figure 6−13   TRICARE—Standard

Figure 6−14   CHAMPVA

Figure 6−15   Workers' Compensation

PRIVATE PAYER
No secondary coverage

PRIVATE INSURANCE COMPANY NAME
MAILING ADDRESS
CITY STATE ZIP CODE

| 1. MEDICARE (Medicare #) | MEDICAID (Medicaid #) | CHAMPUS (Sponsor's SSN) | CHAMPVA (VA File #) | GROUP HEALTH PLAN (SSN or ID) [X] | FECA BLK LUNG (SSN) | OTHER (ID) | 1a. INSURED'S I.D. NUMBER 111704521 | (FOR PROGRAM IN ITEM 1) A482 |

| 2. PATIENT'S NAME (Last Name, First Name, Middle Initial) | 3. PATIENT'S BIRTH DATE | 4. INSURED'S NAME (Last Name, First Name, Middle Initial) |
| FOREHAND HARRY N | MM 01 DD 06 YYYY 1946 SEX M [X] F | SAME |

5. PATIENT'S ADDRESS (No., Street)
1456 MAIN STREET

6. PATIENT RELATIONSHIP TO INSURED
Self [X] Spouse [ ] Child [ ] Other [ ]

7. INSURED'S ADDRESS (No., Street)

CITY WOODLAND HILLS STATE XY

8. PATIENT STATUS
Single [ ] Married [X] Other [ ]

CITY STATE

ZIP CODE 12345 0000 TELEPHONE (include Area Code) (013) 490 9876

Employed [X] Full-Time Student [ ] Part-Time Student [ ]

ZIP CODE TELEPHONE (include Area Code) ( )

9. OTHER INSURED'S NAME (Last Name, First Name, Middle Initial)

10. IS PATIENT'S CONDITION RELATED TO:

11. INSURED'S POLICY GROUP OR FECA NUMBER

a. OTHER INSURED'S POLICY OR GROUP NUMBER

a. EMPLOYMENT? (CURRENT OR PREVIOUS)
YES [ ] NO [X]

a. INSURED'S DATE OF BIRTH MM DD YYYY SEX M [ ] F [ ]

b. OTHER INSURED'S DATE OF BIRTH MM DD YYYY M [ ] F [ ]

b. AUTO ACCIDENT? PLACE (State)
YES [ ] NO [X]

b. EMPLOYER'S NAME OR SCHOOL NAME

c. EMPLOYER'S NAME OR SCHOOL NAME

c. OTHER ACCIDENT?
YES [ ] NO [X]

c. INSURANCE PLAN NAME OR PROGRAM NAME

d. INSURANCE PLAN NAME OR PROGRAM NAME

10d. RESERVED FOR LOCAL USE

d. IS THERE ANOTHER HEALTH BENEFIT PLAN?
YES [ ] NO [X] If yes, return to and complete item 9 a-d.

READ BACK OF FORM BEFORE COMPLETING AND SIGNING THIS FORM.
12. PATIENT'S OR AUTHORIZED PERSON'S SIGNATURE I authorize the release of any medical or other information necessary to process this claim. I also request payment of government benefits either to myself or to the party who accepts assignment below.

SIGNED *Harry N. Forehand* DATE March 3, 20XX

13. INSURED'S OR AUTHORIZED PERSON'S SIGNATURE I authorize payment of medical benefits to the undersigned physician or supplier for services described below.

SIGNED *Harry N. Forehand*

14. DATE OF CURRENT: MM 03 DD 01 YYYY 20XX ILLNESS (First symptom) OR INJURY (Accident) OR PREGNANCY (LMP)

15. IF PATIENT HAS HAD SAME OR SIMILAR ILLNESS GIVE FIRST DATE MM DD YYYY

16. DATES PATIENT UNABLE TO WORK IN CURRENT OCCUPATION FROM MM DD YYYY TO MM DD YYYY

17. NAME OF REFERRING PHYSICIAN OR OTHER SOURCE
PERRY CARDI MD

17a. I.D. NUMBER OF REFERRING PHYSICIAN
6780502700

18. HOSPITALIZATION DATES RELATED TO CURRENT SERVICES FROM MM DD YYYY TO MM DD YYYY

19. RESERVED FOR LOCAL USE

20. OUTSIDE LAB? YES [ ] NO [X] $ CHARGES

21. DIAGNOSIS OR NATURE OF ILLNESS OR INJURY (RELATE ITEMS 1,2,3 OR 4 TO ITEM 24E BY LINE)
1. 38200
2.
3.
4.

22. MEDICAID RESUBMISSION CODE ORIGINAL REF. NO.

23. PRIOR AUTHORIZATION NUMBER

24. A. DATE(S) OF SERVICE						B. Place of Service	C. Type of Service	D. PROCEDURES, SERVICES, OR SUPPLIES (Explain Unusual Circumstances) CPT/HCPCS	MODIFIER	E. DIAGNOSIS CODE	F. $ CHARGES		G. DAYS OR UNITS	H. EPSDT Family Plan	I. EMG	J. COB	K. RESERVED FOR LOCAL USE
From MM	DD	YYYY	To MM	DD	YYYY												
030320XX						11		99203		1	70	92	1			12	45897700

25. FEDERAL TAX I.D. NUMBER 74 1064090 SSN [ ] EIN [X]

26. PATIENT'S ACCOUNT NO. 010

27. ACCEPT ASSIGNMENT? (For govt. claims, see back) YES [X] NO [ ]

28. TOTAL CHARGE $ 70 92

29. AMOUNT PAID $

30. BALANCE DUE $ 70 92

31. SIGNATURE OF PHYSICIAN OR SUPPLIER INCLUDING DEGREES OR CREDENTIALS (I certify that the statements on the reverse apply to this bill and are made a part thereof.)
CONCHA ANTRUM MD 030320XX
SIGNED *Concha Antrum MD* DATE

32. NAME AND ADDRESS OF FACILITY WHERE SERVICES WERE RENDERED (if other than home or office)
SAME

33. PHYSICIAN'S, SUPPLIER'S BILLING NAME, ADDRESS, ZIP CODE AND PHONE #
COLLEGE CLINIC
4567 BROAD AVENUE
WOODLAND HILLS XY 12345 0001
013 486 9002
PIN# GRP# 3664021CC

reference initials

Figure 6–6. Front side of the scannable (red ink) Health Insurance Claim Form approved by the American Medical Association's Council on Medical Service. This form is also known as the HCFA-1500 and is shown illustrating completion to a private insurance company with no secondary coverage. Third party payer, state, and local guidelines vary and may not always follow the visual guide presented here. Screened blocks do not need to be completed for this type of case.

BECAUSE THIS FORM IS USED BY VARIOUS GOVERNMENT AND PRIVATE HEALTH PROGRAMS, SEE SEPARATE INSTRUCTIONS ISSUED BY APPLICABLE PROGRAMS.

NOTICE: Any person who knowingly files a statement of claim containing any misrepresentation or any false, incomplete or misleading information may be guilty of a criminal act punishable under law and may be subject to civil penalties.

REFERS TO GOVERNMENT PROGRAMS ONLY

MEDICARE AND CHAMPUS PAYMENT: A patient's signature requests that payment be made and authorizes release of any information necessary to process the claim and certifies that the information provided in Blocks 1 through 12 is true, accurate and complete. In the case of a Medicare claim, the patient's signature authorizes any entity to release to Medicare medical and nonmedical information, including employment status, and whether the person has employer group health insurance, liability, no-fault, worker's compensation or other insurance which is responsible to pay for the services for which the Medicare claim is made. See 42 CFR 411.24(a). If item 9 is completed, the patient's signature authorizes release of the information to the health plan or agency shown. In Medicare assigned or CHAMPUS participation cases, the physician agrees to accept the charge determination of the Medicare carrier or CHAMPUS fiscal intermediary as the full charge determination of the Medicare carrier or CHAMPUS fiscal intermediary if this is less than the charge submitted. CHAMPUS is not a health insurance program but makes payment for health benefits provided through certain affiliations with the Uniformed Services. Information on the patient's sponsor should be provided in those items captioned in "Insured', i.e., items 1a, 4, 6, 7, 9, and 11.

BLACK LUNG AND FECA CLAIMS

The provider agrees to accept the amount paid by the Government as payment in full. See Black Lung and FECA instructions regarding required procedure and diagnosis coding systems.

SIGNATURE OF PHYSICIAN OR SUPPLIER (MEDICARE, CHAMPUS, FECA AND BLACK LUNG)

I certify that the services shown on this form were medically indicated and necessary for the health of the patient and were personally furnished by me or were furnished incident to my professional service by my employee under my immediate supervision, except as otherwise expressly permitted by Medicare or CHAMPUS regulations.

For services to be considered as "incident" to a physician's professional service, 1) they must be rendered under the physician's immediate personal supervision by his/her employee, 2) they must be an integral, although incidental part of a covered physician's service, 3) they must be of kinds commonly furnished in physician's offices, and 4) the services of nonphysicians must be included on the physician's bills.

For CHAMPUS claims, I further certify that I (or any employee) who rendered services am not an active duty member of the Uniformed Services or a civilian employee of the United States Government or a contract employee of the United States Government, either civilian or military (refer to 5 USC 5536). For Black-Lung claims, I further certify that the services performed were for a Black Lung-related disorder.

No Part B Medicare benefits may be paid unless this form is received as required by existing law and regulations (42 CFR 424.32).

NOTICE: Any one who misrepresents or falsifies essential information to receive payment from Federal funds requested by this form may upon conviction be subject to fine and imprisonment under applicable Federal laws.

NOTICE TO PATIENT ABOUT THE COLLECTION AND USE OF MEDICARE, CHAMPUS, FECA, AND BLACK LUNG INFORMATION
(PRIVACY ACT STATEMENT)

We are authorized by HCFA, CHAMPUS and OWCP to ask you for information needed in the administration of the Medicare, CHAMPUS, FECA, and Black Lung programs. Authority to collect information is in section 205(a), 1862, 1872 and 1874 of the Social Security Act as amended, 42 CFR411.24(a) and 424.5(a) (6), and 44 USC 3101; CFR 101 et seq and 10 USC 1079 and 1086; 5 USC 8101 et seq; and 30 USC 901 et seq; 38 USC 613; E.O. 9397.

The information we obtain to complete claims under these programs is used to identify you and to determine your eligibility. It is also used to decide if the services and supplies you received are covered by these programs and to insure that proper payment is made.

The information may also be given to other providers of services, carriers, intermediaries, medical review boards, health plans, and other organizations or Federal agencies, for the effective administration of Federal provisions that require other third parties payers to pay primary to Federal program, and as otherwise necessary to administer these programs. For example, it may be necessary to disclose information about the benefits you have used to a hospital or doctor. Additional disclosures are made through routine uses for information contained in systems of records.

FOR MEDICARE CLAIMS: See the notice modifying system No. 09-70-0501, titled 'Carrier Medicare Claims Record,' published in the Federal Register, Vol. 55 No. 177, page 37549, Wed., Sept. 12, 1990, or as updated and republished.

FOR OWCP CLAIMS: Department of Labor, Privacy Act of 1974, "Republication of Notice of Systems of Records," Federal Register, Vol. 55 No. 40, Wed., Feb. 28, 1990, See ESA-5, ESA-6, ESA-12, ESA-13, ESA-30, or as updated and republished.

FOR CHAMPUS CLAIMS: PRINCIPLE PURPOSE(S): To evaluate eligibility for medical care provided by civilian sources and to issue payment upon establishment of eligibility and determination that the services/supplies received are authorized by law.

ROUTINE USE(S): Information from claims and related documents may be given to the Dept. of Veterans Affairs, the Dept. of Health and Human Services and/or the Dept. of Transportation consistent with their statutory administrative responsibilities under CHAMPUS/CHAMPVA; to the Dept. of Justice for representation of the Secretary of Defense in civil actions; to the Internal Revenue Service, private collection agencies, and consumer reporting agencies in connection with recoupment claims; and to Congressional Offices in response to inquiries made at the request of the person to whom a record pertains. Appropriate disclosures may be made to other federal, state, local, foreign government agencies, private business entities, and individual providers of care, on matters relating to entitlement, claims adjudication, fraud, program abuse, utilization review, quality assurance, peer review, program integrity, third-party liability, coordination of benefits, and civil and criminal litigation related to the operation of CHAMPUS.

DISCLOSURES: Voluntary; however, failure to provide information will result in delay in payment or may result in denial of claim. With the one exception discussed below, there are no penalties under these programs for refusing to supply information. However, failure to furnish information regarding the medical services rendered or the amount charged would prevent payment of claims under these programs. Failure to furnish any other information, such as name or claim number, would delay payment of the claim. Failure to provide medical information under FECA could be deemed an obstruction.

It is mandatory that you tell us if you know that another party is responsible for paying for your treatment. Section 1128B of the Social Security Act and 31 USC 3801-3812 provide penalties for withholding this information.

You should be aware that P.L. 100-503, the "Computer Matching and Privacy Protection Act of 1988," permits the government to verify information by way of computer matches.

MEDICAID PAYMENTS (PROVIDER CERTIFICATION)

I hereby agree to keep such records as are necessary to disclose fully the extent of services provided to individuals under the State's Title XIX plan and to furnish information regarding any payments claimed for providing such services as the State Agency or Dept. of Health and Humans Services may request.

I further agree to accept, as payment in full, the amount paid by the Medicaid program for those claims submitted for payment under that program, with the exception of authorized deductible, coinsurance, co-payment or similar cost-sharing charge.

SIGNATURE OF PHYSICIAN (OR SUPPLIER): I certify that the services listed above were medically indicated and necessary to the health of this patient and were personally furnished by me or my employee under my personal direction.

NOTICE: This is to certify that the foregoing information is true, accurate and complete. I understand that payment and satisfaction of this claim will be from Federal and State funds, and that any false claims, statements, or documents, or concealment of a material fact, may be prosecuted under applicable Federal or State laws.

Public reporting burden for this collection of information is estimated to average 15 minutes per response, including time for reviewing instructions, searching existing date sources, gathering and maintaining data needed, and completing and reviewing the collection of information. Send comments regarding this burden estimate or any other aspect of this collection of information, including suggestions for reducing the burden, to HCFA, Office of Financial Management, P.O. Box 26684, Baltimore, MD 21207; and to the Office of Management and Budget, Paperwork Reduction Project (OMB-0938-0008), Washington, D.C. 20503.

Figure 6–7. Back side of the Health Insurance Claim Form HCFA-1500 approved by the American Medical Association's Council on Medical Service.

MEDICAID
No secondary coverage

MEDICAID FISCAL INTERMEDIARY NAME
MAILING ADDRESS
CITY STATE ZIP CODE

1.	MEDICARE	MEDICAID	CHAMPUS	CHAMPVA	GROUP HEALTH PLAN	FECA BLK LUNG	OTHER	1a. INSURED'S I.D. NUMBER	(FOR PROGRAM IN ITEM 1)
	☐ (Medicare #)	☒ (Medicaid #)	☐ (Sponsor's SSN)	☐ (VA File #)	☐ (SSN or ID)	☐ (SSN)	☐ (ID)	276835090	

2. PATIENT'S NAME (Last Name, First Name, Middle Initial)	3. PATIENT'S BIRTH DATE	4. INSURED'S NAME (Last Name, First Name, Middle Initial)
ABRAMSON ADAM	MM 02 DD 12 YYYY 1995 SEX M ☒ F ☐	

5. PATIENT'S ADDRESS (No., Street)
760 FINCH STREET

6. PATIENT RELATIONSHIP TO INSURED
Self ☐   Spouse ☐   Child ☐   Other ☐

7. INSURED'S ADDRESS (No., Street)

CITY WOODLAND HILLS	STATE XY	8. PATIENT STATUS Single ☐ Married ☐ Other ☐	CITY	STATE

| ZIP CODE 12345 | TELEPHONE (include Area Code) (013) 482 6789 | Employed ☐ Full-Time Student ☐ Part-Time Student ☐ | ZIP CODE | TELEPHONE (include Area Code) ( ) |

9. OTHER INSURED'S NAME (Last Name, First Name, Middle Initial)

10. IS PATIENT'S CONDITION RELATED TO:

11. INSURED'S POLICY GROUP OR FECA NUMBER

a. OTHER INSURED'S POLICY OR GROUP NUMBER

a. EMPLOYMENT? (CURRENT OR PREVIOUS)   ☐ YES   ☒ NO

a. INSURED'S DATE OF BIRTH MM DD YY   SEX M ☐ F ☐

b. OTHER INSURED'S DATE OF BIRTH MM DD YYYY   SEX M ☐ F ☐

b. AUTO ACCIDENT?   ☐ YES   ☒ NO   PLACE (State)

b. EMPLOYER'S NAME OR SCHOOL NAME

c. EMPLOYER'S NAME OR SCHOOL NAME

c. OTHER ACCIDENT?   ☒ YES   ☐ NO

c. INSURANCE PLAN NAME OR PROGRAM NAME

d. INSURANCE PLAN NAME OR PROGRAM NAME

10d. RESERVED FOR LOCAL USE

d. IS THERE ANOTHER HEALTH BENEFIT PLAN?   ☐ YES   ☐ NO   *If yes,* return to and complete item 9 a-d.

READ BACK OF FORM BEFORE COMPLETING AND SIGNING THIS FORM.
12. PATIENT'S OR AUTHORIZED PERSON'S SIGNATURE I authorize the release of any medical or other information necessary to process this claim. I also request payment of government benefits either to myself or to the party who accepts assignment below.

SIGNED _____   DATE _____

13. INSURED'S OR AUTHORIZED PERSON'S SIGNATURE I authorize payment of medical benefits to the undersigned physician or supplier for services described below.

SIGNED _____

14. DATE OF CURRENT: MM DD YYYY	◄ ILLNESS (First symptom) OR INJURY (Accident) OR PREGNANCY (LMP)	15. IF PATIENT HAS HAD SAME OR SIMILAR ILLNESS GIVE FIRST DATE MM DD YYYY	16. DATES PATIENT UNABLE TO WORK IN CURRENT OCCUPATION FROM MM DD YYYY TO MM DD YYYY

17. NAME OF REFERRING PHYSICIAN OR OTHER SOURCE	17a. I.D. NUMBER OF REFERRING PHYSICIAN	18. HOSPITALIZATION DATES RELATED TO CURRENT SERVICES FROM MM DD YYYY TO MM DD YYYY

19. RESERVED FOR LOCAL USE	20. OUTSIDE LAB? ☐ YES ☒ NO $ CHARGES

21. DIAGNOSIS OR NATURE OF ILLNESS OR INJURY (RELATE ITEMS 1,2,3 OR 4 TO ITEM 24E BY LINE)
1. 931   3.
2.   4.

22. MEDICAID RESUBMISSION CODE ___ ORIGINAL REF. NO. ___

23. PRIOR AUTHORIZATION NUMBER

24. A. DATE(S) OF SERVICE From MM DD YYYY To MM DD YYYY	B. Place of Service	C. Type of Service	D. PROCEDURES, SERVICES, OR SUPPLIES (Explain Unusual Circumstances) CPT/HCPCS MODIFIER	E. DIAGNOSIS CODE	F. $ CHARGES	G. DAYS OR UNITS	H. EPSDT Family Plan	I. EMG	J. COB	K. RESERVED FOR LOCAL USE
071420XX	23	1	99282	1	37	02	1	X		
071420XX	23	2	69200	1	49	93	1	X		

25. FEDERAL TAX I.D. NUMBER SSN EIN 71 3206151 ☐ ☒	26. PATIENT'S ACCOUNT NO. 030	27. ACCEPT ASSIGNMENT? (For govt. claims, see back) ☒ YES ☐ NO	28. TOTAL CHARGE $ 86 95	29. AMOUNT PAID $	30. BALANCE DUE $ 86 95

31. SIGNATURE OF PHYSICIAN OR SUPPLIER INCLUDING DEGREES OR CREDENTIALS (I certify that the statements on the reverse apply to this bill and are made a part thereof.) PEDRO ATRICS MD 071420XX SIGNED *Pedro Atrics MD* DATE	32. NAME AND ADDRESS OF FACILITY WHERE SERVICES WERE RENDERED (if other than home or office) COLLEGE HOSPITAL 4500 BROAD AVENUE WOODLAND HILLS XY 12345 0001 HSC 43700F	33. PHYSICIAN'S, SUPPLIER'S BILLING NAME, ADDRESS, ZIP CODE AND PHONE # COLLEGE CLINIC 4567 BROAD AVENUE WOODLAND HILLS XY 12345 0001 013 486 9002 PIN# GRP# HSC12345F

reference initials

Figure 6–8. A Medicaid case with no secondary coverage emphasizing basic elements and screened blocks that do not require completion.

MEDICARE
NO SECONDARY COVERAGE

MEDICARE FISCAL INTERMEDIARY NAME
MAILING ADDRESS
CITY STATE ZIP CODE

1. MEDICARE	MEDICAID	CHAMPUS	CHAMPVA	GROUP HEALTH PLAN	FECA BLK LUNG	OTHER	1a. INSURED'S I.D. NUMBER	(FOR PROGRAM IN ITEM 1)
[X] (Medicare #)	☐ (Medicaid #)	☐ (Sponsor's SSN)	☐ (VA File #)	☐ (SSN or ID)	☐ (SSN)	☐ (ID)	123 45 6789A	

2. PATIENT'S NAME (Last Name, First Name, Middle Initial)
HUTCH   BILL

3. PATIENT'S BIRTH DATE
MM 05 DD 07 YYYY 1910   SEX M [X] F ☐

4. INSURED'S NAME (Last Name, First Name, Middle Initial)

5. PATIENT'S ADDRESS (No., Street)
8888 MAIN STREET

6. PATIENT RELATIONSHIP TO INSURED
Self ☐ Spouse ☐ Child ☐ Other ☐

7. INSURED'S ADDRESS (No., Street)

CITY
WOODLAND HILLS   STATE XY

8. PATIENT STATUS
Single [X] Married ☐ Other ☐
Employed ☐ Full-Time Student ☐ Part-Time Student ☐

CITY   STATE

ZIP CODE 12345   TELEPHONE (include Area Code) (013) 732 1544

ZIP CODE   TELEPHONE (include Area Code) (   )

9. OTHER INSURED'S NAME (Last Name, First Name, Middle Initial)

10. IS PATIENT'S CONDITION RELATED TO:

11. INSURED'S POLICY GROUP OR FECA NUMBER
NONE

a. OTHER INSURED'S POLICY OR GROUP NUMBER

a. EMPLOYMENT? (CURRENT OR PREVIOUS)
☐ YES [X] NO

a. INSURED'S DATE OF BIRTH
MM DD YY   M ☐ SEX F ☐

b. OTHER INSURED'S DATE OF BIRTH
MM DD YYYY   M ☐ SEX F ☐

b. AUTO ACCIDENT?   PLACE (State)
☐ YES [X] NO

b. EMPLOYER'S NAME OR SCHOOL NAME

c. EMPLOYER'S NAME OR SCHOOL NAME

c. OTHER ACCIDENT?
☐ YES [X] NO

c. INSURANCE PLAN NAME OR PROGRAM NAME

d. INSURANCE PLAN NAME OR PROGRAM NAME

10d. RESERVED FOR LOCAL USE

d. IS THERE ANOTHER HEALTH BENEFIT PLAN?
☐ YES ☐ NO   *If yes,* return to and complete item 9 a-d.

READ BACK OF FORM BEFORE COMPLETING AND SIGNING THIS FORM.
12. PATIENT'S OR AUTHORIZED PERSON'S SIGNATURE I authorize the release of any medical or other information necessary to process this claim. I also request payment of government benefits either to myself or to the party who accepts assignment below.

SIGNED   SOF   DATE

13. INSURED'S OR AUTHORIZED PERSON'S SIGNATURE I authorize payment of medical benefits to the undersigned physician or supplier for services described below.

SIGNED

14. DATE OF CURRENT: ◄ ILLNESS (First symptom) OR INJURY (Accident) OR PREGNANCY (LMP)
MM DD YYYY

15. IF PATIENT HAS HAD SAME OR SIMILAR ILLNESS GIVE FIRST DATE MM DD YYYY

16. DATES PATIENT UNABLE TO WORK IN CURRENT OCCUPATION
FROM MM DD YYYY   TO MM DD YYYY

17. NAME OF REFERRING PHYSICIAN OR OTHER SOURCE
GERALD PRACTON MD

17a. I.D. NUMBER OF REFERRING PHYSICIAN
4627889700

18. HOSPITALIZATION DATES RELATED TO CURRENT SERVICES
FROM MM DD YYYY   TO MM DD YYYY

19. RESERVED FOR LOCAL USE

20. OUTSIDE LAB? $ CHARGES
☐ YES [X] NO

21. DIAGNOSIS OR NATURE OF ILLNESS OR INJURY (RELATE ITEMS 1,2,3 OR 4 TO ITEM 24E BY LINE)
1. 487 0   3. _____
2. _____   4. _____

22. MEDICAID RESUBMISSION CODE   ORIGINAL REF. NO.

23. PRIOR AUTHORIZATION NUMBER

24. A. DATE(S) OF SERVICE						B. Place of Service	C. Type of Service	D. PROCEDURES, SERVICES, OR SUPPLIES (Explain Unusual Circumstances) CPT/HCPCS	MODIFIER	E. DIAGNOSIS CODE	F. $ CHARGES		G. DAYS OR UNITS	H. EPSDT Family Plan	I. EMG	J. COB	K. RESERVED FOR LOCAL USE
From MM	DD	YYYY	To MM	DD	YYYY												
03	10	20XX				11		99205		1	132	28	1			64	21106700

25. FEDERAL TAX I.D. NUMBER   SSN ☐ EIN [X]
75 6732101

26. PATIENT'S ACCOUNT NO.
040

27. ACCEPT ASSIGNMENT?
(For govt. claims, see back)
[X] YES ☐ NO

28. TOTAL CHARGE
$ 132 | 28

29. AMOUNT PAID
$

30. BALANCE DUE
$

31. SIGNATURE OF PHYSICIAN OR SUPPLIER INCLUDING DEGREES OR CREDENTIALS
(I certify that the statements on the reverse apply to this bill and are made a part thereof.)
BRADY COCCIDIOIDES   031020XX
SIGNED *Brady Coccidioides MD* DATE

32. NAME AND ADDRESS OF FACILITY WHERE SERVICES WERE RENDERED (if other than home or office)

SAME

33. PHYSICIAN'S, SUPPLIER'S BILLING NAME, ADDRESS, ZIP CODE AND PHONE #
COLLEGE CLINIC
4567 BROAD AVENUE
WOODLAND HILLS XY 12345 0001
013 486 9002
PIN#   GRP# 3664021CC

reference initials

Figure 6–9. Example of a completed HCFA-1500 Health Insurance Claim Form for a basic Medicare case with no other insurance coverage. The physician has accepted assignment. Screened blocks do not need to be completed for a Medicare case with no other insurance.

MEDICARE/MEDICAID
(primary) (secondary)
Crossover claim

MEDICARE FISCAL INTERMEDIARY NAME
MAILING ADDRESS
CITY STATE ZIP CODE

1. MEDICARE	MEDICAID	CHAMPUS	CHAMPVA	GROUP HEALTH PLAN	FECA BLK LUNG	OTHER	1a. INSURED'S I.D. NUMBER	(FOR PROGRAM IN ITEM 1)
X (Medicare #)	X (Medicaid #)	(Sponsor's SSN)	(VA File #)	(SSN or ID)	(SSN)	(ID)	660 46 2715A	

2. PATIENT'S NAME (Last Name, First Name, Middle Initial)
JOHNSON KATHRYN

3. PATIENT'S BIRTH DATE
MM 09 DD 07 YYYY 1937   SEX M☐ F☒

4. INSURED'S NAME (Last Name, First Name, Middle Initial)

5. PATIENT'S ADDRESS (No., Street)
218 VEGA DRIVE

6. PATIENT RELATIONSHIP TO INSURED
Self☐ Spouse☐ Child☐ Other☐

7. INSURED'S ADDRESS (No., Street)

CITY
WOODLAND HILLS   STATE XY

8. PATIENT STATUS
Single☐ Married☒ Other☐

CITY   STATE

ZIP CODE
12345

TELEPHONE (include Area Code)
(013) 482 9112

Employed☐ Full-Time Student☐ Part-Time Student☐

ZIP CODE   TELEPHONE (include Area Code)
( )

9. OTHER INSURED'S NAME (Last Name, First Name, Middle Initial)

10. IS PATIENT'S CONDITION RELATED TO:

11. INSURED'S POLICY GROUP OR FECA NUMBER
NONE

a. OTHER INSURED'S POLICY OR GROUP NUMBER

a. EMPLOYMENT? (CURRENT OR PREVIOUS)
YES☐ NO☒

a. INSURED'S DATE OF BIRTH
MM DD YY   SEX M☐ F☐

b. OTHER INSURED'S DATE OF BIRTH
MM DD YYYY   M☐ SEX F☐

b. AUTO ACCIDENT?   PLACE (State)
YES☐ NO☒

b. EMPLOYER'S NAME OR SCHOOL NAME

c. EMPLOYER'S NAME OR SCHOOL NAME

c. OTHER ACCIDENT?
YES☐ NO☒

c. INSURANCE PLAN NAME OR PROGRAM NAME

d. INSURANCE PLAN NAME OR PROGRAM NAME

10d. RESERVED FOR LOCAL USE
MCD016745289

d. IS THERE ANOTHER HEALTH BENEFIT PLAN?
YES☐ NO☐ *If yes*, return to and complete item 9 a-d.

READ BACK OF FORM BEFORE COMPLETING AND SIGNING THIS FORM.

12. PATIENT'S OR AUTHORIZED PERSON'S SIGNATURE I authorize the release of any medical or other information necessary to process this claim. I also request payment of government benefits either to myself or to the party who accepts assignment below.

SIGNED *Kathryn Johnson*   DATE *10/1/XX*

13. INSURED'S OR AUTHORIZED PERSON'S SIGNATURE I authorize payment of medical benefits to the undersigned physician or supplier for services described below.

SIGNED

14. DATE OF CURRENT: ◄ ILLNESS (First symptom) OR INJURY (Accident) OR PREGNANCY (LMP)
MM DD YYYY

15. IF PATIENT HAS HAD SAME OR SIMILAR ILLNESS GIVE FIRST DATE MM DD YYYY

16. DATES PATIENT UNABLE TO WORK IN CURRENT OCCUPATION
FROM MM DD YYYY   TO MM DD YYYY

17. NAME OF REFERRING PHYSICIAN OR OTHER SOURCE
BRADY COCCIDIOIDES MD

17a. I.D. NUMBER OF REFERRING PHYSICIAN
6421106700

18. HOSPITALIZATION DATES RELATED TO CURRENT SERVICES
FROM MM DD YYYY   TO MM DD YYYY

19. RESERVED FOR LOCAL USE

20. OUTSIDE LAB? $ CHARGES
YES☐ NO☒

21. DIAGNOSIS OR NATURE OF ILLNESS OR INJURY (RELATE ITEMS 1,2,3 OR 4 TO ITEM 24E BY LINE)
1. 172 7
2.
3.
4.

22. MEDICAID RESUBMISSION
CODE   ORIGINAL REF. NO.

23. PRIOR AUTHORIZATION NUMBER
7680560012

24. A. DATE(S) OF SERVICE From MM DD YYYY To MM DD YYYY	B. Place of Service	C. Type of Service	D. PROCEDURES, SERVICES, OR SUPPLIES (Explain Unusual Circumstances) CPT/HCPCS MODIFIER	E. DIAGNOSIS CODE	F. $ CHARGES	G. DAYS OR UNITS	H. EPSDT Family Plan	I. EMG	J. COB	K. RESERVED FOR LOCAL USE
100120XX	24		11600	1	195 06	1			50	30711700

25. FEDERAL TAX I.D. NUMBER   SSN☐ EIN☒
74 6078992

26. PATIENT'S ACCOUNT NO.
050

27. ACCEPT ASSIGNMENT? (For govt. claims, see back)
YES☒ NO☐

28. TOTAL CHARGE
$ 195 06

29. AMOUNT PAID
$

30. BALANCE DUE
$

31. SIGNATURE OF PHYSICIAN OR SUPPLIER INCLUDING DEGREES OR CREDENTIALS (I certify that the statements on the reverse apply to this bill and are made a part thereof.)
COSMO GRAFF MD
SIGNED *Cosmo Graff, MD* DATE 100320XX

32. NAME AND ADDRESS OF FACILITY WHERE SERVICES WERE RENDERED (if other than home or office)
WOODLAND HILLS AMBULATORY CENTER
1229 CENTER STREET
WOODLAND HILLS XY 12345 0001
95 0513700

33. PHYSICIAN'S, SUPPLIER'S BILLING NAME, ADDRESS, ZIP CODE AND PHONE #
COLLEGE CLINIC
4567 BROAD AVENUE
WOODLAND HILLS XY 12345 0001
013 486 9002
PIN#   GRP# 3664021CC

reference initials

Figure 6–10. Example of a Medicare/Medicaid crossover claim. The HCFA-1500 claim form is sent to Medicare (primary payer) and then processed automatically by Medicaid (secondary payer). Screened blocks do not need to be completed for this type of case.

MEDICARE/MEDIGAP
(primary) (secondary)
Crossover claim

MEDICARE FISCAL INTERMEDIARY NAME
MAILING ADDRESS
CITY STATE ZIP CODE

1. MEDICARE	MEDICAID	CHAMPUS	CHAMPVA	GROUP HEALTH PLAN	FECA BLK LUNG	OTHER	1a. INSURED'S I.D. NUMBER	(FOR PROGRAM IN ITEM 1)
[X] *(Medicare #)*	[ ] *(Medicaid #)*	[ ] *(Sponsor's SSN)*	[ ] *(VA File #)*	[X] *(SSN or ID)*	[ ] *(SSN)*	[ ] *(ID)*	419 16 7272A	

2. PATIENT'S NAME (Last Name, First Name, Middle Initial)	3. PATIENT'S BIRTH DATE	4. INSURED'S NAME (Last Name, First Name, Middle Initial)
BARNES AGUSTA E	MM 08 DD 29 YYYY 1917 M [X] F [ ]	

5. PATIENT'S ADDRESS (No., Street)
356 ENCINA AVENUE

6. PATIENT RELATIONSHIP TO INSURED
Self [ ] Spouse [ ] Child [ ] Other [ ]

7. INSURED'S ADDRESS (No., Street)

CITY WOODLAND HILLS   STATE XY

8. PATIENT STATUS
Single [X] Married [ ] Other [ ]
Employed [ ] Full-Time Student [ ] Part-Time Student [ ]

CITY   STATE

ZIP CODE 12345 0000   TELEPHONE (include Area Code) (013) 467 2646

ZIP CODE   TELEPHONE (include Area Code) ( )

9. OTHER INSURED'S NAME (Last Name, First Name, Middle Initial)
SAME

10. IS PATIENT'S CONDITION RELATED TO:

11. INSURED'S POLICY GROUP OR FECA NUMBER
NONE

a. OTHER INSURED'S POLICY OR GROUP NUMBER
MEDIGAP 419167272

a. EMPLOYMENT? (CURRENT OR PREVIOUS)
YES [ ] NO [X]

a. INSURED'S DATE OF BIRTH
MM DD YY   M [ ] SEX F [ ]

b. OTHER INSURED'S DATE OF BIRTH
MM DD YYYY   M [ ] SEX F [ ]

b. AUTO ACCIDENT?   PLACE (State)
YES [ ] NO [X]

b. EMPLOYER'S NAME OR SCHOOL NAME

c. EMPLOYER'S NAME OR SCHOOL NAME

c. OTHER ACCIDENT?
YES [ ] NO [X]

c. INSURANCE PLAN NAME OR PROGRAM NAME

d. INSURANCE PLAN NAME OR PROGRAM NAME
CALFCA002

10d. RESERVED FOR LOCAL USE

d. IS THERE ANOTHER HEALTH BENEFIT PLAN?
YES [ ] NO [ ]   *If yes,* return to and complete item 9 a-d.

READ BACK OF FORM BEFORE COMPLETING AND SIGNING THIS FORM.

12. PATIENT'S OR AUTHORIZED PERSON'S SIGNATURE I authorize the release of any medical or other information necessary to process this claim. I also request payment of government benefits either to myself or to the party who accepts assignment below.

SIGNED *Agusta E. Barnes*   DATE *11/21/XX*

13. INSURED'S OR AUTHORIZED PERSON'S SIGNATURE I authorize payment of medical benefits to the undersigned physician or supplier for services described below.

SIGNED *Agusta E. Barnes*

14. DATE OF CURRENT: ILLNESS (First symptom) OR INJURY (Accident) OR PREGNANCY (LMP)
MM DD YYYY

15. IF PATIENT HAS HAD SAME OR SIMILAR ILLNESS GIVE FIRST DATE   MM DD YYYY

16. DATES PATIENT UNABLE TO WORK IN CURRENT OCCUPATION
FROM MM DD YYYY   TO MM DD YYYY

17. NAME OF REFERRING PHYSICIAN OR OTHER SOURCE
GASTON INPUT MD

17a. I.D. NUMBER OF REFERRING PHYSICIAN
3278312700

18. HOSPITALIZATION DATES RELATED TO CURRENT SERVICES
FROM MM DD YYYY   TO MM DD YYYY

19. RESERVED FOR LOCAL USE

20. OUTSIDE LAB? $ CHARGES
YES [ ] NO [X]

21. DIAGNOSIS OR NATURE OF ILLNESS OR INJURY (RELATE ITEMS 1,2,3 or 4 TO ITEM 24E BY LINE)
1. 78659
2.
3.
4.

22. MEDICAID RESUBMISSION CODE   ORIGINAL REF. NO.

23. PRIOR AUTHORIZATION NUMBER

24. A DATE(S) OF SERVICE From MM DD YYYY	To MM DD YYYY	B Place of Service	C Type of Service	D PROCEDURES, SERVICES, OR SUPPLIES (Explain Unusual Circumstances) CPT/HCPCS MODIFIER	E DIAGNOSIS CODE	F $ CHARGES	G DAYS OR UNITS	H EPSDT Family Plan	I EMG	J COB	K RESERVED FOR LOCAL USE
112120XX		11		93350	1	183 31	1			67	80502700
112120XX		11		93017	1	68 90	1			67	80502700

25. FEDERAL TAX I.D. NUMBER   SSN EIN
70 6421710   [ ] [X]

26. PATIENT'S ACCOUNT NO.
060

27. ACCEPT ASSIGNMENT? (For govt. claims, see back)
[X] YES [ ] NO

28. TOTAL CHARGE
$ 252 21

29. AMOUNT PAID
$

30. BALANCE DUE
$

31. SIGNATURE OF PHYSICIAN OR SUPPLIER INCLUDING DEGREES OR CREDENTIALS (I certify that the statements on the reverse apply to this bill and are made a part thereof.)
PERRY CARDI MD
SIGNED *Perry Cardi, MD*   112220XX   DATE

32. NAME AND ADDRESS OF FACILITY WHERE SERVICES WERE RENDERED (if other than home or office)
SAME

33. PHYSICIAN'S, SUPPLIER'S BILLING NAME, ADDRESS, ZIP CODE AND PHONE #
COLLEGE CLINIC
4567 BROAD AVENUE
WOODLAND HILLS XY 12345 0001
013 486 9002
PIN#   GRP# 3664021CC

reference initials

Figure 6–11. Example of a completed HCFA-1500 Health Insurance Claim Form for a Medicare (primary) and Medigap (secondary) crossover claim. Shaded blocks do not need to be completed for this type of case.

OTHER INSURANCE/MEDICARE-MSP
(primary)   (secondary)

OTHER INSURANCE COMPANY NAME
MAILING ADDRESS
CITY STATE ZIP CODE

1.								1a. INSURED'S I.D. NUMBER	(FOR PROGRAM IN ITEM 1)

1. MEDICARE [X] (Medicare #) MEDICAID [ ] (Medicaid #) CHAMPUS [ ] (Sponsor's SSN) CHAMPVA [ ] (VA File #) GROUP HEALTH PLAN [X] (SSN or ID) FECA BLK LUNG [ ] (SSN) OTHER [ ] (ID)

1a. INSURED'S I.D. NUMBER (FOR PROGRAM IN ITEM 1)
609 24 5523A

2. PATIENT'S NAME (Last Name, First Name, Middle Initial)
BLAIR GWENDOLYN

3. PATIENT'S BIRTH DATE MM 09 DD 01 YYYY 1931 SEX M [ ] F [X]

4. INSURED'S NAME (Last Name, First Name, Middle Initial)
BLAIR GWENDOLYN

5. PATIENT'S ADDRESS (No., Street)
416 RICHMOND STREET

6. PATIENT RELATIONSHIP TO INSURED
Self [X] Spouse [ ] Child [ ] Other [ ]

7. INSURED'S ADDRESS (No., Street)
SAME

CITY
WOODLAND HILLS STATE XY

8. PATIENT STATUS
Single [ ] Married [X] Other [ ]

CITY   STATE

ZIP CODE
12345 0000 TELEPHONE (include Area Code) (013) 459 1519

Employed [X] Full-Time Student [ ] Part-Time Student [ ]

ZIP CODE   TELEPHONE (include Area Code) (   )

9. OTHER INSURED'S NAME (Last Name, First Name, Middle Initial)

10. IS PATIENT'S CONDITION RELATED TO:

11. INSURED'S POLICY GROUP OR FECA NUMBER
7845931Q

a. OTHER INSURED'S POLICY OR GROUP NUMBER

a. EMPLOYMENT? (CURRENT OR PREVIOUS)
[ ] YES [X] NO

a. INSURED'S DATE OF BIRTH MM DD YY SEX M [ ] F [ ]

b. OTHER INSURED'S DATE OF BIRTH MM DD YYYY M [ ] SEX F [ ]

b. AUTO ACCIDENT? PLACE (State)
[ ] YES [X] NO

b. EMPLOYER'S NAME OR SCHOOL NAME
CITY LIBRARY

c. EMPLOYER'S NAME OR SCHOOL NAME

c. OTHER ACCIDENT?
[ ] YES [X] NO

c. INSURANCE PLAN NAME OR PROGRAM NAME
ABC INSURANCE COMPANY

d. INSURANCE PLAN NAME OR PROGRAM NAME

10d. RESERVED FOR LOCAL USE

d. IS THERE ANOTHER HEALTH BENEFIT PLAN?
[ ] YES [ ] NO If yes, return to and complete item 9 a-d.

READ BACK OF FORM BEFORE COMPLETING AND SIGNING THIS FORM.

12. PATIENT'S OR AUTHORIZED PERSON'S SIGNATURE I authorize the release of any medical or other information necessary to process this claim. I also request payment of government benefits either to myself or to the party who accepts assignment below.

SIGNED SOF   DATE

13. INSURED'S OR AUTHORIZED PERSON'S SIGNATURE I authorize payment of medical benefits to the undersigned physician or supplier for services described below.

SIGNED SOF

14. DATE OF CURRENT: ILLNESS (First symptom) OR INJURY (Accident) OR PREGNANCY (LMP) MM DD YYYY

15. IF PATIENT HAS HAD SAME OR SIMILAR ILLNESS GIVE FIRST DATE MM DD YYYY

16. DATES PATIENT UNABLE TO WORK IN CURRENT OCCUPATION FROM MM DD YYYY TO MM DD YYYY

17. NAME OF REFERRING PHYSICIAN OR OTHER SOURCE
GERALD PRACTON MD

17a. I.D. NUMBER OF REFERRING PHYSICIAN
4627889700

18. HOSPITALIZATION DATES RELATED TO CURRENT SERVICES FROM MM DD YYYY TO MM DD YYYY

19. RESERVED FOR LOCAL USE

20. OUTSIDE LAB? [ ] YES [X] NO $ CHARGES

21. DIAGNOSIS OR NATURE OF ILLNESS OR INJURY (RELATE ITEMS 1,2,3 OR 4 TO ITEM 24E BY LINE)
1. 110 1
2.
3.
4.

22. MEDICAID RESUBMISSION CODE   ORIGINAL REF. NO.

23. PRIOR AUTHORIZATION NUMBER

24. A DATE(S) OF SERVICE From MM DD YYYY	To MM DD YYYY	B Place of Service	C Type of Service	D PROCEDURES, SERVICES, OR SUPPLIES (Explain Unusual Circumstances) CPT/HCPCS | MODIFIER	E DIAGNOSIS CODE	F $ CHARGES	G DAYS OR UNITS	H EPSDT Family Plan	I EMG	J COB	K RESERVED FOR LOCAL USE
031520XX		11		99243 | 25	1	103 51	1			54	02228700
031520XX		11		11750 |	1	193 45	1			54	02228700

25. FEDERAL TAX I.D. NUMBER 62 7410931 SSN [ ] EIN [X]

26. PATIENT'S ACCOUNT NO. 070

27. ACCEPT ASSIGNMENT? (For govt. claims, see back) [X] YES [ ] NO

28. TOTAL CHARGE $ 296 96

29. AMOUNT PAID $ 100 00

30. BALANCE DUE $

31. SIGNATURE OF PHYSICIAN OR SUPPLIER INCLUDING DEGREES OR CREDENTIALS (I certify that the statements on the reverse apply to this bill and are made a part thereof.)
NICK PEDRO DPM   031620XX
SIGNED Nick Pedro, DPM DATE

32. NAME AND ADDRESS OF FACILITY WHERE SERVICES WERE RENDERED (if other than home or office)
SAME

33. PHYSICIAN'S, SUPPLIER'S BILLING NAME, ADDRESS, ZIP CODE AND PHONE #
COLLEGE CLINIC
4567 BROAD AVENUE
WOODLAND HILLS XY 12345 0001
013 486 9002
PIN#   GRP# 3664021CC

reference initials

Figure 6–12. Template for a case in which another insurance company is the primary and Medicare is the secondary payer (MSP).

TRICARE
No secondary coverage

TRICARE FISCAL INTERMEDIARY
MAILING ADDRESS
CITY STATE ZIP CODE

1. MEDICARE MEDICAID CHAMPUS CHAMPVA GROUP HEALTH PLAN FECA BLK LUNG OTHER	1a. INSURED'S I.D. NUMBER (FOR PROGRAM IN ITEM 1)
☐ (Medicare #) ☐ (Medicaid #) ☒ (Sponsor's SSN) ☐ (VA File #) ☐ (SSN or ID) ☐ (SSN) ☐ (ID)	581147211

2. PATIENT'S NAME (Last Name, First Name, Middle Initial)	3. PATIENT'S BIRTH DATE MM DD YYYY SEX	4. INSURED'S NAME (Last Name, First Name, Middle Initial)
SMITH SUSAN J	03 16 1976 M ☐ F ☒	SMITH WILLIAM D

5. PATIENT'S ADDRESS (No., Street)	6. PATIENT RELATIONSHIP TO INSURED	7. INSURED'S ADDRESS (No., Street)
420 MAPLE STREET	Self ☐ Spouse ☒ Child ☐ Other ☐	SAME

CITY	STATE	8. PATIENT STATUS	CITY	STATE
WOODLAND HILLS	XY	Single ☐ Married ☒ Other ☐		

ZIP CODE	TELEPHONE (include Area Code)		ZIP CODE	TELEPHONE (include Area Code)
12345 0000	(013) 789 9898	Employed ☐ Full-Time Student ☐ Part-Time Student ☐		( )

9. OTHER INSURED'S NAME (Last Name, First Name, Middle Initial)	10. IS PATIENT'S CONDITION RELATED TO:	11. INSURED'S POLICY GROUP OR FECA NUMBER
a. OTHER INSURED'S POLICY OR GROUP NUMBER	a. EMPLOYMENT? (CURRENT OR PREVIOUS) ☐ YES ☒ NO	a. INSURED'S DATE OF BIRTH MM DD YYYY SEX 06 12 1974 M ☒ F ☐
b. OTHER INSURED'S DATE OF BIRTH MM DD YYYY M ☐ SEX F ☐	b. AUTO ACCIDENT? ☐ YES ☒ NO PLACE (State)	b. EMPLOYER'S NAME OR SCHOOL NAME USN
c. EMPLOYER'S NAME OR SCHOOL NAME	c. OTHER ACCIDENT? ☐ YES ☒ NO	c. INSURANCE PLAN NAME OR PROGRAM NAME
d. INSURANCE PLAN NAME OR PROGRAM NAME	10d. RESERVED FOR LOCAL USE	d. IS THERE ANOTHER HEALTH BENEFIT PLAN? ☐ YES ☒ NO *If yes*, return to and complete item 9 a-d.

READ BACK OF FORM BEFORE COMPLETING AND SIGNING THIS FORM.

12. PATIENT'S OR AUTHORIZED PERSON'S SIGNATURE I authorize the release of any medical or other information necessary to process this claim. I also request payment of government benefits either to myself or to the party who accepts assignment below. SIGNED SOF DATE	13. INSURED'S OR AUTHORIZED PERSON'S SIGNATURE I authorize payment of medical benefits to the undersigned physician or supplier for services described below. SIGNED

14. DATE OF CURRENT: MM DD YYYY ILLNESS (First symptom) OR INJURY (Accident) OR PREGNANCY (LMP) 10 28 20XX	15. IF PATIENT HAS HAD SAME OR SIMILAR ILLNESS GIVE FIRST DATE MM DD YYYY	16. DATES PATIENT UNABLE TO WORK IN CURRENT OCCUPATION MM DD YYYY MM DD YYYY FROM 07 21 20XX TO 09 17 20XX
17. NAME OF REFERRING PHYSICIAN OR OTHER SOURCE ADAM LANGERHANS MD	17a. I.D. NUMBER OF REFERRING PHYSICIAN 60 5783128	18. HOSPITALIZATION DATES RELATED TO CURRENT SERVICES MM DD YYYY MM DD YYYY FROM 08 06 20XX TO 08 08 20XX
19. RESERVED FOR LOCAL USE		20. OUTSIDE LAB? ☐ YES ☒ NO $ CHARGES

21. DIAGNOSIS OR NATURE OF ILLNESS OR INJURY (RELATE ITEMS 1,2,3 OR 4 TO ITEM 24E BY LINE)	22. MEDICAID RESUBMISSION CODE ORIGINAL REF. NO.
1. 650 3.	
2. 4.	23. PRIOR AUTHORIZATION NUMBER

24. A DATE(S) OF SERVICE From To MM DD YYYY MM DD YYYY	B Place of Service	C Type of Service	D PROCEDURES, SERVICES, OR SUPPLIES (Explain Unusual Circumstances) CPT/HCPCS MODIFIER	E DIAGNOSIS CODE	F $ CHARGES	G DAYS OR UNITS	H EPSDT Family Plan	I EMG	J COB	K RESERVED FOR LOCAL USE
080620XX	21	1	59400	1	1864 30	1				A018174

25. FEDERAL TAX I.D. NUMBER SSN EIN	26. PATIENT'S ACCOUNT NO.	27. ACCEPT ASSIGNMENT? (For govt. claims, see back)	28. TOTAL CHARGE	29. AMOUNT PAID	30. BALANCE DUE
72 5713051 ☐ ☒	080	☒ YES ☐ NO	$ 1864 30	$	$ 1864 30

31. SIGNATURE OF PHYSICIAN OR SUPPLIER INCLUDING DEGREES OR CREDENTIALS (I certify that the statements on the reverse apply to this bill and are made a part thereof.) BERTHA CAESAR MD 081020XX SIGNED *Bertha Caesar, MD* DATE	32. NAME AND ADDRESS OF FACILITY WHERE SERVICES WERE RENDERED (if other than home or office) COLLEGE HOSPITAL 4500 BROAD AVENUE WOODLAND HILLS XY 12345 0001 95 0731067	33. PHYSICIAN'S, SUPPLIER'S BILLING NAME, ADDRESS, ZIP CODE AND PHONE # COLLEGE CLINIC 4567 BROAD AVENUE WOODLAND HILLS XY 12345 0001 013 486 9002 PIN# 3664021CC GRP#

reference initials

Figure 6–13. Example of a completed HCFA-1500 claim form, used when billing for professional services rendered in a TRICARE Standard case. Screened blocks do not need to be completed for this type of case.

CHAMPVA
No secondary coverage

CHAMPVA INSURANCE COMPANY NAME
MAILING ADDRESS
CITY STATE ZIP CODE

1. MEDICARE MEDICAID CHAMPUS CHAMPVA GROUP HEALTH PLAN FECA BLK LUNG OTHER	1a. INSURED'S I.D. NUMBER (FOR PROGRAM IN ITEM 1)
(Medicare #) (Medicaid #) (Sponsor's SSN) X (VA File #) (SSN or ID) (SSN) (ID)	560 12 4444

2. PATIENT'S NAME (Last Name, First Name, Middle Initial)
DEXTER BRUCE R

3. PATIENT'S BIRTH DATE MM 03 DD 13 YYYY 1934   SEX M X F

4. INSURED'S NAME (Last Name, First Name, Middle Initial)
DEXTER BRUCE R

5. PATIENT'S ADDRESS (No., Street)
226 IRWIN ROAD

6. PATIENT RELATIONSHIP TO INSURED
Self X Spouse Child Other

7. INSURED'S ADDRESS (No., Street)
SAME

CITY
WOODLAND HILLS   STATE XY

8. PATIENT STATUS
Single X Married Other
Employed Full-Time Student Part-Time Student

CITY   STATE

ZIP CODE 12345 0000   TELEPHONE (include Area Code) (013) 497 1338

ZIP CODE   TELEPHONE (include Area Code) (   )

9. OTHER INSURED'S NAME (Last Name, First Name, Middle Initial)

10. IS PATIENT'S CONDITION RELATED TO:

11. INSURED'S POLICY GROUP OR FECA NUMBER
023

a. OTHER INSURED'S POLICY OR GROUP NUMBER

a. EMPLOYMENT? (CURRENT OR PREVIOUS)
YES X NO

a. INSURED'S DATE OF BIRTH MM DD YY   SEX M F

b. OTHER INSURED'S DATE OF BIRTH MM DD YYYY M F

b. AUTO ACCIDENT? PLACE (State)
YES X NO

b. EMPLOYER'S NAME OR SCHOOL NAME
USAF

c. EMPLOYER'S NAME OR SCHOOL NAME

c. OTHER ACCIDENT?
YES X NO

c. INSURANCE PLAN NAME OR PROGRAM NAME

d. INSURANCE PLAN NAME OR PROGRAM NAME

10d. RESERVED FOR LOCAL USE

d. IS THERE ANOTHER HEALTH BENEFIT PLAN?
YES X NO *If yes,* return to and complete item 9 a-d.

READ BACK OF FORM BEFORE COMPLETING AND SIGNING THIS FORM.

12. PATIENT'S OR AUTHORIZED PERSON'S SIGNATURE I authorize the release of any medical or other information necessary to process this claim. I also request payment of government benefits either to myself or to the party who accepts assignment below.

SIGNED SOF   DATE

13. INSURED'S OR AUTHORIZED PERSON'S SIGNATURE I authorize payment of medical benefits to the undersigned physician or supplier for services described below.

SIGNED

14. DATE OF CURRENT: MM DD YYYY ◄ ILLNESS (First symptom) OR INJURY (Accident) OR PREGNANCY (LMP)

15. IF PATIENT HAS HAD SAME OR SIMILAR ILLNESS GIVE FIRST DATE MM DD YYYY

16. DATES PATIENT UNABLE TO WORK IN CURRENT OCCUPATION FROM MM DD YYYY TO MM DD YYYY

17. NAME OF REFERRING PHYSICIAN OR OTHER SOURCE
GERALD PRACTON MD

17a. I.D. NUMBER OF REFERRING PHYSICIAN
70 3459766

18. HOSPITALIZATION DATES RELATED TO CURRENT SERVICES MM DD YYYY FROM 07 29 20XX TO 07 31 20XX

19. RESERVED FOR LOCAL USE

20. OUTSIDE LAB? YES X NO $ CHARGES

21. DIAGNOSIS OR NATURE OF ILLNESS OR INJURY (RELATE ITEMS 1,2,3 OR 4 TO ITEM 24E BY LINE)
1. 600
2.
3.
4.

22. MEDICAID RESUBMISSION CODE   ORIGINAL REF. NO.

23. PRIOR AUTHORIZATION NUMBER

24. A DATE(S) OF SERVICE From To	B Place of Service	C Type of Service	D PROCEDURES, SERVICES, OR SUPPLIES (Explain Unusual Circumstances) CPT/HCPCS MODIFIER	E DIAGNOSIS CODE	F $ CHARGES	G DAYS OR UNITS	H EPSDT Family Plan	I EMG	J COB	K RESERVED FOR LOCAL USE
072920XX	21	2	52601	1	1193 53	1				C064303

25. FEDERAL TAX I.D. NUMBER SSN EIN
77 8653124   X

26. PATIENT'S ACCOUNT NO.
090

27. ACCEPT ASSIGNMENT? (For govt. claims, see back)
X YES NO

28. TOTAL CHARGE
$ 1193 53

29. AMOUNT PAID
$

30. BALANCE DUE
$ 1193 53

31. SIGNATURE OF PHYSICIAN OR SUPPLIER INCLUDING DEGREES OR CREDENTIALS (I certify that the statements on the reverse apply to this bill and are made a part thereof.)
GENE ULIBARRI MD
SIGNED *Gene Ulibarri* DATE 073020XX

32. NAME AND ADDRESS OF FACILITY WHERE SERVICES WERE RENDERED (if other than home or office)
COLLEGE HOSPITAL
4500 BROAD AVENUE
WOODLAND HILLS XY 12345 0001
95 0731067

33. PHYSICIAN'S, SUPPLIER'S BILLING NAME, ADDRESS, ZIP CODE AND PHONE #
COLLEGE CLINIC
4567 BROAD AVENUE
WOODLAND HILLS XY 12345 0001
013 486 9002
PIN# 3664021CC GRP#

reference initials

Figure 6–14. An example of a completed HCFA-1500 Health Insurance Claim Form for a CHAMPVA case with no secondary coverage. Screened blocks do not need to be completed for this type of case.

WORKERS' COMPENSATION

WORKERS' COMPENSATION INSURANCE COMPANY NAME
MAILING ADDRESS
CITY STATE ZIP CODE

1. MEDICARE MEDICAID CHAMPUS CHAMPVA GROUP HEALTH PLAN FECA BLK LUNG OTHER	1a. INSURED'S I.D. NUMBER (FOR PROGRAM IN ITEM 1)
☐ (Medicare #) ☐ (Medicaid #) ☐ (Sponsor's SSN) ☐ (VA File #) ☐ (SSN or ID) ☐ (SSN) ☒ (ID)	667289

2. PATIENT'S NAME (Last Name, First Name, Middle Initial)	3. PATIENT'S BIRTH DATE MM DD YYYY SEX	4. INSURED'S NAME (Last Name, First Name, Middle Initial)
BARTON PETER A	11 14 1976 M ☒ F ☐	D F CONSTRUCTION

5. PATIENT'S ADDRESS (No., Street)	6. PATIENT RELATIONSHIP TO INSURED	7. INSURED'S ADDRESS (No., Street)
14890 DAISY AVENUE	Self ☐ Spouse ☐ Child ☐ Other ☒	1212 HARDROCK PLACE

CITY	STATE	8. PATIENT STATUS	CITY	STATE
WOODLAND HILLS	XY	Single ☐ Married ☐ Other ☐	WOODLAND HILLS	XY

ZIP CODE	TELEPHONE (include Area Code)		ZIP CODE	TELEPHONE (include Area Code)
12345 0000	(013) 427 7698	Employed ☒ Full-Time Student ☐ Part-Time Student ☐	12345 0000	(013) 427 8200

9. OTHER INSURED'S NAME (Last Name, First Name, Middle Initial)	10. IS PATIENT'S CONDITION RELATED TO:	11. INSURED'S POLICY GROUP OR FECA NUMBER

a. OTHER INSURED'S POLICY OR GROUP NUMBER	a. EMPLOYMENT? (CURRENT OR PREVIOUS) ☒ YES ☐ NO	a. INSURED'S DATE OF BIRTH MM DD YY SEX M ☐ F ☐

b. OTHER INSURED'S DATE OF BIRTH MM DD YYYY SEX M ☐ F ☐	b. AUTO ACCIDENT? PLACE (State) ☐ YES ☒ NO	b. EMPLOYER'S NAME OR SCHOOL NAME

c. EMPLOYER'S NAME OR SCHOOL NAME	c. OTHER ACCIDENT? ☐ YES ☒ NO	c. INSURANCE PLAN NAME OR PROGRAM NAME

d. INSURANCE PLAN NAME OR PROGRAM NAME	10d. RESERVED FOR LOCAL USE	d. IS THERE ANOTHER HEALTH BENEFIT PLAN? ☐ YES ☐ NO If yes, return to and complete item 9 a-d.

READ BACK OF FORM BEFORE COMPLETING AND SIGNING THIS FORM.

12. PATIENT'S OR AUTHORIZED PERSON'S SIGNATURE I authorize the release of any medical or other information necessary to process this claim. I also request payment of government benefits either to myself or to the party who accepts assignment below.

SIGNED _____ DATE _____

13. INSURED'S OR AUTHORIZED PERSON'S SIGNATURE I authorize payment of medical benefits to the undersigned physician or supplier for services described below.

SIGNED _____

14. DATE OF CURRENT: ◄ ILLNESS (First symptom) OR INJURY (Accident) OR PREGNANCY (LMP) MM DD YYYY 01 04 20XX	15. IF PATIENT HAS HAD SAME OR SIMILAR ILLNESS GIVE FIRST DATE MM DD YYYY	16. DATES PATIENT UNABLE TO WORK IN CURRENT OCCUPATION FROM MM DD YYYY 01 04 20XX TO MM DD YYYY 03 27 20XX

17. NAME OF REFERRING PHYSICIAN OR OTHER SOURCE	17a. I.D. NUMBER OF REFERRING PHYSICIAN	18. HOSPITALIZATION DATES RELATED TO CURRENT SERVICES FROM MM DD YYYY TO MM DD YYYY

19. RESERVED FOR LOCAL USE	20. OUTSIDE LAB? $ CHARGES ☐ YES ☐ NO

21. DIAGNOSIS OR NATURE OF ILLNESS OR INJURY (RELATE ITEMS 1,2,3 OR 4 TO ITEM 24E BY LINE) 1. 71831 3. 2. 4.	22. MEDICAID RESUBMISSION CODE ORIGINAL REF. NO.
	23. PRIOR AUTHORIZATION NUMBER

24. A. DATE(S) OF SERVICE				B. Place of Service	C. Type of Service	D. PROCEDURES, SERVICES, OR SUPPLIES (Explain Unusual Circumstances) CPT/HCPCS MODIFIER	E. DIAGNOSIS CODE	F. $ CHARGES	G. DAYS OR UNITS	H. EPSDT Family Plan	I. EMG	J. COB	K. RESERVED FOR LOCAL USE
From MM DD YYYY		To MM DD YYYY											
022720XX				11	1	29055	1	150 51	1				

25. FEDERAL TAX I.D. NUMBER SSN EIN 74 6541270 ☐ ☒	26. PATIENT'S ACCOUNT NO. 100	27. ACCEPT ASSIGNMENT? (For govt. claims, see back) ☐ YES ☐ NO	28. TOTAL CHARGE $ 150 51	29. AMOUNT PAID $	30. BALANCE DUE $ 150 51

31. SIGNATURE OF PHYSICIAN OR SUPPLIER INCLUDING DEGREES OR CREDENTIALS (I certify that the statements on the reverse apply to this bill and are made a part thereof.) RAYMOND SKELTON MD 022820XX SIGNED *Raymond Skelton, M.D.*	32. NAME AND ADDRESS OF FACILITY WHERE SERVICES WERE RENDERED (if other than home or office) SAME	33. PHYSICIAN'S, SUPPLIER'S BILLING NAME, ADDRESS, ZIP CODE AND PHONE # COLLEGE CLINIC 4567 BROAD AVENUE WOODLAND HILLS XY 12345 0001 013 486 9002 PIN# GRP# 3664021CC

reference initials

Figure 6–15. An example of a completed HCFA-1500 Health Insurance Claim Form for a workers' compensation case. Screened blocks do not need to be completed for this type of case.

STUDENT ASSIGNMENT LIST

✔ Study Chapter 6.

✔ Answer the review questions in the *Workbook* to reinforce the theory learned in this chapter and to help prepare you for a future test.

✔ Complete the assignments in the *Workbook* to give you hands-on experience in abstracting information from case histories and ledger cards as well as completing insurance claim forms.

✔ Study the claim sample in the *Workbook* and try to locate as many errors as possible based on the instructions you have been given in this chapter.

✔ Turn to the Glossary at the end of this textbook for a further understanding of the Key Terms used in this chapter.

COMPUTER ASSIGNMENT

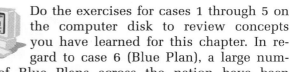

Do the exercises for cases 1 through 5 on the computer disk to review concepts you have learned for this chapter. In regard to case 6 (Blue Plan), a large number of Blue Plans across the nation have been bought by private insurance companies. Since each company has different requirements for completion of the HCFA-1500 claim form, written instructions have been omitted from this edition of the *Handbook*. However, basic Blue Plan instructions are incorporated into the computer disk software. For case 6, most block instructions are the same as for private carriers except blocks 1a, 11, 11a, 11b, 11c, 24E, and 24G. Check Block Help for Private/Blue Plan instructions for these blocks and leave Blocks 13 and 27 blank.

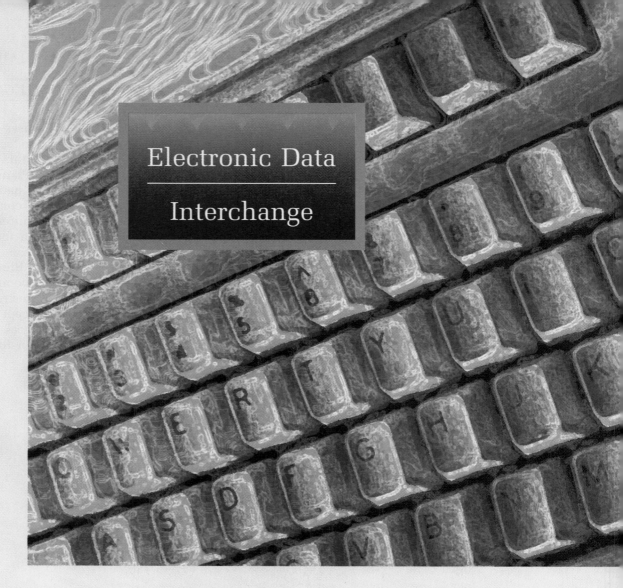

Electronic Data
Interchange

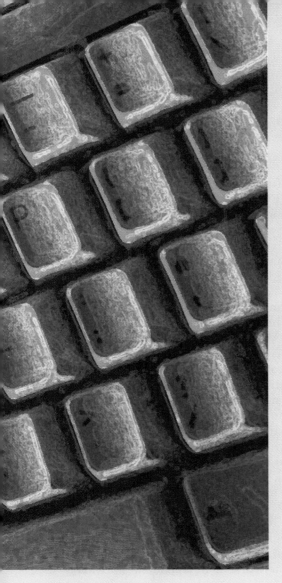

■ Describe what is needed when adopting a computer system.
■ Explain the difference between carrier-direct and clearinghouse electronically transmitted claims.
■ State the job duties of an electronic claims professional.
■ Describe the use of patient encounter forms, crib sheets, and scannable encounter forms in electronic claim submission.
■ Indicate some computer transmission problems.
■ Name some types of interactive computer transactions.

OBJECTIVES*

After reading this chapter you should be able to:

■ Specify differences between manual and electronic claim submission.
■ Identify components of a computer system.
■ Define computer terminology and interpret abbreviations.
■ Explain how to manage and store computer data.
■ List prevention measures to retain computer confidentiality.

KEY TERMS

audit trail

back up

batch

bit

bug

byte

carrier-direct system

central processing unit (CPU)

clearinghouse

debug

down time

electronic claims processor (ECP)

electronic claim submission (ECS)

electronic data interchange (EDI)

electronic mail (e-mail)

encryption

file

format

gigabyte

hard copy

hardware

input

interactive transaction

interface

Internet

keypad

kilobyte

local area network (LAN)

megabyte

memory

continued

---

*Performance objectives and exercises for hands-on practical experience for this chapter appear in the *Workbook*.

History of an Electronic Claim

In the 1960s and early 1970s, large hospitals began submitting electronic claims for payment to insurance carriers. An *electronic claim* is one that is submitted by means of central direct wire, dial-in-telephone, or personal computer upload or download. The transmission of such claims became known as **electronic data interchange (EDI).** This is a process by which understandable data are sent back and forth via computer linkages between two or more entities that function alternatively as sender and receiver. Electronic transmissions are sent encrypted so that they cannot be easily read if they are intercepted by a wrong individual. **Encryption** is to assign a code to represent data and is done for security purposes. In encrypted (encoded) versions, the data look like gibberish to unauthorized users and must be decoded to be used or read.

In the mid 1970s, the Medicare program expanded, thereby increasing the number of covered individuals. To reduce the number of paper claims and administrative costs, the Health Care Financing Administration (HCFA) began to emphasize electronic claims submission (ECS). This system of transmission was practical only for hospitals and large medical practices, because some carriers required 25 or more claims per batch. A **batch** is a group of claims for different patients sent at the same time from one facility.

In 1981, the National Electronic Information Corporation (NEIC) was formed by 11 major insurance companies. This provided a national network to receive, process, edit, sort, and transmit electronic claims to insurers. The NEIC system allowed the physician to use one version of software to communicate with different insurers. Claims can be submitted directly to NEIC for routing or through a network of independent software vendors, clearinghouses, and billing centers. A **clearinghouse,** also referred to as a third party administrator (TPA), is an entity that receives transmission of claims, separates the claims by carrier, performs software edits on each claim to check for errors, and sends claims electronically to the correct insurance payer.

HCFA has a Medicare Transaction System (MTS) that is for Part A (hospital services) and Part B (outpatient medical services) claims processing. This system replaces the numerous software processing programs formerly used by Medicare's claims contractors with a national electronic standard program. The system is used for nearly all Medicare transactions, including claims submission called electronic media claims (EMC), payment, direct deposit, online eligibility verification, coordination of benefits, and claims status.

Advantages of Electronic Claim Submission

Currently almost all insurance companies participate in electronic claims submission. Claims sent electronically require no signing or stamping, no searching for an insurance carrier's address, no postage fees or trips to the post office, and no storing or filing of claim forms in a file cabinet. Also, they leave an **audit trail** that is a chronological record of submitted data that can be traced to their source to determine the place of origin.

Generally, cash flow is improved and less time is spent processing claims, thereby freeing staff for other duties. Because information is going from one computer to another, this also reduces overhead by decreasing labor costs and human error. Payment from electronically submitted claims is received in 2 weeks or less. In comparison, payment from claims completed manually and sent by mail takes 4 to 6 weeks to receive. A proof of receipt is generated at the carrier's end, thus eliminating the insurance carrier's excuse, "We never received the claim, please resubmit."

Another important advantage of **electronic claims submission (ECS)** is the online error-edit process that may be incorporated into the software in the physician's office, clearinghouse, or insurance company. This allows the person processing the claim to know of an error immediately so a correction can be made. The insurance carrier either writes a check, returns the claim for more information, or sets it aside for manual review. Information regarding problem claims can be telecommunicated immediately, allowing quicker submission of corrected data.

Computer Components

When working in a business, whether it be at an in-home office or at a facility, you will be working with equipment that may, at times, have mechani-cal or technical problems. Thus, it is important to know the workings of the *computer* as well as some of the *peripheral* devices. A computer is a machine that uses electricity to maneuver information according to programmed instructions in a larger volume and at a lower cost, faster and more efficiently than can be done by hand (Fig. 7–1). Peripherals are input, output, and storage units that are attached to the computer by cables, such as zip drives, speakers, printer, and a modem. A **modem** is a device (internal or external peripheral) used to transmit electronic information over a dedicated telephone line. When an electronic claim is transmitted to the insurance carrier, a modem accomplishes this task.

Hardware

Hardware represents the physical components of a computer system (e.g., display screen, hard disk, keyboard, mouse) (Fig. 7–2). First data must be **input** using a keyboard, which resembles a typewriter keyboard, and/or a **keypad,** which is used for numeric computation. A **mouse,** *trackball,* or scanning device can also be used to input information. The computer has a television-like screen attached to it, called a **video display terminal (VDT),** which displays the output of data, or **soft copy.** It is also known as a monitor, cathode ray tube (CRT), or liquid crystal display (LCD). The computer is set up to **interface** with a computer **output** device, a printer,

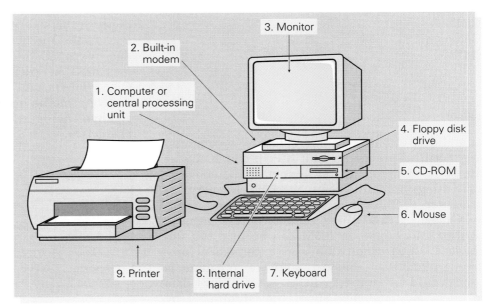

Figure 7–1. Illustration of the hardware components of a computer system. The system consists of input devices (keyboard [7], and mouse [6]), a central processing device (inside the system unit [1]), output devices (monitor [3] and printer [9]), auxiliary storage devices (disk drives and CD-ROM [4, 5, 8], also located within the system unit), and a transmission device or modem (inside the system unit [2]).

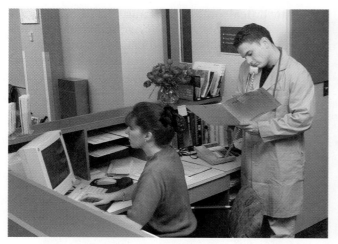

Figure 7–2. Insurance billing specialist's workstation.

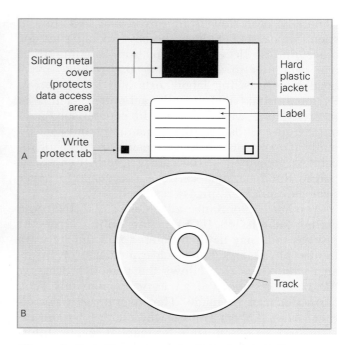

Figure 7–3. *A,* Components of a 3.5-inch disk. *B,* Components of a compact disk–read-only memory (CD-ROM) showing one of the concentric circles in which data are recorded.

which produces **hard copy** of data in readable form. Printer output can be produced by dot matrix, laser-generated copy, or ink jet.

Software

Software represents the **program** (computer instructions) required to make hardware perform a specific task. Although each insurer has different software, physicians typically select one that can interface with the insurance companies they deal with most. Software programs can be purchased or leased. There are many types of software used to perform the function of medical insurance billing. Some common software programs include

Avanta
Lytec
Medical Manager
Medisoft
Meditech
PMW
PRIME

Memory

In addition to hardware and software, a computer has a **central processing unit (CPU)**, which acts as the brain of the computer system. It includes the computing capability and working memory. A computer contains two types of **memory: read-only memory (ROM)** and **random access memory (RAM).** Data stored in ROM can be read but not changed. ROM usually contains a permanent program. Whichever medical software program is used would be stored in ROM. RAM allows data to be stored randomly and retrieved directly by

specifying the address location. The data entered into the medical software would be stored in RAM. If the computer is turned off and the data have not been saved, then the data are erased in RAM. Data should always be saved on the hard disk. It can also be saved on a magnetic storage device, such as a CD-ROM recordable disk, zip disk, or 3.5-inch disk (Fig. 7–3).

Computer storage capacity to save data in memory is measured in **bytes,** each of which consists of a group of eight **bits** (from "*bi*nary digi*ts*"), the smallest unit of storage possible (see Box 7–1). One byte of storage capacity will hold one piece of information. Memory capacity is measured in kilobytes, megabytes, or gigabytes. One **kilobyte** will store 1024 bytes or characters, and one **megabyte** is equal to 1000 kilobytes. A **gigabyte** holds approximately 1 billion bytes or characters.

Computer Storage Memory

Bit	0 and 1 (smallest storage unit)
Byte	8 bits
Kilobyte	1024 bytes
Megabyte	1000 kilobytes
Gigabyte	1000 megabytes or 1 billion bytes

Networks

Local Area Network

Many business sites have more than one or two computer stations and there is a type of system setup that is used to interlink multiple computers. It may be found in hospitals, clinics, and large medical practices and is referred to as a **local area network (LAN)**. In a LAN setup, computers that are contained within a room or building are connected by cables allowing them to share files and devices such as printers.

Installing software on a LAN computer has different installation instructions then when installing software on a single computer terminal. In fact, many schools have the computers networked so you may encounter this type of system setup before you actually begin to work as an insurance biller.

Wide Area Network

A *wide area network (WAN)* is a communications network that covers a wide geographic area. Examples of wide area networks are America Online, CompuServe, the worldwide airline reservation system, and in the medical field, MEDLINE and Physicians Online. MEDLINE was developed by the National Library of Medicine and is a database with access fees that provides 7 million references from about 4000 medical journals published worldwide.

Internet/World Wide Web

The **Internet** is a large interconnected message-forwarding system linking academic, commercial, government, and military computer networks all over the world. Applications available are electronic mail (e-mail), online conversations (one-on-one or in chat rooms), information retrieval, and bulletin board systems (BBS) where messages may be posted via the World Wide Web facility on the Internet. Some insurers offer incentives to practitioners for using the Web to process medical claims, make referrals, and check claim status, patient eligibility, and deductibles. Incentives can consist of faster payment of claims, payment of claim transaction fees, and direct deposit of claim payments to the practice's bank account. A Uniform or Universal Resource Locator (URL) is the web address or location of an organization, government or military network, commercial business, or academic or research site on the Internet (e.g., http://www.ama-assn.org [American Medical Association]).

Electronic Mail

Electronic mail (e-mail) is the transmitting, receiving, storing, and forwarding of text, voice messages, attachments, or images by computer from one person to another. Every computer user subscribing to an on-line service may establish an e-mail address (see Example 7–1).

EXAMPLE 7–1

Electronic Mail (e-mail) Address mason@aol.com means:

Mason	Individual user (Mason)
@	at
aol	site (America Online, an online service provider)
com	type of site (commercial business)

Because this is a more cost-effective and efficient method of sending a message to someone and obtaining a quicker response, you may be composing, forwarding, and responding by means of e-mail with staff in other locations, with patients, and with insurance billers (Fig. 7–4). It is important to set some standards to follow when communicating via e-mail. The

Figure 7–4. Electronic mail message to *The APCs Weekly Monitor* asking a question about use of modifiers.

Subj: **anesthesia modifiers**
Date: Thursday, August 17, 2000
To: apcmonitor@shore.net

Question: Is conscious sedation considered anesthesia in relationship to modifier -73 and -74? A speaker at a recent conference said "yes" but another said it had not yet been clarified by HCFA. Our fiscal intermediary manual has an example that said modifier -52 would be used in conjunction with a colonoscopy with conscious sedation. What is correct?
brownm@aol.com

messages you send are a reflection of your professional image.

1. Identify yourself and the reason for the message.
2. Compose the message in a clear and concise manner using good grammar and proper spelling. Make sure it cannot be misconstrued.
3. Include a descriptive subject line. If a reply changes the topic, then change the subject line.
4. Do not put confidential information in an e-mail message (e.g., patient-identifiable information).
5. Encrypt (code) all files about patients and e-mail attachments and limit the size of attachments. Some users pay a per minute connect time and will be downloading the attachment.
6. Recognize that all e-mail is discoverable in legal proceedings so be careful with content and choice of words.
7. Do not use all capital letters for more than a word.
8. Insert a blank line between paragraphs.
9. Surround URLs (long web addresses) with angle brackets [ ] to avoid problems occurring at the end of a line with the word wrap feature.
10. Do not use variable text styles (bold or italic) or text colors.
11. Quote sparingly when automatically quoting the original message in replies. Some programs allow you to select some text in the original message by pressing a keyboard shortcut, and only that text appears quoted in the reply. Quote marks should be inserted to differentiate original and new text.
12. Avoid sending junk messages (e.g., welcome messages, congratulation messages, jokes, chain messages).
13. Avoid "emoticons," a short sequence of keyboard letters and symbols used to convey emotion, gestures, or expressions (e.g., "smiley" (☺; :–)).
14. Do not respond immediately if someone's e-mail makes you angry or emotional. Put the message aside until the next day and then answer it diplomatically.
15. Do not write anything racially or sexually offensive.
16. Insert a short signature at the end of the message that includes your name, affiliation, and e-mail and/or URL address.

Web Search Engine

You may also be accessing the Internet and using a web browser (search engine) to go to a specific address to obtain current legal and regulatory information from insurance programs and federal agencies. You may be downloading data or attachments from the web. Some web sites to contact for current information about insurance regulations and code updates for insurance billing are given at the end of the chapter.

Computer Confidentiality

Confidentiality Statement

The majority of information in patients' medical records and physicians' financial records is considered confidential and sensitive. Employees who have access to such computer data should have integrity and be well chosen because he or she will have a high degree of responsibility and accountability. It is wise to have those handling sensitive computer documents sign an annual confidentiality statement, as recommended by the Alliance of Claims Assistance Professionals (Fig. 7–5). In this way, the statement can be updated when an individual's responsibilities increase or decrease. The statement should contain the following:

▶ Written or oral disclosure of information pertaining to patients is prohibited.
▶ Disclosure of information without consent of the patient results in serious penalty (e.g., immediate dismissal).

An additional example of an employee confidentiality agreement that may be used by an employer when hiring an insurance biller is shown in Chapter 1, Figure 1–7.

Prevention Measures

Employees can take a number of preventive measures to maintain computer security. Follow these guidelines:

1. Obtain a software program that stores files in coded form.
2. Never leave disks or tapes unguarded on desks or anywhere else in sight.
3. Use a privacy filter over the computer monitor so data may be read only when one is directly in front of the computer.
4. Log off the computer terminal before leaving a work station, especially if working in a local area network (LAN) environment, which is used in most hospitals, clinics, or large offices.
5. Check and double check the credentials of any consultant hired.
6. Read the manuals for the equipment, especially the sections entitled "Security Controls," and follow all directions.
7. Store confidential data on diskettes or zip disks rather than only to the computer's hard

YOUR COMPANY NAME
ADDRESS
PHONE/FAX

CONFIDENTIALITY STATEMENT

I, _____ , understand and acknowledge that as a
(Type in individual's name)
principle/employee of _____(company name)_____ my position
as __(job title)_____ requires that I access and use computer equipment and
software applications owned or leased by____(company name)_____ .
I understand that my position as a principle/employee of this company obligates me to abide by
the purchase, lease or rental agreements applicable to this equipment and software.

I understand and acknowledge that my position may require that I handle information regarding
the physicians and medical suppliers who are clients of____company name_____ . I
understand and acknowledge that such client information, including financial data, fees,
corporate structure, etc., is privileged and confidential and that I am not at liberty to divulge or
discuss such information with unauthorized individuals within this company or to anyone outside
this company.

I understand and acknowledge that my duties may require me to access and/or process specific
patient data for individuals under the care of____company name_____ client
physicians and/or medical suppliers. I understand and acknowledge that all patient's data is
protected under federal privacy legislation and that discussion or release of this information in any
form without the patient's express permission is prohibited by federal law and subject to
prosecution and civil monetary penalties for any violation.

I further understand that violations of this confidentiality agreement will result in termination of
employment with____company name_____ .

My signature below is to verify my understanding and acceptance of the above data
confidentiality requirements and to signify my explicit agreement to abide by these requirements.

_____   _____ Date
Signature

_____   _____
Type Name   Title

Figure 7–5. Sample of confidentiality statement for an employee using computer equipment and software. (Originally developed by the National Association of Claims Assistance Professionals, Inc., Downers Grove, IL.)

drive. Diskettes should be stored in a locked, secure location, preferably one that is fireproof and away from magnetic fields.

8. Turn off the modem when the office is closed. This can keep amateurs, but not professional hackers, from accessing your electronic system. Hackers can access digital copiers, laser printers, fax machines, and other electronic equipment that have internal memories. Some offices transmit and receive data during low-cost, low-volume hours. This means the modem would be left on.

9. Develop passwords for each individual user and access codes to protect the data. A **password** is a combination of letters, numbers, or symbols that each individual is assigned to access the system. Passwords should be changed at regular intervals and never written down. A good password is composed of more than five characters and is case sensitive. *Case sensitive* means that the password must be entered exactly as stored using upper and/or lower case characters. Delete obsolete passwords from the system. Change any passwords known by an employee who is fired or resigns. Individuals with their own passwords allow the employer to distinguish work done by each employee. If errors or problems occur, focus may then be directed toward correcting the individual user who can learn from the mistakes.

10. Send only an account number (not the patient's name) when e-mailing a colleague with specific questions (e.g., regarding coding).

Records Management

Data Storage

A paperless office requires an organized and efficient system for keeping **files** that have been saved to the hard drive against accidental destruction. Keep financial records on disks or tapes and store in an area that does not have temperature extremes or magnetic fields.

When keyboarding data, it is wise to **back up** (save data) frequently. Automated back up is possible, and the computer regularly initiates the process. Most financial software programs display a screen prompt instructing the operator to back up before quitting the program. If there is no automated back up, remember to always back up files at the end of the day or several times a week so information is not lost during a power outage (e.g., surge, spike, blackout, brownout, lightning), computer breakdown, or head crash. *Head crash* is when the read-write head on a disk drive strikes the surface of the disk, causing damage at the point of impact.

About once a week a verification process should be done that compares the original records with the copies. This can take 20% to 30% longer than ordinary back up, but if a comparison is not made there is no way to ensure that the data have been backed up. Store back-up copies away from the office in case of fire, flood, or theft.

Maintain a notebook (log) of the documents you have on your disks/tapes with an index located at the front of the book. The log enables you to keep track of files and should list when you backed up the files last so they can be located quickly. Be sure another employee knows where this notebook is kept and is familiar with how to track down files through this system. Note the code for accessing these documents and date your revisions when updating old documents.

Electronic Power Protection

Plug equipment into power surge suppressors or, preferred, one with an uninterruptible power supply (UPS) to prevent computer and data file damage. In addition, the entire office should be protected by a surge suppressor installed near the electric circuit breaker panel. This device is called an all-office or whole-office surge suppressor.

Selection of an Office Computer System

A medical practice wishing to use an in-office computer or an individual wishing to set up his or her own business should consider the following:

1. What is the cost of the basic equipment and will it be purchased or leased?
2. What accessories will be needed, and what are their costs?
3. How much space will be needed for the equipment and accessories for the office or home office business?
4. What type of electrical installation should be done to handle electronic transmission of data?
5. Should a computer fax/modem be obtained, or should there be a separate fax line installed?
6. How much electrical energy will be used, and how much additional cost will be required?
7. If the computer is on a time-sharing system with other users, how much will the telephone line cost when communicating on-line or directly to the computer?
8. What are the hardware maintenance costs, and who will do the repair work?
9. What initial software will be required, and will it be compatible with the operating system?
10. What is the estimated cost of software upgrades and will upgrades require an expanded operating system?
11. What are the software maintenance costs, and who will provide technical support?
12. Should a document scanner be obtained?
13. What forms will be used as output from the computer? Also, consider their size, design, acquisition, storage, waste, and cost.
14. What other supplies will be needed, and what will their costs be?
15. How many on the staff will operate the computer? Will recruitment be necessary? Who will train employees, and how much training time is required?
16. Will there be financing when the equipment is purchased and, if so, what type?
17. Will there be insurance and a warranty on the system?
18. How much will the consulting costs be?
19. What is the backup support and response time when there is a system crash (software or hardware)? Who will respond to software problems, and who will respond to hardware problems?
20. How much time will it take to convert the present accounting system to the computerized system, and who will be doing the conversion?

Computer Claims Systems

For a better understanding of how insurance claims are transmitted, it is important to know the two types of systems and how they work (i.e., carrier-direct and clearinghouse).

Carrier-Direct

Fiscal agents for Medicaid, Medicare, TRICARE, and many private insurance carriers use the **carrier-direct system.** With this system, either the medical practice must have its own computer and software or the physician must lease a terminal from the carrier to key-in claim data directly. The data are then transmitted via modem over a dedicated telephone line.

Clearinghouse

If the physician's system cannot be linked with the insurance carrier or the insurers do not accept claims directly from the physician's office, then the physician may use a *clearinghouse*, which forwards a batch of claims to the insurers. The insurance carrier may stipulate that the claims be sent on diskette or tape to a clearinghouse, which reformats the claims, performs an edit check, transmits them to the carrier, and charges the physician a fee.

As mentioned in earlier chapters, when using this system the medical practice submits either paper claims (typed or computer generated) or electronic claims. Claims are submitted every day or once a week, dictated by need or volume.

Some clearinghouses have additional services, such as manually processing claims to carriers that are not on-line. This means that the physician's office can send all claims electronically to the clearinghouse rather than processing half electronically and printing and mailing the rest. Sufficient volume must exist with a particular insurer to make using a clearinghouse cost effective. Clearinghouses may charge a flat fee per claim or charge a percentage of the claim's dollar volume. Some clearinghouses will advance a certain amount determined by the contract before the carrier has paid the claims and then keep whatever it recovers. Figure 7–6 is a flow sheet illustrating electronic claim submission.

Electronic Claims Processor

An individual who converts insurance claims to standardized electronic format and transmits electronic claims data is known as an **electronic claims processor (ECP).** This individual can work in a physician's office, clinic setting, billing center, or be self-employed. A knowledgeable and efficient ECP can expedite payment to the physician and reduce the number of rejected claims. One of the duties of an ECP is to perform a front-end edit (online error checking) to correct any errors before the claim is transmitted to the insurance carrier. A good software program can edit claims and indicate areas where data are missing.

An important responsibility of an ECP is to make sure the software is always up to date. Diagnostic and procedural codes need to be updated annually in the software as well as on the encounter form. This ensures that claims are always correctly submitted. Failure to do this can result in claims that are refused, denied, or downcoded.

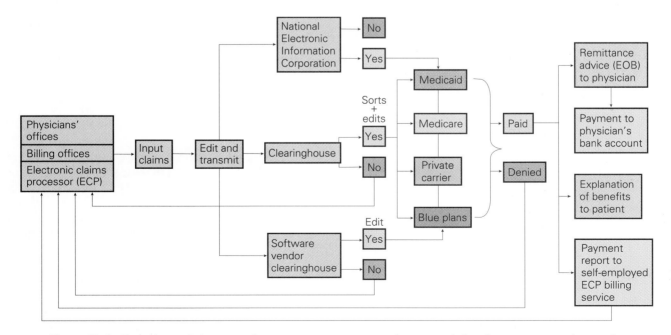

Figure 7–6. Flow sheet of electronic claims transmission systems showing path for claim payment and route for a denied claim.

The Alliance of Claims Assistance Professionals (ACAP) offers an examination to those eligible and interested in being certified as an ECP. Those who pass receive the title certified electronic claims professional (CECP). Information about certification is given in Chapter 17.

Electronic Data Interchange

A physician who plans to begin electronic billing must contact all major insurers and the fiscal intermediaries for each government and/or state program for a list of vendors approved to handle ECS. Each carrier has special electronic billing requirements and knows which systems can meet their criteria and are compatible in format. The field data requested is almost identical to that required on the HCFA-1500 claim form. It is also important to request information from insurance carriers about how to submit an electronic bill for patients who have secondary coverage. Some carriers, such as Medicare fiscal intermediaries, may provide the software and training to encourage electronic submission.

Carrier Agreements

It is necessary to have a signed agreement with each carrier with whom the physician wishes to submit electronic claims. Look over the agreement carefully to make sure it will be accepted for ECS.

Signature Requirements

Physician

The physician's signature on the agreement is a substitute for his or her signature on the claim form.

Patient

For assigning benefits and release of medical information, each patient's signature must be obtained either once a month, once a year, or on a one-time basis, depending on the circumstance of each case, because there are no signatures on electronic claims (Fig. 7–7). An authorization and assignment release may be designed specifically for the purpose of obtaining signatures for transmitting electronic claims. The HCFA-1500 Health Insurance Claim form may also be used for this pur-

Figure 7–7. Examples of patients' Medicare electronic signature authorization forms. A, Monthly form. B, One-time form.

PATIENT'S MEDICARE ELECTRONIC SIGNATURE MONTHLY AUTHORIZATION FORM

I authorize any holder of medical or other information about me to release to the Social Security Administration and Health Care Financing Administration or its intermediaries or carriers any information needed for this or a related Medicare claim. I permit a copy of this authorization to be used in place of the original, and request payment of medical insurance benefits either to myself or to the party who accepts assignment.

_____   _____
Signature of Patient   Date

A

PATIENT'S MEDICARE ELECTRONIC SIGNATURE ONE-TIME AUTHORIZATION FORM

I request that payment of authorized Medicare benefits be made either to me or on my behalf to _____ for services furnished me by that physician or supplier. I permit a copy of this authorization to be used in place of the original and authorize any holder of medical information about me to release to the Health Care Financing Administration or its agents any information needed to determine these benefits or the benefits payable for related services.

_____   _____
Signature of Patient   Date

B

pose, and the patient should sign in Block 12 and/or Block 13. Some software programs ask a question whether the patient's signature is on file and require a "yes" or "no" answer. Other software systems do not have this requirement so it depends on how the software is set up.

Signatures must be maintained on file in the physician's record for 72 months (6 years) after the month in which the claim was submitted. Some Medicare fiscal intermediaries require annual renewal of signatures, so check with the local carrier.

Multipurpose Billing Forms

As mentioned in Chapter 2, a **multipurpose billing form** (also known as charge slip, communicator, encounter form, fee ticket, patient service slip, routing form, superbill, or transaction slip) is a form used to record information about the service rendered to a patient. It is personalized and custom-printed to the specialty of the physician. These forms may be printed by the computer and customized with specific patient information, thus saving outside printing expenses and time filling in patient data.

Crib Sheet Encounter Form

In 1992 when the CPT Evaluation and Management procedure codes were introduced, another routing slip method was designed by physicians. An abbreviated style is used, and the form is known as a crib sheet or charge slip. A *crib sheet* is a summary form listing key components of the Evaluation and Management (E/M) codes (Fig. 7–8). It aids the physician in determining the correct level of E/M service, ensures each component is addressed in the physician's dictation, and expedites data entry of professional services. The physician circles the codes, and the insurance billing specialist can easily take that information and enter it into the computer system. Because crib sheets are abbreviated and not in detail, they, along with other types of billing forms, cannot be used in place of documentation in the patient record and may not withstand an external audit.

Scannable Encounter Form

Some encounter forms are designed so that they may be scanned to input charges and diagnoses into the patient's computerized account (Fig. 7–9). Time is saved and fewer errors occur because no keystrokes are involved.

Keying Insurance Data for Claim Transmission

Initially, you have learned that manual claim completion is accomplished by obtaining patient and insurance data, looking up a diagnosis and procedure in an index, referring to medical and financial records, and following block by block guidelines for the HCFA-1500 insurance claim form. Much of this source information is found on an encounter form that is used to post charges and payments.

When operating computer software, the encounter form may also be used to obtain information. A screen **prompt** (question) appears on the monitor, and the data are keyed in reply to the prompt. Reusable data are entered initially in a file and identified by a number. Each treating physician, referring physician, patient, and insurance carrier has a computer code number assigned; for example, Dr. Jones might be keyed in as 010; a patient, Jane Doe, might be input as an account number; and the ABC Insurance Company might be 003. This information is stored in the database and is the same as that required when completing a claim manually. It is automatically retrieved by the system when a computer code number is keyed in and used to generate a computerized claim and/or electronic claim. Because there are computer code numbers and prompts for each item, there is less chance for error or omitting mandatory information. The program checks to see that data are complete and in proper **format.**

Some entries are made using a *macro*. This technique involves a series of menu selections, keystrokes, and/or commands that have been recorded into memory and assigned a name or key combination. When the macro name is keyed in, the steps and/or characters in the macro are executed from beginning to end, saving time and key strokes.

Here are some general guidelines for keying in data and billing electronic claims:

▶ Do not use special characters (dashes, spaces, or commas).
▶ Use the patient account numbers to differentiate between patients with similar names.
▶ Use correct numeric locations of service code, valid *Current Procedural Terminology* (CPT), or HCFA Common Procedure Coding System (HCPCS) procedure codes.
▶ Do not bill codes using modifiers -21 or -22 electronically unless the carrier receives documents (called attachments) to justify more payment.
▶ Print out an insurance billing worksheet or perform a front-end edit (on-line error checking) to

MC2 NAME:		CHARGE SLIP				DATE:
CODE	HIST	EXAM	DEC	CODE	HIST	EXAM	DEC
99201	* NEW PAT. OFF.			99261	+ F. UP CONSULT — INPATIENT		
99202	* EPF	EPF	SF	99262	+ EPF	EPF	MC
99203	* D	D	LC	99263	+ D	D	HC
99204	* C	C	MC	99281	* EMERG. DEP.		
99205	* C	C	HC	99282	* EPF	EPF	LC
99211	+ EST. PAT. OFF.			99283	* EPF	EPF	L-MC
99212	+ PF	PF	SF	99284	* D	D	MC
99213	+ EPF	EPF	LC	99285	* C	C	HC
99214	+ D	D	MC	99291	CRITIC. CARE 1st Hr.		
99215	+ C	C	HC	99292	ADDIT. 30 MIN		
99221	* INIT. HOSP. VIS — NEW or ESTAB.			99301	* NURSING FACIL.		
99222	* C	C	MC	99302	* D	C	M-HC
99223	* C	C	HC	99303	* C	C	M-HC
99231	+ SUBSQ. HOSPIT.			99311	+ SNF SUBSEQ.		
99232	+ EPF	EPF	LC	99312	+ EPF	EPF	MC
99233	+ D	D	HC	99313	+ D	D	M-HC
99238	HOSPIT. DISCH.			99341	* HOME SERVICES — NEW PAT.		
99241	* CONSULT. OFF.			99342	* PF	PF	SF-LC
99242	* EPF	EPF	SF	99343	* EPF	EPF	MC
99243	* D	D	LC	99351	+ ESTAB. PATIENT		
99244	* C	C	MC	99352	+ EPF	EPF	MC
99245	*C	C	HC	99353	+ D	D	HC
99251	* INIT. CONSULT. — INPATIENT			DIAGNOSIS:			CPT CODES:
99252	* EPF	EPF	SF				
99253	* D	D	LC				
99254	* C	C	MC				
99255	* C	C	HC				

KEY: PF: Probl.Foc.　EPF: Expand.Probl.Foc　D: Detail.　C: Comprehens.
LC: Low Complex.　MC: Moder.Complex.　HC: High Complex.
Requirem.: *: 3 Key Components req. + : 2 out of 3 Key Compon. req.

Figure 7–8. Example of a crib sheet. This system of abbreviations has cut in half the time the physician spends in choosing the correct Evaluation and Management CPT codes. The format shown here can be adapted to any specialty. (Reprinted with permission from Helmut O. Haar, MD, Ventura, CA.)

look for and correct all errors before the claim is transmitted to the insurance carrier.
▶ Request electronic-error reports from the insurance carrier to make corrections to your system.
▶ Obtain and cross-check the electronic status report against all claims transmitted.

After input is complete, the information is stored in memory and a claim may be transmitted individually or in batches. Batched claims can be divided according to insurance type or date(s) of service and are ideally sent during low volume times.

Electronically Completing the Claim

Coding Requirements

When electronically transmitting insurance claims you may need Medicare HCPCS national and regional procedural codes for services, supplies, and procedures; CPT codes with modifiers; and *International Classification of Diseases, Ninth Revision, Clinical Modification* (ICD-9-CM) diagnostic codes. Most insurers require the physician to be responsible for assigning diagnostic and procedural codes. Refer to Appendix B for the names and addresses of publishers of the code books.

CFR

PAT 4140.0

( ) 985-6575 01/22/1936 F63
PRI: (Y) BLUE SHIELD ENVOY
201-XX-9969
SEC:

DOCTOR:	**2 FRANK CHI, M.D.**
ROOM:	
APPTLOC:	
APPTCD:	
REASON:	OX, F/U visit
LAST DX:	000.0 No diagnosis applicable
SSN/STA:	201-XX-9969, 1 Active
OVERLAY:	1 INTERNAL MEDICINE

APPT DATE:	**05/27/XX**
APPT TIME:	2:30 PM
APPT LEN:	10 min.
DEPT/LOC:	0, n/a
DSET/PRT:	1, 12
ACCT BAL:	75.00
PAT DUE:	0.00
VOUCHER:	7887

Each line below is preceded by selection bubbles: ①②③④Ⓟ/Ⓛ

NEW PT OFFICE VISITS
99203 NP LEVEL THREE
99204 NP LEVEL FOUR
99205 NP LEVEL FIVE
EST PT OFFICE VISIT
99211 EST PT LEVEL ONE
99212 EST PT LEVEL TWO
99213 EST PT LEVEL THREE
99214 EST PT LEVEL FOUR
99215 EST PT LEVEL FIVE
00003 GLOBAL VISIT

OTHER PROCEDURES
99000 COLL & PREP/PAP TEST
93000 EKG WITH INTERPRETATION
82270 HEMOCCULT
81000 URINALYSIS

INJECTIONS
~FLU, FLU INJ/ADMIN/MCR
~9065 FLU INJ/NON MCR
~PNEU PNEUMO/ADMIN/MCR
~9073 PNEUMO INJ NON MCR

UNLISTED PROCEDURES

_____

STOP FOR VERIFICATION
BREASTS
610.2 FIBROADENOSIS, BREAST
611.72 LUMP OR MASS IN BREAST

CARDIOVASCULAR
441.4 ABDOM AORTIC ANEURYSM
411.1 ANGINA
424.1 AORTIC VALVE DISORDER
427.31 ATRIAL FIBRILLATION
427.32 ATRIAL FLUTTER
427.61 ATRIAL PREMATURE BEATS
426.11 ATRIOVENT BLOCK-1ST DE
785.2 CARDIAC MURMURS NEC
429.3 CARDIOMEGALY
428.0 CONGESTIVE HEART FAILU
425.1 HYPERTR OBSTR CARDIOMY
414.01 ISCHEMIC CHR HEART DIS
426.2 LEFT BB HEMIBLOCK
424.0 MITRAL VALVE DISORDER
785.1 PALPITATIONS
427.0 PAROX ATRIAL TACHYCARD
427.1 PAROX VENTRIC TACHYCAR

CHEST
466.0 BRONCHITIS, ACUTE
491.0 BRONCHITIS, CHRONIC
493.20 CH OB ASTH W/O STAT AS
493.00 EXT ASTHMA W/O STAT AS

491.21 OBS CHR BRNC W ACT EXA
491.20 OBS CHR BRNC W/O ACT E

ENDOCRINE
250.61 DMI NEURO CMP CONTROLL
250.01 DMI WO CMP CONTROLLED
250.03 DMI UNCONTROLLED
250.60 DMII NEURO CMP CONTROL
250.00 DMII WO CMP CONTROLLED
250.02 DMII UNCONTROLLED
272.0 HYPERCHOLESTEROLEMIA
272.1 HYPERGLYCERIDEMIA
245.2 HYPOTHYROIDISM
278.01 MORBID OBESITY
241.0 THYROID NODULE

EXTREMITIES
782.3 EDEMA
440.22 LOWER EXT EMBOLISM
451.0 PHLEBITIS-LEG
440.21 PVD W/CLAUDICATION
454.9 VARICOSE VEIN OF LEG

GI
789.06 ABDMNAL PAIN EPIGASTRI
789.02 ABDMNAL PAIN LFT UP QU
789.04 ABDMNAL PAIN LT LWR QU
789.05 ABDMNAL PAIN PERIUMBIL
789.03 ABDMNAL PAIN RT LWR QU
789.01 ABDMNAL PAIN RT UPR QU
578.1 BLOOD IN STOOL
575.12 CHOLECYSTITIS, ACUTE
564.0 CONSTIPATION
787.91 DIARRHEA
562.11 DIVERTICULITIS
562.10 DIVERTICULOSIS
574.20 GALLSTONE(S), CHRONIC
535.00 GASTRITIS
530.81 GERD
455.3 HEMORRHOID, EXT W/O COM
455.0 HEMORRHOID, INT W/O COM
564.1 IRRITABLE COLON
787.01 NAUSEA WITH VOMITING
569.3 RECTAL & ANAL HEMORRHA
530.11 REFLUX ESOPHAGITIS
V76.41 SCREEN COLORECTAL

GU
601.0 ACUTE PROSTATITIS
600 BPH
592.0 CALCULUS OF KIDNEY
592.1 CALCULUS OF URETER
595.0 CYSTITIS, ACUTE
595.1 CYSTITIS, CHRONIC
599.7 HEMATURIA
607.84 IMPOTENCE, ORGANIC ORI
791.0 PROTEINURIA

HEENT
380.4 CERUMEN, IMPACTED
372.02 CONJUNCTIVITIS
784.7 EPISTAXIS
784.0 HEADACHE
464.0 LARYNGITIS/TRACHEITI
465.0 LARYNGOPHARYNGITIS, A
780.4 LIGHT-HEADEDNESS
346.00 MIGRAINE
460 NASOPHARYNGITIS, ACUT
381.01 OTITIS MEDIA
462 PHARYNGITIS, ACUTE
477.0 RHINITIS ALLERGIC
461.0 SINUSITIS, ACUTE
780.2 SYNCOPE/VERTIGO

HEMATOLOGIC
280.0 CHR BLOOD LOSS ANEMI
280.1 IRON DEF ANEMIA DIET
281.0 PERNICIOUS ANEMIA

HYPERTENSION
404.12 BEN HY HT/REN/CHF
403.10 BEN HTN REN W/O REN
403.11 BEN HYP WITH REN FAI
401.1 BENIGN HYPERTENSION
401.0 MALIGNANT HYPERTENSI
458.0 ORTHOSTATIC HYPOTENS

NEURO
345.10 GEN CNV EPIL W/O INT
435.3 TIA
433.10 CAROTID STENOSIS
437.0 CEREBRAL ATHEREOSCLER

OB GYN
112.1 CANDIDAL VULVOVAGINI
627.2 MENOPAUSAL SYMPTOMS
V76.2 SCREEN MAL NEOP-CERV

RHEUMATOLOGIC
723.1 CERVICAL PAIN
274.0 GOUT
724.2 LUMBAGO/BACK PAIN
729.5 PAIN IN LIMB
724.1 PAIN IN THORACIC SPI
714.0 RHEUMATOID ARTHRITIS
724.3 SCIATICA
710.0 SYST LUPUS ERYTHEMAT

MISC
780.6 FEVER UNKN ORGIN
054.9 HERPES SIMPLEX NOS
786.05 SHORTNESS OF BREATH

UNLISTED DIAGNOSIS
STOP FOR VERIFICATION

①②③④Ⓟ/Ⓛ **REFERRALS**	①②③④Ⓟ/Ⓛ **LOCATIONS**	①②③④Ⓟ/Ⓛ **DOCTORS**	①②③④Ⓟ/Ⓛ **NEXT VISIT**
①②③④Ⓟ/Ⓛ	①②③④Ⓟ/Ⓛ	①②③④Ⓟ/Ⓛ	①②③④Ⓟ/Ⓛ ____ DAYS
①②③④Ⓟ/Ⓛ	①②③④Ⓟ/Ⓛ	①②③④Ⓟ/Ⓛ F. CHI, MD	①②③④Ⓟ/Ⓛ _1_ WEEKS
①②③④Ⓟ/Ⓛ	①②③④Ⓟ/Ⓛ	①②③④Ⓟ/Ⓛ A. SWERD, MD	①②③④Ⓟ/Ⓛ ____ MONTHS
①②③④Ⓟ/Ⓛ	①②③④Ⓟ/Ⓛ	①②③④Ⓟ/Ⓛ J. STEVEN, MD	①②③④Ⓟ/Ⓛ

Figure 7–9. Scannable encounter form. (Form template only ©2000 NCS Pearson, Inc., Eden Prairie, MN. Form data are fictitious and not a part of the template copyrighted by NCS Pearson, Inc.)

Because the insurance billing specialist inputs the codes, claims examiners do not need to recode. This eliminates transposition of numbers or missing or added digits on transmitted claims. During the edit/error process, software code editors identify invalid codes, age conflicts, gender conflicts, procedural and diagnostic code conflicts, and other data before issuing payment. If certain information is submitted incorrectly (e.g., patient's name or insurance identification number is incorrect, a diagnosis code is missing a fifth digit, or a provider's identification number is omitted), the claim is rejected and must be resubmitted with correct data. Incorrect coding may be keying errors, or it may be a deliberate attempt to obtain fraudulent payment. The edit check allows immediate feedback regarding the status of an electronically transmitted claim.

Beginning April 1, 1996, Medicare requires certain information when submitting paper and electronic claims for some blocks of the HCFA-1500 claim form. Carriers may return claims if this information is omitted. A list of mandatory information and conditional requirements is shown in Table 7–1.

TABLE 7–1	**Medicare Requirements When Submitting Paper and Electronic Claims**	
	Mandatory Information	
Block No.	*Paper Claims*	**Electronic Claims**
IA.	Insured ID number	Insured ID number
2.	Patient name	Patient last and first names
II.	Insured's policy group number	Group number/Source of payment
13.	Patient signature source	Patient signature source/Release of information indicator
24a.	Dates of service	Service from/through dates
24b.	Place of service	Place of service
24d.	Procedures, services, and so on	HCPCS procedure code
24f.	$ charges	Line charges
24g.	Days or units of service	Units of service
31.	Provider signature indicator	Provider signature indicator
33.	Provider's billing name and address	Provider last and first names
		Payer organization, name
		Provider Medicare number (batch level)
		Provider's pay-to address I
		Provider's pay-to city
		Provider's pay-to state
		Provider's pay-to ZIP code
		Provider's pay-to telephone number
	Conditional Requirements	
4.	Insured name	Insured last and first names
6.	Patient relationship to insured	Patient relationship to insured
7.	Insured's address	Insured address-line I Insured city, state, ZIP code and telephone number
9c.	Employer's or school name	Insured employer name
9d.	Insurance plan or program name	Group name
14.	Date of current illness, and so on	Accident/symptom date
17.	Name or refer/ordering	Refer/ordering provider last name
17a.	ID no. of refer/ordering	Refer/ordering provider NPI, referring provider NPI
19.	Reserved for local use	Date last seen, supervising provider NPI, date of last x-ray
20.	Outside lab	Laboratory indicator, lab charges, purchased service indicator, purchased service charge
21.	Diagnosis	Diagnosis I, 2, 3, 4
24d.		HCPCS modifier I, 2, 3, 4
24k.	Reserved for local use	Rendering provider NPI
32.	Facility name and address	Facility/laboratory name and/or facility/laboratory NPI number, mammography certification no.

The physician or the medical insurance billing specialist may revise coding on the medical record and on the claim to reflect the services more accurately up until the time at which the claim is transmitted for payment.

Encoder and Grouper

When hospitals or large medical practices/clinics are transmitting an electronic claim, encoders and groupers may be used. A computer-assisted *encoder* (computer software program that assigns a code to represent data) helps users assign the most accurate code by prompting them with a series of questions or choices leading to a specific code assignment or by affecting code assignment by displaying code-specific edits. However, there are cases in which an encoder would not accurately assign codes, so never be completely dependent on code-assist software. For example, if a patient has three thorns incised and extracted (removed), the CPT code 10120 *incision and removal of foreign body, subcutaneous tissue; simple* (integumentary system) might be generated by the encoder. But if internally audited, the case may warrant CPT code 27372 *removal of foreign body, deep, thigh region in knee* area (musculoskeletal system). Thus, one learns that not all procedures involving the skin are found in the integumentary system and, if deeper skin layers are affected, a code may be found in another system. A *grouper* is software designed for use in a network that serves a group of users working on a related project that allows access to the same data.

Automated Coding

Still in its infancy but being developed is *automated coding*. This system does not make the coder go through questions or steps to assign a code. Instead, the system pulls data (diagnoses, procedures, patient care information) that is linked to a code and the code is assigned automatically. Thus, complete and accurate documentation of clinical information must be input into the patient's medical record to ensure an accurate code is generated.

Electronic Processing Problems

Some problems can occur in electronic claims submission. Usually a status report of claims is received electronically from the insurance company consisting of an acknowledgment report and indicating assigned and not assigned claims, crossed over and not crossed over claims, claims accepted with errors, and rejected claims (Fig. 7–10). Data transmission problems arise periodically owing to hardware or software problems.

Bug

An error in a program is called a **bug;** to remove the error is to **debug.** A static telephone line can impair transmitted claims by delaying transmission and can result in rejected claims. Sometimes the computer is malfunctioning, resulting in a period known as **down time.** Peak load problems may occur, delaying access to the insurance carrier's computer. Submit claims early in the morning or after hours to avoid "traffic jams" (logjams).

Virus

A **virus** is a destructive program that attaches and copies itself to other programs in the computer system. Some viruses destroy programs and data after a precise lapse of time. To help prevent a virus from infecting the computer, install software designed to display a warning message when an infected disk has been found. Antiviral utility software programs must be updated frequently. Never bypass the virus scan software when booting up the computer. As an additional prevention measure, never download public domain software files from electronic bulletin boards or other communication systems. Never download e-mail from unfamiliar sources or questionable files from the Internet. Avoid bringing in a disk from outside the office (or classroom) because it may be infected by a virus. If a networked computer station becomes infected with a virus, it can infect all of the other networked stations.

Facsimile Communication Transmission

Insurance claims as well as supporting documentation on a claim may be sent to the carrier via a fax machine if the carrier's guidelines allow this. Even clearer transmission is accomplished if the office computer has fax capabilities. The process is simple, fast, and accurate.

Claims sent by fax used to be considered to be "electronically submitted." However, beginning January 1, 1996, "digital fax" claims are no longer considered as electronic claims. *Digital fax* is a claim that arrives at the insurance carrier via fax but is never printed on paper. The fax is encoded by optical character recognition (OCR) and

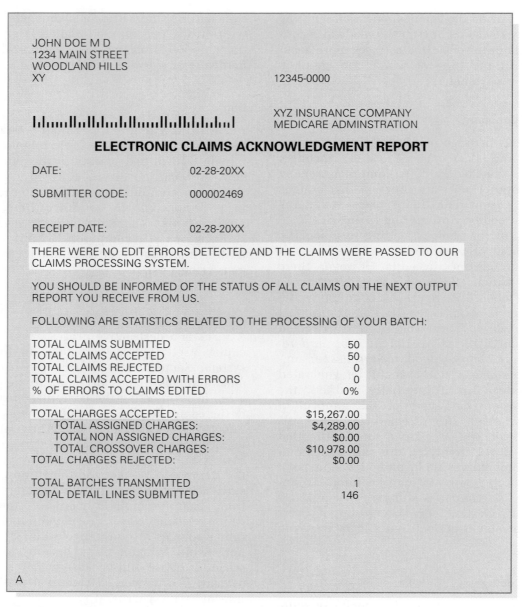

JOHN DOE M D
1234 MAIN STREET
WOODLAND HILLS
XY   12345-0000

|ılı....ıllııllılıııllıllıı...ıllıllılılılıl   XYZ INSURANCE COMPANY
                                                        MEDICARE ADMINSTRATION

ELECTRONIC CLAIMS ACKNOWLEDGMENT REPORT

DATE: 02-28-20XX

SUBMITTER CODE: 000002469

RECEIPT DATE: 02-28-20XX

THERE WERE NO EDIT ERRORS DETECTED AND THE CLAIMS WERE PASSED TO OUR
CLAIMS PROCESSING SYSTEM.

YOU SHOULD BE INFORMED OF THE STATUS OF ALL CLAIMS ON THE NEXT OUTPUT
REPORT YOU RECEIVE FROM US.

FOLLOWING ARE STATISTICS RELATED TO THE PROCESSING OF YOUR BATCH:

TOTAL CLAIMS SUBMITTED	50
TOTAL CLAIMS ACCEPTED	50
TOTAL CLAIMS REJECTED	0
TOTAL CLAIMS ACCEPTED WITH ERRORS	0
% OF ERRORS TO CLAIMS EDITED	0%
TOTAL CHARGES ACCEPTED:	$15,267.00
TOTAL ASSIGNED CHARGES:	$4,289.00
TOTAL NON ASSIGNED CHARGES:	$0.00
TOTAL CROSSOVER CHARGES:	$10,978.00
TOTAL CHARGES REJECTED:	$0.00
TOTAL BATCHES TRANSMITTED	1
TOTAL DETAIL LINES SUBMITTED	146

A

Figure 7–10. A, Weekly status report (Electronic Claims Acknowledgment Report) of electronically transmitted claims.

transmitted into the claims processing system, bypassing manual data entry.

Some carriers require the medical office to complete a short test phase and, after approval, claims may be faxed and processed. A cover sheet may or may not be required, and some carriers may allow multipage claims or claims with attachments.

Although most procedure codes no longer require reports, a few codes still need them. If the claim is transmitted electronically, indicate "Report Sent" or "Report Faxed" in the "Comments" field of the EMC claim format. Then immediately mail or fax the documentation to the insurance carrier. Some insurance carriers set

up a fax line specifically for electronic billers and may require an agreement form completed and signed (Fig. 7–11).

After receiving the claims, some carriers send a faxback report verifying acceptance of the submitted claims (Fig. 7–12). However, the fax machine needs to be left on to ensure receiving the report. Payment after claims have been faxed will be quicker than a paper claim sent via mail.

For legal information in regard to faxing documents and confidentiality issues, see Chapters 1 and 3.

Here are some general fax guidelines for insurance claims.

XYZ INSURANCE COMPANY
MEDICARE ADMINISTRATION

ELECTRONIC CLAIMS BILLER OUTPUT REPORT ** DUE TO SYSTEM CHANGES THIS REPORT SHOWS ONLY ASSIGNED CLAIMS THIS WEEK **

CURRENT DATE: 03/04/20XX

SUBMITTER CODE: 000002469 MAIL

TAPE VOL. SER. NO.:

	ASSIGNED (NOT CROSSOVER)	ASSIGNED CROSSOVER	NOT ASSIGNED	TOTAL
CLAIMS:	105	114	0	219
TOTAL CHARGES	$47,647.00	$14,551.00	$0.00	$62,198.00
COMPLETED CLAIMS:	93	106	0	199
CLAIMS SETTLED BUT NOT PAID	0	0	0	0
CLAIMS PAID	88	51	0	139
CLAIMS APPLIED TO DEDUCTIBLE	5	2	0	7
CLAIMS DENIED	0	0	0	0
CLAIMS TRANSFERRED	0	0	0	0
CLAIMS SENT TO MEDICAID	0	53	0	53
TOTAL AMOUNT PAID	$15,493.57	$5,817.48	$0.00	$21,311.05
PENDING CLAIMS:	12	8	0	20
CLAIMS PENDING MANUAL REVIEW	9	4	0	13
CLAIMS PENDING CWF RESPONSE	0	4	0	4
CLAIMS PENDING DEVELOPMENT	3	0	0	3
TOTAL AMOUNT PENDING	$6,005.00	$1,500.00	$0.00	$7,505.00

INSURANCE BILLING COMPANY
230 MAIN STREET, SUITE J
WOODLAND HILLS XY 12345-0000

B

Figure 7–10 *Continued.* **B,** Weekly report (Electronic Claims Biller Output Report) of assigned claims.

Illustration continued on following page

▶ Purchase light blue-green or white unlined—NOT red—versions of the HCFA-1500 claim form and NOT photocopies containing claim form lines.
▶ Use dark, distinct print.
▶ Select a fixed pitch font, such as sans serif, with a font size of between 10 and 14 points.
▶ Properly align and center claim data.
▶ Do not use stamps or stickers or handwrite information on the claim.
▶ Do not submit claims on continuous-feed paper unless the pages are separated.

Electronic Inquiry or Claims Status Review

Eligibility Verification

Smart Card

Cards similar to plastic credit cards are beginning to make their way into the insurance scene. A *smart card* is a wallet-sized, machine-readable card containing computer chips that allows the card to store a variety of information, such as payer information, coverage limits, eligibility status, and precertification requirements. As an extra service, some hospitals supply cards for patients containing the patient's medical record and history. This service is especially helpful for patients who have complex health histories, such as heart conditions, or for patients with serious allergies and those requiring special medication. These cards can function like a self-contained mini-computer. For information on how smart cards are used as credit and debit cards, refer to Chapter 9.

Swipe Card

A *swipe card* is a plastic, machine-readable wallet-sized card with a magnetic strip containing small memory capacity. This card is used to hold small amounts of information, such as patient's eligibility and coverage.

Both a smart card and a swipe card allow information to be transferred electronically and may be used for eligibility verification.

XYZ INSURANCE COMPANY
MEDICARE ADMINISTRATION

CLAIMS ACCEPTED WITH ERRORS
(PLEASE CORRECT FOR FUTURE TRANSMISSIONS)

REPORT DATE: 02-28-20XX
SUBMITTER CODE: 000005905
SUBMITTER NAME: COLLEGE CLINIC
RECEIPT DATE: 02-28-20XX

PROVIDER CODE: 3664021CC
PROVIDER NAME: COLLEGE CLINIC
PROVIDER ADDR: 4567 BROAD AVENUE
                    WOODLAND HILLS XY 12345-0001

BENE'S NAME HIC NUMBER	DATE OF SVC	SUBMITTER FIELD DATA	LINE NO.	ERROR MESSAGE
KIRKORIAN C	02/19/20XX	KIRKOR0001	04	MODIFIER IS MISSING OR INVALID FOR DIAGNOSTIC TEST BILLED BY A PHYSICIAN
FOLEY D	02/27/20XX	FOLEY00001	01	SERVICE FROM DATE IS INVALID (093099)
			01	PLACE OF SERVICE IS INVALID (31)
				SUM OF THE DETAIL LINE CHARGES DOES NOT EQUAL TOTAL CHARGES FIELD (90.00)

C

Figure 7–10 *Continued.* C, Weekly report showing claims accepted with errors to be corrected before retransmission.

Computer Verification

Some insurance carriers can be accessed directly by computer and can give information electronically about patient eligibility. Simply type demographic and insurance information about a patient into the computer and push a button. The information received on the computer screen is the same as what the insurance company's employee uses to verify and determine the patient's eligibility, insurance coverage, and benefits.

Interactive Transaction

Interactive transaction is back-and-forth communication between two computer systems. One requests information, and the other provides information during what is referred to as on-line real time. It can involve eligibility verification, deductible status, claim inquiries, status of claims, and other insurance claim data. The patient's deductible status can be tracked from all providers the patient has seen during the year.

Other information may also be accessed such as limiting charges, fee schedules, procedure codes, and postoperative days for specific procedures. Many insurance companies, such as Medicare fiscal intermediaries, provide access to information on assigned pending and paid claims. Additional information that may be determined includes whether the individual has other coverage and which insurance carrier should be billed as primary. In addition, some insurance carriers will deposit payments into the physician's bank account automatically via electronic funds transfer (EFT).

Remittance Advice Statements

An on-line transaction about the status of a claim is called an *electronic remittance notice.* This gives information on charges paid or denied and automatically posts the information to patients' accounts without data entry if the software has this feature. The computer tests the claims computer data against various guidelines or parameters

XYZ INSURANCE COMPANY
MEDICARE ADMINISTRATION

REJECTED ELECTRONIC CLAIMS
(PLEASE CORRECT FOR FUTURE TRANSMISSIONS)

REPORT DATE: 02-28-20XX
SUBMITTER CODE: 000005905
SUBMITTER NAME: COLLEGE CLINIC
RECEIPT DATE: 02-28-20XX

PROVIDER CODE: 3664021CC
PROVIDER NAME: COLLEGE CLINIC
PROVIDER ADDR: 4567 BROAD AVENUE
                                    WOODLAND HILLS XY 12345-0001

BENE'S NAME HIC NUMBER	DATE OF SVC	SUBMITTER FIELD DATA	LINE NO.	ERROR MESSAGE
LOREN B 278-26-6487-A	02/02/20XX	LOREN0000	2	DATE SUBMITTED IN THE FIELD BELOW WAS NOT IN EIGHT DIGIT FORMAT. FROM DATE OF SERVICE (9990420)
MARTINEZ A 550-10-0414-A	02/19/20XX	MARTINEZ	2	MEDICARE IS NOT IDENTIFIED AS A PAYOR ON THIS CLAIM
MOSS E 248-06-9870-A	02/22/20XX	MOSS0000	2	MEDICARE IS NOT IDENTIFIED AS A PAYOR ON THIS CLAIM

D

Figure 7–10 *Continued. D,* Weekly report showing rejected electronic claims to be corrected and resubmitted.

known as *screens*. If the services billed on the claim exceed the screens, the claim is either denied, returned to the physician for more information, or sent for review. If a claim is denied or rejected, the ECP receives a printout stating the reason. Simply add or correct the missing, miscoded, or incomplete information and resubmit the claim instead of remaining on a telephone on hold or resubmitting a claim via mail.

The Medicare electronic Remittance Advice (RA), formerly known as Explanation of Medicare Benefits (EOMBs) is based on the American National Standards Institute (ANSI) Accredited Standards Committee X12 (ASCX12) Health Care Claim Payment/Advise (837), or "ANSI 837." A subcommittee, X12N, has developed standards for a variety of electronic transactions between third party payers and health care providers.

The use of ANSI 837 Version 4010 generates an electronic Medicare remittance advice instead of the paper RA. To improve cash flow, ANSI 837 also allows electronic fund transfer (EFT) of Medicare payments to the physician's bank account, which is called *direct deposit.*

RESOURCES ON THE INTERNET

American Association of Professional Coders
   www.aapcnatl.org
   American Health Information Management Association's Clinical Coding Forum
   www.ahima.org
American Medical Association
   www.ama-assn.org
Blue Cross Blue Shield Association
   www.bluecares.com
CHAMPVA
   www.va.gov/hac/champva/champva/html

PROVIDER AGREEMENT

This Agreement is made by and between Blue Shield of California, herein called "Carrier" and_____, herein called "Provider".
(Provider Name/Provider Number)

It is understood that this Agreement is subject to modification, revision, or termination due to changes in the prime contract between the Carrier and the Department of Health and Human Services or changes in federal laws or regulations pertaining to Medicare. This Agreement will be deemed modified, revised, or terminated, to comply with any change in the federal law or regulations or change in the aforesaid prime contract on the effective date of such change.

In consideration of the Carrier agreeing to permit Provider to Fax claims in lieu of written requests for payment, Provider agrees:

(1)   That claims will be submitted to the Carrier in the specific format required by the Carrier, as is described in the Blue Shield of California instructions to billers as they may be amended from time to time.

(2)   That the Secretary of Health and Human Services, his or her designee(s) or agent(s), or the Carrier has the right to audit and confirm for any purposes any information submitted by the Provider and shall be permitted access to claim documentation records and original source documentation, including patient signatures, medical and financial records in the office of the Provider or any other place for that purpose. Any and all incorrect payments discovered, as a result of such audit, will be adjusted according to the applicable provisions of Title XVIII of the Social Security Act, as amended, Federal Regulations, or Supplementary Medical Insurance (Medicare Part B) Guidelines.

(3)   That the Provider accepts responsibility for any and all Medicare claims submitted to the Carrier to research and correct any and all billing or claim discrepancies submitted under this agreement and that the Carrier will be held harmless for any claims, costs, or damages incurred as a result of such discrepancies.

Figure 7–11. Example of a fax agreement between a physician and an insurance carrier.

BLUE SHIELD OF CALIFORNIA FAX SUBMISSION   DATE: 01/19/20XX
450 W EAST AVE, CHICO, CA 95926
916-896-7195

PROVIDER RID (FAX) NUMBER: XXX-XXXX

CONTROL NUM	PATIENT NAME	HIC NUMBER	DATES OF SVC	TOTAL AMOUNT	PHYSICIAN
1094003000000	Herman, Louise	123456789A	1201XX123120	161.10	xxAxxxxxx
1094003000010	Hope, Hortense	951847623B	1201XX121720	91.29	xxAxxxxxx
1094003000020	Kamb, Charles	753869421C1	1229XX122920	128.88	xxAxxxxxx

Figure 7–12. Example of a faxback report verifying receipt of three transmitted insurance claims.

(4)   That all original source documents and source records (e.g., medical/financial records and/or billing statements) will be maintained in such a way that all faxed claims can be readily associated and identified by source documents, including patient's signatures or signatures on behalf of patient. All original source documents will be retained for a period of seventy-two months following the date of submission to the Carrier. Medical records shall be retained pursuant to applicable state law.

(5)   That all claims represent services or supplies actually furnished by the Provider identified on the faxed claims; that all claims have corresponding original source documents as referenced in this Agreement; and that no claims will be submitted to the Carrier which the Provider knows or has reason to know conflict with the Social Security Act, as amended, Federal Regulations, or Medicare guidelines.

(6)   That the submission of a faxed claim to the Carrier is a claim for Medicare payment, and that anyone who misrepresents or falsifies any record or other information essential to that claim or that is required pursuant to this Agreement may, upon conviction, be subject to fine and imprisonment under Federal law. That the required patient signatures or appropriate signatures on behalf of patients are on file in accordance with prescribed procedures. If assignment is accepted, the Provider agrees to accept the reasonable charge, as determined by the Carrier, as the full charge for services on the claim and to bill the patient for deductible, co-insurance, and noncovered services.

Figure 7–11 *Continued*

PROVIDER NAME _____   PROVIDER NUMBER _____

PROVIDER ADDRESS _____   TELEPHONE NUMBER _____

_____   PROVIDER FAX NUMBER _____

BY _____

DATE _____

Federal Register
   http://ssdc.ucsd.edu/gpo/glossary/help.fed.html
Health and Human Services Office of Inspector General
   www.dhhs.gov/progorg/oig
Health Care Financing Administration
   www.hcfa.org
Medicaid
   http://158.73.248.10/medicaid/obs5.htm
Medicare
   www.medicare.gov
TRICARE
   www.tricare-on@csdmail.medcom.amedd.army.mil
TRICARE Support Office
   www.tso.osd.mil

Workers' Compensation related links
   www.dwd.state.wi.us/wc/WCLinks.htm

STUDENT ASSIGNMENT LIST

✔ Study Chapter 7.
✔ Answer the review questions in the *Workbook* to reinforce the theory learned in this chapter and to help prepare you for a future test.
✔ Complete the assignments in the *Workbook* to edit and correct insurance claims that have been transmitted and rejected with errors.
✔ Turn to the Glossary at the end of this textbook for a further understanding of the Key Terms used in this chapter.

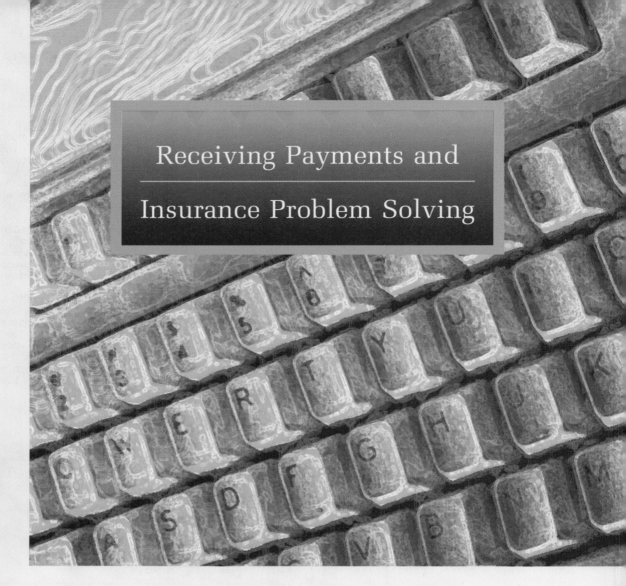

Receiving Payments and
Insurance Problem Solving

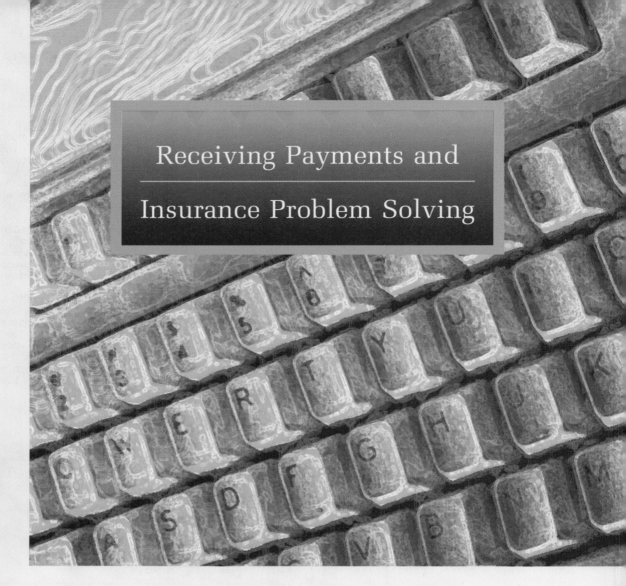

8

CHAPTER OUTLINE

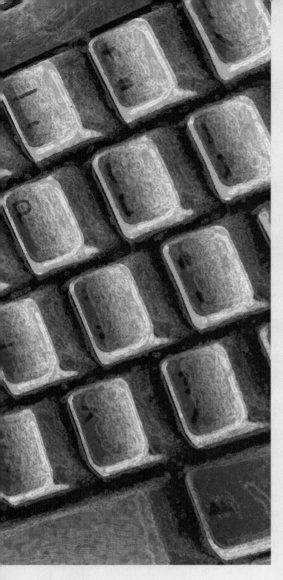

- Define terminology pertinent to problem claims.
- State solutions for problem claims.
- Identify reasons for rebilling a claim.
- List four objectives of state insurance commissioners.
- Mention seven problems to submit to insurance commissioners.
- Describe situations for filing appeals.
- Name three levels of review under the TRICARE appeal process.
- State six levels of review and appeal in the Medicare program.
- Determine which forms to use for the Medicare review and appeal process.

KEY TERMS

appeal

delinquent claim

denied claim

explanation of benefits (EOB)

inquiry

lost claim

overpayment

peer review

rebill

rejected claim

remittance advice (RA)

review

suspense

tracer

two-party check

OBJECTIVES*

After reading this chapter you should be able to:

- Identify three health insurance payment policy provisions.
- Name three claim management techniques.
- Identify purposes of an insurance company history reference file.
- Indicate time limits for receiving payment for manually versus electronically submitted claims.
- Explain reasons for claim inquiries.

*Performance objectives and exercises for hands-on practical experience for this chapter appear in the *Workbook*.

Follow-Up After Claim Submission

For an overall picture of where and when insurance claim problems occur after submission, you must study all aspects of the insurance picture from beginning to end. This chapter begins with the provisions for payment in the insurance contract and explains how this affects the timeliness for payment. Then you learn to interpret the document that accompanies the payment and acquire knowledge on how to manage and organize financial records. To improve cash flow, you are presented with numerous problems that can occur and some solutions to put into action. Finally, you learn about the review and appeal process for various programs.

With the development of proficient skills and experience in following up on claims, you will become a valuable asset to your employer and can bring in revenue that might otherwise become lost to the business.

Claim Policy Provisions

Insured

Each health insurance policy has provisions relating to insurance claims. There is a provision that the claimant has an obligation to notify the insurance company of a loss within a certain period of time or the insurer has the right to deny benefits for the loss.

If the insured is in disagreement with the insurer for settlement of a claim, a suit must begin within 3 years after the claim was submitted. Another provision states that an insured person cannot bring legal action against an insurance company until 60 days after a claim is submitted to the insurance company.

Payment Time Limits

The health insurance policy also has a provision regarding the insurance company's obligation to pay benefits promptly when a claim is submitted. However, time limits vary in this provision from one insurance carrier or program to another. Read and note specific time limits mentioned in insurance contracts. It is reasonable to expect payment as shown in Table 8–1. If a payment problem develops and the insurance company is slow, ignores, denies, or exceeds time limits to pay a claim, then it is prudent to contact the insurance company. In the letter, state the contracted time limit, ask why the claim has not been paid, and retain a copy for the physician's files. If the problem persists and there is no favorable response, then contact the state insurance commissioner and mail a copy of the correspondence to see whether he or she can take action to improve the situation.

Managed care plans usually process claims on a daily basis, but some plans release payments quarterly. There are plans that withhold a percentage that is reserved in a pool and distributed at the end of the fiscal year. In some states, managed care plans do not come under the jurisdiction of the state insurance commissioner but another agency. Contact your state medical society to find out who the responsible entity is. Because managed care plans vary considerably in payment policies and administrative procedures, Chapter 10 details follow up on procedures and problem-solving techniques.

Explanation of Benefits

An **explanation of benefits (EOB)/remittance advice (RA)** is a document issued stating the status of the claim: whether it is paid, suspended (pending), rejected, or denied. If benefits have been as-

TABLE 8–1	Time Limit for Receiving Insurance Reimbursement	
Program	**From Date Claim Was Manually Submitted**	**From Date Claim Was Electronically Submitted**
Private insurance companies	4 to 6 weeks by mail	2 weeks or less
TRICARE standard	8 to 12 weeks by mail	2 weeks or less
Medicare	4 to 6 weeks by mail	$2\frac{1}{2}$ weeks for participating physicians $3\frac{1}{2}$ weeks for nonparticipating physicians
Workers' compensation	4 to 8 weeks by mail	2 weeks or less

signed, the physician receives a copy of the EOB/RA along with a payment check, also called a voucher. If benefits have not been assigned, payment goes to the patient and the physician may have a difficult time in obtaining this payment and EOB.

Components of an EOB

At first glance, the form may seem difficult to understand. Unfortunately, there is no standardization of format for EOBs from one carrier to the next, but information contained in each one is usually the same. If you read one line at a time, you can easily understand the description and calculations for each patient. The EOB breaks down how payment was determined and contains the following information in categories or columns:

1. Insurance company's name and address
2. Provider of services
3. Dates of services
4. Service or procedure code numbers
5. Amounts billed by the providers
6. Reduction or denial codes. Comment codes (reason, remarks, or notes) indicating reasons payments were denied, asking for more information to determine coverage and benefits, or stating amounts of adjustment because of payments by other insurance companies (coordination of benefits)
7. Claim control number
8. Subscriber's and patient's name and policy numbers
9. Analysis of patient's total payment responsibility (amount not covered, copayment amount, deductible, coinsurance, other insurance payment, and patient's total responsibility)
10. Copayment amount(s) due from the patient
11. Deductible amounts subtracted from billed amounts
12. Total amount paid by the insurance carrier

Refer to Figure 8–1, which illustrates an EOB for a private insurance carrier, and identify each component mentioned in the preceding list.

Interpretation of an EOB

Reading and interpreting an EOB has become a complicated procedure for a number of reasons. If several patients' claims are submitted to an insurance carrier, the EOB may reflect the claim status of all of those claims and one check is issued. If the physician has signed a contract agreeing to discount fees with a number of insurance carriers and managed care plans, payment amounts may vary along with the percentage of the fee that is adjusted off of the account. In addition, if more than one physician is in the medical practice and the practice is submitting claims using one group tax identification number, more than one physician's patients claims may appear on a single EOB. Read the explanation of benefits shown in Figure 8–1 line by line to see if you can interpret the meanings under each category or column, referring to the numbered explanations when needed.

Posting an EOB

On receipt of an EOB in the physician's office, pull the claim(s) or refer to the patient's computerized account and check every payment against the applicable insurance contract to find out whether the amount paid is correct. Refer to the step-by-step directions for posting to a patient's ledger in Chapter 2 and see Figure 2–17.

If services are reimbursed and are not clearly described on an EOB, ask the patient to send you a copy of the EOB he or she received from the carrier. The patient's copy often differs from the physician's copy and may have a better explanation of what was or was not paid.

Claims paid with no errors are put into a file designated for closed claims. An EOB for a single payment may be stapled to the claim form and then filed with the closed claims according to the date the payment was posted. EOBs that have many patients' payments listed may be filed in an EOB file. Some offices prefer to make copies of each multiple EOB, highlight the appropriate patient account, and attach the copy to the individual claim or file it in each patient's financial record.

Additional information and examples of documents may be found in the following chapters: Chapter 10 explains a Statement of Remittance for managed care systems, Chapters 7 and 11 explain both a Medicare electronic Remittance Advice (RA) and a hard copy RA, and Chapter 13 shows a Summary Payment Voucher for the TRICARE program.

State Insurance Commissioner

Commission Objectives

The insurance industry is protected by a special exemption from the Federal Trade Commission (FTC) under the McCarran Act (named for the late Senator Pat McCarran of Nevada). Under the exemption, the FTC cannot attack unfair or decep-

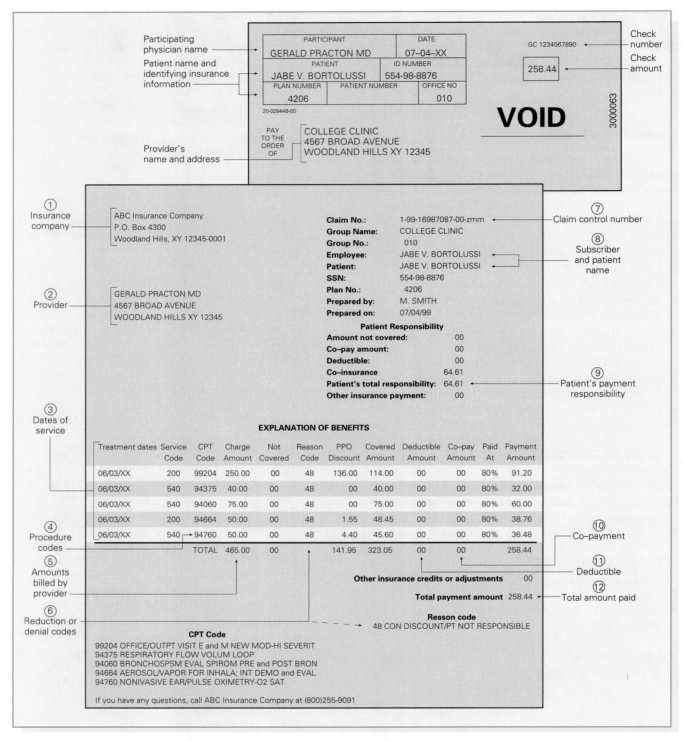

Figure 8–1. Example of an explanation of benefits document with accompanying check that provider received from a private insurance company.

tive practices if there is any state law regarding such practices. The regulations vary widely from state to state, and by no means are all 50 states equally strict. If a complaint arises about an insurance policy, medical claim, or insurance agent or broker, contact the insurance department of the state you reside in or the state where the insurance company's corporate office is headquartered. Sometimes this department is referred to as the insurance commission of the state. State insurance departments usually have various objectives, including the following:

▸ To make certain that the financial strength of insurance companies is not unduly diminished.

▸ To monitor the activities of insurance companies to make sure the interests of the policyholders are protected.

▸ To verify that all contracts are carried out in good faith.

▸ To make sure that all organizations authorized to transact insurance, including agents and brokers, are in compliance with the insurance laws of that state.

▸ To release information on how many complaints have been filed against a specific insurance company in a year.

▸ To help explain correspondence related to insurance company bankruptcies and other financial difficulties.

▸ To assist if a company funds its own insurance plan.

▸ To help to resolve insurance conflicts.

The insurance commissioner can hold a hearing to determine whether licensed insurers, agents, or brokers are in compliance with the insurance laws of the state, but the commissioner does not have the authority vested in a court of law to order an insurance company to make payment on a specific claim.

The insurance commissioner will review the policy to see whether the denial of a claim by the insurance company was based on legal provisions of the insurance contract and will advise the patient if there is an infraction of the law. If there is an infraction, the patient should consult an attorney to determine whether the claim should be submitted to a court of law.

Types of Problems

The types of problems that should be submitted to the insurance commissioner are as follows:

1. Improper denial of a claim or a settlement of an amount less than that indicated by the policy, after proper appeal has been made.
2. Delay in settlement of a claim, after proper appeal has been made.
3. Illegal cancellation or termination of an insurance policy.
4. Misrepresentation by an insurance agent or broker.
5. Misappropriation of premiums paid to an insurance agent or broker.
6. Problems about insurance premium rates.
7. Two companies that cannot determine who is primary.

Commission Inquiries

Requests to the insurance commissioner must be submitted in writing. An example of an insurance complaint form showing pertinent required information when making a request for assistance from the state insurance commissioner is shown in Figure 8–2. In some states, the insurance commissioner requires that the complaint come from the patient even if an assignment of benefits form has been signed. In such cases, prepare a letter or form for the patient to sign and then send it in. Depending on the situation of the case, you may wish to send copies to the state medical association and/or an attorney. Mail may be sent certified, return receipt requested. The request should contain the following information:

1. The inquiring person's (patient) or policyholder's name because the commissioner's responsibility is to the patient (the consumer), not the physician
2. The policyholder's address
3. The policyholder's telephone number
4. The insured's name
5. Name, address, and title of the insurance agent or official of the insurance company
6. A statement of the complaint including, if possible, a copy of the policy, medical bills, unpaid medical insurance claim, canceled checks, and any correspondence from the company pertaining to the claim
7. The patient's signature
8. The name and address of the insurance company, agent, or broker and/or name and address of the finance company if the premium was financed
9. The policy or claim number
10. The date of loss
11. The date the patient signed the complaint form

If an insurance company is continually a slow payer, a method to speed up payments is to include a note to the carrier that reads: "Unless this claim is paid or denied within 30 days, a formal written complaint will be filed with the state insurance commissioner."

Or, a letter may be sent to the insurance commissioner with a copy notation inserted at the end to the insurance company. It might read: "The attached claim has been submitted to the XYZ Insurance Company. It has not been paid or denied. Please accept this letter as a formal written complaint against the XYZ Insurance Company."

Insurance companies are rated according to the number of complaints received about them, so they do not want the insurance commissioner to

INSURANCE COMPLAINT FORM

To: State Insurance Commissioner
Address
City, State, ZIP code

1. ——→ Your Name _____Grace T. O'Neal_____   _____XYZ Insurance Company_____   ←—— **8.**
                                                    (Agent or Company Complaint Against)

2. ——→ Address _____4572 Southport St._____   Policy No. _____531 78 492_____   ←—— **9.**

        _____Woodland Hills, XY 12345_____   Date of Loss: _____10-11-20XX_____   ←—— **10.**

3. ——→ Day Telephone No. _013-421-0733_____   Claim or File No. _____

4. ——→ Insured: _____Grace T. O'Neal_____

        Is this the only complaint you have filed with the insurance commissioner concerning this matter?
        Yes ___X___   No _____

5. ——→ Have you taken up this problem with an official of the company, agent, or broker: If yes, give name,
        address, and title.   Yes ___X___   No _____

        _John Knave, Insurance Agent_____

        _____

        The following is a brief statement of what the agent or company has done, or failed to do:

6. ——→ Insurance payment has been denied by insurance company, as a noncovered service
        but policy covers professional procedure performed.

7. ——→ *Grace T. O'Neal*   _____12-15-20XX_____   ←—— **11.**
        Signature of Patient   Date

        Attach a copy of the insurance policy, related documents, correspondence, etc.

Figure 8–2. Insurance Complaint Form, showing pertinent information required when stating a complaint and making a request for assistance from the state insurance commissioner.

be alerted to any problems. Some states have information available to the public on how many claims have been submitted against a company if you need this information. To contact the state insurance commissioner for assistance or information regarding state laws, refer to Appendix A.

Claim Management Techniques

Insurance Claims Register

In Chapter 2 you learned to establish a follow-up procedure for insurance claims by logging the completed claims onto an insurance claims register (see Chapter 2, Fig. 2–23). A log like this could also be developed and updated with little effort using a spreadsheet software program, which would allow statistical data to be retrieved quicker and easier. Most medical software programs offer practice management reports that can be used to track in-

surance payments. Regardless of what method is used, the ease of tracking quickly and accurately should be the goal in setting up a system.

After logging into a register, place a copy of all insurance claims in a pending file labeled for each month of service so that the unpaid claims can be retrieved for easy follow-up. Or, place a copy of the insurance claim in an alphabetical file by insurance company name. This method permits an inquiry on multiple outstanding claims in one letter to the insurance carrier each month rather than many letters covering individual claims. Place the insurance claims register in a loose-leaf notebook indexed according to the various insurance companies. When referring to a claims register, you can quickly locate delinquent claims by simply looking through the book under the Date Claim Paid column. If that column is blank, check the Date Claim Submitted column and follow up as needed.

When referring to a report generated by a medical software program, claims will be aged according to date submitted, allowing easy reference for timely follow up. You can send a claim tracer when no payment has been received from the insurance company.

When a payment is received, pull all copies of claims that correspond with the payments and attach the EOB/RA. Post payment received and the contracted adjustment to the patient's ledger and to the day sheet or the computerized financial record. File the EOB/RA and deposit the payment check in the physician's bank account. Draw a line through the pertinent information in the claim register, but do not obscure data. When all claims on the page have been paid, draw a diagonal line across the page. Pages may be retained for future reference.

Tickler File

An alternate method used to track pending or resubmitted insurance claims is a *tickler file*. This file is also called a *suspense* or *follow-up file*. A type of tickler file is also used to remind patients of upcoming or missed appointments (see Chapter 2, Fig. 2–21). Tickler files can also be set up in computer systems that prompt the insurance billing specialist to telephone or send inquiries about unpaid insurance claims.

To set up this reminder system, divide active claims by month and file them in chronologic order by date of service. Subdivisions can also be made by patient name or in numerical order by account number. Maintain the active file (unpaid claims) for the calendar year and put inactive resolved claims (older than 1 year) in storage that is accessible.

To incorporate this system into the billing process, start by printing two completed HCFA-1500 claim forms or copy completed claim forms. Send the original to the payer and file the copy in the tickler file by date of service. After receiving the payment check and EOB/RA, pull all claims noted on the EOB/RA from the tickler file. Post the payment to the patient's account (ledger) and day sheet or financial record in the computer system. Compare the charges made on each claim to the payments listed on the EOB/RA. Refer to the insurance contract, if necessary. If a patient has received many services and the claim was submitted on several forms, determine whether services on all forms were processed for payment. After performing this reconciliation process, attach a copy of the EOB/RA to the claim and put it in a paid file. Each claim should be referenced with the date of payment posted to the patient's account.

Delinquent claims remaining in the tickler file and exceeding the contract time limits should be traced. Complete the insurance claim tracer form shown in Figure 8–3 or if a claim has been denied, send a letter to the appeals division of the insurance company as shown in Figure 8–4. Attach a copy of the tracer or letter to the claim and re-file it in the tickler file. It is recommended to send a copy of correspondence marked "For your information," to the patient. Follow-up procedures for claim inquiries are discussed next in detail.

Insurance Company Payment History

Medical practices that employ computer software to handle the financial end of the their business refer to monthly computerized reports to track payment history of insurance companies. This is an easy method to discover which companies are slow pay or pay less on certain services as well as providing excellent reports for tax purposes.

To manually obtain this information, make a file of 3×5-inch index cards or $8\frac{1}{2} \times 11$-inch three-hole punched sheets in a loose-leaf binder listing the insurance companies or managed care plans that send claim payments directly to the physician. Every time a payment is received, pull out the card or the loose-leaf sheet for that company and update the information. The following information is necessary for tracking:

▶ Insurance company name and regional office addresses
▶ Claims filing procedures
▶ Payment policies (provisions) for each plan
▶ Time limits to submit claims
▶ Time limit for receiving payments
▶ Dollar amount for each procedural code number
▶ Names of patients covered and their policy and group numbers

If the patients' names and group policy numbers are listed, this file is helpful when discussing with the patient what the insurance company may be expected to pay for certain services. Remember, group numbers may change annually as benefits increase or decrease so be sure to keep the policy numbers current.

An insurance company payment history system can help avoid potential problems and pinpoint requirements that must be met to help secure additional payment on a reduced or denied claim.

Claim Inquiries

An **inquiry**, sometimes called a **tracer** or follow-up, is made to an insurance company to locate the status of an insurance claim or to inquire about payment determination shown on the EOB/RA. As previously mentioned, claim status can be easily

---

INSURANCE CLAIM TRACER

INSURANCE COMPANY NAME XYZ Insurance Co.　　　　　　　　　DATE 8-5-20XX

ADDRESS: 20 Main Street, Woodland Hills, XY 12345

PATIENT NAME Brendan O'Brien　　　　　　　　INSURED: Brendan O'Brien

POLICY/CERTIFICATE NUMBER 432076122　　　GROUP NAME/NUMBER P40213

EMPLOYER NAME AND ADDRESS: M B Auto

DATE OF INITIAL CLAIM SUBMISSION 6-11-20XX　　　　AMOUNT: $2001.00

An inordinate amount of time has passed since submission of our original claim as described above. We have not received a request for additional information and still await payment of this assigned claim. Please review the attached duplicate and process for payment within seven (7) days.

If there is any difficulty with this claim, please check one of these below and return this letter to our office.

Claim pending because: _____
Payment of claim in process: _____
Payment made on claim:　　Date: _____ To whom: _____
Claim denied: (Reason) _____
Patient notified: Yes _____ No _____
Remarks: _____

Thank you for your assistance in this important matter. Please contact _____ in our office if you have any questions regarding this claim.

　　　　Office of: _____Perry Cardi_____ M.D.

Address: College Clinic, 4567 Broad Avenue
Woodland Hills, XY 12345-0001　　　　TELEPHONE NUMBER: ___013-486-9002___

Figure 8–3. Insurance Claim Tracer. An example of how a form may be set up to follow up on a delinquent claim.

---

accessed by means of computer or teledigital response systems, thus speeding up inquiry time. It may also be accessed with a telephone call or by mail. Here are some reasons for making inquiries.

▸ There was no response to a submitted claim.
▸ Payment was not received within the time limit for the plan or program.
▸ Payment is received but the amount is incorrect.
▸ Payment is received but the amount allowed and the patient's responsibility are not defined.
▸ Payment received was for a patient not seen by the physician. It is possible to receive a payment check made out to a payee's name that is different from the patient's name. Making a call may quickly clarify whom the payment is for.

In addition to nonpayment or reduced payment, there are other reasons for inquiries to an insurance company. These might include the following:

▸ EOB/RA shows that a professional or diagnostic code was changed from what was submitted.

▸ EOB/RA shows that the service was disallowed. The claim should be revised and resubmitted. Check to see whether the procedure codes were correct and that the services listed were described fully enough to justify the maximum, allowable benefits.
▸ Error on the EOB/RA.
▸ Check received was made out to the wrong physician.

If any of these situations occurs, inquire about the claim. If the inquiry is submitted in writing, some programs require special forms completed with a copy of the claim attached. Figure 8–4 is an example of a letter used when asking for a review about a denied claim that was submitted to a managed care plan. If you need to have a claim reviewed after payment has been rendered, send in the letter as shown in Figure 8–5. When calling, document the name of the person spoken to, date and time of call, department or extension of person, and an outline of the conversation.

ABC MEDICAL GROUP, INC.

123 Main Street
Woodland Hills, XY 12345-0239
Tel. 013/487-4900
Fax. No. 013/486-4834

September 12, 20XX

Ms. Jane Hatfield
Appeals Division
XYZ Managed Care Plan
100 South H Street
Anytown, XY 12345-0001

Dear Ms. Hatfield:

Re: Claim number: A0958
         Patient: Carolyn B. Little
         Dates of service: August 2–10, 20XX

Recently I received a denied claim from your office (see enclosure). A review of the contract I have with your managed care plan shows that these services should have been approved and paid according to your fee schedule.

Enclosed is a photocopy of my chart notes for the professional services rendered to the patient on these dates. I have seen Ms. Hatfield five times in the last nine days and each service was medically necessary by the specific complaints expressed by the patient.

On examination, I found the complaints by the patient were valid.

If after review of this claim you still feel reimbursement is not appropriate, please forward this request to the Peer Review Committee for a final determination.

If you need additional information, please telephone, fax, or write my office.

Sincerely,

John Doe, MD

mtf
Enclosures

Figure 8–4. Example of a letter asking for a review about a claim submitted and denied by a managed care plan.

Problem Claims

Types of Problems

There are many types of problem claims (e.g., delinquent, in suspense [pending], lost, rejected, denied, downcoding, partial payment, payment lost in the mail, payment paid to patient, and overpayment). These problems require some type of follow-up action. The claim status may be indicated on an EOB; however, sometimes a claim is submitted and no status is reported. As mentioned earlier, sending a claim inquiry form (tracer) is often the quickest way of determining the status of a claim (see Fig. 8–3).

To prevent repeated claims errors, the office manager should identify the source of the errors within the medical office. Often, a claim may be denied because of an error that occurred when collecting registration information at the front desk or when posting charges to the account. Other errors occur due to wrong procedure or diagnostic codes, incorrect provider numbers, and a variety of situations previously mentioned in prior chapters. A large number of claims are denied for wrong gender and wrong year of birth. The more unusual or foreign sounding a name is, the more denials occur based on gender.

The individual handling the front desk must collect insurance information accurately and update this information routinely (e.g., insurance identifi-

Cosmo Graff, M.D.
4567 Broad Avenue
Woodland Hills, CA 91364
213/486-9002

Committee on Physician's Services

Re: Underpayment	
Identification No.:	M18876782
Patient:	*Peaches Melba*
Type of Service:	Plastic & Rec. Surgery
Date of Service:	1 - 3 - XX
Amount Paid:	$ 75.00
My Fees:	$ 180.00

Dear Sirs:

Herewith a request for a committee review of the above-named case, since I consider the allowance paid very low having in mind the location, the extent, the type and the necessary surgical procedure performed: *The skin graft, only one inch in diameter, included the lateral third of eyebrow and was full thickness to preserve hair follicles.*

Operative report for the surgery has been sent to you with the claim.

Considering these points I hope that you will authorize additional payment in order to bring the total fee to a more reasonable amount.

Sincerely,

Cosmo Graff, M.D.

Cosmo Graff, M.D.

mf

Figure 8–5. Appeal of Fee Reduction. This letter may be sent to an insurance company after payment has been received that the physician believes should be increased. This simple form requires little time and effort. It has helped physicians to win back many fee cuts made by insurers.

cation number, address). The person posting to accounts must be certain to post to the correct account and see that supplemental insurers are billed after the primary insurance carrier has paid. Identified errors should be brought to the attention of the individual(s) responsible to improve accuracy of outgoing claims and avoid future problems.

Delinquent, Pending, or Suspense

The following are specific claim problems and possible solutions.

Problem: The term **delinquent claim** means payment is overdue from a nonpayer. The nonpayer can be an insurance company, a managed care plan, or an intermediary for the Medicaid, Medicare, or TRICARE programs. Sometimes nonpayment is due to a claim in review or in **suspense** (pending) due to an error or the need for additional information. The carrier may be investigating a claim due to pre-existing conditions or possibly because the patient may have a work-related injury.

Solution: To keep on top of delinquent claims, use claim management techniques (i.e., insurance claims register, tickler file, insurance company payment history), so that follow-up can be accomplished in a timely manner. If the office handles a large volume of claims, divide the unpaid claims into four groups, one for each of the three largest insurers and the fourth for all others. Work on one group each week so the work is spread out over the 4 weeks in the month. You can either write a follow-up letter to the insurance company asking for payment and enclose a copy of the original claim form or complete and send in the insurance claim tracer shown in Figure 8–3.

Lost Claims

Problem: When an insurance claim is received by the insurance company, the claim is date stamped usually within 24 hours, assigned a claim number, and logged into the payer system. However, if there is a backlog of claims it may take 7 to 15 days or longer to be logged into the system. If you call to find out the status of the claim during that time, you may be told it has not been received or it may be considered a **lost claim.**

Solution: To resolve the situation, ask if there is a backlog of claims. This will indicate to you that the claim probably has not been logged into the system. Always verify that the patient is insured by the insurance carrier and is covered for the basic benefits claimed. If it is determined to be lost, then submit a copy of the original claim referencing it "copy of the original claim submitted on *(date)*." Before sending it, verify the correct mailing address (e.g., post office box number, zip code). If you have had several problems with the same insurance company, there are several ways to track the claim. Either send it by certified mail with return receipt or fax the claim and ask for a confirmation. Another method available to show proof that a special communication was sent by a deadline is to obtain and complete a Certificate of Mailing form from the post office. The form is initialed and postmarked at the post office and returned to the insurance biller for office file records. Because the post office does not keep a record of the mailing, this certificate costs less than certified mail. If you have verifiable information of a lost claim, call or write to the provider relations department or member services and explain the problem. You may want to check the time limit in the contract with the payer in question. Some contracts have a clause that specifies any claims not paid within a certain number of days (e.g., 30 days) after receipt will be paid at an increased rate or in full. If you believe there is mishandling of claims, gather documentation and

send a letter to the state insurance commission with a letter to the insurance carrier about the action taken.

Rejected Claims

In Chapter 6 you learned some common reasons why claims are rejected or delayed. A **rejected claim** is one submitted that does not follow specific insurance carrier instructions or contains a technical error (Fig. 8–6). Such claims may be disproved or discarded by the system and returned to the biller. Technical errors consist of missing or incorrect information and are found through computer edits, screening processes for benefit provisions, and proofreading. Medicare-mandated prepayment screens are discussed in Chapter 11.

Problem: Claim rejections occur because of the following:

- Transposed numbers
- Missing, invalid, or incorrect procedure codes and modifiers
- Missing or invalid place of service
- Mismatch of place of service to type of service
- Missing referring physician when billing tests
- Missing or invalid provider number when the patient was referred
- Incorrect, invalid, nonspecific, or missing diagnostic code numbers
- Incorrect dates of service
- Incorrect year of service
- Incorrect number of days in the month (e.g., February)
- Code description does not match services rendered
- Duplicate dates of service
- Duplicate charges

Solution: If a claim is rejected and returned, add the missing or incomplete information and resubmit a corrected claim for regular claims processing. Do not send a corrected claim for review or appeal.

Problem: Claim submitted for several services and one service is rejected for incomplete information and other services are paid.

Solution: Complete a new HCFA-1500 claim form including all information and resubmit for the rejected services only. Note in Block 19 that it is a resubmission.

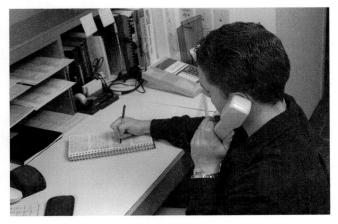

Figure 8–6. Insurance billing specialist troubleshooting a rejected claim.

Problem: Insurance carrier requests further information or information about another carrier.

Solution: Verify primary and secondary insurance information with the patient and call or mail the information to the insurance company. Identify the subscriber, subscriber number, and date of service on all correspondence.

Problem: Resubmitted claim is returned a second time.

Solution: Review the EOB/RA statement to see if there is a denial code or narrative explanation. Examine the claim for missing, incomplete, or incorrect information and, if found, correct it. Evaluate the claim to determine if it is a candidate for the appeal process. Determine if a specific appeal form must be submitted. Submit chart notes, a detailed summary, or a copy of the operative or pathology report, as applicable, to clearly identify the procedure or service. Enclose a cover letter with the resubmitted data.

Denied Claims

A **denied claim** is one that may be denied due to medical coverage policy issues or program issues. Insurance companies save money when a claim is denied, and only a small percentage of individuals pursue appeals. State laws require insurance companies to notify the insured of a denial and state why the claim was denied. It is possible that payment can be received even after a claim has been denied in whole or in part.

When a claim is denied and the patient has not been contacted by the insurance company, notify the patient by telephone or mail as soon as possible to keep him or her informed. Always retain the correspondence from the insurance company so it can be quickly retrieved in the event a patient inquires and has additional questions. The recourse to a denied claim is to appeal and request a review in writing. The appeals process varies between insurance carriers. A Medicare claim may be appealed by requesting a review in writing, and federal laws require that an explanation be given for each denied service. In Medicare Part B hearing cases, carriers have been instructed to pay an appealed claim if the cost of the hearing process is more than the amount of the claim.

Some reasons why claims are not paid because of denial include the following:

- Payable only for selected diagnoses
- Frequency limitations or restrictions per benefit period
- Procedure performed by ineligible specialty provider (e.g., podiatrist would not be paid for neurosurgery)
- Bundled with other services
- Payable only in certain locations (e.g., outpatient only)
- Prior approval needed and not obtained
- Diagnosis did not justify the service or procedure rendered

To resolve the problem, you cannot simply change the information and resubmit. Some additional examples with suggested solutions are as follows:

Problem: Service was not a policy or program benefit (e.g., routine physical examination, routine tests, routine foot care, routine dental care, cosmetic surgery, custodial care, eye or hearing examinations for glasses or hearing aids, and some immunizations). Plastic surgery may be considered a general exclusion in many insurance policies.

Solution: Send the patient a statement with a notation of the response from the insurance company. Better yet, always verify coverage for routine physical examinations or tests and services that are in question as to whether they will be paid by the insurance policy.

Problem: Treatment given for a preexisting condition (currently some policies do not include this exclusion).

Solution: When a patient is referred, ask the referring physician to forward information on all preexisting conditions that may be relevant to the surgery or procedure to be performed. Request verification of insurance coverage from the insurer for the surgery or procedure with regard to preexisting conditions. Request authorization for the surgical procedure and/or diagnostic tests. If authorization is denied, have the physician discuss other treatment/payment options with the patient (e.g., rendering minimum level of interim care until the preexistence period, usually 6 months, has expired). If the physician believes that the patient's condition is not preexisting, send an appeal to the insurance company. Otherwise, bill the patient, noting the insurance company's response on the statement.

Problem: Insurance coverage canceled before service.

Solution: Send the patient a statement with notation of the insurance determination on the bill.

Problem: Insurance coverage lapsed beyond renewal date for service rendered.

Solution: Send the patient a statement with notation of the response from the insurance company on the bill.

Problem: Service provided before coverage was in effect.

Solution: Send the patient a statement with notation of the response from the insurance company on the bill.

Problem: Service provided when the patient was no longer a member of the insurance plan.

Solution: Send the patient a statement with notation of the response from the insurance company on the bill.

Problem: Insurance company indicates provided service was not medically necessary.

Solution: Determine under what circumstances the insurance carrier considers the service medically necessary. The problem may be that the diagnostic code does not properly support the procedural codes being reported. It is vital that the physician's documentation be specific enough to support the necessity of the services provided. If the physician believes the patient's condition supported the medical necessity for the service, send an appeal for review to the insurance company, explaining in detail the reasons why. Or have the insurance physician write to the patient and advise what might have been a better course of treatment. Keep a list of codes that have been denied for medical necessity and what further determinations were made in the insurance company payment history. Check the insurance contract to determine if the patient may be billed. Consider asking patients to sign a "Waiver of Liability" form before treatment—if payment is in question of being denied, then bill the patient.

Problem: Service was for an injury that is being considered as compensable under workers' compensation.

Solution: Locate the carrier for the industrial injury, request permission to treat, and send the carrier a report of the case with a bill. Notify the patient's health insurance carrier monthly about the status of the case.

Problem: Service was not precertified for a surgery, hospitalization, or diagnostic procedure.

Solution: Ask the patient to bring in his or her insurance policy for review to determine whether precertification was required for the service or whether any sanctions are imposed. If there were problems or difficulties about the case leading to why precertification was not obtained, write a letter of appeal noting the history.

Problem: Patient did not pay premium.

Solution: Verify insurance coverage before treatment begins, especially for procedures and surgery. Change patient's account to "cash" if insurance is not in force.

Problem: Service or procedure is experimental.

Solution: Verify if procedure is approved by the insurance company before procedure is done.

Problem: Deductible was not met.

Solution: Ask patient when he or she arrives at the office about status of deductible. If deductible has not been met, collect from patient. If several services are performed during the same time period and the patient paid the deductible at another office but it has not been recorded by the insurance company, you might consider holding the claim.

Problem: Services are considered cosmetic.

Solution: Appeal claim if the problem was treated because of medical condition, not for cosmetic reasons.

Denied Claims Summary

Remember, prevention measures to avoid denied claims are as follows:

1. Include progress notes and orders for tests for extended hospital services.
2. Submit a letter from the prescribing physician documenting necessity when ambulance transportation is used.
3. Clarify the type of service (e.g., primary surgical services versus assist-at-surgery services).
4. Use modifiers to further describe and identify the exact service rendered.
5. Keep abreast of the latest policies for the Medicare, Medicaid, and TRICARE programs by reading local newsletters.
6. Obtain current provider manuals for Medicaid, Medicare, and TRICARE so these are available for quick reference. When bulletins or pages are

received from these programs during the year, keep the manuals up to date by inserting the current material.

Downcoding

Lowered reimbursement is the result of downcoding. As mentioned in Chapter 5, downcoding occurs for the following reasons:

Problem: Coding system used on a claim does not match the coding system used by the insurance carrier receiving the claim. Computer software is designed to convert the code submitted to the nearest code in use. However, payment may be less.

Solution: Monitor reimbursements and monitor downcodes to discover which codes are affected. Then, telephone the insurance carrier and ask which code system is in use, obtain the proper book, and use the appropriate system.

Problem: Insufficient diagnostic information on a claim.

Solution: Be sure each procedure listed on the claim form is linked to an appropriate diagnosis. Refer to the medical record, if necessary.

Problem: Unspecified diagnoses are listed on the claim form. Routine use of too many nonspecific diagnostic codes (ICD-9-CM codes that have number "9" as the fourth or fifth digit) result in denials or downcoding, especially if extensive or specific surgery is involved.

Solution: Make sure the physician is dictating specific diagnoses and not circling nonspecific diagnoses on an encounter form. Always code to the highest level of specificity. Refer to the patient's medical record when necessary.

Payment Paid to Patient

Problem: Sometimes, an insurance payment may be sent in error to the patient after an assignment of benefits has been signed and sent in with the insurance claim. In some cases, a clause may be in the insurance policy that payment may only be made to the insured.

Solution: Call the insurance company to verify whether the payment was made and to whom. If the account is substantially overdue, ask for a copy of the endorsed check or EOB/RA statement that indicates where payment was sent. If the carrier refuses, ask for help from the supervisor of the provider or customer relations department. There are two different courses of action to take after this has been verified.

1. Call the patient explaining that the insurance company sent payment to him or her in error and ask when you can expect full payment. Document the commitment in the patient's financial record. If not able to reach the patient by telephone, send a letter by certified mail to the patient. If the patient still refuses to pay, inform the patient that the provider is forced to write off the debt, that the money is considered taxable income to the patient, and that you will report the undeclared income the patient received to the Internal Revenue Service on the 1099 form. This may assist in getting the debt paid. If not, discuss with the physician whether he or she wishes to discharge the patient from the practice. It is also advisable to send the information to the credit bureau.

2. Send a letter to the insurance company including a copy of the claim with EOB/RA indicating payment was made to the patient and a copy of the assignment of benefits. Demand payment from the insurance company stating the need to honor the assignment. The insurance company must recover the payment from the patient. If after pursuing reimbursement from the insurance company you run into a dead end, then file a complaint with the state insurance commissioner. After receiving the physician's complaint, the commissioner will write to the insurance company and request a review of the claim. If the insurance company admits that there is an assignment of benefits and that it inadvertently paid the patient, the insurance company must pay the physician within 2 to 3 weeks and honor the assignment even before it recovers its money from the patient. The insurance company will then file for payment from the patient.

Two-Party Check

Problem: Patient cashes a two-party check. A **two-party check** is a check that is made out to the physician and the patient. Although not legal, the patient may be successful in cashing it without the endorsement of the physician.

Solution: Do not allow time to pass. Immediately advise the insurance company of the fraud so it may recover the money from whomever accepted the check without proper endorsement.

Problem: A check is received made out to both the physician and the hospital and only part of the sum is the physician's payment.

Solution: Call the insurance company and ask how much should be retained by the physician. Ask whose tax identification number will be used on the 1099 form for reporting income to the Internal Revenue Service. The hospital's income should not be reflected on the physician's 1099 form. To avoid another problem like this, inquire why the insurance company paid in this manner. Sometimes a participating agreement may exist that the physician did not know about.

Overpayment

An **overpayment** is a sum of money paid by the insurance carrier or patient to the provider of service that is more than the bill or more than the allowed amount. Overpayments may be discovered immediately, called to your attention by the patient or insurance carrier, or not discovered for several months or years. First, determine if an overpayment exists by reviewing the available financial documents on the case in question. Then decide how to handle the overpayment.

It is wise to develop an overpayment policy and procedure for each type of insurer, program, or managed care plan and for every type of overpayment situation that may occur.

Problem: Overpayment. Scenarios that may occur are as follows:

- Receiving more than your fee from an insurance carrier
- Receiving more than the contract rate from a managed care plan
- Receiving payments that should have been paid to the patient
- Receiving duplicate payments from two or more insurance carriers or from the patient and one or more third party payers
- Receiving payment made for someone who is not the provider's patient

Solution: In any type of overpayment situation, always cash the third party payer's check and make out a provider's refund check. In case of an audit, this establishes documentation showing the problem has been resolved.

Refund checks are usually written once a month by the bookkeeper. Make sure this office policy is clearly stated and adhered to in all cases. If the

patient pays and a third party pays and the overpayment must be refunded to the patient, always write a check—never refund in cash. If the patient pays by credit card, wait until the charges have cleared to draft a check.

If the patient cannot be located to return the money, send a check by registered mail to the patient's last known address. When it comes back marked "undeliverable," retain this as legal proof that you did your best in trying to return the overpayment. The money should be listed as taxable income and put in the bank.

Commercial Carriers

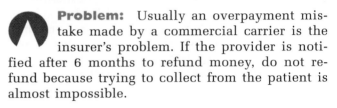 **Problem:** Usually an overpayment mistake made by a commercial carrier is the insurer's problem. If the provider is notified after 6 months to refund money, do not refund because trying to collect from the patient is almost impossible.

Solution: First call and notify the patient; then proceed cautiously before refunding money. If two or more insurance carriers send duplicate payments, write a letter to each explaining the situation and let them straighten it out. Then, send a refund to the correct insurance carrier after receiving a letter explaining who to refund the money to.

Managed Care Plan

 Problem: Discovering an overpayment from a managed care plan.

Solution: Develop a policy regarding overpayments and have it documented in the provider's contract. Allow the plan 60 days to audit its payments.

Medicare

 Problem: If you discover that an overpayment has been made from Medicare, it is important to refund the money immediately. If it is not paid back, future claims may be held up and past claims may be reviewed.

Solution: Check the billing and medical records to see whether the provider made any mistakes. If you feel an error has been made by the insurance carrier, send a letter with documentation to appeal and prove the provider's case.

Rebilling

If a claim has not been paid, *do not* **rebill** the insurance carrier by sending in a monthly claim. Such claims will be considered as duplicate claims, and the insurance company may audit the physician's practice for trying to collect duplicate payment. Instead, follow up on the claim as indicated in the previous section. If it is discovered that an error has been made in billing a case, send in a *corrected* claim.

Generally, if a bill has not been paid, the physician rebills the patient every 30 days. It is important to bill patients on a monthly basis, even when insurance payment is expected. Clearly identify on the statement that the insurance biller has submitted an insurance claim as well as what action is expected from the patient. If collection becomes a problem, action can be referenced to the date of service if the patient has been billed consistently. See Chapter 9 for how to word notations on statements and the collection process.

Review and Appeal Process

An **appeal** is a request for payment by asking for a review of an insurance claim that has been inadequately or incorrectly paid or denied by an insurance company. Usually there is a time limit for appealing a claim. Always check every private insurance carrier, Medicare, TRICARE, and workers' compensation payment against the appropriate fee schedule or customary profile to determine whether the benefits were allowed correctly. To find out this information, read the EOB/RA document or refer to provider manuals for the various programs.

You should base appealing a claim not only on billing guidelines but also on state and federal insurance laws and regulations. A bimonthly newsletter that links to regulatory information online is available at www.integsoft.com/appeals/tal. A software program designed to help providers generate effective insurance appeal letters is available from Appeal Solutions. To locate this company, see Appendix B, Collections.

There may be a discrepancy in the way the physician or physician's staff and insurance company interpret a coding guideline. The decision to appeal a claim should be based on several factors. The provider should determine that there is sufficient information to back up his or her claim, and the amount of money in question should be sufficient in the physician's opinion. Ultimately, the decision to appeal often rests in the physician's hands, not the insurance billing specialist. It takes a team

effort to successfully appeal a claim. To proceed, you may want to make a telephone call to the insurance company. It may save time and money, and you may reach an expert who is able to solve the problem. Here are some basic guidelines to follow:

▶ Assemble all documents needed (e.g., patient's medical record, copy of the insurance claim form, and EOB/RA).
▶ Remain courteous at all times.
▶ Obtain the name and extension number of the insurance claims representative or adjuster and keep this with your telephone records. After developing rapport, you may wish to call on him or her in the future for help. Ask for any toll-free numbers that the company may have, and keep these for future reference.
▶ Listen carefully. Jot down the date and take notes of how to solve the problem. This may be of help if another problem of the same type occurs again.

An appeal would be filed in the following circumstances:

▶ Payment is denied and the reason for denial is not known.
▶ Payment is received but the amount is incorrect. Perhaps there was an excessive reduction in the allowed payment.
▶ Physician disagrees with the decision by the insurance carrier about a preexisting condition.
▶ Unusual circumstances warranted medical treatments rendered that are not reflected in payment.
▶ Precertification was not obtained within contract provisions due to extenuating circumstances, and the claim was denied.
▶ Inadequate payment was received for a complicated procedure.
▶ "Not medically necessary" is stated as the reason for denial and the physician disagrees.

PROCEDURE: Filing an Official Appeal

The following are basic steps to file an official appeal:

1. Send a letter explaining the reason why the provider does not agree with the claim denial listed on the EOB/RA.
2. Abstract excerpts from the coding resource book and attach a photocopy of the article or pertinent information showing the name of the article, coding resource, and date of publication.
3. Send copies of similar cases with increased reimbursement from the same insurance company,

if available from the insurance company payment history file.

4. Call the insurance company and speak to the individual responsible for appeals, explaining what you are trying to accomplish with the resubmission. Direct the correspondence to this person.

5. Retain copies of all data sent for the physician's files.

If you win the appeal but must submit copies of the same documents each time this issue arises, ask the insurance carrier how future claims with the same issue may be handled.

Appeals must be in writing, but some programs require completion of special forms. Always send a copy of the original claim, EOB/RA, and any other documents to justify the appeal.

Remember, it is always important to keep track of the status after inquiry or appeal until payment for the case is resolved. Use the insurance claims register as shown in Chapter 2 or a separate active file labeled "Appeals Pending."

If an appeal is not successful, the physician may want to proceed to the next step, which is a peer review. A **peer review** is a review done by a group of unbiased practicing physicians to judge the effectiveness and efficiency of professional care rendered. This group determines the medical necessity and subsequent payment for the case in question. Some insurance companies send a claim for peer review routinely for certain procedures that have been done for certain diagnoses.

Additional information on tracing delinquent claims, appealing or reviewing a claim, or submitting a claim for a deceased patient can be found in the chapters on Medicaid, Medicare, TRICARE, and workers' compensation.

Medicare Review and Appeal Process

 After payment or denial, a physician or beneficiary has the right to appeal a claim. The Medicare program has six levels of appeal and special guidelines to follow. The steps (levels) are

1. Inquiry
2. Review
3. Fair hearing
4. Administrative law judge (ALJ) hearing
5. Appeals council review
6. Federal district court hearing

Table 8–2 illustrates the Medicare Part B appeals process.

Inquiry (Level 1)

If the claim was denied because of a simple error made by the insurance biller, such as omission of the National Provider Identifier (NPI) of the referring physician or failure to code a diagnosis, then resubmit a corrected claim. Include only the denied services and indicate in Block 19 "resubmission, corrected claim." In the event the insurance carrier made an error—for example, a pro-

TABLE 8–2	Medicare Part B Appeals Process

Step (Level)	Time Limit for Request	Amount in Controversy	Jurisdiction	Form
1. Inquiry		None	Carrier	HCFA 1500 (possible attachment)
2. Review	6 months from date of initial determination	None	Carrier	HCFA 1964
3. Fair Hearing	6 months from date of review determination	$100	Fair Hearing Officer, Medicare Fiscal Agent	HCFA 1965
4. Administrative Law Judge Hearing	60 days from receipt or review decision	>$500	Carrier Social Security Bureau of Hearings and Appeals	HCFA 1965
5. Appeals Council Review	60 days from receipt of hearing decision/dismissal	$500	Bureau of Hearings and Appeals	HA 520
6. Federal District Court Review	60 days from receipt of Appeals Council decision	$1000	U.S. District Attorney Court	

cedure code was different from what was submitted or the date of service was entered incorrectly from the paper claim into the carrier's computer—then resubmit the claim with an attachment explaining the error. If response to the resubmission indicates that the claim has been "processed" previously, then go to the next appeal level.

Review (Level 2)

When a claim is assigned, the physician may ask for a **review.** The request must be within 6 months from the date of the original determination shown on the RA. Figure 8–7 shows Form HCFA-1964, which may be used in requesting a review of Medicare Part B claims. However, some carriers have developed their own request forms. Contact the carrier to find out the form required. Review the RA for the denial code or narrative stating why the claim has been denied. Check the claim for accuracy of diagnostic, procedural, or HCPCS codes or missing modifiers as well as any other item that might be incorrect or missing.

If you are developing a form on the physician's letterhead, it must include the following information:

1. Current date
2. Medicare provider number
3. RA number or claim number
4. Date of RA
5. Patient's name
6. Patient's health insurance claim number (HICN)
7. Date of service
8. Place of service
9. Procedure code(s)
10. Amount billed
11. Amount approved
12. Amount paid
13. Denial reason (action code description from the RA)
14. Brief statement of why service should be reviewed

With the review request, attach the following:

15. Copy of the original insurance claim
16. Copy of the RA showing the denial
17. Photocopy of other documents, such as operative or pathology report or detailed summary about the procedure with appropriate words highlighted to help the reviewer
18. Cover letter explaining the procedure, indicating justification for the services and why the provider should receive more reimbursement. Include the physician's NPI in the letter (Fig. 8–8).

Mail the documents by certified mail with return receipt requested, and retain copies of all documents sent to the carrier in the provider's pending file.

If a claim is unassigned, the beneficiary (patient) can pursue the review or appoint the physician as an authorized representative. The patient completes forms HCFA-1964 and SSA-1696 (Fig. 8–9; see also Fig. 8–7) and obtains the physician's acceptance signature. Decisions on unassigned claims are sent to the patient.

Send all requests to the review department. Most insurance carriers have an address or post office box for review requests that is different from initial claim submissions, so be sure to send it to a correct current address. A review is usually completed by the insurance carrier within 30 to 45 days. Make a follow-up inquiry if no response is received in that time frame.

If certain procedures are consistently denied, ask the carrier what information is necessary to process the claim. If the provider is not satisfied with the results of the review, move to the next level and request a fair hearing.

Fair Hearing (Level 3)

If the physician feels the review is unfair and wishes to request a hearing, obtain and complete the HCFA-1965 form Request for Hearing Part B Medicare Claim (Fig. 8–10) from either the Medicare carrier or local Social Security Administration office. Two conditions must be met to proceed to this level:

1. A fair hearing must be requested within 6 months from the date of the Medicare review determination letter.
2. The amount in controversy (AIC) must be at least $100. This amount may represent a single claim or a combination of several smaller claims involving common billing issues.

The request for an appeal must include the patient's name, Medicare health insurance card number, all carrier control numbers involved, date of review determination, NPI, reason for requesting the hearing, and type of hearing (in-person, by telephone, or on-the-record). Address the request to the fair hearing officer in care of the Medicare fiscal agent. The mailing address of the hearing is usually different from the review request address. The provider may request that a physician of his or her specialty review the case to offer advice or opinion to the fair hearing officer.

An acknowledgment should be received within 10 days, and the provider may either attend the

DEPARTMENT OF HEALTH AND HUMAN SERVICES
HEALTH CARE FINANCING ADMINISTRATION

Form Approved
OMB No. 0938-0033

REQUEST FOR REVIEW OF PART B MEDICARE CLAIM
Medical Insurance Benefits–Social Security Act

NOTICE—Anyone who misrepresents or falsifies essential information requested by this form may upon conviction be subject to fine and imprisonment under Federal Law.

1 Carrier's Name and Address

Medicare Blue Cross and
Blue Shield of Texas, Inc.
P.O. Box 660031
Dallas, TX 75266-0031

2 Name of Patient

Jose F. Perez

3 Health Insurance Claim Number

032-07-6619

4 I do not agree with the determination you made on my claim as described on my Explanation of Medicare
Benefits dated: 3-2-20XX

5 MY REASONS ARE: (Attach a copy of the Explanation of Medicare Benefits, or describe the service, date of service, and physician's name—NOTE.—If the date on the Notice of Benefits mentioned in item 3 is more than six months ago, include your reason for not making this request earlier.)

01-21-20XX Electrocardiographic monitoring; 24 hours (93224)

Physician: Gerald Practon, MD

6 Describe Illness or Injury: Heart palpitations, tachycardia, & light headedness (near syncopal episode). Although patient

had a previous Holter monitor within the 6 mo time limitation, it did not provide any clinical evidence of disease.

Patient underwent recent monitoring after experiencing additional symptoms that were more severe than the initial

symptoms.

7 [X] I have additional evidence to submit. (Attach such evidence to this form.)

[ ] I do not have additional evidence.

See attached rhythm
strip & chart note for
documentation.

COMPLETE ALL OF THE INFORMATION REQUESTED. SIGN AND RETURN THE FIRST COPY AND ANY ATTACHMENTS TO THE CARRIER NAMED ABOVE. IF YOU NEED HELP, TAKE THIS AND YOUR NOTICE FROM THE CARRIER TO A SOCIAL SECURITY OFFICE, OR TO THE CARRIER. KEEP THE DUPLICATE COPY OF THIS FORM FOR YOUR RECORDS.

8   SIGNATURE OF **EITHER** THE CLAIMENT **OR** HIS REPRESENTATIVE

Representative	Claimant
Gerald Practon, MD	
Address 4567 Broad Avenue	Address
City, State, and ZIP Code Woodland Hills, XY 12345	City, State, and ZIP Code
Telephone Number 013-486-9002	Date 6-5-20XX	Telephone Number	Date

FORM HCFA-1664 (8-85)   DESTROY PRIOR EDITIONS   (over)

CARRIER'S COPY

Figure 8–7. Request for Review of Part B Medicare Claim Form HCFA-1964. This form can be used by the Medicare beneficiary and/or physician when requesting a review of a submitted claim.

hearing or waive the right to appear. When choosing the latter, inform the fair hearing officer in writing and enclose any additional documents that should be considered at the hearing. The fair hearing officer will send a written decision based on Medicare regulations, which may be full reversal of the initial claim ruling; adjustment of the review level decision giving more reimbursement; or complete denial. If not satisfied, proceed to the next level.

PHYSICIAN'S LETTERHEAD

January 2, 20XX

Committee on Physician's Services
Medicare
Street address of fiscal intermediary
City, State, ZIP Code

Dear Madam or Sir:

Re: Underpayment

Identification No.:	1910-2192283-101
Patient:	Mrs. Sarah C. Nile
Type of Service:	Exploratory laparotomy
Date of Service:	December 1, 20XX
Amount Paid:	$000.00
My Fees:	$0000.00

Herewith a request for a committee review of the above-named case, since I consider the allowance paid very low having in mind the patient's condition prior to surgery, the location, the extent, the type, and the necessary surgical procedure performed.

Enclosed are photocopies of the history and physical showing the grave status of the patient prior to surgery, operative report, pathology report, and discharge summary. The Medicare Remittance Advice and the Medicare HCFA-1500 claim originally submitted are also enclosed.

Considering these points, I hope that you will authorize additional payment in order to bring the total fee to a more reasonable amount.

Sincerely,

Hugh R. Aged, MD
NPI# 7354210907

mf

Enclosures (6)

Figure 8–8. Example of a cover letter for a Medicare review request to be sent with photocopies of documents pertinent to a claim.

Administrative Law Judge Hearing (Level 4)

A request for a hearing before an administrative law judge (ALJ) may be made if the amount still in question is $500 or more (usually in combined claims). The request must be made within 60 days of receiving the fair hearing officer's decision. It may take 18 months to receive an ALJ assignment. Proof of the claim represents an unusual case and warrants special consideration may lead to a successful conclusion. However, the decision might be reversed, might allow partial adjustment of the carrier's payment, or might deny payment. If the final judgment is not satisfactory, then proceed to the next level.

Appeals Council Review (Level 5)

The Appeals Council is part of the Office of Hearings and Appeals of the Social Security Administration. A request must be made within 60 days of the ALJ decision. Or, if there is a question that the final judgment was not made in accordance with the law, the council by its own election may review the ALJ decision. If the council denies a review, the provider may file a civil action for a federal district court hearing.

Federal District Court Hearing (Level 6)

At this highest level, the amount in controversy must be $1000 or more, and an attorney must be hired to represent the provider and manage the case. The case may be filed where the physician's business is located. Contact the local medical society for suggestions of names of attorneys experienced at this level of the appeals process.

HCFA Regional Offices
One final suggestion, and this can be done with steps for a hearing or a review, is to write or telephone the medical director at one of the 10 HCFA regional offices. Sometimes a regional officer will intercede or take steps to correct problems or inequities. HCFA regional office addresses with the states they serve are listed in the following box.

Medigap
Insurance companies that sell Medigap policies must be certified before being allowed to sell in

---

HCFA Regional Offices

Region I—Boston
Connecticut, Maine, Massachusetts, New Hampshire, Rhode Island, and Vermont

Associate Regional Administrator,
 HCFA Program Operations
John F. Kennedy Federal Building, Room 2325
Government Center
Boston, Massachusetts 02203-0003

Region II—New York
New Jersey, New York, Puerto Rico, and Virgin Islands

Associate Regional Administrator,
 HCFA Program Operations
Jacob K. Javits Federal Building, Room 3811
26 Federal Plaza
New York, New York 10278-0063

Region III—Philadelphia
Delaware, District of Columbia, Maryland, Pennsylvania, Virginia, and West Virginia

Associated Regional Administrator,
 HCFA Medicare
3535 Market Street
P.O. Box 7760
Philadelphia, Pennsylvania 19101

Region IV—Atlanta
Alabama, Florida, Georgia, Kentucky, Mississippi, North Carolina, South Carolina, and Tennessee

Associate Regional Administrator,
 HCFA Program Operations
Atlanta Federal Center
61 Forsythe Street, SW
Atlanta, Georgia 30303-8909

Region V—Chicago
Illinois, Indiana, Michigan, Minnesota, Ohio, and Wisconsin

HCFA Program Operations
105 West Adams Street
15th Floor
Chicago, Illinois 60603-6201

Region VI—Dallas
Arkansas, Louisiana, New Mexico, Oklahoma, and Texas

Associate Regional Administrator,
 HCFA Program Operations
1301 Young Street, 8th floor
Dallas, Texas 75202

Region VII—Kansas City
Iowa, Kansas, Missouri, and Nebraska

Associate Regional Administrator,
 HCFA Program Operations
601 East 12th Street, Room 235
Kansas City, Missouri 64106-2808

Region VIII—Denver
Colorado, Montana, North Dakota, South Dakota, Utah, and Wyoming

Associate Regional Administrator,
 HCFA Medicare
1961 Stout Street, Room 522
Denver, Colorado 80294-3538

Region IX—San Francisco
Arizona, California, Nevada, Guam, Hawaii, and American Samoa

Associate Regional Administrator,
 HFCA Program Operations
Federal Office Building
75 Hawthorne Street, 4th Floor
San Francisco, California 94105-3905

Region X—Seattle
Alaska, Idaho, Oregon, and Washington

HCFA Program Operations
2201 Sixth Avenue
Mail Stop RX-42
Seattle, Washington 98121-2500

DEPARTMENT OF
HEALTH AND HUMAN SERVICES
SOCIAL SECURITY ADMINISTRATION

NAME (Claimant) (Print of Type)	SOCIAL SECURITY NUMBER
Carol T. Usner	432-86-9821
WAGE EARNER (if different)	SOCIAL SECURITY NUMBER

Section I APPOINTMENT OF REPRESENTATIVE

I appoint this individual Gene Ulibarri, MD 4567 Broad Ave., Woodland Hills, XY 12345
_____
(Name and Address)

to act as my representative in connection with my claim or asserted right under:

☐ Title II   ☐ Title XVI   ☐ Title IV FMSHA   ☒ Title XVIII
(RSDI)   (SSI)   (Black Lung)   (Medicare Coverage)

I authorize this individual to make or give any request or notice; to present or elicit evidence; to obtain information; and to receive any notice in connection with my pending claim or asserted right wholly in my stead.

SIGNATURE (Claimant)	ADDRESS
Carol T. Usner	530 Hutch Street, Woodland Hills, XY 12345
TELEPHONE NUMBER 013-386-0122 (Area Code)	DATE August 3, 20XX

Section II   **ACCEPTANCE OF APPOINTMENT**

I, Gene Ulibarri, MD , hereby accept the above appointment. I certify that I have not been suspended or prohibited from practice before the Social Security Administration; that I am not, as a current or former officer or employee of the United States, disqualified from acting as the claimant's representative; and that I will not charge or receive any fee for the representation unless it has been authorized in accordance with the laws and regulations referred to on the reverse side hereof. In the event that I decide not to charge or collect a fee for the repesentation, I will notify the Social Security Administration. (Completion of Section III satisfies this requirement.)

I am a/an medical doctor medical doctor
_____
(Attorney, union representative, relative, law student, etc.)

SIGNATURE (Representative)	ADDRESS
Gene Ulibarri, MD	4567 Broad Ave., Woodland Hills, XY 12345
TELEPHONE NUMBER (Area code) 013-486-9002	DATE August 3, 20XX

Section III (Optional)   **WAIVER OF FEE**

I waive my right to charge and collect a fee under Section 206 of the Social Security Act, and I release my client (the claimant) from any obligations, contractual or otherwise, which may be owed to me for services I have performed in connection with my client's claim or asserted right.

SIGNATURE (Representative)	DATE

WAIVER OF DIRECT PAYMENT

I ONLY waive my right to direct certification of a fee from the withheld past-due benefits of my client (the claimant). I do NOT, however, waive my right to petition for and be authorized to charge and collect a fee directly from my client.

SIGNATURE (Representative)	DATE

Form SSA-1696-U4 (3-88)   (See Important Information on Reverse)   FILE COPY

Figure 8–9. Form SSA-1696-U4 completed by a Medicare patient appointing the physician as his or her authorized representative.

HOW TO COMPLETE THIS FORM

Print or type your full name and your Social Security Number.

Section I—APPOINTMENT OF REPRESENTATIVE

You may appoint as your representative an attorney or any other qualified individual. You may appoint more than one person, but see "The Fee You Owe The Representative(s)." You may NOT appoint as your representative an organization, the law firm, a group, etc. Example, you go to a law firm or legal aid group for help with your claim, you may appoint any attorney or other qualified individual from that firm or group, but NOT the firm or group itself.

Check the block(s) for the program in which you have a claim. Title II, check if your claim concerns disability or retirement benefits, etc. Title XVI, check if the claim concerns Supplemental Security Income (SSI) payments. Title IV FMSHS (Federal Mine Safety and Health Act), check if the claim is for black lung benefits. Title XVIII, check only in connection with a proceeding before the Social Security Administration involving entitlement to medicare coverage or enrollment in the supplementary medical insurance plan (SMIP). More than one block may be checked.

Section II—ACCEPTANCE OF APPOINTMENT

The individual whom you appoint in Section I above, completes this part. Completion of this section is desirable in all cases, but it is mandatory only if the appointed individual is not an attorney.

Section III—WAIVER OF FEE

This section may be completed by your representative if he/she will not charge any fee for services performed in this claim. If you had appointed a co-counsel (second representative) in Section I and he/she will also not charge you a fee, then the co-counsel should also sign this section or give a separate waiver statement.

GENERAL INFORMATION

1. When you have representative:

   We will deal directly with your representative on all matters that affect your claim. Occasionally, with the permission of your representative, we may deal directly with you on the specific issues. We will rely on your representative to keep you informed on the status of your claim, but you may contact us directly for any information about your claim.

2. The authority of your representative:

   Your representative has the authority to act totally on your behalf. This means he/she can (1) obtain information about your claim the same as you; (2) submit evidence (3) make statements about facts and provisions of the law; and (4) make any request (including a fee request). It is important, therefore, that you are represented by a qualified individual.

3. When will the representative stop:

   We will stop recognizing or dealing with your representative when (1) you tell us that he/she is no longer your representative; (2) your representative does any one of the following; (a) submits a fee petition, or (b) tells us that he/she is withdrawing from the claim, or (c) he/she violates any of our rules and regulations, and a hearing is held before an administrative law judge (designated as hearing officer) who orders your representative disqualified or suspended as representative of any Social Security claimant.

4. The fee you owe the representative(s):

   Every representative you appoint has a right to petition for a fee. To charge you a fee, a representative must first file a fee petition with us. Irrespective of your fee agreement, you never owe more than the fee we have authorized in a written notice to you and representative(s). (Out-of-pocket expenses are not included). If your claim went to court, you may owe an additional fee for your representative's service before the court.

5. How we determine the fee:

   We use the criteria on the back of the fee petition (Form SSA 1560-U4), a copy of which your representative must send you.

6. Review of the fee authorization:

   If you or your representative disagrees with the fee authorization, either of you may request a review. Instructions for filing this review are on the fee authorization notice.

7. Payment of fees:

   If past-due benefits are payable in your claim, we generally withhold 25 percent of the past-due benefits toward possible attorney fees. If no past-due benefits are payable or this is an SSI claim, then payment of the fee we have authorized is your responsibility.

8. Penalty for charging an unauthorized fee:

   If your representative wants to charge and collect from you a fee that is greater than what we had authorized, then he/she is in violation of the law and regulations. Promptly report this to your nearest Social Security office.

Form SSA-1696-U4 (3-88)

Figure 8–9 *Continued*

each state. The certification can be lifted from any insurer that does not honor its contract agreements. Only the state insurance commissioner can exert pressure on Medigap insurance companies. If payment is slow in coming or is not received from a Medigap insurer, tell the insurer, "If I do not receive payment, I will have no alternative but to contact the state insurance commissioner."

Document complete follow-up information on each Medigap insurer (firm name, address, tele-

DEPARTMENT OF HEALTH AND HUMAN SERVICES
HEALTH CARE FINANCING ADMINISTRATION

Form Approved
OMB No. 0938-0034

REQUEST FOR HEARING–PART B MEDICARE CLAIM
Medical Insurance Benefits–Social Security Act

NOTICE—Anyone who misrepresents or falsifies essential information requested by this form may upon conviction be subject to fine and imprisonment under Federal Law.

Carrier's Name and Address	**1** Name of Patient
Medicare Blue Cross Blue Shield of North Dakota 4510 13th Avenue, S.W. Fargo, ND 58121-0001	Deborah P. Sawyer
	2 Health Insurance Claim Number
	481-32-6491

3 I disagree with the review determination on my claim and request a hearing before a hearing officer of the insurance carrier named above.

MY REASONS ARE: *(Attach a copy of the Review Notice. NOTE.—If the review decision was made more than 6 months ago include your reason for not making this request earlier.)*

Complications arose during the surgical procedure requiring additional procedures performed. See attached chart notes and medical reports.

4 Check one of the Following:

[X] I have additional evidence to submit. (Attach such evidence to this form or forward it to the carrier within 10 days.)

[ ] I do not have additional evidence.

Check Only One of the Statements Below:

[ ] I wish to appear in person before the Hearing Officer.

[X] I do not wish to appear and hereby request a decision on the evidence before the Hearing Officer.

5 EITHER THE CLAIMANT OR REPRESENTATIVE SHOULD SIGN IN THE APPROPRIATE SPACE BELOW:

Signature or Name of Claimant's Representative	Claimant's Signature
Gaston Input, MD	*Deborah P. Sawyer*
Address	Address
4567 Broad Avenue	*1065 Evans Road*
City, State, and ZIP Code	City, State, and ZIP Code
Woodland Hills, XY 12345	*Woodland Hills, XY 12345*
Telephone Number 013-486-9002	Date 10-11-20XX	Telephone Number *013-742-1821*	Date *10-11-20XX*

(Claimant should not write below this line)

ACKNOWLEDGEMENT OF REQUEST FOR HEARING

Your request for a hearing was received on _____. You will be notified of the time and place of the hearing at least 10 days before the date of the hearing.

Signed	Date

FORM HCFA-1965 (8-79)

CARRIER'S COPY

Figure 8–10. Request for Hearing—Part B Medicare Claim Form HCFA-1965.

TRICARE CLAIM INQUIRY

Date: _____

TO: TRICARE
                Address of fiscal intermediary
                City, State, Zip Code

FROM: Provider's name   Telephone number
                Address   Fax number
                City, State, Zip Code

RE: Sponsor's Social Security Number _____

        Sponsor's Name _____

        Patient's Name _____

        Patient's Mailing Address:

        _____
        Street   City   State   Zip Code

        Dates of service claim: _____

        Total charges billed on claim: _____

        Claim number that appears on TRICARE Explanation of Benefits
        (leave blank if the claim has not been paid and information is not available)

        _____

A. _____   I have submitted a claim, but have not received any payment
                    or other notification from you.

B. _____   I have received notification or payment concerning the claim,
                    but feel it may have been processed incorrectly.

C. _____   Deductible Status. Please confirm that individual and family
                    deductibles have been applied correctly.

D. _____   Coverage for this patient is under

                    _____ **TRICARE**   _____ **CHAMPVA**

E. _____   Additional information or explanation which will assist
                    reviewing or processing the claim is attached to this letter or
                    written in this area.

Figure 8–11. Example of a TRICARE Standard claim inquiry form that may be completed to obtain a quick reply. Mail to the TRICARE fiscal intermediary for your region.

phone number, and policy numbers) of every patient seen.

TRICARE Review and Appeal Process

 Before appealing a TRICARE claim, an inquiry should be sent to verify claim status and attempt to resolve the problem. Fig-

ure 8–11 shows an example of a form that may be used for inquiring about a TRICARE Standard claim. TRICARE appeals procedures applicable to the routine processing of TRICARE Standard claims are described here. However, TRICARE managed care contracts have been adopted throughout the United States and the appeals procedures that TRICARE contractors use in these ar-

eas may vary. For information on how to file reviews and appeals for those contracts, ask the contracting insurance carrier for instructions and forms.

Three levels for review under TRICARE Standard appeal procedures exist:

1. *Reconsideration* (conducted by the claims processor or other TRICARE contractor responsible for the decision in a particular case).
2. *Formal review* (conducted by TRICARE headquarters).
3. *Hearing* administered by TRICARE headquarters but conducted by an independent hearing officer.

Reconsideration

Participating providers may appeal certain decisions made by TRICARE, requesting reconsideration. Providers who do not participate may not appeal, but TRICARE Standard patients and parents or guardians of patients younger than 18 years of age who seek care from nonparticipating providers may file appeals. Providers who do not participate may not receive any information regarding a particular claim without the signed authorization of the patient or the patient's parent or guardian.

Matters that can be appealed include the following:

1. Medical necessity disagreements (inappropriate care, level of care, investigational procedures)
2. Factual determinations (hospice care, foreign claims, provider sanction cases)
   a. Denials or partial denials of requests for preauthorization for certain services or supplies
   b. Coverage issues—notification that TRICARE will not pay for services before or after a certain date

Matters that cannot be appealed include the following:

1. Denial of services received from a provider not authorized to provide care under TRICARE
2. A specific exclusion of law or regulation
3. Allowable charges for particular services
4. Issues relating to the establishment and application of diagnosis-related groups
5. Decisions by the claims processor to ask for additional information on a particular case
6. A determination of a person's eligibility as a TRICARE beneficiary

The TRICARE department handling appeals collects and organizes all information necessary to review the case effectively. Usually a determination decision is made within 60 days from receipt of the appeal. Disagreements regarding the amount allowed for a particular claim may be reviewed by the claims processor to determine whether it was calculated correctly. However, an individual cannot appeal the amount that the TRICARE contractor determines to be the allowable charge for a certain medical service.

Requests must be sent to the claims processor of the state in which services were provided and must be postmarked within 90 days of the date the provider receives the Summary Payment Voucher (formerly referred to as an EOB). Include photocopies of the claim, Summary Payment Voucher, and other supporting documents with the request form or letter. The claim identification number assigned by the claims processor should be included in any inquiry concerning payment of the claim. If TRICARE denies the initial request, then the other two levels of review, formal review and hearing, may be pursued.

Formal Review

A formal review must be done within 60 days from the date on the reconsideration decision notice. Include photocopies of the notice as well as any other information or documents to support why there is a disagreement in the TRICARE decision. The case will be reviewed again and a formal review decision will be issued. If the amount of dispute is less than $300, the formal review decision is final.

Hearing

If the amount in dispute is $300 or more, an independent hearing may be pursued. The request must be postmarked or received within 60 days from the date of the formal review decision. A hearing is conducted by an independent hearing officer at a location convenient to both the requesting party and the government.

VIDEO RESOURCE

MEDICAL ASSISTANT VIDEO SERIES, TAPE 6: "The HCFA Files: A Case for Medical Billing Accuracy."

This video is an interesting and entertaining presentation about what happens to rejected claim forms. It gives reasons why claims are denied and gives solutions to avoid such problems. It is an excellent enhancement when used at the conclusion to this chapter. An assignment is presented in the *Workbook* for completion after viewing this video.

RESOURCES ON THE INTERNET

A bimonthly newsletter that links to regulatory information online:
www.integsoft.com/appeals/tal

STUDENT ASSIGNMENT LIST

✔ Study Chapter 8.

✔ Answer the review questions in the *Workbook* to reinforce the theory learned in this chapter and to help prepare you for a future test.

✔ Complete the assignments in the *Workbook* to fill in a form for tracing a delinquent claim, to locate errors on returned claims, and to complete a form to appeal a Medicare case.

✔ Turn to the Glossary at the end of this textbook for a further understanding of the Key Terms used in this chapter.

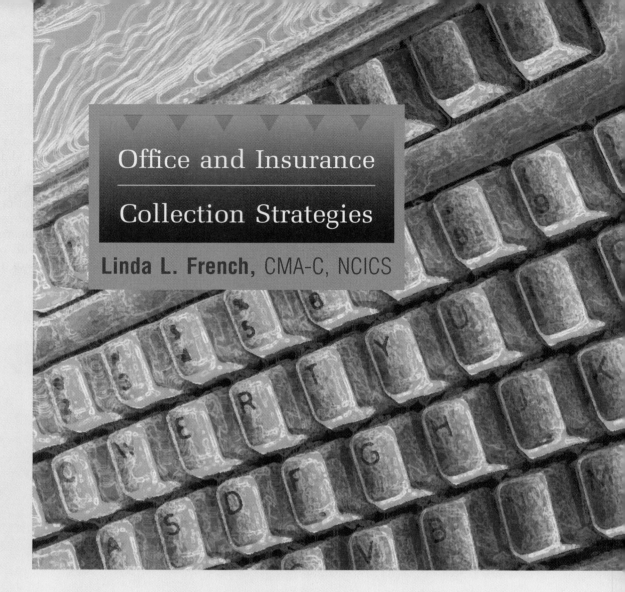

Office and Insurance
Collection Strategies

Linda L. French, CMA-C, NCICS

9

CHAPTER OUTLINE

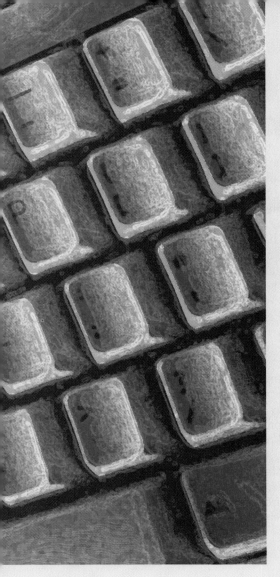

- Define accounts receivable and explain how it is handled.
- Recite types of fee adjustments available to patients.
- Enumerate credit options available to patients.
- Perform oral and written communication collection techniques.
- State the role of a billing service, collection agency, and credit bureau in the collection process.
- List possible solutions to collection problems.
- Explain the purpose of small claims court in the collection process.
- Name basic actions in tracing a debtor who has moved and left no forwarding address.

OBJECTIVES*

After reading this chapter, you should be able to:

- Define credit and collection terminology.
- Translate collection abbreviations.
- Describe office billing procedures.
- Define aging analysis.
- Discuss ways to determine fees and describe an office's fee policies.
- Summarize credit laws applicable to a physician office setting.

KEY TERMS

accounts receivable

age analysis

automatic stay

balance

bankruptcy

cash flow

collateral

collection ratio

computer billing

credit

credit card

creditor

cycle billing

debit card

debt

debtor

discount

dun message

estate administrator

estate executor

fee schedule

garnishment

insurance balance billing

itemized statement

ledger card

lien

manual billing

netback

no charge (NC)

nonexempt assets

professional courtesy

reimbursement

secured debt

continued

*Performance objectives and exercises for hands-on practical experience for this chapter appear in the *Workbook*.

287

Cash Flow Cycle

The practice of medicine is both a profession and a business. Although the physician decides what type of medicine he or she will practice, it is often the multiskilled health practitioner (MSHP) who is responsible for the business portion of the practice. It is extremely important for the physician and the insurance specialist to work together to provide all patients the best possible medical care and to ensure that the physician is paid fairly for services that are rendered.

Today, this process has become increasingly difficult. Physician office and billing practices have evolved from the barter system of days past; and since the Great Depression, the availability of credit and credit cards have become a common feature of the financial marketplace. The word **credit** comes from the Latin credere, which means "to believe" or "to trust." This trust is in an individual's business integrity and his or her financial ability to meet all obligations when they become due. For many, the idea of credit has changed and may simply mean to put off paying today what one can pay tomorrow.

A large percentage of **reimbursement** to physicians' offices is generated from third party payers (private insurance, government plans, managed care contracts, and workers' compensation). It is important for the physician, the MSHP responsible for financial affairs, and the patient to understand these insurance contracts, which list reimbursement provisions, medical services not covered, the portion of the bill the patient is responsible for, and the process for reimbursing the office.

Accounts Receivable

Accounts receivable (A/R) include the unpaid balances due from patients for services that have been rendered. Each medical practice has a policy about handling A/R. The effectiveness of this policy and its enforcement is reflected in the practice's **cash flow.** The cash flow is the ongoing availability of cash in the medical practice. When charges are collected at the time of service, the A/R is zero. In an ideal situation, all outstanding balances are paid within 60 days; however, this is not possible for the following reasons:

1. Health care expenses have increased and exceed the expenses the patient pays for everyday living.
2. The public feels it is a right, rather than a privilege, to receive the best possible health care. The care of the indigent, therefore, becomes an unreimbursable expense in the medical office.
3. Legal proceedings often delay the payment of medical expenses.
4. Insurance carriers do not pay claims in a timely manner, resulting in further delays in the collection of patient copayments.

By monitoring the A/R, the insurance billing specialist will be able to evaluate the effectiveness of the collection process. The formula for finding out the A/R ratio is to divide the month-end

A/R balance by the monthly average charges for the prior 12-month period. An average total A/R (all monies not collected at the time of service) should be one and one-half to two times the charges for 1 month of services (see Example 9–1).

firmation letter (Fig. 9–1) may be sent to welcome the new patient to the practice. This letter will inform the patient about the practice, clearly outline payment expectations, provide collection policies and procedures in printed form, establish a

---

EXAMPLE 9–1

Formula

Physician's Charges Monthly Total	$50,000 × 1.5 = $75,000 or $50,000 × 2.0 = $100,000	Total Outstanding Accounts Receivable

Total outstanding A/R should range from $75,000 to $100,000.

Accounts that are 90 days or older should not exceed 15% to 18% of the total A/R. To calculate this figure, divide the total amount of A/R by the amount of accounts that are 90 days old and older (see Example 9–2).

EXAMPLE 9–2

Formula

Accounts Receivable Total	$75,000 ÷ $5,000 = 15%	Amount of A/R Over 90 Days

---

The **collection ratio** is the relationship of the amount of money owed to a physician and the amount of money collected on the physician's A/R. A collection rate of 90% to 95% should be a goal for the MSHP managing collections in the physician's office. To calculate the collection rate for a 1-month period, divide the amount of monies collected during the current month by the total amount of the A/R.

Patient Education

During the initial contact with the patient, information should be provided about office fees and payment policies. This will decrease the number of billing statements sent and increase collections. Never allow a patient to believe that he or she is not responsible for the bill. Discuss copayment requirements (see Chapter 2) with patients who are enrolled in managed care plans, and convey the office policy of collecting this amount when registering the patient for the office visit. A new patient information pamphlet or brochure and con-

contact person, invite questions, and confirm all specific details discussed.

Patient Registration Form

There is no substitution for good information gathering techniques at the time of initial patient registration. Always obtain a complete and accurate registration from the patient on the first visit. Chapter 2 describes what data should be obtained from the patient and Figure 2–7 is an example of a patient registration information form, also called a patient information sheet. Have the guarantor agree in writing to pay for all medical treatment. By obtaining the guarantor's signature, he or she is then bound by contract to pay the bill.

Learn as much as possible about the patient before any services are provided. This is when the patient is likely to be the most cooperative. Information provided on the patient information sheet will prove critical to any billing and collection efforts. The patient should be instructed to answer all questions and indicate any spaces on the form that do not apply by marking "N/A" (not applicable). Review of the completed patient information sheet will ensure that all blanks have been addressed and accurate information has been collected. It will also alert office staff of an account that may be a future problem. Items often overlooked are the street address, when a post office box is given; an apartment or mobile home number; and a business telephone number with department and extension. These will help to trace a patient who has moved. If a patient refuses to divulge any information, invoking the privacy laws, it should be policy to require payment for services at the time care is rendered. A potential nonpaying patient may be recognized at this time. Here are some clues to look for:

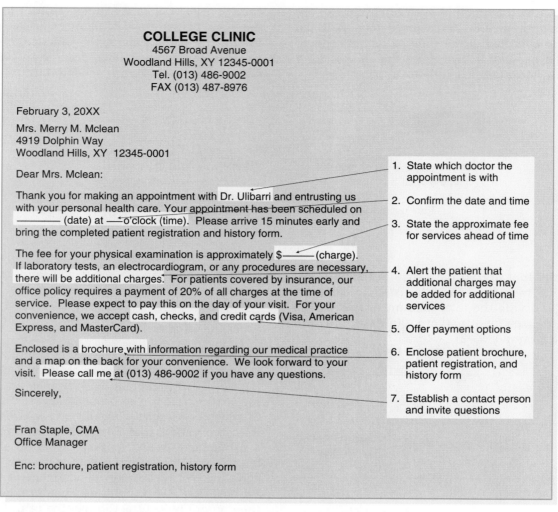

Figure 9–1. New patient confirmation letter emphasizing information to incorporate when writing to a new patient.

- Incomplete information on the registration form
- Multiple changes of residence
- Questionable employment record
- No business or home telephone
- Post office box listed with no street address
- Motel address
- Incomplete insurance information
- No referral information or authorization from a primary care physician for patients enrolled in a managed care plan

Employers are changing health plans with increasing frequency and patients are more transient than ever, so update this form whenever the patient is seen or every 6 months. This can be done by printing out a data sheet or having the patient review a copy of his or her registration form and inserting changes or corrections with a red pen. New information can also be ob-

tained using an updated or abbreviated form (see Chapter 2, Figure 2–9).

Fees

Fee Schedule

Most medical practices operate with more then one fee schedule. As discussed in Chapter 5, a **fee schedule** is a listing of accepted charges or established allowances for specific medical procedures. It is important to determine which fee schedule applies to a patient before quoting fees and stating policies regarding the collection of fees. Under federal regulations, a list of the most common services the physician offers, including procedure code numbers, with a description of each service and its price, must be available to all patients, and a sign must be posted in the office advising patients of this.

Occasionally, a physician assigns a fee for a service that is not on the fee schedule, such as an uncanceled appointment (referred to as a "no show"), completion of an insurance form, a long-distance telephone consultation, a narrative medical report for an insurance company, or interest assessed on a delinquent account. It is advisable to inform patients before billing for any such services to preserve the patient/physician relationship. If the fee schedule is increased at a later date, a notice should be placed in the reception room and communicated to patients via their monthly billing statement.

Fee Adjustments

Discounted Fees

A physician may choose to discount his or her fees for various reasons. A **discount** is a reduction of the normal fee based on a specific amount of money or a percentage of the charge. When a physician offers a discount, it must apply to the total bill, not just the portion that is paid by the patient (copayment or coinsurance amount). By following this rule, the physician is giving a discount to the patient and to the insurance company. This practice could reduce the physician's profile with the insurance company and trigger a reduction in the physician's allowable reimbursement schedule; therefore, the physician should consider the outcome of discounting fees. All discounts must be noted on the patient's **ledger card** (Fig. 9–2), and any financial reasons or special circumstances need to be documented in the patient's medical record. This will ensure complete record keeping and safeguard any questions that may be brought up during a financial audit.

Cash Discounts

Cash discounts may be offered (5%–20%) to patients who pay the entire fee, in cash, at the time of service. If a cash discount system is offered, this policy should be posted in the office and every active patient sent notification.

Financial Hardship

Financial hardship cases are the most difficult for the physician to determine. The insurance billing specialist should never assume anything about a patient's financial status nor judge a patient's ability to pay by his or her appearance. The Department of Health and Human Services has published a 1999 guideline on poverty income (Fig. 9–3), which is used to determine eligibility for uncompensated services under the Hill-Burton program, the Community Services Block Grant program, and the Head Start program. Physicians may choose to follow these guidelines to direct patients to government-sponsored programs, to obtain public assistance, and to determine who is eligible for a hardship waiver. A hardship waiver can vary from 25% to 100% of the bill. Various financial forms are available to obtain this information, and a copy of the patient's wage and tax statement (W2) or tax return needs to be examined to make a reliable decision. The patient should also sign a written explanation to verify true financial hardship. This will help in the collection process and allow the physician to accept the insurance as payment in full, in certain circumstances, without being suspected of insurance fraud. The reason for a fee reduction must be noted in the patient's medical record.

Write-off or Courtesy Adjustment

Write-off, or preferred term, *courtesy adjustment,* is an asset or debt that has been determined to be uncollectable and is therefore taken off (subtracted/credited) the accounting books. It is considered lost income but may not be claimed as a loss for tax purposes. The insurance specialist should obtain financial information on all patients who request a "write-off." Office policies regarding adjustments and all discounts should be in writing, and all staff members should be informed. The physician must approve the portion of the charge to be credited to the financial record before the debt is forgiven.

Professional Courtesy

Professional courtesy is a concept attributed to Hippocrates, but the foundations are actually derived from Thomas Percival's Code of Medical Ethics written in 1803. The American Medical Association Code of Ethics, formulated and adopted in 1847, closely mirrored Percival's code. The practice of professional courtesy served to build bonds between physicians and to reduce the incentive for physicians to treat their own families. Most physicians agree that one of the greatest honors and privileges in the practice of medicine is to be asked to care for a physician and his or her family members. The practice of professional courtesy was often extended to others in the health care profession and to members of the clergy. Most

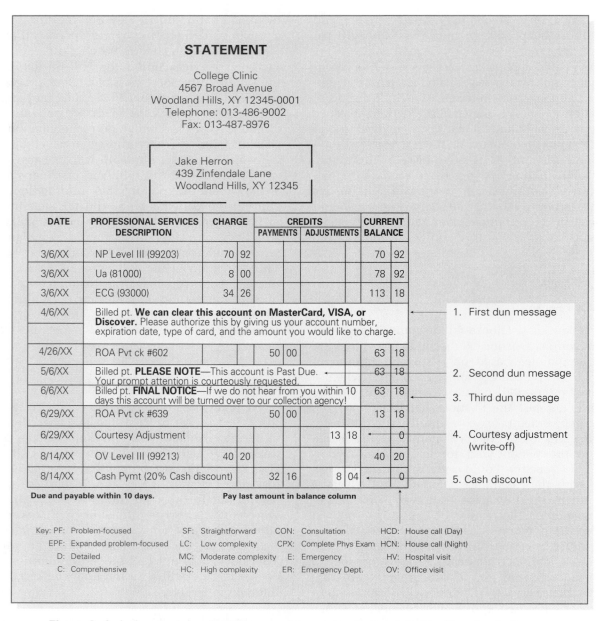

STATEMENT

College Clinic
4567 Broad Avenue
Woodland Hills, XY 12345-0001
Telephone: 013-486-9002
Fax: 013-487-8976

Jake Herron
439 Zinfendale Lane
Woodland Hills, XY 12345

DATE	PROFESSIONAL SERVICES DESCRIPTION	CHARGE		CREDITS				CURRENT BALANCE	
				PAYMENTS		ADJUSTMENTS			
3/6/XX	NP Level III (99203)	70	92					70	92
3/6/XX	Ua (81000)	8	00					78	92
3/6/XX	ECG (93000)	34	26					113	18
4/6/XX	Billed pt. **We can clear this account on MasterCard, VISA, or Discover.** Please authorize this by giving us your account number, expiration date, type of card, and the amount you would like to charge.								
4/26/XX	ROA Pvt ck #602			50	00			63	18
5/6/XX	Billed pt. **PLEASE NOTE**—This account is Past Due. Your prompt attention is courteously requested.							63	18
6/6/XX	Billed pt. **FINAL NOTICE**—If we do not hear from you within 10 days this account will be turned over to our collection agency!							63	18
6/29/XX	ROA Pvt ck #639			50	00			13	18
6/29/XX	Courtesy Adjustment					13	18		0
8/14/XX	OV Level III (99213)	40	20					40	20
8/14/XX	Cash Pymt (20% Cash discount)			32	16	8	04		0

Due and payable within 10 days.   Pay last amount in balance column

1. First dun message

2. Second dun message

3. Third dun message

4. Courtesy adjustment (write-off)

5. Cash discount

Key: PF: Problem-focused   SF: Straightforward   CON: Consultation   HCD: House call (Day)
      EPF: Expanded problem-focused   LC: Low complexity   CPX: Complete Phys Exam HCN: House call (Night)
        D: Detailed   MC: Moderate complexity   E: Emergency   HV: Hospital visit
        C: Comprehensive   HC: High complexity   ER: Emergency Dept.   OV: Office visit

Figure 9–2. Ledger card showing dun messages, courtesy adjustment (write-off), and cash discount.

hospitals and many surgeons have since given up the practice of free care. Today, most physicians have insurance coverage for medical expenses.

Professional courtesy means making no charge to anyone, patient or insurance, for medical care. The law does not provide exceptions that allow professional courtesy to physicians in situations where the same courtesy could not be extended to all patients. Physicians must examine their policies on professional courtesy to ensure that they do not violate either the contractual terms in private or managed care insurance policies or Medicare/Medicaid laws and regulations. If the treating physician does not bill the physician-patient for services rendered, the third party payer is relieved of its contractual obligation. If the treating physician waives the deductible and copayment, the physician may be accused of not treating others with the same insurance coverage in an equal manner. Although there may be some situations in which it is defensible to "no charge" for services to health care professionals, the physician should ensure that this professional courtesy is not linked to patients who have been referred to the practice. There are laws that prohibit any inducement or kickbacks from physicians (or others) that could influence the decision of a physician (or other) to refer patients or that may affect a patient's decision to seek care.

2000 GUIDELINES ON POVERTY INCOME			
Size of family unit	48 contiguous states and D.C.	Alaska	Hawaii
1	$ 8,350	$10,430	$ 9,590
2	$11,250	$14,060	$12,930
3	$14,150	$17,690	$16,270
4	$17,050	$21,320	$19,610
5	$19,950	$24,950	$22,950
6	$22,850	$28,580	$26,290
7	$25,750	$32,210	$29,630
8	$28,650	$35,840	$32,970
For each additional person add:	$ 2,900	$ 3,630	$ 3,340

Figure 9–3. Department of Health and Human Services 2000 guidelines on poverty income; published in the *Federal Register.*

Copayment Waiver

Waiving copayments is another way physicians have reduced the cost of medical care for patients in the past. By doing this, the physician accepts the insurance payment only. In most situations, both private insurers and the federal government ban waiving the copayment. It is, therefore, not recommended. There is one exception to this rule in that Medicare recognizes a courtesy discount, doctor to doctor.

No Charge

No charge (NC) means waiving the entire fee for professional care. This is permitted as long as it is not part of a fraudulent scheme and is offered to all patients. All "NC" visits must be fully documented in the clinical portion of the patient's medical record and in the financial record. A physician or insurance specialist cannot assess a fee for services for which the insurance company does not approve as a way of trying to satisfy a patient's deductible.

Another instance when "no charge" would occur on a patient's account is when follow-up visits are posted after a patient undergoes surgery considered under a surgical package or a Medicare global fee structure. When posting such charges in a computer system, CPT procedure code 99024 (postoperative follow-up visit included in global fee) may be used.

Reduced Fee

Precautions need to be taken before reducing the fee of a patient who dies. The doctor's sympathy in this case could be misinterpreted and result in a malpractice suit. A fee reduction should never be based on a poor result in the treatment of a patient.

If a patient is disputing a fee and the physician agrees to settle for a reduced fee, the agreement should be in writing with a definite time limit for payment and the words "without prejudice" inserted. By doing this the physician protects the right to collect the original sum if the patient fails to pay the reduced fee. The physician and the patient should sign the agreement and each receive a copy.

Communicating Fees

People have a difficult time asking each other for money and talking about financial obligations. Financial arrangements should be discussed up front and in great detail before any services are provided (Fig. 9–4). Many medical practices create their own collection problems by not being clear about *how* and *when* they expect to be paid. If you do not tell patients that payment is due at the time of service, most will assume they can pay at a later time. Following are some guidelines to help communicate effectively about money:

1. Be courteous at all times but express a firm, business-like approach that will not offend the patient.
2. Never badger or intimidate a patient into paying; merely state the payment policy and educate the patient.
3. Inform the patient of the fee and any deductible and balance due in a clear manner.
4. Verify the patient's copayment listed on his or her insurance card and collect this amount before the patient's office visit.

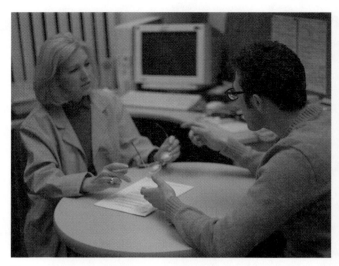

Figure 9–4. Insurance billing specialist discussing fees with the patient.

5. Make it easier for the patient to pay, rather than to leave without making payment.
6. Do not give patients an option by asking if they would like to pay now or have a bill sent.
7. Motivate the patient to pay by appealing to his or her honesty, integrity, and pride.

Following are examples of communicating in a positive manner and letting the patient know exactly what is expected:

▶ "The office visit is $62, Mrs. Smith. Would you like to pay by cash, check, or credit card?"
▶ "Your copayment will be $10, Mr. Jones. I will be collecting it prior to your office visit."
▶ "Your insurance policy shows a deductible of $100 that is your responsibility and currently has not been met, Miss Rodriguez. You will need to pay the full fee today, which is $75."
▶ "Mrs. Merryweather, I need to collect $4.77 today for your vitamin B$_{12}$ injection. The injection is not covered by your insurance policy."
▶ "We look forward to seeing you on Tuesday, March 3, at 10 A.M. Mr. Gillespie; the consultation will be approximately $150 and payment is expected at the time of service. We accept cash, check, or credit cards for your convenience."

Collecting Fees

Payment at the Time of Service

Do not miss the opportunity to ask for payment at the time of service. Collect all fixed copayments before the patient is seen to alleviate billing for small amounts. Patients do not make health care bills a priority, so the importance of collecting outstanding bills, coinsurance amounts, and money from cash

paying patients up front should be communicated to office staff. One-on-one communication is the best way to motivate a **debtor.** Each patient's account **balance** (amount due) should be reviewed before his or her appointment. If the appointment schedule is on a computer system, print the account balance by each patient's name. If an appointment book is used, make a copy of the page showing the day's schedule. Write overdue balances by the patient's name after obtaining overdue amounts from each patient's ledger card. This information should also be recorded on the transaction slip for that day's visit and may be "flagged" when the transaction slips are printed or written. Treat this information confidentially and keep it out of view of other patients. When a patient arrives whose name is "flagged," alert the Patient Accounts Manager.

To do effective pre-appointment collection counseling, the patient should be led to a quiet area away from the general activity of the office. Sit down with the patient and discuss the situation. Use an understanding attitude and a helpful nature while verbalizing phrases such as "I understand" and "I can help." Ask direct questions to learn exactly what problems the patient is facing. Answers to questions such as "When do you expect your next paycheck?" and "How much are you able to pay today?" will help determine your strategy. Your goal should be to try and collect the full amount. If that is not possible, try to collect a portion of the balance. Get a promise to pay for the remaining balance by a specific date. If the patient is unable to comply, then set up a payment plan. The chances of reaching a mutually satisfactory resolution are greatly improved when the two parties are face to face.

A personal interview is preferential to a telephone interview, because when the debtor is present a financial agreement can be signed (Fig. 9–5), resulting in a better follow-up response. It is important to let the patient know that the practice is willing to help and that if he or she runs into further problems in making the payment, the debtor should inform the insurance specialist. This personal contact helps if a renegotiation of the agreement is needed. A medical practice cannot refuse to let an established patient see the doctor because of a **debt,** but the office staff has every right to ask for payment while the patient is in the office (Fig. 9–6).

Encounter Forms

Multipurpose billing forms (see Chapter 2) known by many names, including encounter form, are helpful when collecting fees at the time of service. Encounter forms can be given to patients to bill

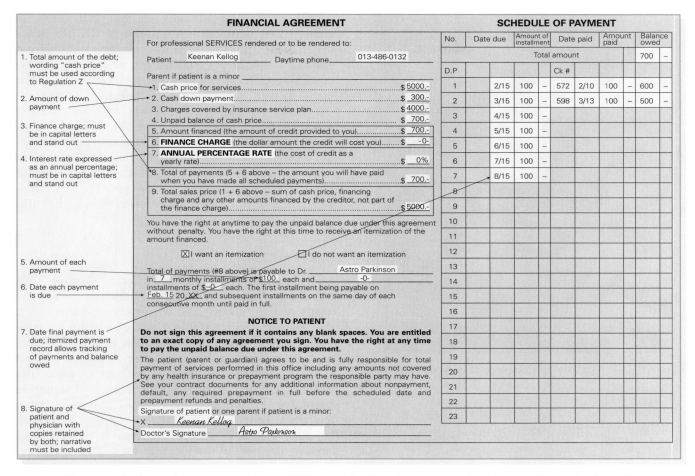

Figure 9–5. Financial Agreement Form (#1826) used for financial payment plans; by completing this form the physician provides full disclosure of all information required by the Truth in Lending Act, Regulation Z. (Reprinted with permission of SYCOM, A Division of New England Business Service, Inc., Groton, MA. Phone: 800-356-8141.)

their insurance companies, used to inform patients of current charges and any outstanding balances, and used as receipts for payment (Fig. 9–7).

Patient Excuses

Nonpayers show a tendency to dismiss financial arrangements with curt remarks. Look directly at the patient, confidently expecting payment. Demonstrate to the patient that you feel secure in knowing you have the right to request payment. If excuses are offered, be ready for them. Table 9–1 shows some examples of patients' excuses and possible responses.

When a patient chatters nervously it may be a way of setting up reasons to rationalize not paying. Do not let this distract you. Pause after asking for payment and do not say another word until the patient responds. Many people feel uncomfortable with silence, but pauses may work to your advantage and help you complete a transaction. By taking this approach you will help increase cash flow and the collection ratio, while decreasing billing chores and collection costs. You will also be able to get a quick identification of nonpayers and notify the person responsible for collections.

Payment by Check

Check Verification

Check verification requires the insurance specialist to become familiar with the appearance of a good check. A personal check is the most common method of payment in most medical offices, but it is not a personal guarantee of payment. A driver's license and one other form of identification should always be required. Check these against existing records. Call the bank to verify all out-of-state and suspicious checks. A verification service, which is a private company with resources to quickly identify patient information over the telephone, or a check authorization

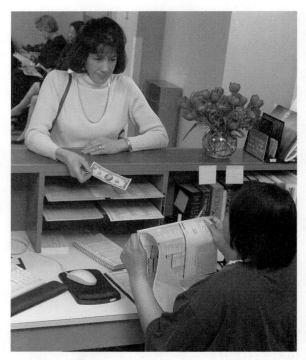

Figure 9–6. Receptionist collecting copayment from the patient.

system, may be worthy of consideration for clinics and larger group practices.

Check Forgery

Forgery is false writing or alteration of a document to injure another person or with intent to deceive (e.g., signing, without permission, another person's name on a check to obtain money or to pay off a debt). To guard against forgery, always check to be sure the endorsement on the back of the check matches the name on the front. Be suspicious if the beneficiary or provider states that he or she did not receive the check but the insurance company shows it as being cashed, or if the payee of the check claims that the signature is not his or hers.

Payment Disputes

Problem checks appear in many forms. One is the check for partial payment when the debtor (the patient) writes "payment in full" on the check. If the **creditor** (the physician) cashes the check, it may be argued that the debt is "paid in full." A legal theory called *"accord and satisfaction"* may apply to this situation if the debt is *truly disputed* by the debtor. If the check is retained (and cashed) by the physician, it can be considered "accord and satisfaction," and the physician cannot go after the patient for the balance. The operative words are "truly disputed." If there is a legitimate, genuine

dispute over the amount of the bill, and an amount less than the full amount of the bill is accepted, the physician could be precluded from seeking the balance. Acceptance of payment, however, does not necessarily mean acceptance of the "paid in full" remark. A good safeguard is to cross out "paid in full" on the check and note on the patient's financial record that the patient wrote "paid in full" on his or her check. Post and deposit the check, then notify the patient that the account is not paid in full and clarify the current state of the account. It is generally in the provider's best interest to resolve billing disputes quickly, amicably, and accurately.

Unsigned Checks

Another problem is unsigned checks. First you can ask the patient to come to the office and sign the check or send a new one. If you are unable to reach the patient or if there is a transportation or time limitation problem, you can write the word "over" or "see reverse" on the signature line on the front of the check. On the back of the check, where the endorsement would appear, write "lack of signature guaranteed," your practice's name, and your name and title. Your endorsement is, in effect, a guarantee that you will absorb the loss if the patient's bank or the patient does not honor the check.

Returned Checks

When the physician's office receives notice that a check was not honored, the reason should be stated on the back of the check. The most common reason is nonsufficient funds (NSF). Call the bank or patient to see if they suggest redepositing it. It may be an oversight or miscalculation by the patient. If it is not worth redepositing, or you receive a second NSF notice, call the patient immediately. Be courteous but straight to the point. Inform the patient that payment is due by cash, money order, or a certified check within 3 days. If you do not receive restitution within 3 days, you need to start the legal process of notifying the patient in writing. Send a NSF demand letter (Fig. 9–8) by certified mail with return receipt requested, and include the following:

1. Check date
2. Check number
3. Bank the check is drawn on
4. To whom the check was payable
5. Check amount
6. Any allowable service charge
7. Total amount due
8. Number of days the checkwriter has to take action

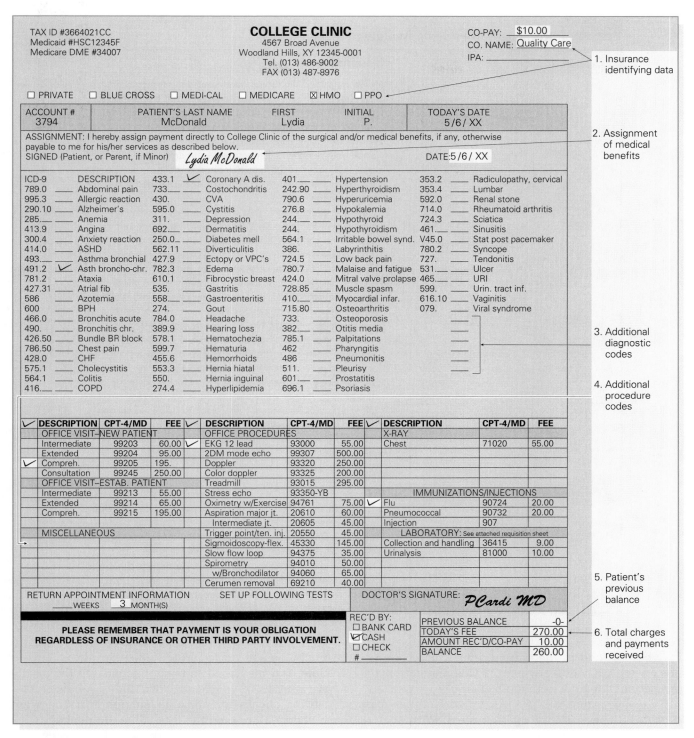

Figure 9–7. Encounter form; diagnostic codes are taken from the *International Classification of Diseases, 9th revision, Clinical Modification* (ICD-9-CM) book, and procedural codes for professional services are taken from the *Current Procedural Terminology* (CPT) book. (Courtesy of Bibbero Systems, Inc., Petaluma, CA. Phone: 800-242-2376; FAX 800-242-9330.)

Once a patient has been informed of the returned check, explain that your facility will no longer be able to accept checks as payment. Future payments need to be in the form of cash, money order, or a cashier's check. If the patient wishes the check returned, be sure to photocopy it and keep it in the financial record because it serves as an acknowledgment of the debt. The bad check

TABLE 9–1	**Responses to Patients Avoiding Payment**
Excuse	**Response**
"Just bill me"	"As we explained when we made your appointment, Mr. Barkley, our practice bills for charges over $50. Amounts under $50 are to be paid at the time of the visit. That will be $25 for today's visit please."
"I have insurance to cover this."	"We will be billing your insurance for you, Miss Butler, but your policy shows a deductible in the amount of $300 that still needs to be met. We need to collect the full fee for today's visit, which is $150 to meet that deductible responsibility."
"I get paid on Friday; you know how it is."	"I understand. Why don't you write the check today and postdate it for Saturday. We will hold the check and deposit it on the next business day" (depending on office policy).
"If I pay for this I won't be able to pay for the prescription."	"Our payment policy is very much like the pharmacy; we expect payment at the time of service. Let me check and see if the doctor can dispense some medication samples to last you until you can get your prescription filled."
"I don't have that much with me."	"How much can you pay, Mrs. Fish? I can accept $10 now and give you an envelope to send us the balance within the week, or I can put it on your credit card." (Get a commitment and write the balance due under the sealing flap of the envelope. Also write the date on a tickler calendar or the patient's ledger while the patient is watching.)
"I'll take care of it."	"I know you will, Mr. Stone; I just need to know when that will be so I can document your intentions for our bookkeeper." (Get a commitment and write down the date on a tickler calendar or on the patient's ledger card while in view of the patient. Hand him an envelope with the amount due written under the sealing flap.)
"I forgot my checkbook."	"We take Visa, MasterCard, and American Express, Mr. Storz." (If the patient still does not pay, provide him with a self-addressed envelope and write the patient's name, account number, date of service, amount due, and expected payment date under the sealing flap. Restate the expected payment date as you hand the patient the envelope. Note the date on a tickler calendar or on the patient's ledger card while the patient is watching.)

may be returned to the patient after it has been replaced with a valid payment. Place a notation on the patient's record to this effect.

To guard against bad checks, larger facilities may consider a check authorization system. With such a system, the company supplies a terminal that will give an approval number for each check that is taken in and guarantees payment on the checks they authorize. If no approval is given, another form of payment will be required. The check guarantee service receives a percentage for the checks that they approve and collects all bad check charges from the patient. One way to help discourage bad checks is to charge a penalty for returned checks. This information should be included in the new patient brochures and posted in the office for all patients to view. You may need to make reference to the particular section of your state Civil Code's provisions regarding checks for nonsufficient funds if you want to collect more then the face value of the check.

If you are notified that the checking account is closed, do not waste time trying to contact the patient. Send a demand letter immediately. In most states if the patient has not responded in 30 days, legal action can be taken. Consider filing a claim in small claims court. Most states have written codes or statutes pertaining to bad checks. Often legislation allows the creditor to add punitive damages to the amount of the debt being collected, sometimes up to three times the amount of the check.

COLLEGE CLINIC
4567 Broad Avenue
Woodland Hills, XY 12345-0001
Tel. (013) 486-9002
FAX (013) 487-8976

August 15, 20XX

Mrs. Maxine Holt
444 Labina Lane
Woodland Hills, XY 12345-0001

Dear Mrs. Holt:

The following check has been dishonored by the bank and returned without payment:

Date: 08/04/20XX
Check No.:   755
Amount: $106.11
Payable to: Perry Cardi, MD
Bank: Woodland Hills National Bank
Reason: Nonsufficient funds

This is a formal notice demanding payment in the amount of $106.11 within 15 days from today's date or your account will be considered for legal action.

Please make payment immediately by cash, cashier's check, or money order at the above address. Your immediate attention will be appreciated.

Sincerely,

Delores Yee, CMA-A

Patient Accounts Manager
for Perry Cardi, MD

Figure 9–8. Demand letter for returned check. This letter serves as a formal notice to collect payment and notifies a patient of impending legal action.

When a patient stops payment on a check, it is usually done to resolve a good faith dispute. In this case, the patient believes that he or she has legal entitlement to withhold payment. The physician may want to contact a lawyer to discuss his or her legal rights and responsibilities before sending a demand letter and trying to collect.

Itemized Statements

Every patient receives an **itemized statement** (Fig. 9–9) of his or her account showing the dates of service, a list of detailed charges, copayments and deductibles paid, the date insurance claim was filed (if appropriate), applicable adjustments, and the account balance. These items will also be listed on the patient's account or ledger card (see Chapter 2, Fig. 2–17 and Fig. 9–2). When sending itemized statements, timeliness, accuracy, and consistency have a significant effect on the cash flow and the collection process.

Professional bills are a reflection of the medical practice. The billing statement should be patient oriented and easy to read and understand. Avoid technical terms and abbreviations that might lead to misunderstandings and confusion. Enclose a return envelope. Addressed envelopes should contain the statement "Forwarding Service Requested" so the postal service can forward the mail and provide the physician's office with a notice of the patient's new address. When this notice is received in the physician's office, it should be circulated to all necessary departments to record the new information.

Patients can be oriented to the billing process by having the insurance specialist generate a printed statement when they are ready to leave the office and explaining pertinent information, such as account number, dates of service, payments, procedures, interest fees, copayments, and deductibles. Patient information pamphlets about common health concerns such as blood pressure, cholesterol, or back pain can be sent along with the bill to convey a caring attitude.

When statements go out in the mail, the office is likely to experience an increase in telephone

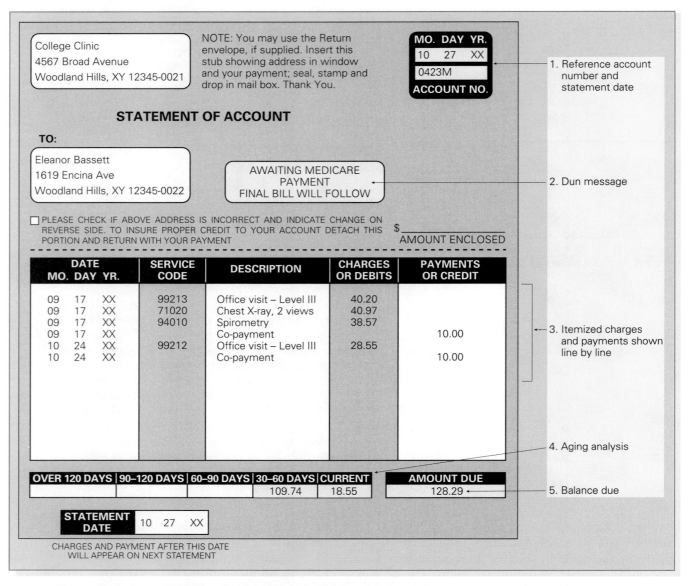

Figure 9–9. Computerized statement. (Courtesy of Bibbero Systems, Inc., Petaluma, CA. Phone: 800-242-2376; FAX 800-242-9330.)

calls from inquiring patients. One person or one department should handle all billing questions, ensuring a consistent response.

Age Analysis

Age analysis is a term used for the procedure of systematically arranging the A/R by age from the date of service. Accounts are usually aged in time periods of 30, 60, 90, and 120 days and older, as shown at the bottom of Figure 9–9. An aging analysis can be automatically done in a computer system. This helps collection follow-up by providing easy recognition of overdue accounts and allows the insurance specialist to determine which

accounts need action in addition to a regular statement. A decision tree showing time frames for sending statements and telephone calls is presented later in this chapter in Figure 9–10 under "Billing Guidelines."

Dun Messages

Dun messages are used on statements to promote payment (see Figs. 9–2 and 9–9). The best and most effective collection statements include a handwritten note; however, this is seldom possible. Dun messages can also be printed by the computer system or applied with brightly colored labels. Some examples of dun messages are:

▶ "If there is a problem with your account, please call me at (013) 486-0000—Marlayn."

▶ "This bill is now 30 days past due. Please remit payment."

▶ "This bill is now 60 days past due. Please send payment immediately."

▶ "Your account is 90 days past due. Please remit payment now to avoid collection action."

▶ "FINAL NOTICE: If we do not hear from you within 10 days, this account will be turned over to our collection agency."

Do not send intimidating, impatient, or threatening statements. These will only serve to antagonize patients. Dun messages should be included in different languages and sent to patients who speak English as a second language. Some examples are as follows:

▶ "No payment yet; your payment by return mail will be appreciated."

▶ "No hemos recibido pago. Agracieramos remita por correo."

▶ "Payment needed now. No further credit will be extended."

▶ "Se requiere pago hoy. No se le estendera mas credito."

Manual Billing

Manual billing is usually done by photocopying the patient's ledger and placing it in a window envelope. The ledger becomes the statement and should be clear and readable with no crossouts or misspellings. Typewritten statements may be used by small offices and are generally typed on continuous form paper. The completed statements are separated, folded, and placed into billing envelopes.

A coding system, with metal clip-on tabs or peel-off labels that are placed on the ledger card, can be used with a manual system. Each time the account is billed, a different color tab or label is placed on the ledger card, which shows, at a glance, how many times the account has been billed. It also provides aging of accounts, although a report, if desired, would have to be manually done in addition to this process.

Computer Billing

Computer billing is made possible by installing software that controls the A/R. All charges, payments, and adjustments are posted into the computer system by a medical assistant and these figures can be used to generate a hard copy, that is, statements and reports (see Fig. 9–9). The computer program usually offers choices of *billing types,* including patient billing, **insurance balance billing,** discounted billing, and no bill. The insurance specialist can instruct the computer to print all bills of a specific type. The computer can also be instructed to print bills according to *specific* accounts, specific dates, and specific insurance types. Accounts are automatically aged, and standard messages can be printed on the statements for each of the aged dates (30, 60, 90, or 120 days). Some systems allow personalized messages to be inserted, which override the standard messages.

Billing Services

Billing services are employed by many medical practices to reduce administrative paperwork by taking over the task of preparing and mailing patient statements. These services may also be employed to prepare and mail insurance claim forms or send them electronically. They may provide data entry of patients' demographic and billing information, charges, receipts, and adjustments; tracking of payments from patients and third party payers; production of management reports, purging of inactive accounts, and collection of accounts.

Some advantages of billing services are advanced technology, professional and understandable bills, experts answering all billing related telephone inquiries, and no downtime due to vacations, medical, or personal leave. This service allows the medical office to have fewer disruptions and the freedom from worry about financial matters when trying to provide medical care.

Billing services are paid by either a flat fee per account or by a percentage of the collection. If a percentage is charged, the billing service is not paid until the account is collected; this adds an additional incentive to promote collection.

The physician's office sends billing and receipt information into the system daily. This may be done in writing or through a computer system. The billing service then prepares the bills, mails them, and may also receive payments. A periodic report is sent to the physician summarizing the transactions. This service may also be called a statement service, centralized billing, or *outsourcing* (when the owner of a medical practice transfers the ownership of a partial or full process [billing, transcription, coding] to a supplier). When choosing a billing service, make a list of important questions and visit the facility. Also, visit a medical practice who has used their service for at least 3 years. The service's past performance is probably the best indicator of what you can expect in the future.

Billing Guidelines

Billing procedures are determined by the size of the practice, the number of accounts, and the number of staff members assigned to the collection process. Adopt a specific method of handling accounts and decide which billing routine best fits the practice. Check insurance and managed care contracts carefully to determine which circumstances allow for patients to be billed. If there is a need to bill managed care patients, be sure and conform to federal guidelines.

PROCEDURE: Seven-Step Billing and Collection Guideline

---

1. Present the *first statement* at the time of service. This can be a formal statement or a multipurpose billing form.
2. Mail the *second itemized statement* within 30 days of treatment. The phrase "due and payable within 10 days" should be printed on each statement. Local paycheck issuing patterns should be considered before selecting a date statements are to be mailed. Choose which billing routine the office will use:

▶ Monthly Billing: Using the monthly billing system, all statements are mailed at the same time during the month. Choose a mail-out day at the beginning of the month, so the patient will receive the bill near the 15th, or send statements near the end of the month, so the patient receives the bill on the 1st.

▶ Cycle Billing: **Cycle billing** is a system of billing accounts at spaced intervals during the month based on a breakdown of accounts by alphabet, account number, insurance type, or date of first service. This relieves the pressure of having to get all the statements out at one time and allows collection at a faster, more organized rate than accounts collected at random. It also allows continuous cash flow throughout the month and distributes the influx of incoming calls from patients about problem accounts. The number of cycles may be determined by how the collector wishes to divide the workload. Using *two cycles* per month, statements would be sent on the 25th to arrive by the 1st, and on the 10th, to arrive by the 15th of the month. Using *four cycles* per month, statements would be sent every Tuesday or Wednesday to arrive at the end of the week. If you use a cycle that was established by the first date of service, and the patient was first seen on the 11th of the month, then every month on the 11th he or she would receive a bill.

3. Send the *third statement* 30 days after the second statement was sent. Indicate the payment is past due.
4. Place the *first telephone* call to the patient. Ask if there is a problem. Ask for a payment commitment and set up a *suspense file.* Accounts are put in a suspense file for active follow-up. Action must be taken within the time frame mentioned, after you have so advised the patient.
5. Check for payment as promised. Allow 1 day for mail delay. Place the *second telephone call* to the patient and ask for payment. Set up a new payment date. Allow 5 days.
6. Check for payment as promised. Send a *10-day notice* advising the patient that unless payment is received in 10 days, the account will be turned over for legal action.
7. Check for payment. Promptly surrender the account for collection/legal action.

Figure 9–10 shows a Collection Decision Tree to be used when determining when to send statements, make telephone calls, send 10-day notices, and send accounts to a collection agency.

Credit Arrangements

Although payment at the time of service is ideal, many patients do not have funds available to pay at the time of the office visit. Alternative payment methods may be offered to help continuous cash flow and reduce collection costs.

Payment Options

Credit Card Billing

Credit card payment is an option that provides patients with an alternative to clear their account balances. Credit cards are issued by organizations that entitle the cardholder to credit at their establishments. This method of payment may be most useful as a down payment on uninsured or elective procedures. According to a survey by American Express, 33% of patients said they would use a credit card to pay for health care–related expenses if the option were given. Credit cards can help manage the A/R by improving cash flow, reducing billing costs, lowering overhead, and reducing the risk of bad debts. If a practice accepts credit cards, advise all patients in the following ways: display a credit card acceptance sign, include an insignia or

COLLECTION DECISION TREE

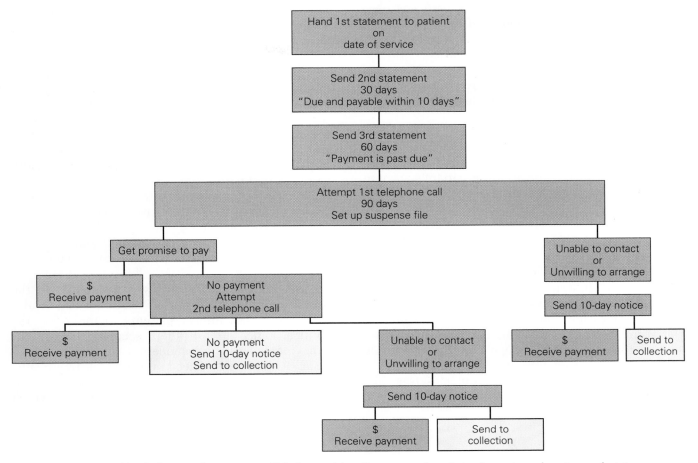

Figure 9–10. Collection decision tree. This is a quick reference used to help determine when to send statements, make telephone calls, and send accounts to a collection agency.

message on the statement, include the credit card policy in the new patient brochure, and have staff members verbalize to patients that this option is available. Patients may prefer to clear a debt immediately and make monthly payments to the credit card company instead of owing money to their doctor.

Verifying Credit Cards

A one- or two-physician office may have a simple credit card imprinter in the office. The insurance specialist should check credit card warning bulletins to make sure that the card has not been canceled or stolen. Large practices may have an electronic credit card machine that allows the insurance specialist to swipe the card through the machine that is linked to the credit card company. Transactions are then approved, processed, and deposited into a bank account, usually in 2 working days. These machines may be rented or purchased.

Verifone terminals are also used for credit card authorization. They are small computers with built-in software and modems for communicating with other computers over telephone lines. They have a small alphanumeric keypad and a small display screen that can show a line or two of data. This device reads the information off the magnetic card as it is swiped through the machine, dials a telephone number, connects with another computer, verifies the patient's credit, and displays a message.

Verifying Credit Cardholders

Always verify the cardholder by asking for a photo identification such as a driver's license. Examine the card carefully and observe the following guidelines:

▶ Accept a credit card only from the person whose name is on the card.

▶ Match the name on the card with the patient's other identification and make sure the expiration date has not passed.

- Look on the back of the card for the word "void." This will alert you if the card has been heated, which is a method used to forge a signature.
- Check the "hot list" for problem cards.
- Verify all charges regardless of the amount and get approval from the credit card company.
- Complete the credit card voucher (Fig. 9–11) before asking for a signature.
- Compare the signature on the credit card voucher against the signature on the card.
- Record the credit card number in the patient's financial file for future use if the patient's account has to be traced or transferred to a collection agency.

Credit Card Fees

Most banks will directly deposit the credit card voucher and subtract the monthly fees from the practice's bank account. A statement from the bank will indicate how much has been credited to the account. The fees can be negotiated based on volume, but will usually range from 2% to 5%. Do not issue cash or check refunds for any payments made by credit card. Credit vouchers (see Fig. 9–11), used for crediting a credit card account, are available at local banks. Patients who want to make payments may have their credit cards charged for each scheduled payment.

Credit Card Options

Other cards are also used for credit in a physician's office. *ATM cards* are sometimes accepted for medical care if the practice has a credit card scanner. *Private-label cards* are credit vehicles that can only be used to pay for health care. Some large practices offer their own private-label health cards. *Smart cards* are also used in some locations. They are small credit or debit cards that contain a computer chip that can store money in the form of electronic data. Special use smart cards for phone calls, gas stations, and fast food are now in use, as are common cards having multiple uses.

Visa offers a credit card service unique to the health care market. It has a Pre-Authorized Health Care Form that allows patients to authorize the medical office to bill their account directly for copayments and the balance not covered by insurance. Patients who need a series of treatments, such as allergy injections or chemotherapy, can fill out one form designating these services, which

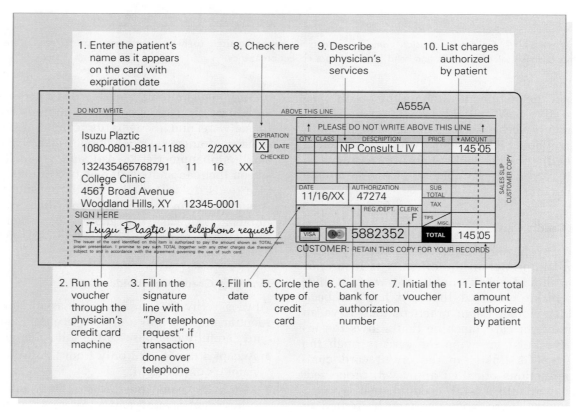

Figure 9–11. Credit card voucher; illustration of completion in a physician's office.

authorizes the staff to charge the patient's account directly.

A national medical card is now available for use by any professional or medical organization and enables the physician to offer a prearranged line of credit or an installment loan agreement by having the company take over the billing, accounting, and collecting for all patients who are approved for this service.

The convenience for patients and amount of reduced A/R should be weighed against the cost of setting up and operating this type of credit before making a decision about the use of credit cards in a medical practice.

Debit Cards

A **debit card** is a card permitting bank customers to withdraw cash at any hour from any affiliated automated teller machine (ATM) in the country. The holder may also make cashless purchases from funds on deposit without incurring revolving finance charges for credit. A small fee is charged to the customer's checking account when the card is used; however, this fee is usually applied only once a month (if the debit card is used) regardless of how many times the card is used during the month. Medical practices offering credit card payment may use the same electronic credit card machine to swipe the debit card for verification and approval. Separate debit card machines are also available for businesses that do not accept credit cards. Debit cards take the place of check writing; however, once the debit card is approved for a certain amount, the bank which issued the debit card is responsible for paying the funds that were approved. There are no returned checks for nonsufficient funds with this method of payment.

Payment Plans

Payment plans are another way of offering the patient a way of paying off an account by spreading out the amount due over a period of time. Caution should be taken when offering patients payment plans. The Truth in Lending Consumer Credit Cost Disclosure law (see Credit and Collection laws), also referred to as Regulation Z, requires and Collection full written disclosure regarding the finance charges for large payment plans involving four or more installments, excluding a down payment. This regulation does not apply, however, if the patient agrees to pay in one sum or in fewer than four payments and then decides independently to make drawn-out partial payments. Patients often think that if they make any amount of

PAYMENT PLAN SCHEDULE		
Balance due amount	Minimum monthly payment	Time frame for full payment
$0 – $200	$35	6 months
$201 – $500	$50	1 year
$500 – $1,000	$100	1 year
$1,001 – $3,000	$125	2 years
$3,001 – $5,000	$150	2 years
>$5,001*	$200	5 years

*Accounts over $5,000 must complete credit card application to certify minimum required payment and are subject to approval by office manager.

Figure 9–12. Payment plan schedule showing balance due amounts, minimum monthly payment, and payment time frames.

payment, the physician is required to accept that payment and not take any additional action. This is incorrect. The physician can take action, including sending the account to a collection agency. It is important to have a written payment plan schedule when working with accounts in which payment plans may be offered. Figure 9–12 illustrates sample guidelines that may be used or revised according to individual practice and management policies (Fig. 9–13).

Credit and Collection Laws

The following laws are important because they provide the legal framework within which the insurance specialist must execute the physician's collection policy. In addition, each state may have specific collection laws that are necessary to research and comply with.

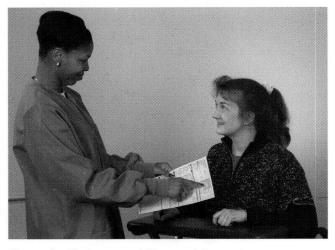

Figure 9–13. Insurance billing specialist setting up a payment plan with a patient.

Statute of Limitations

A formal regulation or law setting time limits on legal action is known as a **statute of limitations.** In regard to collections, the statute of limitations is the maximum time during which a legal collection suit may be rendered against a debtor. However, for a lawsuit to be successful, a concerted effort should be made to collect on an account from the time services are rendered. The patient should receive regular statements indicating that if the insurer does not pay, the patient will be held responsible.

To find out the statute of limitations for your state, refer to Figure 9–14. Statutes vary according to three kinds of accounts:

1. *Open book accounts* (also called open accounts): Accounts that are open to charges made from time to time. Payment is expected within a specific period but credit has been extended without a formal written contract. Physicians' patient accounts are usually open book accounts.
2. *Written contract accounts:* Accounts having a formal written agreement in which a patient signs to pay his or her bill in more than four installments (see Truth in Lending Act).
3. *Single-entry accounts:* Accounts having only one entry or charge; usually these are for a small amount.

Equal Credit Opportunity Act

The Equal Credit Opportunity Act, which is a federal law, prohibits discrimination in all areas of granting credit. If credit is offered, credit is to be available fairly and impartially to all patients who request it. Obtaining detailed credit information before performing services will prevent accusations of credit discrimination. New patients can be informed that payment is due at the time of service and, if they would like to establish credit for possible future treatment, they need to arrive 20 minutes early to fill out a credit application. Check all information with a credit bureau that will verify data such as the patient's address, previous addresses, length of residence, employment history, and approximate wage. The report will also contain the patient's name changes, the patient's bill-paying history, and any history of bankruptcy. If the patient has a poor credit rating, credit may be denied and the patient then has 60 days to request the reason in writing. The law prohibits discrimination against any applicant for credit for the following reasons:

▶ Age, color, marital status, national origin, race, religion, or sex
▶ He or she has exercised rights under consumer credit laws
▶ An applicant is receiving income from any public assistance program

Fair Credit Reporting Act

Agencies who either issue or use reports on consumers (patients) in connection with the approval of credit are regulated by the Fair Credit Reporting Act. The act states that credit reporting agencies can only provide reports when:

▶ A court order is issued
▶ The report is requested by the consumer (patient) or instructions are given by the patient to provide the report
▶ There is a legitimate business need for the information

If credit is refused, the physician must provide the patient with a reason credit was denied. Specific information about what the report contains is not required and should not be given. The provider must also give the name and address of the agency from which the report came. The patient must have an opportunity to correct any inaccuracies if they occur.

Fair Credit Billing Act

This law states that a patient has 60 days from the date a statement is mailed to complain about an error. The creditor must acknowledge the complaint within 30 days of receiving it. If an actual error occurred, the provider is required to correct the mistake within two complete billing cycles, or a maximum of 90 days. If the bill was correct, the accuracy must be explained to the patient.

Truth in Lending Act

The federal Truth in Lending Act (TILA) of 1969 is a consumer protection act that applies to anyone who charges interest or agrees on payment of a bill in more than four installments, excluding a down payment. When a specific agreement is reached between patient and physician, Regulation Z of this act requires that a written disclosure of all pertinent information be made, regardless of the existence of a finance charge (see Fig. 9–5). This full disclosure must be discussed at the time the agreement is first reached between patient and physician and credit is extended. It is essential to include the following items:

STATUTE OF LIMITATIONS*

State	Open Accts.	Contracts Written/Oral
Alabama	3	10
Alaska	6	6
Arizona	3	6/3
Arkansas	3	5/3
California	4	4/2
Colorado	6	6
Connecticut	6	6/3
Delaware	3	3
D.C.	3	3
Florida	4	5/4
Georgia	4	6/4
Hawaii	6	6
Idaho	4	5/4
Illinois	5	10/5
Indiana	6	10/6
Iowa	5	10/5
Kansas	3	5/3
Kentucky	5	15/5
Louisiana	3	10
Maine	6	6
Maryland	3	3
Massachusetts	6	6
Michigan	6	6
Minnesota	6	6
Mississippi	3	3/3
Missouri	5	10/5
Montana	5	8/5
Nebraska	4	5/4
Nevada	4	6/4
New Hamp.	6	6
New Jersey	6	6
New Mexico	4	6/4
New York	6	6
N. Carolina	3	3
N. Dakota	6	6
Ohio	6/15*	15/6
Oklahoma	3	5/3
Oregon	6	6
Pennsylvania	6	6/4
Rhode Island	10	10
S. Carolina	3	3
S. Dakota	6	6
Tennessee	6	6
Texas	4	4
Utah	4	6/4
Vermont	6	6
Virginia	3	5/3
Washington	3	6/3
West Virginia	5	10/5
Wisconsin	6	6
Wyoming	8	10/8

*6 oral/15 written

Figure 9–14. Individual state time limits (Statute of Limitations on Civil Actions) for collection of open accounts and oral/written contracts. (Abstracted from Summary of Collection Laws. Reprinted with permission of the American Collectors Association, Inc., 2000. All rights reserved.)

1. Total amount of the debt
2. Amount of down payment
3. Finance charge
4. Interest rate expressed as an annual percentage
5. Amount of each payment
6. Date each payment is due
7. Date final payment is due
8. Signature of patient and physician with copies retained by both

According to the Federal Trade Commission (FTC), the Truth in Lending provision is not applicable and no disclosures are required if a patient decides on his or her own to pay in installments or whenever convenient.

Late Payment Charges

Medical practices that implement late payment charges that meet the criteria defined in the TILA as a finance charge must comply with a host of requirements that revolve around proper disclosure to patients.

Charges must meet the following criteria to qualify as late payment charges:

1. The account balance must be required to be paid in full at the time of initial billing.
2. The account is treated as delinquent when unpaid.
3. The charge will be assessed to a patient's account *only* because of his or her failure to make timely payments.
4. Installments are limited to no more than three.
5. The creditor (physician/insurance specialist) makes a "commercially reasonable" effort to collect these accounts.

When a physician continues to treat a patient with an overdue account, the courts have viewed this as continuation of care and an *extension of credit*. Patients who fall into this delinquent status should be referred elsewhere. See Chapter 3 (Termination of a Case) for instructions on sending a discharge letter. After the patient has paid the overdue amount, the patient can be taken back and treated on a cash-only basis.

Truth in Lending Consumer Credit Cost Disclosure

The Truth in Lending Consumer Credit Cost Disclosure is similar to the Federal Truth in Lending Act. It requires businesses to disclose all direct and indirect costs and conditions related to the granting of credit. All interest charges, late charges, collection fees, finance charges, and so forth must be explained up front, prior to the time of service. To charge interest and bill the patient monthly, include the following on all statements:

▶ Amount of each payment
▶ Due date
▶ Unpaid balance at the beginning of the billing period
▶ Finance charges
▶ Date balance is due

Fair Debt Collection Practices Act

The Fair Debt Collection Practices Act (FDCPA) was designed to address the collection practices of third party debt collectors and attorneys who regularly collect debts for others. Although this act does not apply directly to physician practices

collecting for themselves, a professional health care collector must avoid the actions that are prohibited for collection agencies. The main intent of the act is to protect consumers from unfair, harassing, or deceptive collection practices. Refer to the guidelines in Table 9–2 which are taken from the FDCPA to help avoid illegalities, enhance collections, and maintain positive patient relations. For more information about collection laws in your state, contact your state attorney general's office. If there is a conflict between state and federal laws, the stricter law prevails.

The Collection Process

For collections to be handled effectively, staff members need to be trained in collection techniques. Most insurance specialists can be trained to be efficient collectors when given the correct tools. New collectors need time to gain confidence, which is an important aspect of being a good collector.

Office Collection Techniques

Telephone Debt Collection

Telephone collections are made easier if the insurance billing specialist is convinced that he or she can collect before trying to convince the patient to pay. Two important factors to consider are the insurance specialist's ability to contact the patient and the patient's ability to pay the bill. Contact the patient in a timely manner at the first sign of payment delay. Prepare before making a telephone collection call by reviewing the account and noting anything unusual. Determine where the patient is employed, or if unemployed. Decide what amount you will settle for if you cannot get payment in full. Make the first call count. Act in a calm, business-like manner and combine empathy with diligence. Be positive and persuasive. Listen to what the patient has to say, even if he or she gets angry and raises his or her voice. Lower the volume of your voice and respond in a composed manner. Try to pick up clues from what the patient is saying; he or she may be giving you the real reason for nonpayment. Ask questions, show interest, and let the patient know that he or she is being listened to. Respond in a respectful manner and carefully word your reply; when patients are distressed they do not always make sense. Your goal is to encourage the patient to pay, not agitate the patient. Use all resources and learn to negotiate.

TABLE 9–2	**Fair Debt Collection Practices Act Guidelines**

1. Contact debtors only once a day; in some states, repeated calls in one day or in the same week could be considered harassment.
2. Place calls after 8 A.M. and before 9 P.M.
3. Do not contact debtors on Sunday or any other day that the debtor recognizes as a Sabbath.
4. Identify yourself and the medical practice you represent; do not mislead the patient.
5. Contact the debtor at work *only* if unable to contact the debtor elsewhere; no contact should be made if the employer or debtor disapproves.
6. Contact the attorney, if an attorney represents the debtor; contact the debtor only if the attorney does not respond.
7. Do not threaten or use obscene language.
8. Do not send post cards for collection purposes; keep all correspondence strictly private.
9. Do not call collect or cause additional expense to the patient.
10. Do not leave a message on an answering machine indicating that you are calling about a bill.
11. Do not contact a third party more than once, unless requested to do so by the party or the response was erroneous or incomplete.
12. Do not convey to a third party that you are calling about a debt.
13. Do not contact the debtor when notified in writing that a debtor refuses to pay and would like contact to stop, except to notify the debtor that there will be no further contact or that there will be legal action.
14. Stick to the facts; do not use false statements.
15. Do not prepare a list of "bad debtors" or "credit risks" to share with other health care providers.
16. Take action immediately when stating a certain action will be taken (e.g., filing a claim in small claims court or sending the patient to a collection agency).
17. Send the patient written verification of the name of the creditor and the amount of debt within 5 days of the initial contact.

Use an organized approach to determine which collection calls to make first. Print out the A/R by age and target the accounts that are in the 60- to 90-day category. The most effective results come from this group. If you use ledger cards, pull all the cards with tabs or labels that indicate the patient has received two or three statements depending on office protocol. Start with the largest amount owed and work the accounts in decreasing amounts owed. After this category has been completed, move on to the 90- to 120-day accounts. Finally, go after accounts that are more than 120 days old.

According to collection experts, the best time to telephone is between 5:30 P.M. and 8:30 P.M. on Tuesdays and Thursdays and 9 A.M. to 1 P.M. on Saturdays. However, regardless of when you call, track the times you are able to contact the most patients and adjust your calling schedule accordingly. The physician's office hours may need to be increased to include one evening a week or Saturday mornings to make collection calls. Another option would be the use of flex time in which the employee can choose his or her own working hours from within a broad range of hours approved by management. Use a private phone away from the busy operations of the office to eliminate interruptions. Patients may be embarrassed about not being able to pay their bills and patient confidentiality must be maintained. Follow the rules stated in the Fair Debt Collection Practices Act.

Be alert for new ideas or approaches to collection by watching how banks and other retailers implement sophisticated collection skills. Decide if any of these could be used to the medical practice's advantage and present the techniques to the office manager. Keep abreast of improvements made to collection software that will improve collection results and allow more collectors to work from their homes. Other advances, such as call block, which is an expanded telephone service, have made it more difficult to make collection calls. This service was originally intended to screen out unwanted telemarketing calls by intercepting blocked, unlisted, or unknown numbers. Standard numbers are usually allowed to go through. The key to averting a block is to make sure the number the call is being placed from is listed and within the patient's area. Telephone company's services vary, so research to discover all expanded services used in your area.

PROCEDURE: Telephone Collection Plan

Following are steps to assist in making the first collection call:

1. Set the mood of the call by the manner in which you speak and the tone of your voice. The first 30 seconds of the call will set the scene for your relationship with the patient.
2. Identify the patient. Be certain you are talking to the debtor before revealing the nature of the call.
3. Identify yourself and your facility.
4. Verify the debtor's address and any telephone numbers.
5. State the reason you are calling.
6. Take control of the conversation and establish urgency by asking for full payment *now;* disclose the full amount owed.
7. Ask when payment will be made, how it will be made, and if it will be sent by' mail or in person.
8. Pause for effect; this turns the conversation back to the patient to respond to the demand or to tell you why payment has not been made. Never assume if a patient does not respond, it means no.
9. Find out if the patient needs clarification of the bill.
10. Inquire if the patient has a problem. Ask if the practice can be of assistance, especially when the patient is unable to give a reason for non-payment.
11. Question the patient by stating "How much are you willing to pay?", "Do you have a regular paycheck?", and "Will payment be made through a checking account?" if the patient is reluctant to agree to an amount.
12. Obtain a promise to pay with an agreeable amount and a due date; be clear how and when payment is expected, but give the patient a choice of action.
13. Ask for one half of the amount if full payment is not possible.
14. Discuss a payment plan if the patient is not able to pay half of the balance owed. Be realistic and reasonable. It is self-defeating to set up payment arrangements the patient cannot afford. Advise the patient that if the payment is even 1 day late, the entire balance becomes due and payable. Ask the patient to please call you before the due date with an explanation if any problems arise that prevent payment.
15. Restate the importance of the agreement.
16. Tell the patient to write down the amount and due date.
17. Document the agreement on the patient's ledger, in the computer, or in a collection telephone log. Note the time you spoke to the patient.
18. Send confirmation of the agreement (Fig. 9–15).
19. Check the account the day after the payment was due; allow 1 day for mail delay. If the patient fails to make payment as promised, make another telephone call and ask the patient if there is still a problem. Get a new commitment to pay and confirm again. If the patient continues to avoid payment, advise the patient that the account will be turned over to a collection agency and follow through as stated.

Telephone "Don'ts"

Following is a list of "DO NOTs" for telephone collections:

◗ Do not raise your voice and antagonize the patient.
◗ Do not accuse the patient of dishonesty or lying.
◗ Do not act like a "tough guy" or threaten a patient.
◗ Do not consent to partial payments until you have asked for payment in full and do not agree to a long string of small partial payments.
◗ Do not engage in a debate.
◗ Do not report a disputed account to a collection agency or bureau until you disclose the patient's dispute as part of the record.

Telephone collection calls are also effective the day before patients are due for their appointments. State the date and time of the appointment and then remind the patient of the balance owed and ask if he or she would please bring payment to the appointment.

Telephone Collection Scenarios

The most difficult part of one-on-one collections is preparing for the many situations you may encounter and the various responses the patient may make. Following are some statements patients make for not paying an account and examples of responses the insurance specialist can make.

Statement: "I can't pay anything now."

Response: "Are you employed? Are you receiving unemployment compensation, welfare, or Social Security benefits?"

You are determining the patient's ability to pay.

"Are you paying some of your bills?" You are uncovering the fact that the

COLLEGE CLINIC
4567 Broad Avenue
Woodland Hills, XY 12345-0001
Tel. (013) 486-9002
FAX (013) 487-8976

October 2, 20XX

Mr. Leonard Blabalot
981 McCort Circle
Woodland Hills, XY 12345-0001

Dear Mr. Blabalot:

I am glad we had an opportunity to discuss your outstanding balance with our practice during our phone conversation on October 1, 20XX. This will confirm and remind you that you agreed to pay $100 on your account on or before October 15, 20XX.

A return envelope is enclosed for your convenience.

Sincerely,

Charlotte Rose Routingham
Business Office

Enc. envelope

Figure 9–15. Telephone confirmation letter sent to remind patient of the terms agreed to in a telephone conversation.

patient is paying certain bills. You can then tell the patient that your bill must be taken care of, also, even if only a small amount at a time.

Statement: "I can't pay the whole bill now."

Response: "How much are you able to pay?" or "Can you pay half of the amount?"
Ask this instead of "How much can you pay?"

Statement: "I can pay, but not until next month."

Response: "When do you get paid?"
Ask for payment the day after payday.
"Do you have a checking account?"
Ask for a postdated check.

Statement: "I have other bills."

Response: "This is also one of your bills that needs to be paid now. Let's talk about exactly how you plan payment."

Statement: "How about $10 a month (on a $350 bill)?"

Response: "I'd like to accept that, but our accountant does not allow us to stretch out payments beyond 90 days, which would be $105 a month."
This adheres to (Truth in Lending Law) regulations for collecting payment in installments without a written agreement. If the patient tries to cooperate, then compromise. If not, turn the account over to a collection agency.

Statement: "I sent in the payment."

Response: "When was the payment sent? To what address was it sent? Was it a check? On what bank was it drawn and for what amount? What is the canceled check number?"
Investigate to see if the check was posted to a wrong account. If not, call the patient back and ask if he or she would call his or her bank to see if it cleared; and if it has not, the patient should stop payment. Ask the patient to call you back and let you know the status of the check. If the patient is lying, he or she will not follow through. Ask for a new check to be sent and

tell the patient a refund will be made if the other one shows up.

Statement: "I cannot make a payment this month."

Response: "The collection agency picks up all our delinquent accounts next Monday. I don't want to include yours, but I need a check today."

Statement: "The check's in the mail."

Response: "May I have the check number and date it was mailed?"
Call back in 3 days if not received.

Statement: "I'm not going to pay the bill because the doctor didn't spend any time with me."

Response: "May I confirm the doctor you saw, the date and time? For what reason did you see the doctor? Do you still have the problem for which you saw the doctor?"
Get as much information as possible and research the office schedule the day the patient was seen. Let the doctor know about the patient's complaint

and inquire how he or she would like to handle the complaint.

Statement: "I thought the insurance company was paying this."

Response: "Your insurance paid most of the bill, now the balance is your responsibility. Please send your check before Friday to keep your account current."
Explain why—deductible, copayment, benefit not covered under the insurance plan.

Collection Letters

Collection letters are another method of reaching patients and reminding them of their debt. Knowledge of the patient base and of individual patients may help determine the effectiveness of collection letters. Every facility is unique, and the number of accounts, the geographic spread of patients, the staff size, and the amount of time collectors have to spend on individual accounts will help determine which collection method best suits the practice.

Some positive aspects of collection letters are the following: they can reach a large number of patients rapidly and the cost is relatively low (especially if form letters are used; Fig. 9–16).

Figure 9–16. Form collection letter sent to all patients who have not responded after two billing cycles.

COLLEGE CLINIC
4567 Broad Avenue
Woodland Hills, XY 12345-0001
Tel. (013) 486-9002
FAX (013) 487-8976

November 13, 20XX

Miss Melanie Markham
1001 Swallow Lane
Woodland Hills, XY 12345-0001

Dear Miss Markham:

It is the office policy of College Clinic to contact patients who have received two billing statements but have not responded. We realize this could be an oversight on your part, not a willful disregard of an assumed obligation. If you have a financial problem or a question about your account, please call me at (013) 486-9002 extension 443 or stop by our office.

We would like to thank you in advance for your cooperation in attending to this matter.

Sincerely,

Shirley Summer, CMA
Clarance Cutler, MD

Some negative aspects of collection letters are that letters usually take 2 or 3 days to reach the patient and may lie unopened for a week or more, letters are one-way communication, thus lacking the ability to provide you with the reason for non-payment, the response and recovery through letters are relatively poor, and manual preparation takes time (especially if a decision must be made before sending each letter).

The insurance specialist is often the one to compose collection letters and devise a plan for collection follow-up. A series of collection letters may be written using varying degrees of forcefulness, starting with a gentle reminder. When you write a collection letter, use a friendly tone and ask why payment has not been made. Imply that the patient has good intentions to pay. You may do this by suggesting that the patient has overlooked a previous statement. Communicate the doctor's sincere interest in the patient. Always invite the patient to explain the reason for nonpayment, either in a letter, telephone call, or a visit to the office. It should sound as though the patient is just as anxious as you are to clear the debt.

When collection letters are sent toward the end of the year, include a statement letting the patient know that if the account is paid in full by the end of the year, the medical expense may be used as an income tax deduction. Another tactic is to send a notice advising the patient that he or she may skip December's payment due to increased expenses during the holidays. This tactic may be used as an opportunity to build patient relations, but the collector must be firm and clear when offering such leeway. Collection letters sent after the first of the year can suggest that the patient clear the debt by using their income tax refund check.

Types of Collection Letters

There are several styles of collection letters. A form letter saves time and can go out automatically at specific times during the billing cycle (see Fig. 9–16). Letters with checklists are a type of form letter (Fig. 9–17) that makes it easier for the patient to choose a payment option. Personally typed letters can be individualized to suit any situation. Collection letters should contain the following information:

▶ Full amount owed
▶ Services performed
▶ What action the patient should take
▶ Time frame in which the patient should respond
▶ How the patient should take care of the bill
▶ Why the patient should take care of the bill
▶ Address to which patients send payment

▶ Telephone number to contact the office
▶ Contact person's name
▶ Signature, which can be listed as "Financial Secretary," "Insurance Specialist," "Assistant to Doctor _____," or your name and title with the physician's name below.

When pursuing collection, the insurance specialist should stay within the authorization of the physician. All letters should be noted on the back of the ledger, in the collection log, or in the computer comment area. Abbreviations can be used to indicate which letter was sent (Table 9–3) along with the date the letter was mailed. Letters can be sent in brightly colored envelopes to attract attention. The envelope should include "Address Service Requested," or "Forwarding Service Requested" on the outside to ensure the letter is forwarded if the patient has moved so that the office will be notified of the patient's new address. Always include a self-addressed stamped envelope.

Collection Abbreviations

Collection abbreviations can be used to save time and space while documenting efforts to collect and patients' responses. A few of the most common abbreviations are listed in Table 9–3. Always use standard abbreviations so anyone working on the account will know exactly what attempts have been made to collect and what action has been taken. Figure 9–18 illustrates some abbreviated collection entries, with interpretations, on the back of a ledger.

Insurance Collection

Most patients carry some form of insurance; however, filing an insurance claim is only the first step in collecting fees owed. Good follow-up techniques (see Chapter 8) are required to ensure payment from the insurance carrier and copayment or coinsurance payment from the patient.

First, affirm that a clean insurance claim was sent with all necessary precertification, preauthorization, and documentation for services. Next, follow up in a timely manner with telephone calls and written tracers. Track all denials to learn what services are being denied and which insurance companies are denying payment. It is worth investing money and staff resources to identify the cause of claim denials. Send all high-dollar claims by certified mail to alleviate the problem of the insurance company saying that "it was never received." This saves time and is cost effective.

COLLEGE CLINIC
4567 Broad Avenue
Woodland Hills, XY 12345-0001
Tel. (013) 486-9002
FAX (013) 487-8976

March 16, 20XX

Mr. Frank Lincoln
3397 Westminster Avenue
Woodland Hills, XY 12345-0001

Account No.   593287
Amount Due: $ _____

Dear Mr. Lincoln:

The care of our patients is more important than writing letters about overdue accounts. Yet, as you must realize, the expense of furnishing care can only be met by payments from appreciative patients.

Your account is seriously past due and has been removed from our current files because of its delinquent status. Our office policy indicates that your account should be placed with a collection agency. However, we would prefer to hear from you regarding your preference in this matter.

Enclosed is a current statement of your account. Please indicate your payment choice.

☐ I would prefer to settle this account immediately. Please find payment in full enclosed.

☐ I would prefer to make monthly payments (up to six months). To exercise this option please call and make arrangements to come into our office to sign a financial agreement.

☐ Please charge the full amount to my credit card. (We accept American Express, MasterCard, and Visa). To exercise this option, please telephone our office or fill in the enclosed form and return it with the envelope provided.

_____   _____
        Signature   Date

Please select one of the three options above, sign the form, and return this notice within 10 days from the date indicated in the letter. A postmarked return envelope is provided. Failure to respond will result in an automatic referral to our collection agency. Please do not hesitate to call if you have any questions regarding this matter.

Sincerely,

Gil Steinberg
Office Manager

Enc. Envelope, Credit Card Agreement Form

Figure 9–17. Multipurpose collection letter with checklist. Advises patient of a seriously past due account, offers the patient three payment options, and warns the patient that failure to respond will result in a referral to a collection agency.

History of Accounts

If the insurance company seems to be ignoring all efforts to trace the claim, an exact history of the account may be the best weapon with which to proceed. A history of the account is a chronologic record of all events that have occurred. Keep all communications received from the insurance company, note all telephone calls, and keep copies of all documents sent. Send a copy of the history of the account directly to the insurance company and demand a reply. This may also be done in the case of an insurance company dispute or a refusal to pay.

Coinsurance Payments

Use a letter or statement to collect from patients who have insurance coverage. Clearly indicate to the patient that the insurance biller has submitted an insurance claim and advise the patient what action is expected. The status of the insurance claim should be noted on all statements.

TABLE 9-3	**Collection Abbreviations**				

ATTY	Attorney		NSN	No such number	
B	Bankrupt		OFC	Office	
Bal	Balance		OOT	Out of town	
Bk*	Bank		OOW	Out of work	
BLG	Belligerent		PA	Payment arrangement	
BTTR	Best time to reach		PH or PH'D	Phoned	
CB	Call back		Ph/Dsc*	Phone disconnected	
CLM	Claim		PIF	Payment in full	
DA*	Directory assistance		PIM	Payment in mail	
DFB	Demand for Balance		PMT	Payment	
DNK	Did not know		POE	Place of employment	
DSC	Disconnected		POLK†	Polk directory	
EMP	Employment		POW	Payment on way	
EOM	End of month		PP	Promise to pay or partial payment	
EOW	End of Week		PT	Patient	
FA	Further action		RCD	Received	
FN	Final notice		R/D*	Reverse directory	
H	He (or husband)		RE	Regarding	
HHCO	Have husband call office		RES	Residence	
HSB	Husband		S	She (or wife)	
HTO	He telephoned office		SEP	Separated	
HU	Hung up		SK*	Skip or skipped	
INS	Insurance		SOS	Same old story	
LI, L2	Letter one, letter two (sent)		SP/DEL*	Special delivery	
LB	Line busy		STO	She telephoned office	
LD	Long distance		T	Telephoned	
LM	Left message		TB	Telephoned business	
LMCO	Left message, call office		TR	Telephoned residence	
LMVM	Left message, voice mail		TT	Talked to	
LTR	Letter		TTA	Turned to agency	
MR	Mail return		UE	Unemployed	
NI, N2	Note one, note two (sent)		U/Emp	Unemployed	
NA	No answer		UTC	Unable to contact	
N/B*	Nearby or neighbors (no phone listing)		VFD	Verified	
NFA*	No forwarding address		Vfd/E	Verified employment	
NHD*	Never heard of debtor		Vfd/I	Verified insurance	
NI	Not in		W/	Will	
NLE	No longer employed		WCO	Will call office	
NPL	No phone listed		WCIO	Will come in office	
NPN	Nonpublished number		W/I	Walk-in	
NR	No record		WVO	Will visit office	
NSF	Not sufficient funds		X	By	

*Used in skip tracing
†Directories used to locate patients by street address or telephone number

Notify patients promptly when insurance payment has been received. Ask patients to get involved in the insurance process or to pay the bill within 10 days if a problem exists. Following are examples of notations on statements for patients with insurance coverage:

▸ "We have received payment from your insurance company. The balance of $_____ is now your responsibility."

▸ "Your insurance company has paid its share of your bill. This statement is for the amount payable directly by you."

▸ "Your insurance company has paid $_____ for the above services. The remaining portion of $_____ is now your responsibility."

▸ "The balance of this account is your share of the cost. Please remit today. For questions, call 486-9002."

Figure 9–18. Back of ledger card showing examples of abbreviated collection entries with interpretation.

Comments:	Interpretation:
3/21/20XX Vfd/E, Vfd/I, LMCO 10:00 am.	Verified employment; verified insurance; left message to call the office
3/22/20XX NA 3:00 p.m.	No answer at 3:00 p.m.
3/23/20XX T, H, PP X 4/1/20XX	Telephoned husband, promised to pay by 4/1/20XX

Due and payable within 10 days.

12-17-20XX NP
1-17-20XX Billed Pt
2-17-20XX Billed Pt–3rd 6
3-17-20XX Billed Pt–4th 90 day
4-1-20XX ROA Pt ck #693

Key: PF: Problem-focused   SF: Straightfo[rward]
EPF: Expanded problem focused   LC: Low complex[ity]
D: Detailed   MC: Moderate compl[exity]
C: Comprehensive   HC: High complexity

▶ "Your insurance company has not responded. The account is due and payable. Please contact your insurance company about payment. Thank you for your assistance."

Insurance Checks Sent to Patients

Send a letter immediately to notify patients who receive insurance checks (see Chapter 8). Advise such patients that you are aware that they have received payment from their insurance company and that their account is due and payable within 10 days. Do not send continuous monthly bills; instead speed up the collection process. If the patient refuses to pay and the physician does not want the patient to return, send a 10-day notification advising the patient that the account will go to a collection agency and if no response discharge the patient from the practice.

Managed Care Organizations

When a medical practice deals with several managed care organizations, it can get confusing trying to remember all the contract information. A managed care desk reference (see Chapter 10) can help staff members find information quickly. "Promised payment date" along with all the other information on the desk reference grid or matrix can be easily referred to by the insurance specialist when trying to collect from managed care organizations.

Make sure all referral authorizations are in place before the patient is to be seen. If a patient shows up without a referral, offer to reschedule or inform the patient that the visit must be paid for, in cash before leaving the office. If the patient has no money, a promissory note may be executed, but this action is not preferred and would be carried out as a last option.

When dealing with managed care contracts, do not sign any contract that holds a third party "harmless." The "hold harmless" clause is a way for one party to shift financial responsibilities to another party. Such "hold harmless" clauses often include phrases that state the third party be "held harmless" to pay claims, liabilities, costs, expenses, judgments, and/or damages awarded by any court to all patients who bring any legal action against the medical practice. If the third party goes out of business or goes bankrupt before the contract is honored, the physician cannot collect any money from the patient that the third party was to have paid. To avoid such possibilities, make sure all managed care organizations keep current on payments.

Check to see that all third party payers are insured by a federal agency. Such insurance would pay the physician in the event the managed care organization could not. In Chapter 10, you will learn more about managed care bankruptcy.

Medicare

A provider must make genuine collection efforts to collect the unpaid deductible and coinsurance amounts from all Medicare patients. Reasonable efforts must include subsequent billings, telephone calls, and in-person collection efforts done in the same manner as with all patients. Accounts may not be written off until sequential statements (spaced 15 to 30 days apart) have been sent with an increasing intensity in the collection message. A telephone call should be placed to the debtor asking for payment, as well as requesting payment when the patient is seen in person.

Medigap Insurance

When a patient has Medigap insurance, make sure the patient's signature appears in Blocks 12 and 13 of the HCFA-1500 insurance claim form. Do not routinely enter "signature on file" unless the insured has signed an insurance specific statement authorizing release of medical information and payment of benefits to the physician named on the claim form. A signed statement allowing the physician to bill for and receive payment on Medigap-covered services until the beneficiary revokes authorization is preferred. A Medicare "signature on file" is not sufficient.

Workers' Compensation

Verify the validity of work-related injury and illness through the patient's employer and obtain accurate billing information. Send timely bills and reports using the correct coding system and fee schedule. Always keep the adjuster assigned to the case informed of ongoing treatment. The patient and employer should both be notified if a problem exists. Document all correspondence, including telephone authorizations for treatment and any tracing efforts. Any disputed or unresolved workers' compensation cases may be revised to self-pay, referred to a Financial Service Representative, or referred to the proper state-level authority. The physician may file for mediation on behalf of the patient if proper authorization was obtained and a claim form sent at the time of the patient's treatment. A claim may also be filed with the state labor board naming the patient's employer and workers' compensation carrier whenever there is difficulty getting full payment. The industrial board will often get the employer to pressure the carrier to resolve the matter. If an insurance company has not paid, or sent a written notice of nonpayment, the provider may file a request for default judgment from the state authority. If the judgment is in the provider's favor, the payer is ordered to pay in full. See Chapter 14 for more information on delinquent workers' compensation claims.

Suing an Insurance Carrier

As stated earlier under Statute of Limitations, there are time periods during which an insured person may sue the insurance company to collect the amount the claimant believes is owed. An insured person may not initiate a legal action against the insurer until 60 days after the initial claim has been submitted. A lawsuit against the insurer must be filed within 3 years of the date the initial claim was submitted for payment.

With regard to the physician's office trying to collect from an insurance plan, when the insurance company does not respond to reason or negotiation, the only alternatives are surrender or litigation. If a high-dollar claim is in question, a lawsuit may be worthwhile. Insurance carriers may be sued for payment under two circumstances: *claim for plan benefits/breach of contract* and *claim for damages.*

Claim for plan benefits is used when the claim is governed by the Employee Retirement Income Security Act (ERISA), a Federal Employee Health Benefit Act (FEHBA). ERISA governs health insurance provided as a benefit of employment. FEHBA governs all health insurance provided as a benefit to federal employees. Under these two federal laws, an insured is entitled to appeal a denied claim. A timely request must be filed to sue for payment. The time limit for ERISA is within 60 days, and for FEHBA it is within 6 months of denial. The federal laws apply across the country and overrule all state laws. Suits based on claims for plan benefits may be made when denial is based on the following:

▶ Medical necessity
▶ Preexisting condition
▶ Usual and customary rate issues
▶ Providers or facilities that are not covered
▶ Services that fall within an exclusion to coverage
▶ Failure to offer COBRA by a plan administrator

When the claim falls outside of the scope of these federal laws, it is possible to sue if the conduct of the payer constitutes a violation of state laws relating to unfair insurance practices.

Suing on the basis of claim for damages falls entirely under state law. This is most likely to occur if the patient has no plan benefit but the patient or physician's office is led to believe so by the insurer or plan administrator. Examples may include the following:

▶ Insurer misquoting benefits during a verification of those benefits
▶ Denial of payment due to lack of medical necessity when preauthorization of treatment was obtained

Collection Agencies

Delinquent accounts should be turned over to a collection agency only after all reasonable attempts have been made to collect by the physician's office. Knowing when to turn accounts over will help determine the success of the collection agency. The longer the unpaid balance remains in the physician's office, the less chance the agency has to collect the account, so the determination that an account is uncollectable needs to be made quickly. Some guidelines are:

▶ When a patient states that he or she will not pay or there is a denial of responsibility
▶ When a patient breaks a promise to pay
▶ When a patient makes partial payments and 60 days have lapsed without payment
▶ When a patient fails to respond to the physician's letters or telephone calls
▶ When payment terms fail for no valid reason
▶ When a check is returned by the bank due to insufficient funds and the patient does not make an effort to rectify the situation within 1 week of notification
▶ When delinquency coexists with marital problems, divorce proceedings, or child support agreements

▶ When a patient is paid by the insurance company and does not forward the payment to the physician (this constitutes fraud and may be pursued with legal action)
▶ When a patient gives false information
▶ When a patient moves and the office has used all resources to locate the patient

Not all accounts should go to a collection agency. Such accounts include those of personal friends, elderly widows or widowers living on pensions, and accounts with balances under $25. Many physicians prefer to adjust small bad debts off of the books rather than to increase administrative costs. All disputed accounts should be reviewed and approved by the physician before going to collection. There should be a systematized approach for turning accounts over to a collection agency that still allows room for an exception, should one occur.

Choosing an Agency

A collection agency should be chosen with great care because it is a reflection of the medical practice. Choose a reputable agency that is considerate and efficient with a high standard of ethics. The agency should specialize in physician accounts and have an attitude toward debtors with which the physician agrees. Find out how long the agency has been in business and request a list of at least 10 references and statistics on their collection effectiveness. The average collection rate varies greatly but falls between 20% to 60% on assigned accounts. Be sure the report rate includes all accounts more than 1 year old and does not exclude accounts with small balances.

An agency's performance can be evaluated by the amount collected, less the agency's fees, which is called the "**netback**." For instance, if the collector recovered 25% of $5,000 ($1,250) and takes a 50% commission, the physician's netback is $625. If the collector recovered 25% of the $5,000 ($1,000) and charged a 30% commission, the netback would be $667. Although the second agency collected less, its lower commission afforded the physician more money.

The biggest key to the agency's effectiveness is the doctor's own credit and collection policy. A comprehensive patient registration form along with verifying employment, turning accounts over quickly when they qualify, and giving the agency all the available information will help the agency pick up the paper trail and secure payment. A good collection agency will have membership in a national collection society and the approval of the local medical society. Review the agency's financial statement and make sure the agency is licensed, bonded, and carries "hold harmless clause" insurance. If a patient should sue because of harassment, this insurance will protect the physician from also being sued. The local bar association and state licensing bureaus can be contacted to see if any complaints have been lodged against the agency or law firm. Find out if the agency reports uncollectable debtors ("deadbeats") to a credit agency, and investigate which one is used.

Types of Agencies

There are local agencies, regional agencies, and national agencies. National agencies and ones that use the Internet may have better results tracing skips. Local agencies are more aware of the socioeconomic status of patients. Some agencies pay their staff commissions and bonuses for high productivity, and others are low key and more customer oriented. Find out the experience level of the staff and make sure the agency values the physician's business.

Another option is to use a collection service such as CollectNet. CollectNet gives small and mid-sized facilities with limited budgets the collection capabilities of large collection systems by connecting to databases. The medical practice is able to make calling lists, print collection letters, search for telephone numbers and addresses, access patient credit reports, write and format reports, monitor collection progress, and set automatic callback reminders. Optional features include BankruptcyNet, SkipNet, LetterNet, and BureauNet. Collection agencies use this service, but it is also available to large groups and clinics.

Agency Operating Techniques

Collection agencies must follow all the laws stated in the Fair Debt Collection Practices Act. They may not "harass" the debtor or make false threats and may not use letters that appear to be legal documents. A provision should be included for the agency to seek permission from the physician's office before suing a debtor in municipal court and charging a percent of the judgment. A progress report should be provided to the physician's office on a regular basis, at least monthly. The agency should also return any uncollectable accounts to the physician's office within a reasonable time and not charge for these accounts. If a debtor moves, ask if the account is forwarded to another collection office. All procedures used to make collections should be shown to the physician's office, including collection letters and telephone script. The physician's office should be aware if the agency uses a personalized approach or a standard approach. A personal visit to the premises of the collection agency can provide a first-hand view of its operating techniques.

Agency Charges

Agencies may be paid a flat rate on all accounts according to volume. Some agencies may leave the accounts in the control of the physician's office where the staff speaks with the patient and posts all delinquent incoming monies. Other agencies charge a commission based on a percentage of an account, and once the account is turned over to the agency, the physician's office refers all calls to the agency. The fixed cost an agency pays to collect on an account is $3.96. A standard rate for most agencies to break even is one third of all monies collected, and an average rate charged is 50%. Make sure the commission is based on how much is collected on the overdue accounts and not the total amount of overdue accounts turned over to the agency.

Agency Assigned Accounts

Patients' accounts turned over to a collection agency should have a letter of withdrawal sent by certified mail (see Chapter 3, Fig. 3-21). Place a note on all ledgers indicating the date the account was assigned. Financial management consultants usually recommend that the patient's balances be written off of the A/R at the time the account is assigned. A portion of the account balance can be written back on if and when the agency collects on the debt. Accounts should also be listed in a separate journal to help track the effectiveness of the agency. Allow enough columns to show the future date, amount, and percentage of an account collected by the agency as well as the total account balance.

Flag or insert a full sheet of brightly colored paper in the patient's chart noting the date the account was assigned to collection. This will alert all medical staff of the situation if the patient calls on short notice or walks in to be seen. If, after the account has been turned over to an agency, the patient sends payment to the physician's office, notify the collection agency immediately. Any calls regarding accounts that have gone to collection should be referred to the agency.

Credit Bureaus

Collection agencies can also offer the services of a credit bureau. Credit bureaus gather credit information from many sources and make it available for a fee to members of a credit bureau service. Credit reports can be issued on new patients enabling the physician's office to verify credit. The information may consist of the patient's residence and moving habits (a measure of permanency), number of dependents, verification of employment and approximate salary, the patient's payment history on other merchant accounts, and any history of bankruptcy or use of an alias. This report can be obtained over the telephone or can be provided in written form.

The Fair Credit Reporting Act of 1971 allows a person to see and correct his or her credit report. The credit report can be checked for negative credit information, disputed information, mistakes, and out-of-date information. If credit is denied based in whole or in part on an adverse credit report, a letter should be sent advising the patient the name and address of the agency and stating that credit has been denied because credit requirements have not been met. The insurance specialist need not reveal data or specify the exact nature of the information obtained from the credit bureau but must name the bureau. A copy of the letter should be kept in the patient's file.

Credit Counseling

A *consumer credit counseling service* is a nonprofit agency that assists people in paying off their debts. The insurance specialist may have to refer patients for this service if continued medical care is being provided and the patient becomes overwhelmed by the cost. The patient may also contact his or her own bank or credit union, which may provide counseling at no charge. Care must be given with such referrals, using only legitimate agencies and warning patients that many private commercial debt consolidators may charge high fees. Dissatisfied patients may blame the physician or the insurance specialist if satisfactory financial arrangements are not made.

A patient seeking medical care who is unable to pay for services and ineligible for state aid should be directed to the local hospital that services recipients under the Hill-Burton Act of 1946. These hospitals obtained federal construction grants to enlarge their facilities in exchange for their provision of health care for needy patients. The Department of Health and Human Services will furnish the names of hospitals in your area participating in this service. Patients must complete financial applications to determine eligibility before care is rendered.

Small Claims Court

Small claims court is a part of our legal system that allows lay people to have access to a court system without the use of an attorney. Some advantages are a modest filing fee, minimal paperwork, exclusion of costly lawyers, and a short time frame from filing the action to trial date. Incorporated physicians must usually be represented by an attorney; and if an account has already been sent to a collection agency, the agency must file in a municipal or justice court.

Most states have small claims courts, also called *conciliation, common-pleas, general-sessions, justice courts, or people's court.* Each state has monetary limits on the amount that can be handled in small claims court, and accounts need to be reviewed for eligibility. The dollar amount varies from state to state and sometimes from one county to another. The average maximum amount generally ranges from $2,000 to $3,000; however, a recent effort has been supported to raise the dollar limit for small claims courts to $20,000. There are several legislative bills being considered by U.S. Senate and House committees that address raising the dollar limit. Several states have already had such bills signed into law. The new limits in these states vary from $3,000 to $10,000. There may also be limits on the number of claims filed per year that are over a specific dollar amount.

When filing a claim, the person filing the petition (the physician's office) is referred to as the *plaintiff* and the party being brought to suit (the patient) is called the *defendant.* It is generally recommended that the plaintiff send a written demand to the defendant before filing a lawsuit to give the defendant a last opportunity to resolve the claim.

PROCEDURE: Filing a Claim

1. Obtain a Claim of Plaintiff or Plaintiffs Original Petition form to notify the patient that action is being filed. This can be obtained from the clerk's office located at the municipal or justice court.
2. File the papers with the small claims court; make sure you have the patient's correct name and street address.

3. Pay the clerk the small filing fee.
4. Make arrangements to serve the defendant. The summons or citation can be served on the patient by a sheriff or court-appointed officer by paying a small fee plus mileage for the constable who serves it. The person serving the defendant must fill out a proof of service form.

A trial date will be set, and both plaintiff and defendant will be ordered to appear before the judge. Often a postcard is sent notifying the plaintiff when the defendant has been served. If the amount of delinquent debt is over the monetary limit for the small claims court, you may "cut your claim to fit" the limit. An example would be a debt amounting to $2,757 and the state limit is $2,500. You may waive, or give up, the $257 (difference) to bring the amount down to the limit. The claim cannot be divided into two different suits of $1,378.50, nor can you sue twice on the same claim.

Claim Resolutions

After the plaintiff is served he or she has four options:

1. *Pay the claim*—the court clerk will receive the money and forward it to the physician's office, but the filing fee or service charges will not be refunded.
2. *Ignore the claim*—the judge may ask the physician representative to state the physician's side, but the physician will win by default and the judgment will be awarded in the physician's favor, usually including court costs.
3. *Answer the petition*—a contested court hearing will be held. The plaintiff (physician) has the burden of proving his or her claim to the court. A counterclaim may be filed by the patient at this time.
4. *Demand a jury trial*—the case will be taken out of small claims court and the physician will be notified by the county clerk to file a formal complaint in a higher court. An attorney must represent the physician if this occurs.

Trial Preparation

On the trial date, the plaintiff and defendant must both appear or the claim will be dismissed and cannot be refiled. The doctor may send his or her assistant or bookkeeper to represent the physician at the trial. If the claim is settled before trial, a dismissal form needs to be dated, signed, and filed with the clerk.

Preparation for the trial is essential and can mean the difference between success and failure.

Decide what the judge needs to hear to conclude in the physician's favor. Although you cannot have a lawyer represent you in court, you can ask a lawyer for advice before you go to court. Following are recommendations to help prepare for trial:

1. Be on time. If you are late, the court may give a judgment in the defendant's favor.
2. Be ready to submit the basic data required by the court; the physician's name, address, and telephone number; the patient's name and address; the delinquent amount being claimed; and a brief summary of the claim.
3. Show all dates of service and amounts owed, the date the physician's bill was due (if a series of treatments is involved), the date of the last visit, the date of the last payment (if any payment was made), and the amount still unpaid.
4. Include all attempts to collect the debt and organize all exhibits in chronologic order. Include documentation such as copies of statements, letters, notes, receipts, contracts, dishonored checks, telephone calls, other discussions with the patient, and other evidence to present to the court. A timeline showing the sequence of events may be useful.
5. Speak slowly and clearly, present the case in a concise manner, and use a business-like approach. Answer all questions accurately but briefly.
6. Present a witness if live testimony is relevant. A notarized statement from a witness is admissible but not as effective.
7. Try and anticipate the opposing party's evidence and arguments so that a rebuttal may be prepared. Keep in mind that a third party will be making the decision.

The judge will question the physician or representative and the patient, review the evidence, and then make a ruling. Winning the case gives the physician the right to attach a debtor's bank assets, salary, car, personal assets, or real property. The small claims office can show the assistant how to execute a judgment. Judgments are usually effective for many years. There is a small charge if the physician decides to execute against the patient's assets, but the charge is recoverable from the defendant.

A losing defendant may appeal and request a new trial in Superior Court. The defendant may ask the judge to make small installment payments, but not all judges will order this alternative. If the defendant fails to pay, a writ of execution may be obtained from the clerk's office to enforce judgment. This writ of execution permits the marshal to obtain funds from a losing party's bank account or take items of the losing party's property to satisfy the judgment.

Federal Wage Garnishment Laws

Federal wage garnishment laws provide a limit on the amount of employee earnings withheld in a work week or pay period when a debtor's future wage is seized to pay off a debt. It also protects the employee from being dismissed if his or her pay is garnished for only one debt regardless of the number of levies that must be made to collect. This law is enforced by the compliance officers of the Wage and Hour Office of the U.S. Department of Labor. The law does not apply to federal government employees, court-ordered support of any person, court orders in personal bankruptcy cases, or state or federal tax levies. The patient's employer becomes involved as the "trustee" because the employer owes money to the debtor for wages earned.

Once a **garnishment** has been ordered by the court, an employer has to honor it by satisfying the terms of garnishment, before wages can be paid to the debtor. Only a percentage of the wage (usually 25%) is garnished and paid to the creditor. This amount is determined from the employee's disposable earnings. *Disposable earnings* is the amount left after Social Security and federal, state, and local taxes are deducted. When state garnishment laws conflict with federal laws, the statute resulting in the smaller garnishment applies. This method of collection should be considered a last resort for the medical office and used only with large bills.

Tracing a Skip

A patient who owes a balance on his or her account and moves but leaves no forwarding address is called a **skip.** In these cases an unopened envelope will be returned to the office marked "Returned to Sender, Addressee Unknown." Instead, place the words "Forwarding Service Requested" below the doctor's return address on the envelope and the post office will make a search and forward the mail to the new address. The physician's office will be informed of this new address for a nominal fee. Complete a Freedom of Information Act Form at the post office if the address is a rural delivery box number, and the United States Postal Service will provide the physical location of a person's residence. When patients send payments by mail, precautions must be taken to avoid discarding envelopes with a change of address. Always match the address on the envelope, along with the check, against the patient's account. One staff person should have the responsibility of updating all patients' addresses in all locations to avoid this problem.

Skip Tracing Techniques

Once it is determined that a patient is a skip, tracing should begin immediately. Office policies should be established stating how the skip should be traced, whether it is to be traced in the office, or at what point the account should be sent to a collection agency. Some offices choose to make only one attempt whereas others prefer to do most of the detective work themselves. Table 9–4 lists techniques that can be used to initiate the search for the debtor.

When trying to make any of these contacts, never state what your business is with the patient. Keep all information confidential. A good skip tracer must be patient and have the ability to pursue all necessary steps with tenacity and tact. A good imagination, a detective's instincts, and the ability to get along with people will help in this tedious job.

Skip Tracing Services

If the medical practice decides to use an outside service, there are several from which to choose. Some agencies offer customized service with several levels of skip tracing available. Each level is more extensive and more costly. The physician's office decides at which level it would like the search conducted. The first level usually involves verifying the patient's information and checking for typographical errors. The highest level uses every resource available to find the patient. The age of the account, the account balance, and the cost of the level of skip tracing service are all considerations when deciding which level to choose. A collection agency or credit bureau (as mentioned earlier) may also offer the services of skip tracing.

Search Via Computer

Another method of skip tracing is to use electronic databases or on-line services. "Information wholesalers" also exist that cater to bill collec-

TABLE 9–4	Search Techniques Used to Trace a Debtor

1. Cross check the address on the returned envelope with the patient registration form and account to ensure it was mailed correctly.
2. Check the ZIP code directory to see if the ZIP code corresponds with the patient's street address or post office box.
3. File a request with the local post office to try and get a new or corrected address.
4. Look in the local telephone directory; call names that are spelled the same; check with information for a new or current listing.
5. Call the primary care physician for updated information when investigating for a physician specialist or any referring practice.
6. Determine if the patient has been seen at the hospital and if so speak to someone in the accounts department.
7. Inquire at the patient's place of employment. If the patient is no longer employed, ask to speak to the personnel department in an effort to locate the patient; do not divulge the reason for the call.
8. Contact persons listed on the patient registration form, including personal referrals.
9. Request information from the Department of Motor Vehicles if a driver's license number is available.
10. Obtain information from street directories, city directories, and cross-index directories (available at many public libraries) for a new address or the names and telephone numbers of neighbors, relatives, or landlords.
11. Telephone the local moving company or moving rental service and ask for the patient's new address.
12. Request information from utility companies.
13. Inquire at the patient's bank to see if he or she is still a customer.
14. Obtain the services of a local credit bureau to check reports and notify you if the patient's Social Security number shows up under a different name or at a new address.
15. Contact the Board of Education, when the patient has children or is a student, to find out the patient's school district and the school closest to his or her former residence. Request a forwarding address.
16. Call the Police Department when you think the patient may have a criminal record.
17. Check public records such as tax records, voter registration, court records, death and probate records, hunting and fishing licenses, and marriage licenses.

tors and similar interested parties. Currently there are a number of bills pending in Congress aimed at restricting the flow of personal data in cyberspace. Perhaps in the future this information will not be so easy to obtain; however, at present, conducting a successful electronic search is relatively easy. Following are several methods used to search electronic databases to locate a debtor's address and home telephone number.

▶ *Surname scan*—can be done locally, regionally, or nationally based on data banks that have been compiled from public source documents.
▶ *Address search*—provides property search and any change of address from all suppliers of data to the database, including the United States Postal Service; names of other adults in the household may also be included who may have the debtor's telephone number listed under their name.
▶ *Electronic directory*—allows access to the regional telephone operating company's screen of information.
▶ *Credit holder search*—used to establish occupation.
▶ *Phone number search*—permits access to the names of other adults within the same household who have a telephone number.
▶ *Neighbor search*—displays the names, addresses, and telephone numbers of the debtor's former neighbors.
▶ *ZIP code search*—provides the names, addresses, and telephone numbers of everyone within that ZIP code who has the same last name as the debtor.
▶ *City search*—locates everyone with the same last and first name within a given city as well as all people who live in that city.
▶ *State search*—finds all people with the same last name or same last and first name within the

state and will list their addresses and telephone numbers.

> *National search*—operates the same way as the state search; recommended for people with unusual last names.
> *Business search*—lists all the names of the businesses in the neighborhood of the patient's last known residence. This search may help find where the patient has relocated or to verify the patient's place of employment.

Refer to the end of the chapter for a listing of some of the larger directories used on the Internet and explore several directories to cross-check results because of frequent data change. Information is not secure when using the Internet. The patient's right to privacy must never be violated.

Special Collection Issues

Bankruptcy

Bankruptcy laws are federal laws applicable in all states that ensure equal distribution of the assets of an individual among the individual's creditors. There are two kinds of bankruptcy petitions: voluntary and involuntary. A *voluntary petition* is one filed by a person asking for relief under the Bankruptcy Reform Act (the Code). An *involuntary petition* is one filed against a person by his or her creditors requesting that a person obtain relief under the Code.

When a patient files for bankruptcy, he or she becomes a ward of the court and has its protection. The patient is granted an **automatic stay** against creditors, which means that the physician may contact patients only for the name, address, and telephone number of their attorney. The insurance specialist should no longer send statements, make telephone calls, or attempt to collect the account. A creditor can be fined for contempt of court if he or she continues to proceed against the debtor. If a collection agency has the account and has been notified of the bankruptcy, the situation is the same as if the physician has been notified. If the physician is notified first, call the collection agency and inform it of the fact. Notification of bankruptcy does not have to be in writing; verbal communication is valid (e.g., if a patient telephones the doctor's office to inform him or her of the bankruptcy). Bankruptcy remains part of the debtor's permanent credit record for 10 years.

After a patient informs the physician's office of the bankruptcy, determine what type of bankruptcy the debtor has filed. Refer to Table 9–5 for a listing of the five types of bankruptcy cases.

Bankruptcy Rules

Under the Bankruptcy Rules, an unsecured creditor must file proof of claim in Chapter 7 or Chapter 13 bankruptcies within 90 days after the first date set for the meeting of creditors. When filing a claim, the proper form may be obtained from a stationery store or by writing to the presiding judge of the bankruptcy court. If a creditor fails to file a claim, the creditor will lose his or her right to any proceeds from the bankruptcy. A plan for payment will be approved by the court. The trustee may be contacted from time to time to check the status of the claim and the payments that should be expected. Once a patient has filed for bankruptcy, there must be a time lapse of 6 years before he or she can file again. The only exception to this is Chapter 13 bankruptcy.

Terminally Ill Patients

Although it may be difficult to collect from patients who are about to die, it is usually harder to collect from the estate after they are gone. When a patient is too sick or scared to communicate necessary information, speak to family members and stress that you want to help. Approximately 50% of the time terminally ill patients will work with you just because they want to do the right thing. Call the patient before he or she comes in to receive service. Make sure the patient is aware of the existing balance and try to work with the patient to eliminate at least a portion of the balance before the next appointment. Estimate costs and prepare a plan that is agreeable to both you and the patient.

Estate Claims

Great care and sensitivity should be taken when trying to collect on a deceased patient's account. The entire probate system was set up to help protect families from painful involvement in estate settlements. Do not offend the deceased's family by making contact during the time of bereavement. After the first or second week, however, a claim should be filed so the physician's name can be added to the list of creditors.

| TABLE 9-5 | **Types of Bankruptcy Cases** |

Chapter 7 Case

This is sometimes called a *straight petition in bankruptcy* or *absolute bankruptcy*. In this case, all of the **nonexempt assets** of the bankrupt person are liquidated and are distributed according to the law to the creditors. Secured creditors are first in line for payment of all **secured debt.** Unsecured creditors are last. A person declares those to whom he or she owes money and is not required to make payment, thus eliminating all of the debtor's outstanding legal obligations for **unsecured debt.** Most medical bills are considered unsecured debt because they are not backed by any form of **collateral.** The only debt that is discharged in Chapter 7 bankruptcy is the debt that had been incurred up to the point of filing for protection under Chapter 7. So, if a patient files before services are rendered, the bankruptcy laws do not apply for the treatment provided. A Chapter 7 bankruptcy does not necessarily result in the discharge of all debts. If the patient lies about his or her financial status, the debt may not be dischargeable. If the debt incurred was for a luxury service (e.g. facelift), immediately preceding the filing, it is possible that it may not be discharged. Consult the practice's attorney before adjusting the debt off the books in such a situation. All creditors are notified by the Administrator in Bankruptcy as to the proceedings and may choose either to attend the proceedings or make a claim against whatever assets remain.

Chapter 9 Case	Chapter 12 Case
This case is used for reorganization proceedings when a city or town is insolvent or unable to meet its debts. A plan is put into effect to adjust such debts.	This case is used for reorganization when a farmer is unable to meet his or her debts.

Chapter 11 Case	Chapter 13 Case
This case is used for reorganization of a business enterprise when the company is unable to meet its debts but would like to continue business and would be unable to do so if creditors took away its assets. A plan of arrangement is confirmed by the court, and each class of creditor must accept the plan or receive at least that which it would receive on liquidation of the company.	This is sometimes called a *wage earner's bankruptcy.* It is designed to protect the wage earner from creditors while allowing the wage earner to make arrangements to repay a portion of his or her bills (about 70%) over a 3- or 5-year period. The debtor pays a fixed amount agreed upon by the court to the trustee in bankruptcy. A claim needs to be filed as directed by the debtor's attorney.

PROCEDURE: Filing an Estate Claim

Following are steps to take when filing a claim on an estate.

1. Confirm the date and place of death with the hospital, nursing home, or funeral home.
2. Pursue payment from all third party payers first.
3. Contact the Register of Wills' office in the county where the patient lived or the probate department of the superior court, County Recorder's Office. Request a Statement of Claim form or the county's proper document to formally register a claim against an estate.

4. File the claim according to the instructions received with the claim form. When probate is filed, a notification will be sent advising the court of probate, the attorney representing the estate, and the **estate executor** or **estate administrator.** A small fee may need to be included for court costs.
5. Send an itemized statement by certified mail, return receipt, to the attorney and copies to the executor and the court. If the physician treated the deceased patient's last illness, that fact should be clearly indicated on the statement.
6. Allow the legal system to take its course. A call to the executor can be made periodically to check on the status of the estate.

The claim will then be denied or accepted. If accepted, an acknowledgment of the debt will be sent to the physician's office. Many delays arise due to the legal complications of settling an estate but when the estate is settled, the debts will be paid according to a priority system. Usually funeral expenses are paid first, then estate administration expenses, third claims due for the deceased person's last illness, and then taxes and other debts. Any amounts left will be divided between family members. In the rare case of a rejection of the claim, a lien or lawsuit may be filed against the estate.

Various state time limits and statutes govern the filing of a claim against an estate. Check with the county court in your state to obtain filing deadlines. Deadlines may range from 2 months to 3 years but must be adhered to for successful collection from an estate.

Litigation

A difficult question arises when the physician is advised that a patient is involved in a pending litigation that is related to the services provided to the patient. It may not be necessary to wait until the litigation is resolved to pursue payment. Assess whether the patient has the ability to pay before possibly receiving a settlement in a lawsuit. Prior to withholding collection activity, the medical practice should get a guarantee that the physician will be paid in full before the patient (debtor) receives money out of a settlement. The agreement must be guaranteed by the lawyer representing the patient. If the patient is working, regular payments should be required pending the settlement of the patient's litigation. It is always advisable to contact a malpractice attorney in such cases.

Liens

A **lien** is a claim on the property of another as security for a debt. This may include a claim on a future settlement of a lawsuit. The physician may be asked to accept a lien by a patient or the patient's attorney when he or she has been involved in an automobile accident and is awaiting a settlement (Fig. 9–19). In litigation cases, it is a legal promise to satisfy a debt owed by the patient to the physician out of any proceeds received on the case. See Chapter 14 for further details regarding industrial cases.

Patient Complaints

It is generally in the physician's best interest to resolve patient complaints and billing disputes quickly, accurately, and amicably. Always address collection complaints seriously. Listen to the patient with an open mind. Note specifically what the patient is saying and what the patient wants to do. Look beyond the complaint to determine what caused the problem. The source of the problem needs to be resolved, not just the result of the problem. To prompt staff to pay close attention to positive customer relations, a patient complaint form may be adapted. This form may help screen poor collection techniques by staff members, pinpoint billing department problems, and identify policies and procedures that need improvement.

If a patient's complaint is not addressed, the patient may refuse to pay the physician. Following are some guidelines to follow when a patient calls or writes a letter complaining about the physician or the medical practice:

1. Listen carefully (or read the letter carefully) and establish exactly what the patient complaint is and what the patient wants you to do about it.
2. Thank the person for calling (or writing); let the patient know you appreciate his or her input into the situation.
3. Apologize, regardless of whether the patient is right or wrong.
4. Answer the complaint. Explain what happened, if applicable, and state what is being done about it.
5. Use a professional and sincere approach. If the patient is wrong, state that the complaint is unjustified. Do not be sarcastic, condescending, or insulting.
6. Take all complaints seriously. Do not respond in a lighthearted manner or use humor; it will only serve to upset the patient.
7. Respond in letter form. Whether the complaint has been received by telephone or letter, take the time to write answering the complaint. It will indicate that you are not taking the matter lightly.
8. Be cordial and sincere. Express to the patient that you hope to continue a friendly relationship, that you want to be on the same side, but that payment is needed. Treat the patient with respect, good will, and sincere appreciation. Often kindness can turn a negative into a positive; the complaint can be turned into a payment.
9. Follow up after the complaint has been resolved by looking at the root of the problem and taking the necessary time to communicate this to the office manager. This will allow for a

To: Attorney
From: Patient
Re: Medical Records and Doctor's Lien

I hereby authorize Dr. _____ to release to you a full report of his findings, diagnosis, treatment, and prognosis for me regarding injuries sustained in the accident in which I was involved on_____.

I direct you as my attorney to pay directly to Dr._____ all monies owed to him in consequence of this accident, as well as any other sums outstanding to him. I authorize that these funds be withheld from any settlement made in this case.

I further give a lien on my case to Dr. _____ against any and all proceeds of the settlement, judgment, or verdict which may be paid to me or to you as my attorney as a result of the injuries sustained in the accident and treated by Dr. _____.

This lien does not supplant my own responsibility for outstanding medical bills, but is given as protection for the doctor and in consideration for his willingness to await delayed payment. I understand that payment of all outstanding fees to Dr. _____ are payable upon demand and are not contingent on the receipt of an award through settlement, judgment or verdict.

_____   _____
Patient's Signature   Date

As the attorney of record for the above-named patient, I hereby agree to observe the terms of this agreement, and to withhold from any award in this case such funds as are required for the adequate protection of Dr._____ .

_____   _____
Attorney's Signature   Date

Figure 9–19. Medical Records and Doctor's Lien. (Reprinted with permission of The Medical Management Institute, Alpharetta, GA.)

plan of action that will help prevent the same type of problem from recurring.

Collection Controls

All collections should be carefully controlled to prevent lost checks and embezzlement. See Chapter 1 for a complete description of the different types of bonding insurance and precautions to take when processing monies and insurance claims in the physician's office.

RESOURCES ON THE INTERNET

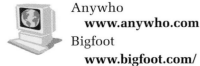

Anywho
   www.anywho.com
Bigfoot
   www.bigfoot.com/

Database America
   www.databaseamerica.com
InfoSpace
   www.infospace.com
Info USA
   www.infousa.com
People Finder
   www.lookupusa.com/
Search-It-All
   www.searchitall.net/peoplefinder.asp
Switchboard
   www.switchboard.com
WhoWhere?
   www.whowhere.com/
Yahoo People Search
   www.yahoo.com/search/people/
411Locate
   www.411locate.com

STUDENT ASSIGNMENT LIST

✔ Study Chapter 9.

✔ Answer the review questions in the *Workbook* to reinforce the theory learned in this chapter and to help prepare you for a future test.

✔ Complete the assignment in the *Workbook* to give you hands-on experience in selecting a dun message, posting a courtesy adjustment and insurance or patient payment, composing a collection letter, and completing a credit card voucher and a financial agreement.

✔ Turn to the Glossary at the end of this textbook for a further understanding of the Key Terms used in the chapter.

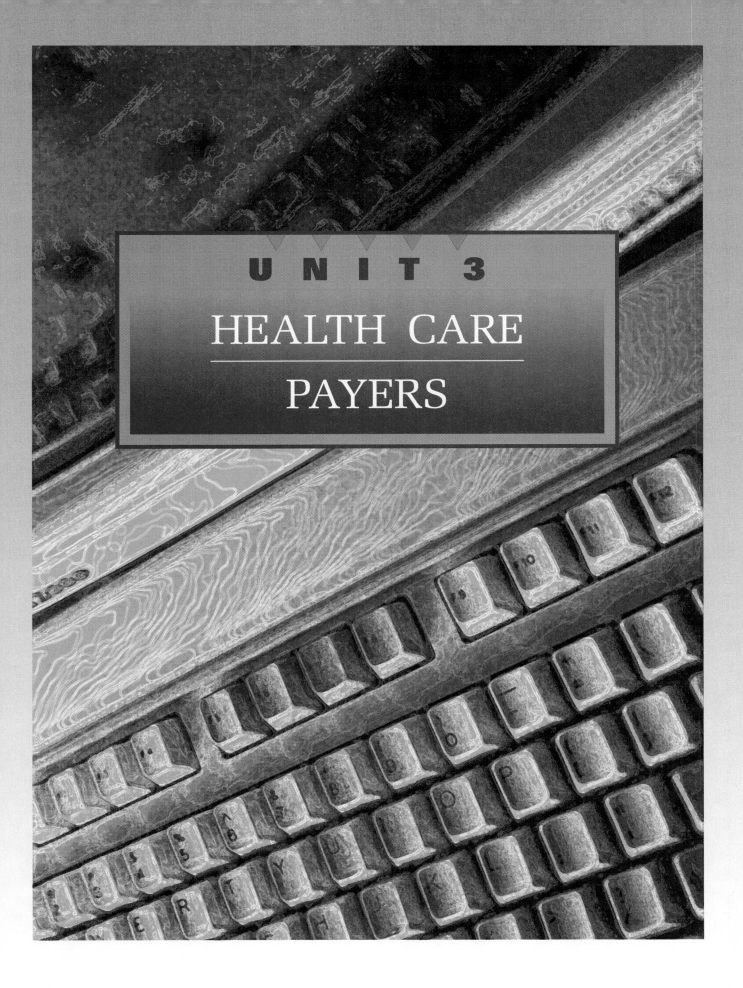

UNIT 3

HEALTH CARE

PAYERS

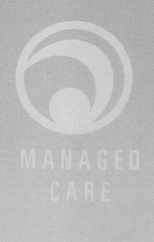

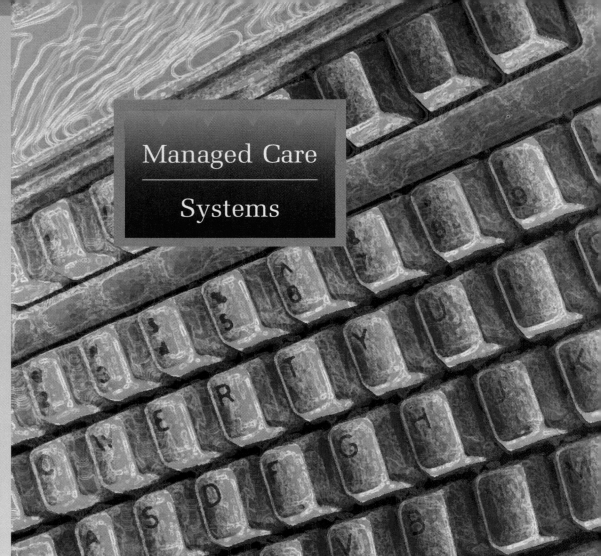

Managed Care
Systems

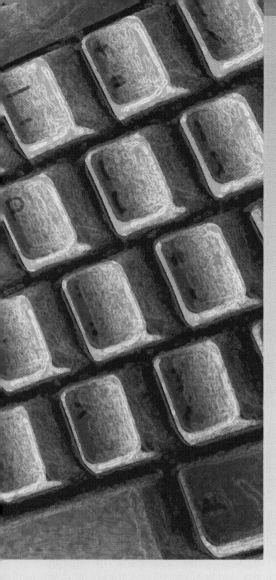

■ State reasons for professional review organizations.
■ Define independent practice associations.
■ Name the elements of preferred provider organizations.
■ Identify four types of authorizations for medical services, tests, and procedures.

OBJECTIVES*

After reading this chapter, you should be able to:

■ Define a prepaid health plan (PHP).
■ Identify types of managed care health plans.
■ List two types and two different functions of foundations.
■ State the provisions of the Health Maintenance Organization Act of 1973.
■ Explain health maintenance organization benefits and eligibility requirements.

*Performance objectives and exercises for hands-on practical experience for this chapter appear in the *Workbook.*

KEY TERMS

ancillary services

buffing

capitation

carve outs

churning

claims-review type of foundation

closed panel program

comprehensive type of foundation

copayment (copay)

deductible

direct referral

disenrollment

exclusive provider organization (EPO)

fee-for-service

formal referral

foundation for medical care (FMC)

gatekeeper

health maintenance organization (HMO)

in-area

independent (or individual) practice association (IPA)

managed care organizations (MCOs)

participating physician

per capita

physician provider group (PPG)

point-of-service (POS) plan

preferred provider organization (PPO)

prepaid group practice model

continued

History

Until the early 1970s, most health insurance was delivered through traditional fee-for-service plans. This scenario has changed from high-cost, old-fashioned indemnity plans to less-expensive managed health care plans, such as health maintenance organizations (HMOs). In this chapter the health care reforms of the past and present are defined and explained. In addition to HMOs, other types of prepaid group practice models operated by **managed care organizations (MCOs)** are discussed that use a managed care approach.

In prepaid group plans, patients join the plan and pay monthly medical insurance premiums individually or through their employer. The physician renders service to the patient, and the patient usually pays a small copayment and occasionally a deductible as required by the plan. Providers that join the plan are paid using the capitation method. **Capitation** is a system of payment used by managed care plans in which physicians and hospitals are paid a fixed, per capita amount for each patient enrolled over a stated period of time, regardless of the type and number of services provided.

Prepaid Group Practice Health Plans

The *Ross-Loos Medical Group* in Los Angeles was America's oldest privately owned, prepaid medical group. It was founded in 1929 by Dr. Donald E. Ross and Dr. H. Clifford Loos and existed only in southern California, where it expanded to 17 medical group locations. In 1975, the Ross-Loos Medical Group formed a corporation and received a federal grant to develop a health care system under the federal Health Maintenance Organization Act of 1973. In 1980, INA Healthplan, Inc., of Philadelphia merged with Ross-Loos. Ross-Loos is now known as CIGNA *Healthplans of California.*

Most CIGNA patients are served under a prepayment group plan by which they pay a monthly premium and receive hospital, surgical, and professional benefits from a CIGNA staff physician or CIGNA Health Care Center. Several thousand other CIGNA patients are private and are treated on a fee-for-service basis. In the case of an emergency when the patient is outside the area of a CIGNA Health Care Center, he or she may seek professional or hospital care in other facilities, but CIGNA must be notified as soon as possible. A dental plan and Medicare supplemental plan are also available through CIGNA.

Another pioneer of the prepaid group practice concept is the *Kaiser Permanente Medical Care Program.* It began in 1933, when Dr. Sidney R. Garfield and a few physicians working for him gave combined industrial accident and personal medical care to approximately 5000 workers building a freshwater aqueduct across the California desert to Los Angeles. Dr. Garfield charged the insurance carriers $1.50 per man per month and the workers 5 cents a day. In return, he provided comprehensive health care. Then, in 1938, Henry J. Kaiser and his son Edgar started a joint venture to complete the Grand Coulee Dam in Washington and invited Dr. Garfield to form a medical group to furnish care to the workers for 7 cents a day prepaid by the employer. The group expanded to include the workers' wives and children.

Kaiser Permanente now has centers in 12 regions covering 16 states. Patients are served under a prepayment group plan and receive hospital, surgical, and professional benefits from physicians located at the Kaiser Permanente Medical Care Centers. In most regions, the Kaiser Permanente Medical Plan is a **closed panel program** composed of multispecialty physicians, and the plan limits the patient's choice of personal physicians to those practicing in 1 of the 12 geographic regions.

In January 1994, Kaiser Permanente announced a venture with Pacific Mutual Life Insurance Company to give Kaiser's 4.6 million California patients a less cost effective option of using physicians and medical facilities outside the vast Kaiser network. This is the first time that Kaiser has allowed certain member groups of its two California health maintenance organizations to seek medical help from non-Kaiser physicians and is termed a point-of-service (POS) option (see discussion later in this chapter). In this option, Kaiser pays up to a specified amount and the patient must pay the rest depending on the contract. Kaiser does not provide care on a fee-for-service or a cost-reimbursement basis.

In emergency situations when patients are out of reach of a Kaiser Center, they may seek the services of outside facilities or physicians. They are then transferred, when their condition is stable, to a Kaiser facility.

Health Maintenance Organization Act of 1973

An HMO is a prepaid group practice that can be sponsored and operated by the government, medical schools, clinics, foundations, hospitals, employers, labor unions, community or consumer groups, insurance companies, hospital-medical plans, or the Veterans Administration.

In 1973, Congress passed the Health Maintenance Organization Act of 1973 (Public Law 93-222), creating authority for the federal government to assist HMO development in a number of ways, including (1) providing grants, loans, and loan guarantees to offset the initial operating deficits of new HMOs that meet federal standards (i.e., are federally qualified) and (2) requiring most employers to offer an HMO to their employees as an alternative to traditional health insurance.

Eligibility

Those who have voluntarily enrolled in an HMO plan from a specific geographic area (**in-area** or **service area**) or who are covered by an employer who has paid an established sum per person to be covered by the plan are eligible. The law states that an employer employing 25 or more persons may offer the services of an HMO as an alternative health treatment plan for employees. Medicare and Medicaid beneficiaries may also become members of managed care plans whether retired or employed. The federal government reimburses the HMOs on a **per capita** basis, depending on the size of the enrollment. This means that the HMO is paid a fixed, per capita amount (also known as capitation) for each patient served without considering the actual number or nature of services provided to each person.

To qualify as an HMO, an organization must present proof of its ability to provide comprehensive health care. To retain eligibility, an HMO must render periodic performance reports to the offices of the Department of Health and Human Services. Thus, accurate and complete medical records are imperative to the survival and cost control of an HMO.

Primary Care Physician

Most managed care plans use a **primary care physician (PCP)** as a gatekeeper. A **gatekeeper** is a physician who controls patient access to specialists and diagnostic testing services. PCPs are usually physicians who practice in the fields of internal medicine, family practice, general practice, or pediatrics. Although obstetrics and gynecology is considered specialty care, the obstetrician/gynecologist may be contracted as a PCP; and when not, it is common for MCOs to allow self-referral by members to obstetricians or gynecologists for certain services (e.g., Pap smears).

Identification Card

Each enrollee of a managed care plan is given an identification card as shown in Chapter 2, Figure 2–10. The card usually lists the patient's name, member number, group number, and primary care physician's name. The name of the MCO and type of plan with the amount of copayment for various outpatient services (e.g., office visit, emergency department, urgent care center, and pharmacy) are also included.

Both sides of the patient's card should be photocopied because the insurance address, telephone numbers used for inquiries and authorizations, or other important information may be listed on the front or back of the card.

Benefits

Benefits under the HMO Act fall under two categories: basic and supplemental health service, which are listed in Table 10–1.

Health Care Reform

Over the past 60 years, leaders of the United States from Presidents Roosevelt to Clinton have announced reforms of the health care system. Medical practices have made transitions from rural to urban, from generalist to specialist, from solo to group practice, and from fee-for-service to capitation and have expanded to a number of health care delivery systems that try to manage the cost of health care. Before capitation, **fee-for-service** was the usual method of billing by physicians in private practice. A professional service was rendered by the

TABLE 10–1	**Health Maintenance Organization Act Benefits of 1973**

Basic Health Services

Alcohol, drug abuse, and addiction medical treatment
Dental services (preventive) for children younger than age 12 years
Diagnostic laboratory, x-ray, and therapeutic radiology services
Emergency health services in or out of the HMO service area
Family planning and infertility services
Health education and medical social services
Home health services
Hospital services (inpatient and outpatient)
Mental health services on an outpatient basis, short-term (not to exceed 20 visits) ambulatory, evaluative, and crisis intervention
Physicians' services and consultant or referral services without time or cost limits
Preventive health services (e.g., physical examinations for adults, vision and hearing tests for children through age 17 years, well-baby care, immunizations, health education)

Supplemental Health Services

Dental care not included in basic benefits
Extended mental health services not included in basic benefits
Eye examinations for adults
Intermediate and long-term care (nursing facilities and nursing homes)
Prescription drugs
Rehabilitative services and long-term physical medicine (e.g., physical therapy)

physician to the patient, and the physician expected to receive a fee for the service provided.

During the 1990s, a major restructuring of the United States health care system was needed for the following reasons:

- A growing percentage of Americans were not covered by private or government insurance.
- Employers were having to pay escalating health care premiums and did not want to cut wages to cover these costs.
- Government needed to reduce the deficit by keeping down increases in the Medicare and Medicaid programs.
- Physicians and hospital costs were soaring with no end in sight due to inflation, high-tech equipment, expensive medications, and so on.
- Patients were spending more and more money for less and less care and coping with a system riddled with inefficiency and fraud.

In the past decade, integrated health care delivery systems have formed in many states to reduce costs. These have included managed care organizations (MCOs), physician-hospital organizations, and group practices accepting a variety of MCOs and fee-for-service patients. These systems allow for better negotiations for contracts with large employers and managed care plans, as well as with medical and office suppliers for discounts. Each type of organization differs in ownership, purpose, governance, management, and type of services provided. Even before the government released its health care reform proposal, some states began establishing laws implementing managed care for the general populations as well as for Medicaid patients and those injured on the job (workers' compensation cases). Hawaii has had a statewide universal health insurance plan since 1974. Many regions have large groups of Medicare-eligible people who have opted to belong to a health maintenance organization or other prepaid plans.

In 1994, California put together a working alliance, the first in the nation, followed by Florida's voluntary purchasing group, the Community Health Purchasing Alliances. In California, the alliance is formally known as the Health Insurance Plan of California. This allows firms with 5 to 50 workers to offer their employees a wide choice of different insurance programs. All plans must offer the same benefits, but some physicians and hospitals are more desirable than others. The company must pay an amount equal to at least half of the cost of the lowest-priced plan; the worker pays the remainder.

In the future, it is foreseen that those on Medicaid, younger than age 65 years, and not receiving either Aid to Families with Dependent Children (AFDC) or Supplemental Security Income (SSI) will no longer be part of Medicaid. They might obtain their health benefits like everyone else. AFDC and SSI recipients would be covered under a Medicaid plan, but Medicaid would pay a capitated premium (payment per capita) to the alliance. The recipient would pick a low-cost plan from the state alliance. Some states have pilot projects in certain communities to determine whether this is feasible for the entire state.

Managed Care Systems

Health Maintenance Organizations

The oldest of all the prepaid health plans is the **health maintenance organization (HMO)**. An HMO is a plan or program by which specified health services are rendered by participating physicians to an enrolled group of persons. Fixed periodic payments are made in advance to providers of services **(participating physicians)** by or on behalf of each person or family. If a health insurance carrier administers and manages the HMO, it contracts to pay in advance for the full range of health services to which the insured is entitled under the terms of the health insurance contract.

HMO Models

There are important differences in the structure of various HMOs that influence the way physicians practice and, perhaps, the quality of medical care delivered. Following are several types of HMO models.

Prepaid Group Practice Model

The **prepaid group practice model** delivers services at one or more locations through a group of physicians who contract with the HMO to provide care or through its own physicians, who are employees of the HMO. For example, Kaiser Permanente is a prepaid group practice model where physicians form an independent group (Permanente) and contract with a health plan (Kaiser) to provide medical treatment to members enrolled by the plan. Although the physicians work for a salary, it is paid by their own independent group, not by the administrators of the health plan. This is designed to permit the physicians to concentrate on medicine.

Staff Model

The **staff model** is a type of HMO in which the health plan hires physicians directly and pays them a salary instead of contracting with a medical group.

Network HMO

A *network HMO* contracts with two or more group practices to provide health services.

For further information on HMOs, write to the Office of Health Maintenance Organizations.*

Exclusive Provider Organizations

An **exclusive provider organization (EPO)** is a type of managed care plan that combines features of HMOs (e.g., enrolled population, limited provider panel, gatekeepers, utilization management, capitated provider reimbursement, authorization system) and PPOs (e.g., flexible benefit design, negotiated fees, and fee-for-service payments). It is referred to as exclusive because employers agree not to contract with any other plan. The member must choose medical care from network providers with certain exceptions for emergency or out-of-area services. If a patient decides to seek care outside the network, generally he or she will not be reimbursed for the cost of the treatment. Technically, many HMOs can be considered EPOs. However, EPOs are regulated under insurance statutes rather than federal and state HMO regulations.

Foundations for Medical Care

A **foundation for medical care (FMC)** is an organization of physicians sponsored by a state or local medical association concerned with the development and delivery of medical services and the cost of health care. The first Foundation for Medical Care was established in 1954 in Stockton, California. Foundations have sprung up across the United States, and some comprehensive foundations have assumed a portion of the underwriting risk for a defined population. Foundations deal primarily with various groups—employer groups, government groups, and county and city employees. Some plans are open to individual subscribers, but this usually is a small percentage of the foundation activity.

There are basically two types of foundations for medical care operations and each functions

---

*Health Care Financing Administration, Room 4350, Cohen Building, 330 Independence Avenue, SW, Washington, DC 20201.

differently: (1) a **comprehensive type of foundation**, which designs and sponsors prepaid health programs or sets minimum benefits of coverage, and (2) a **claims-review type of foundation**, which provides evaluation of the quality and efficiency of services by a panel of physicians to the numerous fiscal agents or carriers involved in its area, including the ones processing Medicare and Medicaid. Reviews are done for services and/or fees that exceed local community guidelines.

A key feature of the foundation is its dedication to an incentive reimbursement system. For a participating physician, income is received in direct proportion to the number of medical services delivered (i.e., fee-for-service) rather than payment through capitation. The FMC offers a managed care plan fee schedule to be used by member physicians. In some areas, foundation physicians agree to accept the foundation allowance as payment in full for covered services. The patient is *not* billed for the balance. However, the patient is billed for nonbenefit items, a deductible, and coinsurance.

The patient may select any member or nonmember physician he or she wishes. Member physicians agree to bill the foundation directly, and a nonmember physician may wish to collect directly from the patient. Many foundations submit claims on the HCFA-1500 form, and others transmit data electronically. The foundation movement has a national society, the American Managed Care and Review Association (AMCRA),* which can give you further information on AMCRA or foundations in your state.

Independent Practice Associations

Another type of MCO is the **independent (or individual) practice association (IPA)** in which the physicians are not employees and are not paid salaries. Instead, they are paid for their services on a capitation or fee-for-service basis out of a fund drawn from the premiums collected from the subscriber, union, or corporation by an organization that markets the health plan. A discount of up to 30% is withheld to cover costs of operating the IPA. IPA physicians make contractual arrangements to treat HMO members out of their own offices. A participating physician may also treat non-HMO patients.

---

*1227 25th Street, NW, #610, Washington, DC 20037 (formerly known as American Association of Foundations for Medical Care).

Preferred Provider Organizations

A **preferred provider organization (PPO)** is another type of managed care plan. A PPO contracts with a group of providers (designated as "preferred") to deliver care to members. PPO members have the freedom to choose any physician or hospital for services, but they receive a high level of benefits if the preferred providers are used. There are usually coinsurance requirements and deductibles, and claims have to be filed. Occasionally, the PPOs pay 100% of the cost, but most do not. As with major medical policies, coinsurance requires the patient to pay 20% to 25% of the allowed amount up to a certain point and then the PPO pays 100% of the balance. Predetermination of benefits may be required as well as fee limits, quality control, and utilization review. Some hospital indemnity plans pay fixed fees for various services. If the charges are higher, the patient pays the difference.

Physician Provider Groups

A **physician provider group (PPG)** is a physician-owned business entity that has the flexibility to deal with all forms of contract medicine and still offer its own packages to business groups, unions, and the general public. One division may function as an IPA under contract to an HMO. Another section may act as the broker or provider in a PPO that contracts with hospitals as well as other physicians to market services or medical supplies to employers and other third parties. And still another portion might participate in joint ventures with hospitals, freestanding imaging centers and laboratories, purchase of diagnostic equipment, retail medical equipment as a corporate subsidiary, and so on. The sideline businesses do not pay dividends but provide income to make future assessments to participating physicians unnecessary. The difference between an IPA and a PPG is that an IPA may not be owned by its member physicians whereas a PPG is physician owned.

The ability of the PPGs to combine services (joint purchasing, marketing, billing, collections, attorneys and accountant fees) is an advantage because it cuts down on the cost of running a business and allows each physician to retain his or her own practice in addition to these joint ventures. The physicians turn over a small percentage of their income to the PPG for expenses. Patients call one telephone number to make appointments and the billing is done in one location.

Point-of-Service Plans

The typical **point-of-service (POS) plan** combines elements of an HMO and a PPO while offering some unique features. It is basically an HMO consisting of a network of physicians and hospitals that provides an insurance company or an employer with discounts on its services. In a POS program, members choose a primary care physician who manages specialty care and referrals. A POS plan allows the covered individual to choose service from a participating or nonparticipating provider, with different benefit levels. The POS program pays members a higher level of benefits when they use program (network) providers. The member may use providers outside the network, but higher deductibles and coinsurance percentages for non-network services give members incentives to stay within the network.

The POS plan may also provide nonparticipating benefits through a supplemental major medical policy. The key advantage of POS programs is the combination of HMO-style cost management and PPO-style freedom of choice.

Triple-Option Health Plan

This type of plan allows members to select from three choices: HMOs, PPOs, or indemnity insurance. Some of these plans allow the employee to change plans more often than under traditional arrangements. They incorporate cost containment measures, such as precertification for hospital admission, hospital stays, and second surgical opinions.

Table 10–2 gives an overview or summary of five of the most common types of managed care plans.

Medical Review

Professional Review Organizations

A *professional review organization* (PRO) determines and assures the quality and operation of health care through a process called *peer review*. *Peer review* is an evaluation of the quality and efficiency of services rendered by a practicing physician or physicians within the specialty group. Practitioners in a managed care program may come under peer review by a PRO. In this type of review, one or more physician(s) working with the federal government under federal guidelines evaluate(s) another physician in regard to the quality and efficiency of professional care. The review may be used to examine evidence for admission and discharge of a hospital patient and to settle disputes on fees (see Figure 8–4 in Chapter 8). PROs are not restricted to MCO programs but also play a role in Medicare inpatient cases.

Utilization Review or Management

In a managed care setting, a management system called **utilization review (UR)** is necessary to control costs. UR is a formal assessment of the cost and use of components of the health care system. The utilization review committee reviews individual cases to determine medical necessity for medical tests and procedures. It also watches over how providers use medical care resources. If medical care, tests, or procedures are denied, then the patient must be informed of the need for the denied service and the risks of not having it. The reasons

---

TABLE 10–2 **Managed Care Plans**					
Plan	**Network** In	**Network** Out	**Copay Deductible**	**Payment Method**	**Authorization Required**
HMO	X		Fixed copay	Capitated Fee-for-service (carve outs)	X
PPO	75/25% 80/20% 90/10%	60/40% 70/30%	Fixed copay Deductible	Fee-for-service	X
IPA	Limit Large group		Fixed copay	Capitated Fee-for-service (carve outs)	X
EPO	X		Fixed copay	Fee-for-service Capitated	X
POS	X	X	Fixed copay Deductible	Fee-for-service Capitated	X

for denial, in writing, let patients know their rights to receive the service and their obligation to pay before obtaining such services.

In a performance-based reimbursement system, emphasis is placed on seeing a high volume of patients. When a physician sees a patient more than is medically necessary, this is termed **churning** and is done to increase revenue through an increased number of services. Churning may be seen in fee-for-service as well as some managed care environments. **Turfing** means to transfer the sickest, high-cost patients to other physicians so the provider appears as a low utilizer. **Buffing** refers to a physician's making this practice look justifiable to the plan. All of these situations may affect utilization review.

Management of Plans

Contracts

To make a knowledgeable financial decision on how a managed care plan will impact an existing medical practice, it is important to obtain nationwide data from Medirisk, Inc.* Data supplied by this company can be used to evaluate existing fees, negotiate with managed care firms, and weigh practice expansions (i.e., add partners or a satellite office). Before signing a contract with a managed care plan, a physician should have the contract reviewed by an attorney. Additional information on managed care contracts is found in Chapter 9 under Managed Care Organizations.

Carve Outs

When an MCO contracts with a physician group several important considerations are:

1. How many patients will the MCO provide?
2. What is the per capita rate (capitation amount per patient)?
3. What services are included in the capitated amount?

Medical services not included in the contract benefits are called **carve outs** (not included within the capitation rate) and may be contracted for separately. For example, if an internist contracts with an MCO, all Evaluation and Management services as well as ECGs, spirometries, hematocrits, fasting blood sugar tests, and urinalyses might be included in the capitation amount that is received

per person, per month regardless of whether any of these services were rendered. However, sigmoidoscopies and hospital visits might be "carved out" of the contract and paid on a fee-for-service basis. Generally, physicians prefer carve outs for expensive procedures when contracting with MCOs.

Preauthorization or Prior Approval

Some managed care plans require preauthorization for certain services or referral of a patient to see a specialist. The following are several types of referrals that a plan may use.

1. **Formal referral**—Authorization request required by the MCO contract to determine medical necessity. This may be obtained via telephone or a completed authorization form mailed or transmitted via fax (Fig. 10-1).
2. **Direct referral**—Authorization request form is completed and signed by the physician and handed to the patient. Certain services may not require completion of a form and may be directly referred (e.g., obstetrical care, dermatology).
3. **Verbal referral**—Primary care physician informs the patient and telephones the referring physician that the patient is being referred for an appointment.
4. **Self-referral**—Patient refers himself or herself to a specialist. The patient may be required to inform the primary care physician.

Patients may be unaware of preapproval requirements. A good precaution is to ask the patient about insurance coverage at the time the appointment is made. If the patient is a member of a managed care plan, carefully review the patient's preauthorization requirements. If approval is required for certain situations, inform the patient of this before he or she sees the physician. If a patient has obtained the written authorization approval, then remind him or her to bring the form at the time of the scheduled visit. Even if preapproved, *the treatment must be medically necessary* or payment may be denied after submission of a claim. If an authorization is delayed and the patient comes in for the appointment, try to call the plan and obtain a verbal authorization. Document the date, time, and name of the authorizing person; otherwise, the patient's appointment may have to be rescheduled. A referral recommendation must be documented in the patient's record and, if applicable, sent to the referring physician.

---

*5901 Peachtree Dunwoody Road, NE, Suite 455, Building B, Atlanta, GA 30328.

MANAGED CARE PLAN
TREATMENT AUTHORIZATION REQUEST

**TO BE COMPLETED BY PRIMARY CARE PHYSICIAN
OR OUTSIDE PROVIDER**

Health Net	☐	Met Life	☐
Pacificare	☐	Travelers	☒
Secure Horizons	☐	Pru Care	☐

Member No._____

Patient Name:_____Louann Campbell_____ Date:_____7-14-20XX_____

M_____ F _X_ Birthdate ____4-7-1952____ Home telephone number ___013-450-1666___

Address ___2516 Encina Avenue, Woodland Hills, XY 12345-0439___

Primary Care Physician ____Gerald Practon, MD____ Provider ID# ____TC 14021____

Referring Physician ____Gerald Practon, MD____ Provider ID# ____TC 14021____

Referred to ____Raymond Skeleton, MD____ Address ____4567 Broad Avenue____

Woodland Hills, XY 12345-0001 ____ Office telephone no.___013-486-9002___

Diagnosis Code ___724.2___ Diagnosis ___Low back pain___

Diagnosis Code ___722.10___ Diagnosis ___Sciatica___

Treatment Plan: ___Orthopedic evaluation of lumbar spine R/O herniated disc L4, 5___

Authorization requested for procedures/tests/visits:

Procedure Code ___99244___ Description ___New patient consultation___

Procedure Code _____ Description _____

Facility to be used: _____ Estimated length of stay _____

Office ☒   Outpatient ☐   Inpatient ☐   Other ☐

List of potential consultants (i.e., anesthetists, assistants, or medical/surgical):

Raymond Skeleton, MD - Orthopedic

Physician's signature *Gerald Practon, MD*

TO BE COMPLETED BY PRIMARY CARE PHYSICIAN

PCP Recommendations: See above _____ PCP Initials *GP, MD*

Date eligibility checked___7-14-20XX___ Effective date____1-15-20XX____

TO BE COMPLETED BY UTILIZATION MANAGEMENT

Authorized _____ Not authorized _____

Deferred _____ Modified _____

Authorization Request#_____

Comments:_____

Figure 10–1. Example of a managed care plan treatment authorization request form completed by a primary care physician for preauthorization of a professional service.

A tracking system, such as a referral tracking log, needs to be in place for pending referrals so care may be rendered in a timely manner and patients do not get lost in the system (Fig. 10–2). This log should include the date the authorization is requested, patient's name, procedure or consul-

AUTHORIZATION REQUEST LOG

Date requested	Patient name	Procedure/ consult	Insurance plan	1st F/U	2nd F/U	3rd F/U	Approved	Scheduled date
2/8/XX	Juan Percy	Bone scan-full body	Health Net	2/20			J. Smith	2/23/XX
2/8/XX	Nathan Takai	MRI-L-knee	Pru-Care	2/20	3/3			
2/9/XX	Lori Smythe	Consult Neuro G. Frankel MD	FHP	2/22			T. Hope	2/26/XX
2/10/XX	Bob Mason	Cervical collar	Secure Horizons	2/22	3/5	3/19		

Figure 10–2. Example of an authorization request log to be used as a system for tracking referral of patients for procedures and consultations.

tant requested, insurance plan, dates of follow-up, name of person who approved or denied request, and appointment date for consult or procedure. Sometimes authorization approvals are sent to the primary care physician and not to the referring/ordering physician. In these cases, follow-up must be made with the primary care physician. Allow a maximum 2-week turnaround time and track all authorization requests.

If a managed care plan refuses to authorize payment for a recommended treatment, tests, or procedures, have the primary care physician send a letter to the plan that is worded similarly to that shown in Figure 10–3. Then, send a letter, such as that shown in Figure 10–4, to the patient informing him or her of this fact and asking the patient to appeal the denial of benefits.

In some managed care plans, when a primary care physician sends a patient to a specialist for consultation who is *not* in the managed care plan, the specialist bills the primary care physician. This is done because the primary care physician receives a monthly capitation check from the plan and any care for the patient must come from the capitation pool. This type of plan encourages primary care physicians not to refer patients in order to retain profits.

If a specialist recommends referral to another specialist (**tertiary care**), be sure the recommendation is in writing. Call the specialist at a later date to see whether the recommendation was acted on. If the patient refuses to be referred, be sure this is documented. If a referral form is required, do NOT telephone or write a letter. The managed care plan may refuse payment if the proper form is not completed.

When receiving a referral authorization form, make a copy of the form for each approved office visit, laboratory test, or series of treatments. Then use the form as a reference to bill for the service.

When all copies are used, this indicates all the services that the patient's plan has approved are completed. Ask the primary care physician or the managed care plan for a new authorization to continue treatment on the patient. The request should be generated in a timely manner so that treatment is not delayed.

Diagnostic Tests

Many managed care plans require that patients have laboratory and radiology tests performed at plan-specified facilities. These are referred to as *network facilities*. Obtain the necessary authorizations for such services and allow sufficient time to receive the test or x-ray results before the patient's return appointment.

When there is doubt about coverage for a test or the managed care plan indicates a test is not covered, inform the patient ahead of time. Disclose the cost and have the patient sign a waiver agreement to pay for the service and then you will be able to bill the patient for the service. If an authorization is denied because a test is deemed "medically unnecessary" and the physician wishes to appeal, the physician can present clinical reasons to the MCO's medical director to receive approval and bring attention to possible expansion of benefits for future patients.

Managed Care Guide

To assist in keeping up with the growth of local managed care plans as well as knowing which physician belongs to which plan in the practice, create a grid or matrix of all MCOs that the practice has contracts with. Use a sheet of paper and list each plan with billing address vertically in a column to the left, then list significant data hori-

Ms. Jane Smith
Chairperson
Utilization Review Committee
ABC Managed Care Plan
111 Main Street
Anytown, XY 12345-0122

Dear Ms. Smith:

On _____ I prescribed_____ for_____ .
     Date   List treatment, test, procedure   Patient's Name

On _____ you refused to authorize for that treatment. I find that I
     Date
must take issue with your determination for the following reasons:

In my medical judgment, the treatment is a very important part of my overall care of_____
_____ . This patient suffers from _____ .The treatment is
Patient's Name   Describe condition
necessary to _____ . Failure to perform the treatment could
                Describe why necessary
result in the following problem(s):

For these reasons, I urge you to reconsider your refusal to authorize payment for the
procedure I have prescribed.

By copy of this letter to_____ I am reiterating my suggestion that
he/she   Patient's Name

obtain the treatment despite your refusal to authorize payment, for the reasons I have set
forth in this letter and in prior discussions with_____ .
                                     Patient's Name
Yours truly,

John Doe, MD

cc: (Name of patient)

Figure 10–3. Example of a letter to a managed care plan when there is a refusal to authorize payment for a recommended treatment, test, or procedure.

zontally across the top. Suggested titles for column categories are: eligibility telephone numbers, copayment amounts, preauthorization requirements, restrictions on tests frequently ordered, participating laboratories, participating hospitals, and the contract's time limit for promised payment. Reference to this guide will give you specifics at a glance about each plan's coverage and copayment amounts (Fig. 10–5).

Plan Administration

Patient Information Letter

Inform managed care subscribers in writing what you expect from them and what they can expect from you. The patient information letter should outline possible restrictions, noncovered items, expectations for copayment, and names of the managed care plans in which your physician is presently participating. Note if the patient neglects to notify the office of any change regarding eligibility status in the plan, such as **disenrollment**, the patient is held personally responsible for the bill. Also, mention that if hospitalization, surgery, or referral to a specialist is required, then the managed care patient must inform the office. State that because of restrictions, failure to do so would make the patient liable for denied services. Post a sign in the waiting room advising managed care patients to check with the receptionist regarding participating plans.

Figure 10–6 is a sample letter of appropriate wording and content. File a copy of the letter given to the patient in the patient's medical

Mr. Avery Johnson
130 Sylvia Street
Anytown, XY 12345-0022

Dear Mr. Johnson:

On _____ I prescribed _____ for you. On _____ ,
         Date   Treatment, test, procedure   Date

_____ refused to authorize for same. On that basis,
    Name of Managed Care Plan

you have informed me of your decision to forego the treatment I have prescribed. I
expressed my concerns regarding your decision during our discussion on _____ about
                                                                        Date

the potential ramifications of your refusal to undergo the treatment.

The purpose of this letter is to recommend that you appeal_____
                                                              Name of Managed Care Plan's

denial of benefits and reconsider your decision to forego the treatment in light of the
potential consequences of your refusal.

Should you wish to discuss this further, please do not hesitate to contact me.

Sincerely yours,

John Doe, MD

Figure 10–4. Example of a letter to inform the patient about refusal of payment for treatment, test, or procedure by the managed care plan.

MANAGED CARE PLAN REFERENCE GUIDE

Plan name/address	Telephone eligibility	Copay	Preauthorization requirements	Test restrictions	Contracted lab(s) radiology	Contracted hospital(s)	Promised payment
Aetna PPO POB 43 WH XY 12345	013-239-0067	$5	hosp/surg/all dx tests	PE 1/yr	ABC Labs	College Hosp	30 days
Blue PPO POB 24335 WH XY 12345	013-245-0899	$8	referral specialist	PE 1/yr	Main St. Lab	St. John MC	30 days
Health Net POB 54000 WH XY 12345	013-408-5466	$5	hosp/surg see check list referrals	Mammo-gram 1/yr	Valley Lab	St. Joseph MC	45 days
Travelers MCO POB 1200 WH XY 12345	013-435-9877	$10	surg/hosp admit referrals	Pap >50 q3yr <50 q1yr	College Hosp. Metro Lab	College Hosp	30 days

Figure 10–5. Managed care plan reference guide to help keep efficient track of specifics for each managed care plan.

XYZ MEDICAL GROUP, INC.
1400 Avon Road, Suite 200
Woodland Hills, XY 12345

January 1, 20XX

TO: OUR PATIENTS

RE: PREFERRED PROVIDER ORGANIZATIONS

The following is a list of the PPOs and health insurance plans that we are members of and, therefore, will bill for you:

1. Georgia County Foundation
2. VIP Health Plan
3. Blue Cross Prudent Buyer Plan
4. Georgia County PPO
5. Northwest PPO
6. Blue Shield PPO

We are participating providers in several different PPOs. In order that we may maintain proper records for referrals and/or hospitalization, we request that each patient who is enrolled in a specific PPO keep our office currently informed regarding his or her eligibility status in that plan. Each time you are in the office for a visit, please verify with the receptionist that we have the correct coverage information.

If you have not informed us of changes in the status of your eligibility within the plan, you will be held responsible for any outstanding balance on your account due to that change.

Additionally, when your physician feels it is necessary to either hospitalize you or refer you to another physician outside this group, it is your responsibility to inform your physician that you belong to a specific PPO, as there may be restrictions imposed by that PPO regarding admission and referrals. If you fail to inform your physician at the time of referral or admission, our group may not be held responsible for noncoverage charges due to these restrictions.

If you have any questions regarding the above, please ask to speak to our insurance specialist.

I have read and understand the above text.

Signed: _____   Date: _____
            Patient (subscriber)

Figure 10–6. Sample letter to PPO subscribers outlining restrictions and noncovered services.

record. If the patient refuses to cooperate regarding managed care policy, document this in the medical record. Reimbursement may depend on the documentation.

Medical Records

Medical record management may differ when handling multiple managed care contracts. Place colored adhesive dots on patient file folder labels or color code managed care files by using a different colored chart for each EPO, HMO, IPA, and PPO patient. This decreases confusion and saves time in identifying individual plans so that coverage, copayment, billing, and authorization requirements are met.

Scheduling Appointments

Screen patients when they call for appointments to determine whether they belong to the same prepaid health plan as the physician. You may ask the patient to read from the insurance card to determine whether the physician's name is listed as the patient's primary care physician. Keep on hand an alphabetical list and profile of all plans with which the practice has a signed contract. It might also be useful to have a list of plans to which the practice does not belong. If the patient is not in a participating plan and still wishes to schedule a visit, inform him or her that payment at the time of the appointment is required and the amount is determined by the private fee schedule.

Encounter Form

Many managed care plans use an internal document on which the services rendered to the patient are checked off (charge ticket, encounter form, routing slip). It may also be used as a billing statement. The original is forwarded to the health plan's administrative office, and one copy is retained in the physician's files. Some plans require such documentation on an HCFA-1500 Health Insurance Claim form. Examples of encounter forms are shown in Chapters 2, 7, and 9, Figures 2–14, 7–9, and 9–7.

Financial Management

Payment

Deductibles

Usually, there is no **deductible** for a managed care plan. However, if there is one, be sure to collect it in the early months of the year (January through April) by asking patients if they have met their deductibles.

Copayments

In a managed care plan, a **copayment** is a predetermined fee paid by the patient to the provider at the time service is rendered. It is commonly referred to as a *copay* and is a form of cost sharing because the managed care plan or insurance company pays the remaining cost. Always collect the copay when the patient arrives for his or her appointment. Billing for small amounts is not cost effective, and it is easy to forget to ask for payment when the patient is leaving the office. Copays are commonly made for office visits, prescription drugs, inpatient mental health services, urgent care visits, and emergency department visits. However, the amount may vary according to the type of service.

Payment Mechanisms

Payment mechanisms in managed care plans vary and can range from fee for service and capitation to salaried physicians. The following are some details about other payment mechanisms.

Contact Capitation

Contact capitation is based on the concept of paying physicians for actual patient visits or "contacts." A scenario under this payment method would be when a patient needs to be referred to a specialist for care. When the patient visits the specialist for treatment, a "contact" occurs. The patient is assigned to the specialist for a defined period of time called the contact period. The length of the contact period is set in advance for each type of specialty by the participating specialty physician panel and MCO and may be tailored to the demographic and practice needs of the group. Each new patient visit during a contact period initiates a "contact point." Contact points determine how much to pay each physician. The average contact point value is determined by dividing the net specialty capitation pool or total amount of money set aside to be used for a particular specialty by the number of contacts in a certain time period. The average contact value is used to determine the amount paid to each specialist during each month in the contact period.

Case Rate Pricing

For specialists, another payment method is *case rate pricing*. This means the specialist contracts with the managed care plan for an entire episode of care. This may be done for certain high-volume, expensive surgical procedures (e.g., knee surgery, cataracts, bypass surgery).

Stop-Loss Limit

Some contracts have a "**stop-loss**" section, which means that if the patient's services go over a certain amount, then the physician can begin asking the patient to pay (fee for service); thus, in those instances, it is important to monitor each patient's ledger.

Contract Payment Time Limits

Usually state laws dictate the time limit within which a managed care plan must pay. The contract may or may not state the terms of payment, time limits, and late payment penalties, all of which can vary from one plan to another. Prompt-payment laws require payment within 30, 45, 55, or 60 days. To diminish late payment of claims, a contract can specify that late claims accrue interest (e.g., 5% interest for claims paid after the payment time limit has elapsed). Some states have enacted laws enforcing interest penalties for late payment for either or both private payers as well as managed care plans. Therefore, it is important to know the laws for your state. A time limit payment provision is an important factor to consider when reviewing a contract before a medical practice participates.

Monitoring Payment

Monitor payments made from all managed care plans, and note whether the payment received is less than the agreed amount as stated in the contract. If payment has been reduced, send a letter to the plan citing, "As per contract see page ___ regarding the fee for the consultation."

Sometimes a procedure (e.g., angioplasty with an assistant) may be done and the plan will not pay for an assistant, stating that it is not usual practice. However, you discover that in your region the standard practice is to always use an assistant for an angioplasty. When this is emphasized, the plan may remit additional payment.

Some states may have screening fees for emergency services and may or may not require prior approval for such services as defined by the Consolidated Omnibus Budget Reconciliation Act of 1985 (COBRA). There are also states that have adjudication laws with penalties if the managed care plan does not pay promptly. If claims are not being paid in a timely manner (30 days), take the following steps.

1. Write to the plan representative and list the unpaid claims, claims paid after the payment time limit, and claims paid in error.
2. Send a statement to the director of the managed care plan notifying him or her that if the bill is not paid you will contact the employer's benefits manager or patient and alert them to outstanding, slow-paying accounts. Say that this will prevent the physician from renewing the plan's contract, and ask the recipient to contact the plan's representative. The consumer has a choice of managed care plans; if the present plan does not fulfill his or her intent to pay, the managed care plan loses members because of dissatisfaction.
3. Take examples and statistics to the next renegotiating session when the physician's contract is expiring.

In Chapters 8 and 9, information is presented on how to handle slow or delinquent managed care plan payers.

Statement of Remittance

Managed care plans pay by either a capitation system (monthly check for the number of patients in the plan) or based on the services given to the patient (monthly check with a statement of remittance or explanation of benefits [EOB]).

In the capitation system, a monthly check arrives written out for the total amount of monthly capitation. The accompanying paperwork lists all eligible patients being paid for on a per capita basis divided into two groups, commercial and senior. Patients categorized as commercial are usually younger than age 65 and are paid at a lesser rate because their risk is lower (i.e., they do not need to see the doctor frequently). The senior patient category includes those older than age 65, and these are paid at a higher rate due to the increased risk. Always verify the individual capitated amounts listed by each name on the accompanying paperwork against the monthly eligibility list to balance the amount of the check. Contact the MCO if an error appears. If a specialist is capitated, there may be thousands of patients on the capitation plan and a list of patients would not be provided. The capitation amount for a specialist may be only a few cents per month calculated according to the risk of the patient needing specialty services.

In the system when payment is based on services rendered and an EOB is generated, such statements itemize services that have been rendered to patients and usually indicate the amount billed, amount allowed, amount paid, and whether there is any copayment to be made by the patient (Fig. 10–7). Generally, patients under managed care plans do not receive an EOB. Payments are checked against the managed care contract for verification and then posted to the patients' accounts. If an error is discovered, it should be brought to the attention of the plan's administrator and, depending on the circumstances, appealed.

Accounting

Managed care plans vary in their financial reimbursement structure, and careful accounting procedures are required. Accounting can become a confusing issue because of mixture of private patients and managed care patients with copayment requirements, coinsurance amounts, deductibles, and withholds.

Fee-for-Service

Some medical practices handle managed care patient accounts the same as fee-for-service patient accounts. If coinsurance payment is required at the time of service, post first the charge and then the coinsurance prepayment, calculated on the percentage of the charge the plan allows. Finally post an adjustment entry of the disallowed amount, which is calculated on a percentage of the MCO's allowable charge to balance the account (Fig. 10–8). If there is an overpayment, this would be shown as a refund or credit to the account.

STATEMENT OF REMITTANCE

PATIENT NAME (ID NUMBER)	SERVICE DATE MO. DAY YR	P O S	NO SVC	PROCEDURE NUMBER AND DESCRIPTION	AMOUNT BILLED	AMOUNT ALLOWED	RISK WITHHELD	CO PAY	AMOUNT PAID	ADJ. CODE
380224171-01 ALAN E.				CLAIM NO. 62730406 ACCOUNT NO.						
	092620XX	03	1 81000 URINALYSIS-ROUTINE		1000	1000	100	0	900	
	092620XX	03	1 82270 OCCULT BLOOD ANY S		1200	1200	120	0	1080	
	092620XX	03	1 99243 COMPRE RE-EXAM OR		6500	6500	650	0	5850	
	092620XX	03	1 36415 VENIPUNCTURE W/CEN		1700	1700	170	0	1530	
				CLAIM TOTALS =	10400	10400	1040	0	9360	
558700321-01 RONALD B.				CLAIM NO. 62730407 ACCOUNT NO.						
	092520XX	03	1 90050 LIM EXAM EVAL A/O		3000	3000	300	300	2400	
				CLAIM TOTALS =	3000	3000	300	300	2400	
473760096-01 DORMA L.				CLAIM NO. 62730408 ACCOUNT NO.						
	092520XX	03	1 90050 LIM EXAM EVAL A/O		3000	3000	300	300	2400	
				CLAIM TOTALS =	3800	3000	300	380	3120	

VENDOR SUMMARY: TOTAL AMOUNT PAID $1,638.96   TOTAL WITHHELD $194.39
AMOUNT PAID YEAR-TO-DATE: $42,411.95   AMOUNT WITHHELD YEAR-TO-DATE $5,109.94

Adjustment Code Legend
A = Adjusted: Billed amount exceeds VIP allowed.
O = Claim for service denied. Charges for this service included in other benefit payment. No patient liability.

Figure 10–7. Statement of remittance or explanation of benefits for noncapitated patients or contracted fee for service indicating the amount billed, amount allowed, amount paid, and if any copayment is to be made by the patient.

Year-End Evaluation

Withhold

Depending on the contract, a managed care plan may retain a percentage of the monthly capitation payment or a percentage of the allowable charges to physicians until the end of the year to cover operating expenses. This is known as **withhold**. A Statement of Remittance from the MCO shows the risk amounts withheld for each patient's visit in Column 8 of Figure 10–7. If the budgeted services for the plan are not overused, the withhold plus interest is returned to the physician at the end of the plan year. However, if services are overutilized, the withhold or a portion of it is retained by the plan. Thus, at year's end, the physicians share in any surplus or pay part of any deficit. This risk sharing creates an incentive for limiting care by the gatekeeper and limiting referrals to specialists, thereby keeping medical costs down. The withhold can cover all services or be specific to hospital care, **ancillary services** (laboratory/x-ray usages), or specialty referrals.

A managed care plan that withholds a percentage of the allowable charge must be tracked in the physician's accounts receivable so it is not prematurely written off as a bad debt. To do this, develop a capitation accounting worksheet listing the dates of service, patients' names, CPT code for the service rendered, fee-for-service charges, withheld amounts and disallowed amounts (Fig. 10–9). Then total all columns. The total of the withheld column is a debit entry that indicates what the managed care plan owes to the medical practice pending its year-end reconciliation. If and when the withheld amount arrives, the accounting worksheet can be compared with what was withheld during the year. The amount of the withholds that are not returned to the physician is adjusted off once withholds are settled. The total of the column for disallowed amounts shows the amount written off by the medical practice. Combine the withheld returned amount with the managed care payment for the year to determine whether it is worthwhile for the practice to participate in the plan. Some practices can use the information to renegotiate increased fees when the managed care contract is to be renewed.

Capitation versus Fee-for-Service

In most medical practices, financial management reports are generated via computer and are the responsibility of the manager and/or accountant. However, it can be an asset for an insurance biller to have some knowledge of what these reports con-

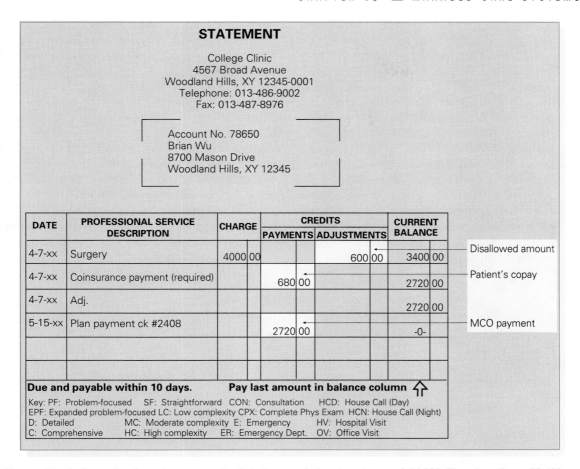

Figure 10–8. Example of posting to a patient's ledger card showing charge of $4,000. The plan allows $3,400, so the patient's prepaid coinsurance amount is $680 (20% of $3,400). The managed care plan sent a check for $2,720 (80% of $3,400), and the disallowed amount ($600) was adjusted off of the account, which brings the account balance to zero.

tain. Most medical practices monitor plan payments for profit or loss by comparing actual income from managed care patients with what would have been received from fee-for-service plans. To do this, one would design a capitation accounting sheet for each capitated plan. This sheet would show a listing of

dates of service and professional service descriptions (procedures, injections, and laboratory work) as well as charges and payments (Fig. 10–10). As managed care plan patients receive services, actual service fees would be posted in a charge column from the office fee schedule as if the patient were a

			DEBIT			
Date	**Patient**	**Service**	**Charge**	**Withhold**	**Disallow**	
5/15/20XX	Mason	99204	106.11	5.94	21.22	Disallowed amounts
5/15/20XX	Mason	93000	34.26	1.92	3.43	
5/15/20XX	Mason	81000	8.00	.38	2.40	
5/15/20XX	Self	93501	1500.00	240.00	300.00	
Total			1648.38	248.24	327.05	Total withheld amount owed by MCO

Figure 10–9. Example of a managed care plan when payment is on a fee-for-service basis. Note disallowed portion of the charge based on the plan's allowable charge. A portion of the allowable charge is withheld.

private payer. In a payment column, office visit, co-payments, and the monthly capitation payment would be posted. Then all columns would be totaled. Because the physician is usually paid on an allowed amount rather than an actual charge, it is necessary to apply a discount to the total charged amount for a realistic comparison. To do this, calculate the difference between the actual charge and the average allowed amount.

At the end of the year, compare the capitated payment amounts plus copayment amounts to the total discounted charges. This gives an accurate idea of whether the capitated payment received is adequate for the services the physician performed. Compiling monthly records and reviewing them at the end of the year helps a medical practice assess the gain or loss of each capitation plan.

Bankruptcy

If an MCO declares bankruptcy, such as a Chapter 11 filing, it is obligated to pay for all bills incurred after the filing. If the patient had treatment before the filing, a delay in getting reimbursed may occur

because the MCO cannot repay debts incurred before its filing until it has worked out a reorganization plan. Physicians under contract with the MCO are obligated to honor their contractual commitments. If their contracts expire or if they have escape clauses, they may be required to continue accepting patients depending on the contract provisions.

Some clauses allow a physician to withdraw from seeing managed care patients or leave if the MCO is in bankruptcy proceedings for more than 4 months. However, bankruptcy courts have broad powers to prevent physicians from leaving MCOs in bankruptcy proceedings if the court deems such actions to be detrimental to the rehabilitation of the debtor.

In some states, laws such as California's Knox-Keene Health Care Service Plan Act of 1975 prohibit hospitals and physicians under contract to an MCO from billing patients. Other states do not have such protection but may have created emergency insurance funds to limit the financial liability of enrollees in bankrupt MCOs. If you write to the insurance commissioner, he or she will refer you back to the MCO. However, your letter makes

CAPITATION ACCOUNTING WORKSHEET

NAME OF PLAN ABC Managed Care Plan

DATE OF SERVICE	PROFESSIONAL SERVICE DESCRIPTION	CHARGES Services Fees	PAYMENTS Capitation	Copay	
20XX 1/15	Capitation (105 members) @ $8 ea		840.00 ←		Capitation payment
2/15	Capitation (115 members)		920.00		
2/20	Sanchez OV/Copay	35.00		5.00 ←	Copayment amount
2/22	Jones OV/Copay	35.00		5.00	
2/23	Davis OV/Copay	35.00 ←		5.00	Actual fee-for-servce charge
3/6	Evans OV/Copay	35.00		5.00	
3/15	Capitation (130 members)		1040.00		
4/10	Wu OV/Copay	35.00		5.00	
4/15	Capitation (135 members)		1080.00		
	May through December are not shown				
END OF YEAR TOTALS		3500.00	6880.00	500.00	

Figure 10–10. Example of an accounting sheet for a capitation plan from January through April showing dates of service, professional service descriptions, members' charges, and capitation payments and copayments received by the medical practice. Charges and payments columns may be totaled at the end of the year to compare capitation with fee-for-service earnings.

insurance commissioners aware of problems that have developed.

Further information on the topic of bankruptcy can be found in Chapter 9.

STUDENT ASSIGNMENT LIST

✔ Study Chapter 10.
✔ Answer the review questions in the *Workbook* to reinforce the theory learned in this chapter and to help prepare you for a future test.

✔ Complete the assignments in the *Workbook* to give you hands-on experience in abstracting information from a medical record to complete treatment authorization forms for prepaid health insurance cases.
✔ Turn to the Glossary at the end of this textbook for a further understanding of the Key Terms used in this chapter.

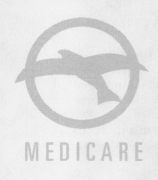

MEDICARE

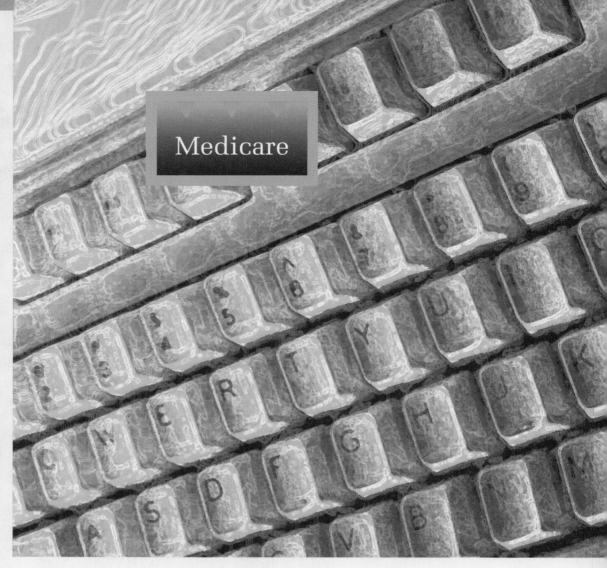

Medicare

11

CHAPTER OUTLINE

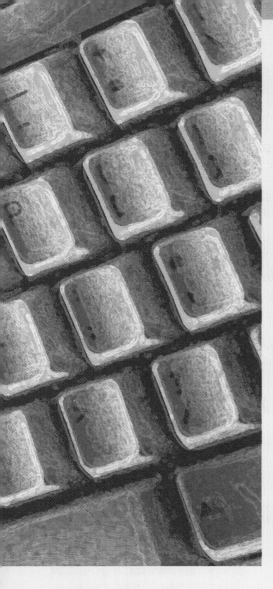

OBJECTIVES*

After reading this chapter, you should be able to:

- Explain eligibility criteria for Medicare.
- Name important information to abstract from a patient's Medicare card.
- Identify the benefits and nonbenefits of Medicare.
- List the federal laws adopted to increase health benefits for employed workers and the elderly.
- Name the conditions when an HMO-Medicare patient can be seen by a nonmember HMO physician.
- Differentiate between an HMO Risk Plan and an HMO Cost Plan.
- Name the federal laws that relate to cost containment of health services and to reduction of fraud and abuse issues.
- Explain when to obtain a patient's signature on a waiver of liability agreement.
- Define a Medicare-mandated prepayment screen.
- State the benefits for a participating versus nonparticipating physician.
- Calculate a payment for a procedure using the current conversion factor.
- List situations for using a lifetime beneficiary claim authorization and information release document.
- Determine the time limit for submitting a Medicare claim.
- Explain claims submission for individuals who have Medicare with other insurance.
- List HCFA-1500 block numbers that require Medigap information when submitting a Medicare/Medigap claim.
- Post information on the patient's ledger after a Medicare payment has been received.

KEY TERMS

approved charges

assignment

benefit period

crossover claim

diagnostic cost groups (DCGs)

disabled

end-stage renal disease (ESRD)

fiscal intermediary (FI)

Health Care Financing Administration (HCFA)

hospice

hospital insurance

intermediate care facilities (ICFs)

limiting charge

medical necessity

Medicare

Medicare/Medicaid (Medi-Medi)

Medicare Secondary Payer (MSP)

continued

---

*Performance objectives and exercises for hands-on practical experience for this chapter appear in the *Workbook* and on the computer disk.

Chartrand's Medicare Laws

Individuals completing claims and working with Medicare patients will rapidly discover the frustration that is captured in writer David Chartrand's humorous poster "Medicare Laws".* These "laws" sometimes refer to the lack of or constant changes in Medicare policy.

There are no rules for properly coding reimbursement forms. There are only penalties for doing it wrong.

Or there are a myriad of required forms for trying to deal with government regulations.

Medicare will always revise its claim forms the week after you have purchased a year's supply of the current ones.

In addition, the patient may be hard of hearing, visually impaired, have poor memory retention, or difficulty in getting around.

There is an inverse relationship between the hours spent treating a nursing-home patient and the fee Medicare thinks you should receive for doing it.

Then there are telephone questions about Medicare rules and hours spent trying to find information in the Medicare manual or getting transferred via voice mail in the Medicare telephone system.

When more than one supervisor at Medicare gives you the same incorrect information, no one will be at fault. If you feel you've finally figured out Medicare's rules, don't worry. The feeling will soon go away.

Finally, there are the denied, rejected, or returned claims and no payment.

Medicare, as a rule, will always expect you to know if the instructions you got from a Medicare representative were correct or incorrect. When the enforcement officer calls, you then will learn whether you guessed right.

Well, you probably guessed by now that everything in this section in italics was written with a sense of humor. It is important to learn about the Medicare program but also just as vital to be able to laugh to relieve some of the stress that occurs while dealing with its intricate policies and contradictions.

Policies and Regulations

Eligibility Requirements

Medicare is run by the **Health Care Financing Administration (HCFA).** Local Social Security Administration (SSA) offices take applications for Medicare and provide information about the program. The eligible person must apply to receive the benefits.

---

*To obtain David V. Chartrand's complete set of "Medicare Laws" in poster form, write him at 130 North Cherry Street, #202, Olathe, KS 66061-3460 or send a fax to (913) 768-4900.

Eligible persons may apply at age 65 to receive full-time retirement benefits and Medicare Parts A and/or B. In the year 2000, the retirement age gradually increased for people born in the year 1938 or later. By 2027, for people born after 1959 full-time retirement age will be 67. Benefits may increase if retirement is delayed beyond full-retirement age. As of this edition, Medicare may still be applied for at age 65. Those who apply for Social Security early (at age 62 years) do not receive Medicare but receive monthly reduced Social Security benefits.

Medicare is a federal health insurance program for the following categories of people:

1. People 65 years of age or older who are retired on Social Security
2. People 65 years of age or older who are retired from the railroad or civil service
3. Blind individuals
4. **Disabled** individuals who are eligible for Social Security disability benefits[*] and are in the following categories:
   a. Disabled workers of any age
   b. Disabled widows of workers who are fully or currently insured through the federal government, civil service, Social Security Administration (SSA), **Supplemental Security Income (SSI),** or the Railroad Retirement Act and whose husbands qualified for benefits under one of these programs
   c. Adults disabled before age 18 whose parents are eligible for or retired on Social Security benefits
5. Children and adults who have chronic kidney disease requiring dialysis or **end-stage renal disease (ESRD)** requiring kidney transplant.
6. Kidney donors (all expenses related to the kidney transplantation are covered)

All persons who meet one of the previously stated eligibility requirements are eligible for Medicare Part A (hospital coverage). Those who qualify for full Medicare benefits may also elect to take Medicare Part B (outpatient coverage). Medicare Part B recipients pay annually increasing basic premiums to the SSA, and some pay a Medicare surtax on federal income tax payments. This premium may be automatically deducted from the patient's monthly Social Security check if he or she wishes. Those individuals not eligible

for Medicare Part A (hospital insurance) at age 65 may purchase Part B from the SSA.

Aliens

An alien on Medicare may be eligible for Part A and/or Part B coverage. To be eligible, the applicant must have lived in the United States as a permanent resident for 5 consecutive years. It is usually not necessary to state on the HCFA-1500 form that the patient is an alien when billing Medicare.

Health Insurance Card

The patient should present his or her Medicare health insurance card indicating the patient's insurance claim number (Figs. 11–1 and 11–2). The claim number is the Social Security number of the wage earner with an alpha suffix. The card indicates hospital and medical coverage, the effective date, and the patient status. When a husband and wife both have Medicare, they receive separate cards and claim numbers. Medicare cards are red, white, and blue, and cards issued after 1990 are plastic.

The letters following the Medicare number on the patient's identification card indicate the patient's status as follows (this is only a partial listing):

A = wage earner (shown in Fig. 11–1)
B = husband's number (wife 62 years or older)
D = widow
HDA = disabled adult
C = disabled child
J, Kl, or Jl = special monthly benefits, never worked under Social Security
M = Part B benefits only
T = uninsured and entitled only to health insurance benefits

A patient whose Medicare card claim number ends in "A" will have the *same* Social Security and claim numbers. A patient whose Medicare card claim number ends in "B" or "D" will have *different* Social Security and claim numbers. A quick check between Social Security and card claim numbers may identify a submission error and forestall a claims rejection.

The letters preceding the Medicare number on the patient's identification card indicate *railroad retirees*:

A   Retired railroad employee
              Examples: A 000000 (6 digits);
                  A 000-00-0000 (9 digits)
MA   Spouse of a retired railroad employee

---

[*]Note: In the disabled categories, a person must be disabled for not less than 12 months to apply for disability benefits. A disabled beneficiary must receive disability benefits for 24 months before Medicare benefits begin. See Chapter 15 for further information on this topic.

WA/WD	Widow or widower of deceased employee (age or disability)
	Examples: WA000000 (6 digits); WA000-00-0000 (9 digits)
CA	Child or student
WCA/WCD	Widow of retiree with child in her care or disabled child of deceased employee
PA/PD	Parent of deceased employee (male or female)
H	Railroad retirement board pensioner before 1937
MH	Wife of railroad retirement board pensioner before 1937
WH	Widowed wife of railroad retirement board pensioner before 1937
WCH	Widow of railroad retirement board pensioner with child in her care
PH	Parent of railroad retirement board pensioner before 1937
JA	Widow receiving a joint and survivor annuity
X	Divorced spouse's annuity, for use on forms AA-3 and AA-7 only
	Example: CA 123-45-6789C

Enrollment Status

An individual is eligible to enroll in Medicare 3 months before his or her 65th birthday, and the enrollment period ends 3 months after the month in which the person turns 65. If the enrollment period is missed, the individual must wait until the next general enrollment period—January 1 through March 31.

A telephone hotline or, in some states, a modem is available to verify the enrollment status.

This is useful because patients can switch coverage to a senior managed care plan on a month-to-month basis. Most carriers also allow information on deductible status. The patient's numeric information (Medicare number and date of birth) is entered into the telephone system, and the digital response indicates how much of the deductible has been satisfied. Contact the Medicare fiscal agent in your location for information about this service.

Benefits and Nonbenefits

Medicare Part A—Hospital Benefits

Part A of Medicare is **hospital insurance** benefits for the aged, disabled, and blind. Funds for this health service come from special contributions from employees and self-employed persons, with employers matching contributions. These contributions are collected along with regular Social Security contributions from wages and self-employment income earned during a person's working years.

A **benefit period** begins the day a patient enters a hospital and ends when the patient has not been a bed patient in any hospital or **nursing facility (NF)** (formerly called skilled nursing facility) for 60 consecutive days. It also ends if a patient has been in a nursing facility but has not received skilled nursing care for 60 consecutive days. A nursing facility offers nursing and/or rehabilitation services that are medically necessary to a patient's recovery. Services provided are not custodial. Custodial services are those that assist the patient

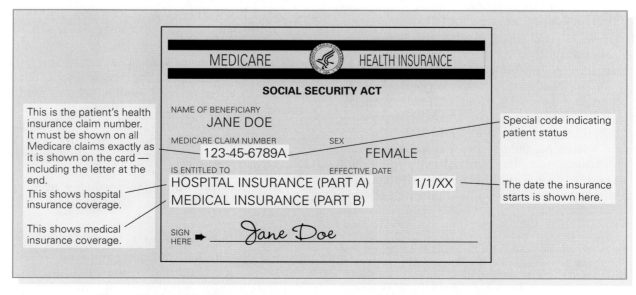

Figure 11–1. Medicare Health Insurance Claim Card. Cards issued since 1990 are plastic.

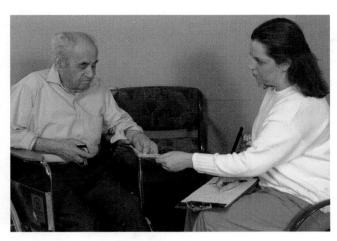

Figure 11-2. Insurance billing specialist welcoming a Medicare patient to obtain the identification card from a disabled patient.

with personal needs (i.e., dressing, eating, bathing, getting in and out of bed). Hospital insurance protection is renewed every time the patient begins a new benefit period. There is no limit to the number of benefit periods a patient can have for hospital or nursing facility care. However, special limited benefit periods apply to hospice care.

Medicare Part A provides benefits to applicants in any of the following situations:

1. A bed patient in a hospital (up to 90 hospital days for each benefit period).
2. A bed patient in a nursing facility (up to 100 extended-care days for each benefit period).
3. A patient receiving home health care services.
4. A patient who needs care in a psychiatric hospital (up to 190 days in a lifetime).
5. A terminally ill patient diagnosed as having 6 months or less to live who needs hospice care. A **hospice** is a public agency or private organization that is primarily engaged in providing pain relief, symptom management, and supportive services to terminally ill people and their families.
6. A terminally ill patient who needs respite care. **Respite care** is a short-term inpatient stay that may be necessary for the terminally ill patient to give temporary relief to the person who regularly assists with home care. Inpatient respite care is limited to stays of no more than 5 consecutive days for each respite period.

Figure 11-3 contains information on five major classifications of inpatient hospital cost-sharing benefits for Medicare Part A. Miscellaneous hospital services and supplies might consist of intensive care unit (ICU) costs, blood transfusions, drugs, x-ray and laboratory tests, medical supplies (casts, surgical dressings, splints), use of wheelchair, op-

erating room (OR) and recovery room costs, and therapy (physical, occupational, speech-language). There are no benefits for personal convenience items (television, radio, telephone), private duty nurses, or a private room unless it is determined medically necessary. Similar benefits also relate to nursing facilities.

Benefits for hospice and respite care consist of nursing and physicians' services, drugs, therapy (physical, occupational, speech-language pathology), home health aide, homemaker services, medical social services, medical supplies and appliances, short-term inpatient care, and counseling.

Medicare Part B—Medical Benefits

Part B of Medicare is **supplementary medical insurance (SMI)** benefits for the aged, disabled, and blind. Funds for this program come equally from those who sign up for it and the federal government. A medical insurance **premium** is automatically deducted from monthly checks for those who receive Social Security benefits, railroad retirement benefits, or a civil service annuity. Others pay the premium directly to the SSA.

Figure 11-4 contains information on five major classifications of medical benefits for Medicare Part B. In addition to medical and surgical services by a doctor of medicine (MD), doctor of osteopathy (DO or MD), or a doctor of dental medicine or dental surgery (DDS), certain services by podiatrists (DPM) and limited services by chiropractors (DC) are paid for. Dental care is covered only for fractures or surgery of the jaw. Optometric examinations are provided if a person has aphakia (absence of the natural lens of the eye).

Preventive care benefits that Medicare will pay for are

❱ Annual mammograms for women age 40 and older, plus a one-time baseline mammogram for women aged 35 to 39.
❱ Papanicolaou tests every 3 years. For women at high risk for cervical and vaginal cancer and those with a recent abnormal Papanicolaou test, Medicare will pay for an annual examination.
❱ Colorectal cancer screening for people age 50 and older. The test covered is dependent on the patient's risk level and the time elapsed from his or her last screening.
❱ Annual prostate cancer screening procedures, including digital rectal examinations and prostate-specific antigen (PSA) blood tests, for men older than age 50.
❱ Purchase of home glucose monitors and testing strips for people with diabetes. Wider range of

MEDICARE (PART A): HOSPITAL INSURANCE-COVERED SERVICES FOR 2001

Services	Benefit	Medicare Pays	Patient Pays
HOSPITALIZATION Semiprivate room and board, general nursing and miscellaneous hospital services and supplies. (Medicare payments based on benefit periods.)	First 60 days	All but $792	$792 deductible
	61st to 90th day 91st to 150th day[1]	All but $198 a day	$198 a day
	60-reserve-days benefit	All but $396 a day	$396 a day
	Beyond 150 days	Nothing	All costs
NURSING FACILITY CARE Patient must have been in a hospital for at least 3 days and enter a Medicare-approved facility generally within 30 days after hospital discharge.[2] (Medicare payments based on benefit periods.)	First 20 days	100% of approved amount	Nothing
	21st to 100th day	All but $99 a day	Up to $99 a day
	Beyond 100 days	Nothing	All costs
HOME HEALTH CARE Part-time or intermittent skilled care, home health aide services, durable medical equipment and supplies, and other services.	Unlimited as long as Medicare conditions are met and services are declared "medically necessary".	100% of approved amount; 80% of approved amount for durable medical equipment.	Nothing for services; 20% of approved amount for durable medical equipment.
HOSPICE CARE Pain relief, symptom management, and support services for the terminally ill.	If patient elects the hospice option and as long as doctor certifies need.	All but limited costs for outpatient drugs and inpatient respite care.	Limited cost sharing for outpatient drugs and inpatient respite care.
BLOOD	Unlimited if medically necessary.	All but first 3 pints per calendar year.	For first 3 pints.[3]

[1] This 60-reserve-days benefit may be used only once in a lifetime.
[2] Neither Medicare nor private Medigap insurance will pay for most long-term nursing home care.
[3] To the extent the blood deductible is met under Part B of Medicare during the calendar year, it does not have to be met under Part A.

Figure 11–3. Five major classifications of Medicare Part A benefits. (Modified from Your Medicare Handbook for Railroad Retirement Beneficiaries. U.S. Government Printing Office, 2001.)

diabetes self-management training and therapeutic shoes for severe diabetic foot disease may also be covered.

▶ Bone mass measurements for women 65 and older at high risk for osteoporosis.
▶ Vaccines (influenza, pneumococcal pneumonia, hepatitis B).
▶ Ambulance service meeting medical necessity requirements.
▶ Rental or purchase of durable medical equipment for home use, prosthetic devices for internal body organs, artificial limbs and eyes, and braces or supports (leg, arm, back, neck).

Nonbenefits consist of routine physical examination, routine foot care, eye or hearing examinations, and cosmetic surgery unless due to injury or performed to improve functioning of a malformed part. A physician may bill a patient separately for noncovered services.

There are many other benefits and nonbenefits too numerous to list here. To find out whether a particular procedure qualifies for payment, refer to Medicare newsletters or contact your Medicare carrier.

Medicare Part C—Medicare Plus (+) Choice Program

The Balanced Budget Act of 1997 created Medicare + Choice. This program increased the number of health care options in addition to those that are available under Part A and Part B. Medicare + Choice plans receive a fixed amount of money from Medicare to spend on their Medicare members. Some plans may require members to pay a premium similar to the Medicare Part B premium.

Plans available under this program may include the following: health maintenance organiza-

MEDICARE (PART B): MEDICAL INSURANCE-COVERED SERVICES FOR 2001

Services	Benefit	Medicare Pays	Patient Pays
MEDICAL EXPENSES Physicians' services, inpatient and outpatient medical and surgical services and supplies, physical and speech therapy, ambulance, diagnostic tests, and other services.	Unlimited if medically necessary.	80% of approved amount (after $100 deductible). Reduced to 50% for most outpatient mental health services.	$100 deductible,[1] plus 20% of approved amount or limited charges.[2]
CLINICAL LABORATORY SERVICES Blood tests, urinalyses, and more.	Unlimited if medically necessary.	100% of approved amount.	Nothing for services.
HOME HEALTH CARE Part-time or intermittent care, home health aide services, durable medical equipment and supplies, and other services.	Unlimited as long as patient meets conditions and benefits are declared medically necessary.	100% of approved amount; 80% of approved amount for durable medical equipment.	Nothing for services; 20% of approved amount for durable medical equipment.
OUTPATIENT HOSPITAL TREATMENT Services for the diagnosis or treatment of illness or injury.	Unlimited if medically necessary.	Medicare payment to hospital based on hospital cost.	$100 deductible, plus 20% of whatever the hospital charges.
BLOOD	Unlimited if medically necessary.	80% of approved amount (after $100 deductible and starting with 4th pint).	First 3 pints plus 20% of approved amounts for additional pints (after $100 deductible).[3]
AMBULATORY SURGICAL SERVICES	Unlimited if medically necessary.	80% of predetermined amount (after $100 deductible).	$100 deductible plus 20% of predetermined amount.

[1]Once the patient has had $100 of expenses for covered services in the year, the Part B deductible does not apply to any further covered services received for the rest of the year.

[2]See Figure 11–8 for an explanation of approved amount for participating physicians and limited charges for nonparticipating physicians.

[3]To the extent the blood deductible is met under Part A of Medicare during the calendar year, it does not have to be met under Part B.

Figure 11–4. Five major classifications of Medicare Part B benefits. (Modified from Your Medicare Handbook for Railroad Retirement Beneficiaries. U.S. Government Printing Office, 2001.)

tion (HMO), point-of-service (POS) plan, preferred provider organization (PPO), private fee-for-service (PFFS) plan, provider sponsored organization (PSO), religious fraternal benefit society (RFBS), and a pilot program, medical savings account (MSA). Most of these are discussed in Chapters 2 and 10, except for PSO, RFBS, and MSA.

A PSO is a managed care plan that is owned and operated by a hospital and provider group instead of an insurance company. An RFBS is a managed care option that is associated with a church, group of churches, or convention. Membership is restricted to church members and is allowed regardless of the person's health status. In an MSA plan, the patient chooses an insurance policy approved by Medicare that has a high annual deductible. Medicare pays the premiums for this policy and deposits the dollar-amount difference between what it pays for the average beneficiary in the patient's area and the cost of the premium into the patient's MSA. The patient uses the MSA money to pay medical expenses until the high deductible is reached. If the MSA money becomes depleted, the patient pays out of pocket until the deductible is reached. Unused funds roll over to the next year.

Railroad Retirement Benefits

Railroad Retirement Board offices take applications for Medicare and provide information about the program for railroad workers and their beneficiaries. Medical insurance premiums are automatically deducted from the monthly checks of people who receive railroad retirement benefits. Those who do not receive a monthly check pay their premiums directly or, in some cases, have premiums paid on their behalf under a state assistance program. If the allowed fees differ from those allowed by your regular Medicare carrier, write or fax the Medicare railroad retiree carrier, asking that fees be based on fee data from your local carrier.

Railroad retirement beneficiaries are generally entitled to benefits for covered services received from a qualified American facility. However, under certain circumstances, a Medicare beneficiary may receive care in Canada or Mexico. Benefits and deductibles under Parts A and B are the same as for other Medicare recipients.

Some railroad retirees are members of a railroad hospital association or a prepayment plan. These members pay regular premiums to the plan and then can receive health services the plan provides without additional charges. In some plans, small charges are made for certain services, such as drugs or home visits. Many prepayment plans make arrangements with Medicare to receive direct payments for services they furnish that are covered under Medicare Part B. Some prepayment plans have contracts with Medicare as HMOs or competitive medical plans and can receive direct payment for services covered by either hospital or medical insurance. After a claim is submitted to the Medicare railroad retiree carrier, a Remittance Advice (RA) document is generated, explaining the decision made on the claim and what services Medicare paid.

A list of fiscal agents or carriers for Medicare railroad retirees appears in Appendix A.

Employed Elderly Benefits

To understand various types of scenerios that may be encountered when submitting claims for elderly individuals, it is important to know about several powerful federal laws that regulate health care coverage of those age 65 and older who are employed. Such individuals may have group insurance or a Medigap (MG) policy and may fall under billing categories of Medicare First payer or Medicare Secondary Payer (all are presented in detail later in this chapter).

Omnibus Budget Reconciliation Act

The Omnibus Budget Reconciliation Act (OBRA) of 1981 required that, in the case of a current or former employee or dependent younger than age 65 and Medicare eligible solely because of end-stage renal disease, the employer's group coverage is primary for up to 12 months. This act applies to all employers regardless of the number of employees. OBRA of 1986, effective in 1987, required that if an employee or dependent younger than age 65 has Medicare coverage due to a disability other than end-stage renal disease, the group coverage is primary and Medicare is secondary. This act applies only to large group health plans having at least 100 full- or part-time employees.

Tax Equity and Fiscal Responsibility Act

The Tax Equity and Fiscal Responsibility Act (TEFRA) of 1982 established that an employee or spouse aged 65 to 69 years is entitled to the same health insurance benefits offered under the same conditions to younger employees and their spouses. The group insurance is primary and Medicare is secondary. TEFRA applies to employers with at least 20 full- or part-time employees.

Deficit Reduction Act

The Deficit Reduction Act (DEFRA) of 1984, effective 1985, was an amendment to TEFRA and stated that a spouse aged 65 to 69 years or an employee of any age is entitled to the same group health plan offered to younger employees and their spouses. The group's coverage is primary and Medicare is secondary. DEFRA applies to employers with at least 20 full- or part-time employees.

Consolidated Omnibus Budget Reconciliation Act

The Consolidated Omnibus Budget Reconciliation Act (COBRA) of 1985, effective 1986, is another amendment to TEFRA eliminating the age ceiling of 69 years. An employee or spouse age 65 or older is entitled to the same group health plan offered to younger employees and their spouses. COBRA requires that third party payers reimburse for certain care rendered in government-run veteran and military hospitals. The group's coverage is primary and Medicare is secondary. COBRA applies to employers with at least 20 full- or part-time employees.

Tax Reform Act

The Tax Reform Act was passed in 1986; it clarified certain aspects of COBRA. A spouse and dependents may elect to receive continued coverage even if the employee does not wish insurance coverage and terminates the plan. However, the spouse and dependents must have been covered under the plan before the covered employee terminates it. Spouses who are widowed or divorced while receiving continued coverage must report such changes to the benefit plan administrator within 60 days of the employee's death to determine how many additional months of coverage are available.

Additional Insurance Programs

Many Medicare recipients have Medicare in combination with other insurance plans. This section explains various coverage combinations. Guidelines for processing claims for these plans are presented later in this chapter.

Medicare/Medicaid

Patients designated as **Medicare/Medicaid (Medi-Medi)** are on both Medicare and Medicaid (in California Medi-Cal) simultaneously and are those who qualify for Old Age Security (OAS) assistance benefits (older than age 65), the severely disabled, and the blind.

Medicare/Medigap

A specialized insurance policy devised for the Medicare beneficiary is called **Medigap (MG)** or *Medifill.* This type of policy is designed to supplement coverage under a fee-for-service Medicare plan. It may cover prescription costs and the deductible and copayment (e.g., 20% of the Medicare allowed amount) that are typically the patient's responsibility under Medicare. These plans are offered by private third party payers to Medicare beneficiaries.

The federal government in conjunction with the insurance industry established predefined minimum benefits for 10 Medigap policies categorized by alpha letters A through J (Fig. 11–5). Basic benefits are found in policy A. Each subsequent letter represents basic benefits plus other coverage, with the most comprehensive benefits in Policy J. Sale of all policies are not available in all states, so individuals in some states have fewer options than others.

A slightly different variation of a Medigap policy is *Medicare Select.* This policy has the same coverage as regular Medigap policies, but there is a restriction in that the beneficiary must obtain medical care from a list of specified network doctors and providers.

Medicare Supplemental Insurance

Many people older than the age of 65 years elect to purchase private insurance to supplement Medicare. This is not to be confused with Medicare Part B, which is referred to as Supplementary Medical Insurance (SMI) because it supplements the hospital coverage (Part A). It helps pay for some of the expenses that Medicare does not cover. There are two types of policies: service benefit or incurred type and indemnity benefit type.

Service benefit policies pay Medicare's Part A deductible and copayments as well as Part B's coinsurance requirements. This type of policy automatically adjusts with cost increases caused by inflation or changes in the Medicare Part A deductible. These policies only supplement what Medicare pays for *covered services* the patient has actually received; they do not cover Medicare noncovered (disallowed) services. However, a comprehensive insurance policy sometimes covers some things Medicare does not pay for, but it usually requires that the patient pass a physical examination.

Indemnity benefit policies pay fixed-dollar benefits and do not necessarily keep up with inflation or changes in Medicare's deductible or copayments. Therefore, the patient has to purchase additional coverage from time to time.

There are also private insurance policies that insure against specific diseases, such as cancer.

When a patient is in an NF and is declared *custodial,* meaning in need of long-term care and with little chance for improvement, Medicare and most private health insurance will not pay. A few insurance policies are written specifically for custodial care. There are three types of long-term care insurance policies:

1. Indemnity plans that pay a set amount per day for care
2. Reimbursement policies that pay a percentage for services
3. Policies that combine indemnity and reimbursement.

Medicare Secondary Payer

In some instances, Medicare is considered secondary and classifies the situation as **Medicare Secondary Payer (MSP).** To identify whether Medicare is primary or secondary and to know what additional benefits the patient might have, follow the suggested steps in the following procedure.

TEN MEDIGAP STANDARDIZED POLICIES

(Not all may be available in all states.)

A	B	C	D	E	F	G	H	I	J
Basic Benefit	Basic Benefit	Basic Benefit	Basic Benefit	Basic Benefit	Basic Benefit	Basic Benefit	Basic Benefit	Basic Benefit	Basic Benefit
		Skilled Nursing Coinsurance	Skilled Nursing Coinsurance	Skilled Nursing Coinsurance	Skilled Nursing Coinsurance	Skilled Nursing Coinsurance	Skilled Nursing Coinsurance	Skilled Nursing Coinsurance	Skilled Nursing Coinsurance
	Part A Deductible	Part A Deductible	Part A Deductible	Part A Deductible	Part A Deductible	Part A Deductible	Part A Deductible	Part A Deductible	Part A Deductible
	Part B Deductible				Part B Deductible				Part B Deductible
					Part B Excess 100%	Part B Excess 100%		Part B Excess 100%	Part B Excess 100%
		Foreign Travel Emergency	Foreign Travel Emergency	Foreign Travel Emergency	Foreign Travel Emergency	Foreign Travel Emergency	Foreign Travel Emergency	Foreign Travel Emergency	Foreign Travel Emergency
			At-Home Recovery			At-Home Recovery		At-Home Recovery	At-Home Recovery
							Basic Drug Benefit ($1,250 Limit)	Basic Drug Benefit ($1,250 Limit)	Extended Drug Benefit ($3,000 Limit)
				Preventive Care					Preventive Care

Figure 11–5. Ten Medigap standardized policies. (Reprinted with permission from Cash C: The Medicare Answer Book. Provincetown, MA, Race Point Press, 1998.)

PROCEDURE: Determining if Medicare is Primary or Secondary/ Determining Additional Benefits

1. Inquire whether the patient is covered under one or more of the following plans or situations:

   ▶ *Automobile liability insurance, no-fault insurance, and self-insured liability insurance.* An individual injured or ill because of an automobile accident may be covered by liability insurance or no-fault insurance.

   ▶ *Disability insurance.* Disability insurance coverage offered through an employer-sponsored large group health plan (LGHP).

   ▶ *Employee group health plan (EGHP).* Insurance policies for individuals aged 65 years or older who are still employed. Employers with 20 or more employees are required to offer workers and their spouses aged 65 through 69 the same health benefits offered to younger workers. Workers may accept or reject the employer's health insurance plan. If they accept it, Medicare becomes the secondary insurance carrier.

   ▶ *Employer supplemental insurance.* A Medicare beneficiary has this plan through a former employer. Some people are covered by employment plans even after retirement, provided the plan allows it and the insured informs the insurance company he or she wishes to maintain coverage. Benefits can vary in these supplemental plans, and these policies are not considered "Medigap" as defined by federal law. *Note:* When an employee retires and Medicare becomes the primary coverage, the company's group health plan coordinates benefits with Medicare. These are known as conversion policies.

▶ *Federal Black Lung Act.* An act was formed to cover employees or former coal miner employees who have illness related to black lung disorder and have acceptable diagnoses that occur on the Department of Labor's list.

▶ *Veterans Affairs.* A Medicare beneficiary is also receiving benefits from the Department of Veterans Affairs.

▶ *Workers' compensation.* An individual suffers a disease or injury connected with employment.

These plans are billed as **primary** (first) **payer** and Medicare second. Payments for these types of policies may not necessarily go to the physician but may go to the insured.

1. Ask to see the Medicare card as well as any other insurance cards and make photocopies of both sides of each card.
2. Inquire from the patient whether the supplemental coverage was carried over (conversion policy) from his or her employer.
3. Call the carrier if the type of plan is not clearly identified.
4. Bill the correct insurance plan.

   ▶ For Medigap cases, nonparticipating physicians may collect copayments and deductibles up to their limiting charge (unless the state forbids collection of more than the allowed amount) from patients at the time of service. Participating physicians may not collect copayments/deductibles from patients covered by Medigap if the patient requests the physician to submit the claim to the Medigap insurer. Collect copayments after receiving the Medicare/Medigap RA document.

   ▶ For other secondary insurance, write the patient's group and policy (or certificate) numbers on the Medicare RA and attach it to a copy of the original Health Insurance Claim Form HCFA-1500 and submit it to the secondary carrier. Then copy the physician's billing statement showing date of treatment, description of service(s) rendered, fees, and diagnosis.

Managed Care and Medicare

When a patient's primary insurance is a managed care plan that requires fixed copayments, it is possible to obtain reimbursement from Medicare for those amounts. An assigned MSP claim must be filed with Medicare after the MCO has paid. When Medicare's copayment reimbursement has been received, the provider must refund to the patient the copayment amount previously collected.

The practice is paid a capitated amount and there will be no Explanation of Benefits (EOB) document. Have the patient sign a statement that explains the situation. Attach the statement and the copayment receipts to the claim. The statement may read as shown in the following box:

Patient Name _____

Medicare Number _____

There is no Explanation of Benefits documentation available for the attached billed services. I am currently enrolled with _____ managed care plan for my health care. My physician, _____ MD, is paid on a capitated basis, and the copayment that I pay is $ _____, for each service or visit.

Patient's signature _____

Date _____

A nonparticipating physician must file an unassigned MSP claim. The patient will be directly reimbursed by Medicare and no refund is necessary.

Automobile or Liability Insurance Coverage

Liability insurance is not secondary to Medicare because there is no contractual relationship between the injured party and the third party payer. A physician who treats a Medicare patient who has filed a liability claim must bill the liability insurer first *unless* the insurer will not pay promptly (e.g., within 120 days after the liability insurance claim is filed). After 120 days have gone by without a payment from the liability insurer and if the services performed are covered Medicare benefits, a par or nonpar physician may seek conditional payment from Medicare. However, if a claim is filed with Medicare, the provider must drop the claim against the liability insurer.

If the payment made by the liability insurer is less than the physician's full charge, the physician may file an assigned claim and must accept as full payment the greater of either the Medicare-approved charge or sum of the liability insurance primary payment and the Medicare secondary payment.

A nonpar physician may file an unassigned claim for Medicare secondary payment only if the payment by the liability insurer is less than the Medicare limiting charge. If the payment equals or exceeds the limiting charge, the physician must accept the payment as full payment.

If Medicare payments have been made but should not have been because the services are excluded under this provision, or if the payments were made on a conditional basis, they are subject to recovery. A Report to Medicare on Automobile or Liability Insurance Coverage Form HCFA-L 365 should be completed and sent to the fiscal agent (Fig. 11–6). The patient must sign and date the form. A copy of the notice of payment or denial form from the other insurer should be included when sending in Form HCFA-L 365, along with the HCFA-1500 claim form. Medicare is secondary even if a state law or a private contract of insurance states that Medicare is primary. The physician must bill the other insurer first. A claim for secondary benefits may be submitted to Medicare only after payment or denial has been made by the primary coverage. Liability insurance is not considered a Medicare secondary payer.

Medicare Managed Care Plans

Health Maintenance Organizations

During the spring of 1984, the Department of Health and Human Services published regulations giving Medicare enrollees the right to join and assign their Medicare benefits to health maintenance organizations (HMOs). HMOs had been in operation for nearly 50 years when they became available as an option for Medicare enrollees. With a Medicare HMO (also known as an HMO senior plan), the patient does not need a Medicare supplemental insurance plan. Medicare cards, however, are not forfeited, and an elderly patient may show two cards, leading to confusion about what their coverage is and who they are covered by.

Medicare makes payments directly to the HMO on a monthly basis for Medicare enrollees who use the HMO option. Enrollees pay the HMO a monthly premium, which is an estimate of the coinsurance amounts for which the enrollee would be responsible plus the Medicare deductible. It appears that HMOs contracting to provide services for Medicare patients will be converted to a Medicare + Choice plan as their contract renewal dates come up.

Some HMOs provide services not usually covered by Medicare, such as eyeglasses, prescription drugs, and routine physical examinations. Once a person has converted from Medicare to an HMO, he or she cannot go back to a former physician of personal choice and expect Medicare to pay the bill. The patient needs to receive services from a physician and hospital facility who is contracted with the HMO plan.

If a Medicare patient has switched over to a managed care plan and wishes to disenroll, the patient must

1. Notify the plan in writing of disenrollment.
2. Complete Medicare form HCFA 566, attach a copy of the disenrollment letter, and take it to the Social Security office.

Many plans allow the patient to enroll and disenroll at any time during the year. It may take the plan 30 days for disenrollment, and Medicare may take as long as 60 days to re-enroll a patient. Patients who disenroll may have to requalify for supplemental coverage at a higher cost.

There are two types of HMO plans that may have Medicare Part B contracts: HMO risk plans and HMO cost plans.

Risk Plan

As a condition of enrollment in an HMO risk plan, beneficiaries receive Medicare-covered services (except emergency, urgent need, and prior authorized services) only from providers who are contracted members of the HMO network. Enrollees of HMO risk plans are referred to as "restricted" beneficiaries. Usually services rendered by "out-of-plan" physicians are not covered when the same services are available through the organization unless a referral or prior authorization is obtained. The only exception is for emergency care. Claims for HMO risk plan beneficiaries must be sent directly to the organization.

A system of Medicare reimbursement for HMOs with risk contracts is called **diagnostic cost groups (DCGs).** The HMO enrollees are classified into various DCGs on the basis of each beneficiary's prior 12-month history of hospitalization, and payments are adjusted accordingly. This payment system does not apply to disabled and hospice patients, those on renal dialysis, or those enrolled only in Medicare Part B. Patients are reclassified each year according to their previous year's use of hospital service.

Cost Plan

Under an HMO cost plan, beneficiaries receive Medicare-covered services from sources in or outside of the HMO network. Enrollees are referred to as "unrestricted" beneficiaries. Claims for cost plan beneficiaries may be sent to the HMO plan or the regular Medicare carrier.

Noncontract Physician

If a noncontract physician treats a Medicare HMO patient, the services are considered "out-of-plan" services. The claim must be submitted to the managed care plan, which will determine whether it is

REPORT TO MEDICARE OF AUTOMOBILE OR LIABILITY INSURANCE COVERAGE

HEALTH INSURANCE CLAIM NUMBER	DATE	SEND COMPLETED FORM TO:
3459876	7-12-20XX	

Fiscal intermediary's
name and address

NAME OF PROVIDER, PHYSICIAN, OR SUPPLIER	DATE OF SERVICES
Gerald Practon, MD	FROM: 7-10-20XX TO: 7-30-20XX

NOTE: SEE REVERSE FOR PRIVACY ACT STATEMENT BEFORE COMPLETING FORM.

This refers to the services you received from the provider, physician or supplier named above.

We have information indicating that the expenses for these services may be payable under automobile insurance or under liability insurance (including automobile liability insurance). The law excludes Medicare payment for expenses which have been paid by such insurance or which such insurance can reasonably be expected to pay. All Medicare payments are made on the condition that the individual is responsible for refunding them if an automobile or liability insurer also makes payment.

Medicare may also recover its payments directly from an automobile or liability insurer or from anyone who has been paid by the insurer. Medicare can be a party to any claim by an individual against an insurer.

To help us determine whether Medicare must pay for these services, we need the information requested below. Please return the completed form in the enclosed self-addressed, postage paid envelope.

PLEASE ANSWER ALL QUESTIONS

1. DATE INJURY OCCURRED OR ILLNESS BEGAN	2. BRIEF DESCRIPTION OF ACCIDENT OR OTHER CAUSE OF INJURY OR ILLNESS
7-10-20XX	automobile accident in which car patient was riding in was rear ended
3. NAME, ADDRESS, AND TELEPHONE NUMBER OF ATTORNEY, IF YOU HAVE ONE	4. YOUR TELEPHONE NUMBER
	013-244-0098

5. MAY THE SERVICES YOU RECEIVED BE COVERED UNDER AN AUTOMOBILE MEDICAL OR NO FAULT INSURANCE POLICY OR PLAN?	NAME, ADDRESS AND TELEPHONE NUMBER OF INSURANCE COMPANY AND THE AUTOMOBILE INSURANCE CLAIM NUMBER
☒ YES ☐ NO IF YES, GIVE: ──────────▶ IF YOU HAVE RECEIVED A DECISION NOTICE FROM THE COMPANY, PLEASE SEND US A COPY.	Speedy Insurance Company 112 Royal Street Woodland Hills, XY 12345 Claim #4580098

6. IF YOU HAVE NOT FILED A CLAIM WITH AN AUTOMOBILE INSURER BUT BELIEVE YOU MAY BE ENTITLED TO DO SO, PLEASE EXPLAIN WHY YOU HAVE NOT FILED

A	(CONTINUED ON REVERSE)	FORM HCFA-L 365 (7-85) PRIOR EDITIONS MAY BE USED

Figure 11–6. *A,* Front of HCFA-L 365 Report to Medicare of Automobile or Liability Insurance Coverage Form.

(Illustration continued on following page)

7. DO YOU FEEL YOU HAVE A RIGHT TO BE COMPENSATED BY A PARTY WHO MAY HAVE CAUSED THE INJURY OR ILLNESS FOR WHICH THESE SERVICES WERE FURNISHED?

[X] YES   [ ] NO

8. HAVE YOU FILED, OR DO YOU INTEND TO FILE, A LIABILITY CLAIM OR LAWSUIT IN CONNECTION WITH THIS INJURY OR ILLNESS?

[X] YES   [ ] NO

9. IF YOU ANSWERED YES TO EITHER QUESTION 7 OR 8, PLEASE FURNISH THE FOLLOWING INFORMATION:

A. NAME, ADDRESS AND TELEPHONE NUMBER OF ANY PARTY THAT YOU BELIEVE WAS RESPONSIBLE FOR INJURY OR ILLNESS

Chloe R. Levine
349 Citrus Drive
Woodland Hills, XY 12345
Telephone No. 013-458-2233

B. NAME, ADDRESS AND TELEPHONE NUMBER OF INSURANCE COMPANY OF PARTY NAMED IN A., AND CLAIM NUMBER ASSIGNED BY THAT INSURANCE COMPANY

Zebra Insurance Company
2400 Central Avenue
Woodland Hills, XY 12345
Claim #3450098

If you have filed or have a right to file a liability claim or lawsuit against another party who you feel was responsible for this injury or illness, Medicare can pay for the service pending a decision on your liability claim. Do not settle your liability claim with the other party or his/her insurance company without first letting us know. If you do receive payment from a liability insurer, you will be responsible for paying Medicare back, or arranging for the insurance company to repay. The refund is the amount Medicare paid for this injury or illness up to the amount of the liability insurance payment less a part of your cost in procuring that payment. If Medicare is not repaid after you receive a liability insurance payment, the amount may be withheld from any social security benefits to which you are entitled.

If you do not at present intend to file a liability claim or lawsuit against any person or insurance company for this injury or illness but later change your mind, you are responsible for notifying us promptly of your decision.

CERTIFICATION: To the best of my knowledge and belief, the above answers are true.

DATE FORM COMPLETED	SIGNATURE OF BENEFICIARY OR REPRESENTATIVE	TELEPHONE NUMBER
August 1, 20XX	*Elizabeth L. Jenkins*	013-560-8798

PRIVACY ACT STATEMENT

We are authorized to collect this information by sections 205(a) and 1862(b) of the Social Security Act (42 USC 405a and 1395y). The information will be used to determine if the services you received are covered by Medicare or whether an automobile, no-fault, or liability insurer or any other persons may be responsible for payment. Section 1877(a)(3) of the Social Security Act (42 USC 405a and 1395nn) provides criminal penalties for withholding this information.

Figure 11–6 *Continued. B,* Back of HCFA-L 365 Report to Medicare of Automobile or Liability Insurance Coverage Form.

responsible to pay for the services. Conditions that must be met are:

1. Service was an emergency and the patient was not able to get to an HMO facility or member physician (patient was out of the HMO area).
2. Service was one covered by Medicare.
3. Service was medically necessary.
4. Service was prior authorized or an approved referral.

If the HMO determines there was no emergency and denies payment, the patient is responsible for the fee. The HMO reimburses according to the Medicare Fee Schedule Allowable Amount, so the physician cannot bill the patient for the balance. If the physician does not receive 100% of the allowable, steps must be taken through the HMO's appeals process. If this fails, contact the Medicare Managed Care Department at your Medicare Regional HCFA Operations Office. Denied services can be billed to the patient (no more than the Medicare fee schedule or limiting charge) after the HMO Explanation of Benefits is received.

Carrier Dealing Prepayment Organization

A Carrier Dealing Prepayment Organization may be set up by a medical practice under contract to the government. Such plans are considered a service contract rather than insurance. In the past, such plans were run by HMOs, but now practices of 12 to 15 physicians are opting to run their own plans. These organizations must be incorporated and have their own Medicare provider number. The organization must furnish physicians' services through employees and partners or under formal arrangement with medical groups, independent practice associations, or individual physicians. Part B services must be provided through qualified hospitals or physicians. When operating this type of organization, the physician accepts Medicare assignment and agrees to deal with the Medicare carrier instead of HCFA. Patients sign a contract agreeing to pay a monthly fee (usually $20 to $25). This is supposed to cover all Medicare copayments, deductibles, and nonreimbursable expenses (annual physical examinations and preventive care). The patient is not responsible to pay for noncovered services.

Utilization and Quality Control

Peer Review Organization

A **peer review organization (PRO)** is a state-based group of physicians working under government guidelines reviewing cases for hospital admission and discharge, extended stay, or extended services. The PRO evaluates physicians in regard to the quality and appropriateness of professional care and settles fee disputes. It is involved in implementing a quality of improvement plan using statistical data. Case reviews focus on admission and discharge, invasive procedures, documentation, extraordinarily high costs (outlier costs), and limitation of liability determinations.

HCFA has assigned a point system for medical documentation as discussed in Chapter 3. If sufficient points are lacking, penalties can lead to fines and/or forfeiture of the physician's license. Therefore, it is extremely important that each patient's care be well documented from the treatment standpoint as well as for justifying maximum reimbursement. A physician who receives a letter from a PRO regarding quality of care should consult his or her attorney before responding by letter or personal appeal. A photocopy of the patient's medical record can be used to substantiate the claim if there is detailed clinical documentation.

Federal False Claims Amendment Act

Another federal law to prevent overuse of services and to spot Medicare fraud is the Federal Claims Amendment Act of 1986. This act offers financial incentives of 15% to 25% of any judgment to informants who report physicians suspected of defrauding the federal government. This is called a *qui tam* **action**. The laws are intended to help catch Medicare and Medicaid cheaters. The health insurance companies that process Medicare claims have a Medicare fraud unit whose job is to catch people who steal from Medicare. The Office of the Inspector General (OIG), Department of Health and Human Services, is the law enforcement agency that investigates and prosecutes people who steal from Medicare. The OIG works closely with Medicare insurance companies, the Federal Bureau of Investigation (FBI), the Postal Inspection Service, and other federal law enforcement agencies. If the physician is on an optical disk retrieval (ODR) A-1000 system, it is possible for the OIG to obtain procedure codes that show comparison billing with peers in the area. The Health Care Financing Administration alerts offices of whom to investigate.

For information on fraud and abuse, see Chapter 1, Tables 1−2 and 1−3. See Chapter 14 for information about fraud in the workers' compensation program.

Health Insurance Portability and Accountability Act

The Health Insurance Portability and Accountability Act of 1996 (HIPAA) has a section that deals with prevention of health care fraud and abuse of patients on Medicare and Medicaid. Insurance billing specialists, coders, physicians, and any individuals who knowingly and willfully break the law could suffer a penalty or a fine, an imprisonment, or both. Civil monetary penalties are assessed for the following:

▶ Intentional incorrect coding that will result in greater payment than appropriate

▶ A pattern of claims being submitted for a service or product that is not medically necessary

▶ Offering remuneration to induce an individual to order from a particular provider or supplier who receives Medicare or state health funds

The federal criminal sanctions of this act are established for those who

▶ Knowingly or willfully defraud a health care program.

▶ Knowingly embezzle, steal, or misapply a health care benefit program.

Civil Monetary Penalties Law

In 1983, the federal government passed the Civil Monetary Penalties Law (CMPL) to prosecute cases of Medicare and Medicaid fraud. The law carries three separate forms of sanction:

1. A penalty of up to $2,000 for each item or service wrongfully listed in a payment request to Medicare or Medicaid.
2. An assessment of up to twice the total amount improperly claimed.
3. Suspension from the programs for whatever period the Department of Health and Human Services determines.

A physician may be penalized when participating in the following violations:

▶ Billing more than once for the same service to obtain greater reimbursement.

▶ Billing for services that were not provided.

▶ Fragmenting billed services that could be accurately described by one procedural code.

▶ Upgrading the reported level or complexity of services, over those services actually furnished, to obtain greater reimbursement.

A physician who fails to practice due care to ensure the accuracy of Medicare and Medicaid claims prepared in his or her office risks enormous financial penalties. The CMPL makes no distinction between outright fraud and negligence in billing. Therefore, if an employee submits billings

that the physician knows nothing about, the physician may be held liable. Reckless disregard of federal and state regulations by the insurance billing specialist can affect the way claims are submitted and possibly cause a physician to incur a civil monetary penalty. Incorrectly coded procedures can affect the penalties imposed on a physician.

The insurance billing specialist should periodically attend Medicare and Medicaid training workshops to keep up-to-date and gain a better understanding of federal and state government claim requirements. Medicare and Medicaid manuals and bulletins should be kept up-to-date and accessible for quick reference. Keep documentation to support claims submission in the event of an audit. If a record is missing, make a written note that it has been lost or destroyed because it might be presumed that the physician deliberately destroyed the documents to conceal evidence. If a billing error is discovered after a claim submission or an overpayment is received, notify the fiscal agent or insurance carrier immediately.

Always document any meetings with representatives of the fiscal agent or state welfare department and include the advice given. If the advice later proves to be erroneous, such records can support the physician's good faith. The Office of the Inspector General of the Department of Health and Human Services and each state's Medicaid fraud control unit investigates violations. Notify the physician's attorney if the physician is advised that he or she is being investigated. Documents should be released only after the attorney's approval. Retain photocopies of all documents given to the investigator.

Stark I and II Regulations—Physician Self-Referrals

On January 1, 1992, Federal legislation, Stark I, took effect, without regulations until they were published in 1995. This law prohibits a physician or his or her family who has a financial relationship with a laboratory from referring patients to that facility. Clinical laboratories must submit financial information to the HCFA, including the names and identification numbers of physicians who hold a financial interest in the business. Stark II, an amendment, took effect on January 1, 1995, and expanded these regulations by prohibiting Medicare and Medicaid payments for treatment that results from the referral of a patient by a physician (or immediate family member of the physician) who has a financial relationship (ownership interest or compensatory arrangement) with providers of designated health services. It also prohibits the provider from billing for the designated health service. These services include:

- Clinical laboratory services
- Durable medical equipment and supplies
- Home health services
- Inpatient and outpatient hospital services
- Occupational therapy services
- Outpatient prescription drugs
- Parenteral and enteral nutrients, related equipment, and supplies
- Physical therapy services
- Prosthetics, orthotics, and prosthetic devices and supplies
- Radiation therapy services and supplies
- Radiology services, including magnetic resonance imaging, computed tomography, and ultrasound services

Many states have passed laws and administrative rules that may apply the same principles to other private payers. Uncovered self-referral deceits or failure of a laboratory to report financial information can lead to hefty fines, sanctions, payment denials, and exclusion from the Medicare/Medicaid programs by the Office of the Inspector General, Department of Health and Human Services. There are some general exceptions related to ownership/investment and compensation arrangements, so it is important to obtain a complete description of this legislation for proper compliance.

Clinical Laboratory Improvement Amendment

The Clinical Laboratory Improvement Amendment (CLIA) of 1988 established federal standards, quality control, and safety measures for all free standing laboratories including physician laboratories. Various laboratory procedures fall within CLIA categories depending on the complexity of each test. Each category level requires a yearly licensing fee to be paid by the physician. A certificate is then issued and must be posted in the laboratory. Various levels of quality control measures are required for each CLIA level and must be performed in a timely manner (e.g., daily, weekly). Fines may be levied if federal standards are not maintained. This has had an impact on office laboratories; and because of the strict requirements, many physicians send patients to independent laboratories for tests (i.e., blood cell counts, cytology specimens, and cultures). However, some physicians prefer to draw blood from a patient, particularly if the patient has a history of difficult venous access.

When submitting claims to Medicare fiscal intermediaries for laboratory services performed in the physician's office, the 10-digit CLIA certificate number needs to be entered in Block 23 of the HCFA-1500 claim form (Fig. 11–7). Physicians billing patients for outside laboratory work are not held to these standards but may charge the patient only what the laboratory charges (based on a fee schedule), plus any additional services the physician provides (e.g., drawing, handling, shipping, and interpretation of the blood or the office visit).

Payment Fundamentals

Provider

Participating Physician

In a **participating physician (par)** agreement, a physician agrees to accept payment from Medicare (80% of the **approved charges**) plus payment from the patient (20% of approved charge) after the

14. DATE OF CURRENT: MM DD YY ◀ ILLNESS (First symptom) OR INJURY (Accident) OR PREGNENCY (LMP)	15. IF PATIENT HAS HAD SAME OR SIMILAR ILLNESS. GIVE FIRST DATE MM DD YY	16. DATES PATIENT UNABLE TO WORK IN CURRENT OCCUPATION FROM MM DD YY TO MM DD YY
17. NAME OF REFERRING PHYSICIAN OR OTHER SOURCE	17a. I.D. NUMBER OF REFERRING PHYSICIAN	18. HOSPITALIZATION DATES RELATED TO CURRENT SERVICES FROM MM DD YY TO MM DD YY
19. RESERVED FOR LOCAL USE		20. OUTSIDE LAB? ☐ YES ☐ NO $ CHARGES
21. DIAGNOSIS OR NATURE OF ILLNESS OR INJURY. (RELATE ITEMS 1,2,3 OR 4 TO ITEM 24E BY LINE) 1. 2.	3. 4.	22. MEDICAID RESUBMISSION CODE ORIGINAL REF. NO. 23. PRIOR AUTHORIZATION NUMBER

24. A DATE(S) OF SERVICE From MM DD YY To MM DD YY	B Place of Service	C Type of Service	D PROCEDURES, SERVICES, OR SUPPLIES (Explain Unusual Circumstances) CPT/HCPCS MODIFIER	E DIAGNOSIS CODE	F $ CHARGES	G DAYS OR UNITS	H EPSDT Family Plan	I EMG	J COB	K RESERVED FOR LOCAL USE

Figure 11–7. Section of the HCFA-1500 claim form with Block 23 emphasized indicating where to insert a certificate number for laboratory services (CLIA No.) or a prior authorization number for a procedure when permission has been granted.

$100 deductible has been met (Fig. 11–8). The Medicare annual deductible is based on the calendar year, January 1 through December 31. This agreement is referred to as accepting **assignment.** The physician must complete and submit the HCFA-1500 claim form to the fiscal intermediary. The assignment of benefits, Block 12, is signed by the patient, the physician indicates that assignment is being accepted by checking "Yes" in Block 27, and the payment goes directly to the physician (Fig. 11–9). Physicians, practitioners, and suppliers who fail to submit claims are subject to civil monetary penalties up to $2,500 for each claim.

Nonparticipating Physician

A **nonparticipating physician (nonpar)** does not have a signed agreement with Medicare and has an option regarding assignment. The physician may not accept assignment for all services or has the option of accepting assignment for some services and collecting from the patient for other services performed at the same time and place. An exception to this policy is mandatory assignment for clinical laboratory tests and services by physician assistants.

If a patient receives medical services from a nonparticipating physician, he or she is responsible for an annual $100 deductible, 20% of the nonpar approved amount, and the difference between the nonpar approved amount and the limiting charge. Medicare pays 80% of the nonpar approved amount. Usually a nonparticipating physician who is not accepting assignment collects the fee from the patient and Medicare sends the payment check to the patient.

Limiting charge is a percentage limit on fees, specified by legislation, that nonpar physicians may bill Medicare beneficiaries above the allowed amount. For assigned claims, nonpar physicians may submit usual and customary fees. Nonpar physicians usually maintain two fee schedules, one with usual fees and one with limiting charges, because of these two situations. Some states have set limiting charges that are more restrictive than Medicare policies. These states are Connecticut, Massachusetts, New York, Ohio, Pennsylvania, Rhode Island, and Vermont. For guidelines, inquire from the fiscal intermediary of those states.

Prior Authorization

Many insurance carrier group plans and MCO senior plans require prior authorization for surgical procedures, diagnostic testing, and referrals to specialists. Some of these procedures requiring authorization are on a mandatory list, whereas others are chosen by the regional carrier. The mandatory list is composed of such procedures as

❯ bunionectomy
❯ carotid endarterectomy

PAYMENT EXAMPLES
The annual Part B deductible has been met

	Doctor's bill	Medicare approved amount*	Medicare pays	Beneficiary responsible for	Medicare courtesy adjustment**
Doctor A accepts assignment	$480	$400	$320 (80% of approved amount)	$80 (20% of approved amount)	$80

Doctor B does not accept assignment and charges no more than the limiting charge	$437	$380	$304 (80% of approved amount)	$ 76 (20% of approved amount)
				+ 57 (difference between $437
				$133 actual charge – which is also
				        the limiting charge – and
				        $380 approved amount)
					None

* The Medicare approved amount is less for non-participating physicians than for participating physicians.

** The courtesy adjustment is the amount posted to the patient's account to zero out the balance. The word "courtesy" implies that Medicare patients are treated well and is preferred to phrases like "not allowed" or "write off."

Note: If Medicare does not cover a service, e.g., cosmetic, hearing aid related, refractions, and so forth, the patient pays for the service whether the doctor accepts the assignment or not.

Figure 11–8. Example of a case showing a physician accepting an assignment versus not accepting an assignment, and the amount the patient is responsible for paying.

PLEASE
DO NOT
STAPLE
IN THIS
AREA

APPROVED OMB-0938-008

CARRIER

HEALTH INSURANCE CLAIM FORM

PICA

PICA

1. MEDICARE MEDICAID CHAMPUS CHAMPVA GROUP HEALTH PLAN FECA BLK LUNG OTHER	1a. INSURED'S I.D. NUMBER (FOR PROGRAM IN ITEM 1)

(Medicare #) (Medicaid #) (Sponsor's SSN) (VA File #) (SSN or ID) (SSN) (ID)

2. PATIENT'S NAME (Last Name, First Name, Middle Inital)

3. PATIENT'S BIRTH DATE
MM   DD   YY   SEX
M   F

4. INSURED'S NAME (Last Name, First Name, Middle Initial)

5. PATIENT'S ADDRESS

6. PATIENT RELATIONSHIP TO INSURED
Self   Spouse   Child   Other

7. INSURED'S ADDRESS (No., Street)

CITY   STATE

8. PATIENT STATUS
Single   Married   Other

CITY   STATE

ZIP CODE   TELEPHONE (Include Area Code)
(   )

Employed   Full-Time Student   Part-Time Student

ZIP CODE   TELEPHONE (Include Area Code)
(   )

9. OTHER INSURED'S NAME (Last Name, First Name, Middle Initial)

10. IS PATIENT'S CONDITION RELATED TO:

11. INSURED'S POLICY GROUP OR FECA NUMBER

a. OTHER INSURED'S POLICY OR GROUP NUMBER

a. EMPLOYMENT? (CURRENT OR PREVIOUS)
YES   NO

a. INSURED'S DATE OF BIRTH
MM   DD   YY   SEX
M   F

b. OTHER INSURED'S DATE OF BIRTH
MM   DD   YY   SEX
M   F

b. AUTO ACCIDENT?   PLACE (State)
YES   NO

b. EMPLOYER'S NAME OR SCHOOL NAME

c. EMPLOYER'S NAME OR SCHOOL NAME

c. OTHER ACCIDENT?
YES   NO

c. INSURANCE PLAN NAME OR PROGRAM NAME

d. INSURANCE PLAN NAME OR PROGRAM NAME

10d. RESERVED FOR LOCAL USE

d. IS THERE ANOTHER HEALTH BENEFIT PLAN?
YES   NO   If yes, return to and complete item 9 a-d.

READ BACK OF FORM BEFORE COMPLETING & SIGNING THIS FORM.
12. PATIENT'S OR AUTHORIZED PERSON'S SIGNATURE I authorize the release of any medical or other information necessary to process this claim. I also request payment of government benefits either to myself or to the party who accepts assignment below.

SOF

SIGNED _____   DATE _____

13. INSURED'S OR AUTHORIZED PERSON'S SIGNATURE I authorize payment of medical benefits to the undersigned physician or supplier for services described below.

SIGNED _____

14. DATE OF CURRENT: ILLNESS (First symptom) OR
MM   DD   YY   INJURY (Accident) OR
PREGNANCY (LMP)

15. IF PATIENT HAS HAD SAME OR SIMILAR ILLNESS. GIVE FIRST DATE   MM   DD   YY

16. DATES PATIENT UNABLE TO WORK IN CURRENT OCCUPATION
MM   DD   YY   MM   DD   YY
FROM   TO

17. NAME OF REFERRING PHYSICIAN OR OTHER SOURCE

17a. I.D. NUMBER OF REFERRING PHYSICIAN

18. HOSPITALIZATION DATES RELATED TO CURRENT SERVICES
MM   DD   YY   MM   DD   YY
FROM   TO

19. RESERVED FOR LOCAL USE

20. OUTSIDE LAB? $ CHARGES
YES   NO

21. DIAGNOSIS OR NATURE OF ILLNESS OR INJURY. (RELATE ITEMS 1,2,3 OR 4 TO ITEM 24E BY LINE)
1.   3.
2.   4.

22. MEDICAID RESUBMISSION
CODE   ORIGINAL REF. NO.

23. PRIOR AUTHORIZATION NUMBER

24. A DATE(S) OF SERVICE		B Place of Service	C Type of Service	D PROCEDURES, SERVICES, OR SUPPLIES (Explain Unusual Circumstances)	E DIAGNOSIS CODE	F $ CHARGES	G DAYS OR UNITS	H EPSDT Family Plan	I EMG	J COB	K RESERVED FOR LOCAL USE
From MM DD YY	To MM DD YY			CPT/HCPCS MODIFIER							
1											
2											
3											
4											
5											
6											

25. FEDERAL TAX I.D. NUMBER   SSN   EIN

26. PATIENT'S ACCOUNT NO.

27. ACCEPT ASSIGNMENT?
(For govt. claims, see back)
[X] YES   NO

28. TOTAL CHARGE
$

29. AMOUNT PAID
$

30. BALANCE DUE
$

31. SIGNATURE OF PHYSICIAN OR SUPPLIER INCLUDING DEGREES OR CREDENTIALS
(I certify that the statements on the reverse apply to this bill and are made a part thereof.)

SIGNED _____   DATE _____

32. NAME AND ADDRESS OF FACILITY WHERE SERVICES WERE RENDERED (If other than home or office)

33. PHYSICIAN'S, SUPPLIER'S BILLING NAME, ADDRESS, ZIP CODE & PHONE #

PIN#   GRP#

(APPROVED BY AMA COUNCIL ON MEDICAL SERVICE 8/88)

FORM HCFA-1500 (12-90)
FORM OWCP-1500   FORM RRB-1500

PATIENT AND INSURED INFORMATION

PHYSICIAN OR SUPPLIER INFORMATION

Figure 11–9. Block 12 of the HCFA-1500 claim form where the patient signs authorizing payment to be sent to the physician and Block 27 marked with an X showing that the physician accepts Medicare assignment of benefits.

- cataract extractions
- cholecystectomy
- complex peripheral revascularization
- coronary artery bypass graft surgery
- hysterectomy
- inguinal hernia repair
- joint replacements (hip, shoulder, knee)
- transurethral prostatectomy

Some carriers have an 800 toll-free line to call for authorization; some require the completion of a preauthorization form; and some require a letter only if there is a dispute over claims payment. Check with your local carrier on its policy for preauthorization.

The prior authorization number is used when billing the Medicare carrier and is entered on the HCFA-1500 claim form in Block 23 (see Fig. 11–7). If the procedure is not approved, the carrier sends a denial to the physician, the patient, and the hospital, if applicable. If the procedure is done as an emergency, notify the carrier within the time frame designated by the insurance plan so an authorization can be arranged.

Waiver of Liability Provision

Limited Liability

When a patient is to receive a service from a participating physician that might be denied for **medical necessity** or because of *limitation of liability* by Medicare, inform the patient and have him or her agree to pay for the denied service in advance. If you do not know what the Medicare guidelines or parameters are for a certain procedure or service, refer to Medicare bulletins or call the Medicare carrier and ask. Instruct the patient to sign a waiver of liability agreement or responsibility statement as shown in Figures 11–10 and 11–11. This form should not be given to someone who is in a medical emergency, confused, legally incompetent, or otherwise under great duress. It cannot be signed after a patient has received the service and must specifically state what service or procedure is being waived. Obtain guidance from the insurance carrier when in doubt about using a waiver of liability form. An office policy should be in place for handling patients who refuse to sign a waiver. When

Name and address of physician
ADVANCE NOTICE MEDICARE BENEFICIARY WAIVER OF LIABILITY AGREEMENT

If Medicare determines that a particular service, although it would be otherwise covered, is not reasonable and necessary under Medicare program standards, Medicare will deny payment for that service. In your case, Medicare might deny payment for:

1. _B12 injection_____
2. _____

for the following reasons:

Medicare does not usually pay for this:

_____ many visits or treatments
_____ service or this many services within this period of time
___✓_____ injection or this many injections
_____ because it is a treatment that is yet to be proved effective
_____ office visit unless it was needed because of an emergency
_____ same services by more than one doctor during the same time period
_____ equipment
_____ laboratory test
_____ visit since it is more than one visit per day
_____ extensive procedure
_____ same service by more than one doctor of the same specialty
_____ nursing home visit since only one is allowed per month

Beneficiary Agreement

I have been notified by my physician that, in my case, Medicare might deny payment for the service(s) checked above. If Medicare denies payment, I agree to be personally and fully responsible for payment.

_Mary Judd_____   ___3/20/20xx_____
Beneficiary's Signature   Date Signed

Figure 11–10. Example of an Advance Notice Medicare Beneficiary Waiver of Liability Agreement, which is also known as a responsibility statement.

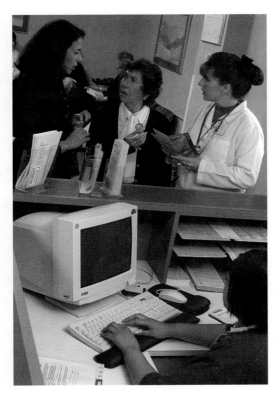

Figure 11–11. Insurance billing specialist instructing an elderly patient to sign an Advance Notice Medicare Beneficiary Waiver of Liability Agreement for services not covered.

sending in a claim, the HCPCS Level II modifier-GA (waiver of liability on file) must be added to pertinent codes to indicate a patient has signed the waiver. The Medicare carrier will inform the patient that he or she is responsible for the fee. Keep this signed waiver with other patient financial documents and not with the patient's medical record.

If you know the service was not reasonable because of Medicare guidelines but the patient thought it was covered and there is no advance notice given with signed waiver of liability agreement, then:

▶ You cannot collect from Medicare or the patient.
▶ The patient does not have to pay the deductible or coinsurance.
▶ Refund to the patient any amount paid to the provider on the item or service.

If assignment is accepted and the physician and patient thought the service was covered under reasonable assumptions, then:

▶ Bill Medicare to pay for the service.
▶ The patient must pay the deductible and coinsurance.
▶ Medicare will not seek a refund of money already paid to the physician.

Nonparticipating providers must refund any amounts collected from the beneficiary when ser-

vices are later found to be not reasonable and necessary.

Noncovered Services

Do not get confused with the issue of *noncovered* Medicare services because these may always be billed to the patient. Some physicians prefer to obtain a Waiver of Liability for noncovered services; however, it is not mandated. Services denied as inclusive of another service (a payment already made for the other service) are not considered a noncovered item and may not be billed to the patient. If you need a formal denial to bill the patient or another insurer, send in a claim with a letter attached stating you need the denial to bill another payer; otherwise, to bill for a noncovered service is inappropriate and may possibly be viewed by some as fraud.

Elective Surgery Estimate

Effective October 1, 1987, under the Tax Reform Act, a nonparticipating physician who does not accept assignment for an *elective surgery* for which the actual charge will be $500 or more must provide the beneficiary in writing (1) the estimated fee for the procedure, (2) the estimated Medicare-approved allowance for the procedure, and (3) the difference in the physician's actual charge and the limiting or allowed charge (Fig. 11–12). *Elective surgery* means a surgical procedure that can be scheduled in advance, is not an emergency, and is discretionary on the part of the physician and the patient. Failure to undergo elective surgery does not pose a mortality threat. Give a copy of the estimation letter to the Medicare patient and keep the original for your files. Document the patient's acknowledgment by obtaining his or her signature at the bottom of the letter.

Prepayment Screens

On some procedures, Medicare limits the number of times a given procedure can be billed during 1 year (e.g., four office visits per month or one treatment every 60 days for routine foot care). This is known as a Medicare Prepayment Screen. The screens or flags are computer triggers that suspend processing. These screens are used to identify and review claims for medical necessity and determine compliance with other appropriate criteria. The suspended claim is checked by a reviewer who decides if the services are medically necessary. If the patient previously submitted a claim for the procedure performed in the same year by another physician and has

**WORKSHEET FOR
ESTIMATED MEDICARE PAYMENT FOR ELECTIVE SURGERY**

1. Physician's actual fee	$ 1248.03
2. Medicare approved or allowed amount	$ 1085.24
3. Difference between physician's fee and Medicare approved or allowed amount (1 - 2 = 0)	- 162.79
4. Twenty per cent coinsurance (0.20 X 2 = 0)	+ 217.05
5. Beneficiary's out-of-pocket expense (3 + 4 + 0) Assume the $100 deductible has been met	$ 379.84

Items 1, 2, and 5 must be included in the letter to the beneficiary

A

Physician's Letterhead

Dear Patient:

Because I do not accept assignment for elective surgery, Medicare requires that I give you certain information before surgery when my charges are $500 or more.

The following information concerns the surgery we have discussed. These estimates assume that you have already met the $100 deductible.

Type of surgery	Osteotomy, proximal left tibia	
Limiting charge	$	1248.03
Medicare estimated payment	$	868.19
Patient's estimated payment	$	379.84

This estimate is based upon our present expectations of what surgical procedure(s) will be required. Please remember that this is only an estimate of charges, we cannot be sure that additional procedures will or will not be necessary.

Sincerely,

John Doe, M.D.
Medicare Provider Number   126785479A

I understand the foregoing physician charges and my financial responsibility with respect to those estimated charges.

Patient's Signature   *Jane Doe*   Date 5-18-20XX
B   Jane Doe

Figure 11–12. Worksheet *(A)* and sample beneficiary letter *(B)* for estimated Medicare payment for elective surgery.

met the limit for the year, then the claim will be down-coded or denied. Refer to your local Medicare fiscal agent's newsletters or bulletins or contact them for a complete list of the Medicare Prepayment Screens applicable in your area.

To avoid problems, use good procedure code guidelines discussed in Chapter 5 and adhere to the following criteria.

▶ Level of service is appropriate to documentation
▶ Procedure is accurate to the gender of the patient
▶ Frequency is appropriate
▶ Diagnosis and procedure match
▶ Provider has certification for performing services (e.g., laboratories)
▶ Fee is within the Medicare-approved charge

Medicare Reimbursement

Chronology of Payment

For many years Medicare payments were based on reasonable fees (i.e., the amounts approved by the Medicare carrier [fiscal agents]). Medicare paid 80% of the approved charge. On October 1, 1983, an important development in the Medicare Part A program, the **prospective payment system (PPS)**, became effective. Under the regulations enacted by the Social Security Amendments of 1983, hospitals treating Medicare patients are reimbursed according to preestablished rates for each type of illness treated based on diagnosis. Payments to hospitals for Medicare services are classified according to 503 diagnosis-related group (DRG) numbers. Beneficiaries (patients) cannot be billed beyond the preestablished DRG rate except for normal deductible and copayment amounts. (See Chapter 16 for an in-depth discussion of DRGs.)

In 1984, the Deficit Reduction Act established a participating physician program that offered incentives to participating physicians and froze the fees of nonparticipating physicians. After this, the 1987 Omnibus Budget Reconciliation Act (OBRA) introduced the maximum allowable actual charge (MAAC) formula, which developed the maximum fee (limiting charge) a nonpar physician could charge Medicare patients for each service.

Reasonable Fee

Reasonable fee means the amount that Medicare participating providers agree to accept. It is listed on the remittance advice (RA), formerly known as Explanation of Benefits (EOB), as an allowed (approved) charge for a procedure. This charge may be higher or lower than the fee the physician lists on the claim. When a physician accepts assignment, he or she may bill the patient only 20% of the Medicare-allowed charge. Charging for completion and submission of a claim form on an assignment claim violates the terms of the assignment. Interest fees cannot be assessed to Medicare patients. It is permissible to collect the deductible at the time of service, but do not collect the Medicare copayment until Medicare pays.

Mandatory assignment laws have been adopted in several states, and legislation is under consideration and pending in many more states. These state laws would require physicians to accept the approved charge for their Medicare patients as a condition for being licensed to practice medicine in the state. Arkansas, Florida, Illinois, Maryland, Montana, and New Hampshire have rejected mandatory assignment proposals.

Resource-Based Relative Value Scale

A **resource-based relative value scale (RBRVS)** system was established as a means to redistribute Medicare dollars among physicians more equitably. This became the basis for physicians' payments nationwide for a 5-year phase-in that began on January 1, 1992. This system consists of a fee schedule based on relative values. The formula for obtaining relative value units is somewhat complex and involves a bit of mathematics in computing three components: a **relative value unit (RVU)** for the service, a geographic adjustment factor (GAF), and a monetary conversion factor (CF).

Relative value unit formula:
RVU × GAF × CF = Medicare $ per service

RVUs are based on the physician work RVU, the practice expense RVU, and the malpractice insurance RVU. To bring the fees in line for the region where the physician practices and to adjust for regional overhead and malpractice costs, each of the RVUs is adjusted for each Medicare local carrier by geographic practice cost indices (GPCIs), pronounced "gypsies."

To convert a geographically adjusted relative value into a payment amount, a CF is used. This CF is updated to a new amount each year. Figure 11–13 provides an example of calculating payment for one procedure code.

The figures to work out this formula in the chart for each service are published annually in the Federal Register.

RVSs help when determining cost accounting because they take into account the practice expense, malpractice expense, work effort, and cost of living. They are also helpful when negotiating the best contract available with managed care plans, so it is important for office managers or individuals assisting physicians to know and understand RBRVS

Figure 11–13. Example of formula showing calculations to determine the fee for a specific procedure.

FORMULA TO CALCULATE PAYMENT FOR EACH SERVICE

Example: CPT code 91000   Esophageal intubation
The medical practice location is Oakland, California.

	Work	**Overhead**	**Malpractice**
RVUs	1.04	0.70	0.06
GPCI*	× 1.028	× 1.258	× 1.370
	1.07 +	0.88 +	0.08 = Total adjusted RVUs, 2.03

For 2001, the Conversion Factor for nonsurgical care is $38.2581 × 2.03 = Allowed amount $77.66

Geographic practice cost indices

TABLE 11–1	RBRVS Crosswalk						
A	**B**	**C**	**D**	**E**	**F**	**G**	**H**
Code	Code Description	RBRVS/RVUs	Conversion Factor	Fee	Contract Conversion Factor	Contract Fee	% Contract Payment
99212	Ofc Visit	0.68	72.06	$49	64.71	$44.00	90%

data. A crosswalk is an effective way to see how the practice may be affected by an RBRVS contract (Table 11–1). To develop one, make several columns using spreadsheet software. In column A, list common procedure codes used by the practice; column B, the code description; and column C, the RBRVS RVUs. Leave column D blank to insert a conversion factor. In column E, put in the present fee-for-service rate (rounded out figure). Divide the fee in column E by column C to get the conversion factor. Leave a blank for column F to insert a conversion factor for the contract. List the managed care contract payment in column G. Divide column G by column C to get the conversion factor for column F. Then, to work out the percentage being paid at the contract rate, divide the plan's contract fee by the physician's fee for column H.

Medicare Fee Schedule

Beginning in 1996, each Medicare local carrier annually sends each physician a Medicare fee schedule for their area or region number listing three columns of figures: participating amount, nonparticipating amount, and limiting charge for each procedure code number. To see an example of this, refer to the Mock Fee Schedule shown in Appendix A of the *Student Workbook for the Insurance Handbook for the Medical Office.*

Health Care Financing Administration Common Procedure Coding System (HCPCS)

As mentioned in Chapter 5, the federal government developed the Health Care Financing Administration Common Procedure Coding System (HCPCS) for the Medicare program. To obtain correct payment for a procedure or service, a code number must be selected from Level I, II, or III of HCPCS coding system. When submitting a claim, be sure to use the Level II HCPCS **national alphanumeric codes** and modifiers rather than CPT procedure codes for certain appliances and procedures when indicated. When billing CPT modifiers, a good reference is presented in Chapter 5, Table 5–4, as helpful hints in italics entitled "Medicare Payment Rule."

Claim Submission

Fiscal Intermediaries and Fiscal Agents

An organization handling claims from hospitals, nursing facilities (NFs), **intermediate care facilities (ICFs)**, long-term care facilities (LTCFs), and home health agencies is called a **fiscal intermediary (FI).** The National Blue Cross Association holds the fiscal intermediary contract for Medicare Part A; it, in turn, subcontracts it out to member agencies.

Organizations handling claims from physicians and other suppliers of services covered under Medicare Part B are called *carriers* or *fiscal agents.* Medicare Part B payments are handled by private insurance organizations under contract with the government. Since January 1, 1992, the rule for where to send a Medicare claim is to bill the carrier who covers the area where the service occurred or was furnished, NOT the carrier who services the physician's office.

See Appendix A for the name and address of where to submit claims in your state and to obtain further information about this program.

Provider Identification Numbers

Another requirement of the Tax Reform Act was the establishment of several types of identification numbers for each physician and nonphysician practitioner providing services paid by Medicare. Because there are so many numbers, they are easily confused and end up being the source of many errors when completing blocks on the HCFA-1500 claim form. The numbers defined and shown in template examples with correct placement in Chapter 6 are:

- Provider identification numbers (PINs); group and individual
- Unique physician identification numbers (UPINs)
- Performing physician identification number (PPINs)
- National provider identifier (NPI)
- Durable Medical Equipment (DME) supplier number

Patient's Signature Authorization

A Medicare patient's signature authorization for release of medical information and assignment of benefits to the insurance carrier is obtained in Block 12 of the HCFA-1500 claim form. This block needs to be signed regardless of whether the physician is a participating or nonparticipating physician. The signed authorization should be kept on file in the patient's medical record for an episode of care or for a designated time frame (e.g., 1 year or lifetime). Subsequent claims may then indicate "Signature on file" or "SOF" in Block 12 of the claim form. The lifetime beneficiary claim authorization and information release form shown in Figure 11–14 is an example that can be used for assigned and nonassigned Medicare claims and kept in the patient's medical record. An original copy of an HCFA-1500 claim form may be used to obtain a lifetime signature authorization. Write across the top of the form "Lifetime Signature Authorization" and file as just described. Further information on this topic may be found in Chapters 3 and 6.

Signature on file situations that may occur in a medical practice are:

- **Illiterate or physically handicapped.** When an illiterate or physically handicapped enrollee signs by mark (X), a witness should sign his or her name and address next to the mark. If the claim is filed for the patient by another person, that person should enter the patient's name and write "By," sign his or her own name and address, indicate relationship to the patient, and state why the patient cannot sign.
- **Confinement in a facility.** Sometimes it is not possible to obtain the signature of a Medicare patient because of confinement in a nursing facility, hospital, or home. In such cases, physicians should obtain a lifetime signature authorization from the patient.
- **Medigap claim.** When submitting a crossover claim to a Medigap carrier, obtain a lifetime signature authorization for the Medigap carrier.
- **Deceased patient.** Refer to section on "Deceased Patient Claims" later in this chapter for signature requirements.
- **Medicare/Medicaid (Medi-Medi) claim.** These claims do not require the patient's signature.

Time Limit

The *time limit* for sending in claims is the end of the calendar year following the fiscal year in which services were furnished. The fiscal year for claims begins October 1 and ends September 30. (*see the following box*).

Hugh R. Aged, M.D.
1000 Any Street
Anytown, XY 12345
013/486-9002

LIFETIME BENEFICIARY CLAIM AUTHORIZATION AND INFORMATION RELEASE

Patient's Name Jane Doe Medicare I.D. number 540-98-8755A

I request that payment of authorized Medicare benefits be made either to me or on my behalf to (name of physician/supplier) for any services furnished me by that physician/supplier. I authorize any holder of medical information about me to release to the Health Care Financing Administration and its agents any information needed to determine these benefits or the benefits payable to related services.

I understand my signature requests that payment be made and authorizes release of medical information necessary to pay the claim. If other health insurance is indicated in Item 9 of the HCFA-1500 claim form or elsewhere on other approved claim forms or electronically submitted claims, my signature authorizes releasing of the information to the insurer or agency shown. In Medicare assigned cases, the physician or supplier agrees to accept the charge determination of the Medicare carrier as the full charge, and the patient is responsible only for the deductible, coinsurance, and noncovered services. Coinsurance and the deductible are based upon the charge determination of the Medicare carrier.

Jane Doe — Patient's Signature

January 3, 20XX — Date

Figure 11–14. Lifetime Assignment of Benefits and Information Release.

For services furnished on:	The time limit for filing is:
Oct. 1, 2000–Sept. 30, 2001	December 31, 2002
Oct. 1, 2001–Sept. 30, 2002	December 31, 2003

On assigned claims, the provider may file without penalty up to 27 months after providing service if reasonable cause for the delay is shown to the insurance carrier. Otherwise, there is a 10% reduction in the reimbursement. On unassigned claims, the provider may be fined for delinquent claim submission up to $2,000 and/or dropped from Medicare. When submitting a late claim, ask the fiscal intermediary for the guidelines HCFA considers reasonable cause for delay.

Manual Claims

The form that physicians use to submit paper claims to Medicare is the HCFA-1500. Refer to Chapter 6 for instructions on how to complete the HCFA-1500 claim form for the Medicare program. The reference templates for Medicare and supplemental coverage shown at the end of that chapter are:

Medicare—No secondary coverage	Figure 6–9
Medicare/Medicaid—Crossover	Figure 6–10
Medicare/Medigap—Crossover	Figure 6–11
Other insurance/Medicare MSP	Figure 6–12

Patients are not allowed to submit claims to Medicare (with four exceptions). Situations when a patient may file a claim are:
- Services covered by Medicare for which the patient has other insurance that should pay first; called Medicare Secondary Payer (MSP)
- Services provided by a physician who refuses to submit the claim
- Services provided outside the United States
- When durable medical equipment is purchased from a private source

Medicare claim status is also explained in detail in Chapter 6 (i.e., clean, incomplete, rejected, invalid, dirty, dingy, and other claims). To obtain the mailing address for the Medicare claim form for your state or county, refer to Appendix A. For further information and booklets, pamphlets, and the annual Medicare Handbook, contact your nearest Social Security office.

Electronic Claims

Medicare requests that all providers submit claims electronically. All electronic transmission formats are scheduled to be standardized by the use of ANSI X12N (837) Version 4010. Refer to Chapter 7 on how to submit claims electronically to your Medicare carrier.

Medicare/Medicaid Claims

Medi-Medi patients qualify for the benefits of Medicare as well as Medicaid. Use the HCFA-1500 claim form and check "Yes" for the assignment in Block 27. If the physician does not accept assignment, then payment goes to the patient and Medicaid (in California Medi-Cal) will not pick up the residual. The HCFA-1500 claim form will be crossed over and processed automatically by Medicaid after processing is completed by Medicare. The fiscal intermediary may refer to this as a **crossover claim** or *claims transfer*. It is not necessary to submit another form. Claims should be sent according to the time limit designated by the Medicaid program in your state. Generally, the Medicare payment exceeds the Medicaid fee schedule and little or no payment is received except when the patient has not met his or her annual Medicare deductible.

In some states the fiscal intermediary for a Medi-Medi claim may have a different address from that used for the processing of a patient who is on Medicare only. Write or call your nearest Medicare fiscal intermediary for the guidelines pertinent to your state.

Medicare/Medigap Claims

In most states, Medicare has streamlined the processing of Medicare/Medigap claims. Medicare carriers transmit Medigap claims electronically for participating physicians, thus eliminating the need to file an additional claim. This is also called a *crossover claim*. Medigap payments go directly to the participating physicians, and a Medicare Summary Notice is sent to the patient that states, "This claim has been referred to your supplemental carrier for any additional benefits."

To assure the crossover of the Medicare/Medigap claim, complete Blocks 9 through 9d of the HCFA-1500 claim form and list the PAYRID number of the Medigap plan in Block 9d. The PAYRID for Medigap plans is referred to as the Other Carrier Name and Address (OCNA) number, and a list of all OCNAs is published in the Medicare newsletter.

If automatic crossover capabilities are not offered in your state, attach the Medicare RA to the claim form and submit a claim to the Medigap plan separately.

Refer to Figure 6–11 for submitting claims when Medicare is primary and the patient has a Medigap (supplemental) policy.

Medicare/Supplemental and MSP Claims

Completing the HCFA-1500 claim form for a Medicare patient who has supplemental insurance can be confusing. First decide whether the case is Medicare primary or secondary payer. If Medicare is primary and the secondary payer is a Medigap policy, follow Medicare/Medigap processing guidelines. After determining who is primary, follow the directions on what should be entered in each block of the HCFA-1500 claim form, depending on the primary payer or follow MSP guidelines.

Templates shown at the end of Chapter 6 make it easier to learn which blocks to complete and which to ignore, depending on the primary and secondary payer. Figure 6–12 is for billing other insurance primary and Medicare secondary (MSP). A copy of the front and back sides of the primary insurance's Explanation of Benefits document must be attached to the claim when billing Medicare.

For general instructions for completing claims in Medicare and Medicare Secondary Payer cases, see Chapter 6.

Deceased Patients Claims

There are two ways in which to submit billing for a patient who has expired. They are:

1. Participating physician accepts assignment on the claim form. This will result in the quickest payment. No signature by a family member is needed on the HCFA-1500 claim form. In Block 12 where the patient's signature is required, type "Patient died on (indicate date)."
2. Nonparticipating physician does not accept assignment, bills Medicare, and submits the following.
   a. A HCFA-1500 claim form signed by the estate representative who is responsible for the bill
   b. A statement or claim for all services provided
   c. Name and address of the responsible party
   d. Provider's statement, signed and dated, refusing to accept assignment

Nothing can be done about the open balance on the account until the estate is settled, and then Medicare will pay. If family members of a deceased Medicare patient need to request reimbursement for services for which they have already paid, the person(s) who paid the bill should complete Form HCFA-1660, shown in Figure 11–15.

Physician Substitute Coverage

There are many times that special substitute coverage arrangements are made between physicians (e.g., on-call, vacation, unavailable due to another commitment). These arrangements are referred to as either reciprocal for on-call situations or *locum tenens* for a vacation situation. Specific modifiers are used to distinguish these situations and special billing guidelines are stated as follows:

▶ *Reciprocal Arrangement.* When submitting Medicare claims, the *regular* physician must identify the service provided by the *substitute* doctor by listing the -Q5 modifier after the procedure code.
▶ *Locum Tenens Arrangement.* When submitting Medicare claims, the *regular* physician must identify the service provided by the *substitute* doctor by listing the -Q6 modifier after the procedure code.

After Claim Submission

Remittance Advice

Medicare sends a payment check and a nationally standardized document to participating physicians called a Medicare **remittance advice (RA)**, formerly known as an Explanation of Medicare Benefits (EOMB). On the front side of the RA are status codes that are the same nationwide representing the reason a claim may not have been paid in full, denied, and so forth. On the reverse side of the RA, these codes are defined. If the patient has Medigap coverage, the "other payer" statement will say whether the claim has been transferred to the supplemental insurer.

Nonparticipating physicians also receive a remittance advice with payment information about unassigned claims. The remittance advice will separate payment information about assigned claims from unassigned claims to avoid posting errors by the practice. Check the payment against the fee schedule to determine whether the benefits are for the correct amount. On each claim form, note the date the payment is posted for reference. Optional

---

DEPARTMENT OF HEALTH AND HUMAN SERVICES
HEALTH CARE FINANCING ADMINISTRATION

Form Approved
OMB No. 0938-0020

REQUEST FOR INFORMATION—MEDICARE PAYMENT FOR SERVICES TO A PATIENT NOW DECEASED

No further monies or other benefits may be paid out under this program unless this report is completed and filed as required by existing law and regulations (20 C.F.R. 405 1683).

When completed, send this form to:	Deceased patient
Fiscal intermediary's name and address	Philip E. Tubes
	Health insurance claim number of deceased patient
	430-12-7651A

For Services Provided By:

Gerald Practon, MD

PART 1—PAID BILL (If The Bill Is Not Paid Go To Part II)

If bills for medical or other health services were paid by or for the deceased person, Medicare benefits may be due. We hope you will be able to help us determine who should receive payment. The person who paid the deceased's bill(s) has first right to any payment due. If the deceased or his estate paid the bill(s), benefits will be paid to the legal representative of the estate. If there is no legal representative, payment will be made to the person who stands highest in the list of relatives below. If the person who paid the bill(s) dies before being reimbursed, payment is also made to the person standing highest in the list of relatives. If there are no living relatives or legal representatives, no payment will be made. Please answer the questions, sign on the reverse side and return this form in the enclosed envelope.

ALWAYS INCLUDE EVIDENCE OF PAYMENT SUCH AS A RECEIPTED BILL OR OTHER RECEIPT

1. Who paid the deceased's bills for medical or other health services?

   ☐ The deceased or his estate (Answer (2) below)   ☒ Yourself (Sign on reverse side and return form)

   ☐ Other person or organization. (Enter the person's or organization's name and address in item 4 below.) If there is more than one person or organization, attach a listing of names and addresses of these persons or organizations to this form.

2. Is there a legal representative of the estate?

   ☐ Yes (If "Yes," print his name and address below, Sign on reverse side and return form). If you are the legal representative, submit a copy of your appointment papers with this form.   ☒ No (If "No," answer item 3 below.

3. This item is answered only if item 2 above is checked "No." Put a check in the box next to the living relative that stands highest on the following list and then write that relative's name and address in item 4 below. (If you check the box for child or children and there is more than one child, attach a listing of the names and addresses of all the children to this form.)

   ☒ Widow or widower living in the same household as the deceased at the time of death, or entitled to a monthly Social Security or Railroad Retirement benefit on the same earnings record as the deceased in the month of death.

   ☐ A child or children of the deceased entitled to monthly Social Security or Railroad Retirement benefits on the same earnings record as the deceased in the month of death (List the names and addresses of all entitled children of the deceased.)

   ☐ A parent or parents of the deceased entitled to monthly Social Security or Railroad Retirement benefits on the same earnings record as the deceased at the time of death.

   ☐ A widow or widower who was neither living with the deceased at the time of death nor at the time entitled on the same earnings record to a Social Security or Railroad Retirement benefit.

   ☐ A child or children of the deceased who were not entitled in the month of death to monthly Social Security or Railroad Retirement benefits on the same earnings record as the deceased. (List the names and addresses of all such children.)

   ☐ A parent or parents not entitled in the month of death to monthly Social Security or Railroad Retirement benefits on the same earnings record as the deceased.

4. Name	Address
Mary Ellen Tubes	4073 Angle St., Woodland Hills, XY 12345-9088

FORM HCFA-1660 (8-81)   DESTROY PRIOR EDITIONS   Continued on Back

Figure 11–15. A, Front of Medicare form HCFA-1660, Request for Information—Medicare Payment for Services to a Patient Now Deceased. This form is completed by the family of the deceased patient.

items to document are amount of payment, RA processing data, and batch number.

Offices transmitting claims electronically receive an Electronic Remittance Advice (ERA) showing payment data, and this may be automatically up-loaded into the office computer system. The ERA electronically posts payments and the provider does not have to manually post them. Paper and electronic remittance notices have the same format.

PART II—UNPAID BILL (If The Bill Is Paid, Complete Part I)

When the beneficiary has died and a physician or supplier does not agree to accept the reasonable charge as the full charge, payment may be made on the basis of an upaid bill to the person who has agreed to assume legal liability to pay the physician or supplier.

If you are assuming such legal liability and want to claim Medicare benefits for the services furnished to the deceased beneficiary, you must furnish the documents listed below to us and sign this form below. Your signature below certifies to the following statement:

I have assumed the legal obligation to pay the physician or supplier named below for services furnished to the deceased beneficiary on the date(s) indicated. I hereby claim any Medicare benefits due for these services.

Name of Physician or Supplier	Name of Deceased Beneficiary	Date(s) of Services
Gerald Practon, MD	Philip E. Tubes	4-2-20XX to 4-30-20XX

In addition furnish the following documents together with this form to us.

1. A completed form HCFA-1490S, PATIENT'S REQUEST FOR MEDICARE PAYMENTS. You must sign item 6 of the HCFA-1490S in lieu of the deceased beneficiary. (You may obtain a copy of the HCFA-1490S from a Social Security Office if you did not receive one with form;) and

2. A signed statement from the physician or supplier which shows that the physician or supplier refuses to accept assignment for the bill; and

3. An itemized bill from the physician or supplier which identifies you as the person to whom the physician or supplier looks for payment.

Sign below and return this form together with the documents specified above to the address shown in the upper left portion of the form on the other side. If no carrier name and address is shown on the other side of this form request the proper addressee information from a Social Security Office.

I certify that if I receive the entire amount due, I will distribute it among other persons if they are legally entitled to it. Knowing that anyone making a false statement or representation of a material fact for use in determining the right to or the amount of Health Insurance benefits commits a crime punishable under the Federal law, I certify that the above statements are true.

If this statement has been signed by mark (X), two witnesses who know the claimant should sign below, giving their full addresses. The signature and title of a Social Security employee will suffice in lieu of signatures of two witnesses.	Name of claiment *(Please print)*
	Mary Ellen Tubes
Name	Signature of claimant *(Write in ink)*
	SIGN HERE ▶ *Mary Ellen Tubes*
Address *(Number and Street, City, State and ZIP Code)*	Mailing Address *(Number and Street, P.O. Box or Route)*
	4073 Angle Street
Name	City, State and ZIP Code
	Woodland Hills, XY 12345
Address *(Number and Street, City, State and Zip Code)*	Date *(Month, Day and Year)* 5-10-20xx	Telephone number 013-732-1500

If you wish assistance in completing this request, please take it to a Social Security Office. The people there will help you.
PLEASE RETURN THIS REQUEST IN THE ENCLOSED ENVELOPE

HCFA-1660 (8-81)   * U S G P O 1966- 491-258/53795

Figure 11–15 *Continued. B,* Back of Medicare form HCFA-1660, Request for Information—Medicare Payment for Services to a Patient Now Deceased.

Medicare Summary Notice

A patient is mailed a similar document called a **Medicare Summary Notice (MSN).** This document is designed to be easier for the patient to under- stand, but because many patients do not know what is meant by *amount charged, Medicare ap- proved, deductible,* and *coinsurance,* it often be- comes necessary for the insurance billing special- ist to educate the patient. First photocopy an RA

STATEMENT

College Clinic
4567 Broad Avenue
Woodland Hills, XY 12345-0001
Telephone: 013-486-9002
Fax: 013-487-8976

Account No. 946
John Smith
100 James Street
Woodland Hills, XY 12345-0001

| DATE | PROFESSIONAL SERVICE DESCRIPTION | CHARGE | | CREDITS | | | | CURRENT BALANCE | |
				PAYMENTS		ADJUSTMENTS			
2-15-xx	Surgery	800	00					800	00
2-17-xx	Medicare/Medigap billed (2-15-xx)							800	00
4-2-xx	Medicare payment voucher #12498 (2-15-xx)			440	00			360	00
4-12-xx	Medigap payment voucher #45500 (2-15-xx)			110	00			250	00
4-12-xx	Medicare courtesy (adjustment 2-15-xx)					250	00	-0-	

Due and payable within 10 days   **Pay last amount in balance column** ⇧

Key: PF: Problem-focused   SF: Straightforward   CON: Consultation   HCD: House Call (Day)
     EPF: Expanded problem-focused LC: Low complexity   CPX: Complete Phys Exam   HCN: House Call (Night)
     D: Detailed   MC: Moderate complexity   E: Emergency   HV: Hospital visit
     C: Comprehensive   HC: High complexity   ER: Emergency Dept.   OV: Office Visit

Figure 11–16. Sample ledger card illustrating how payments and courtesy adjustments should be posted. In the case illustrated, the Medicare allowed amount is $550.

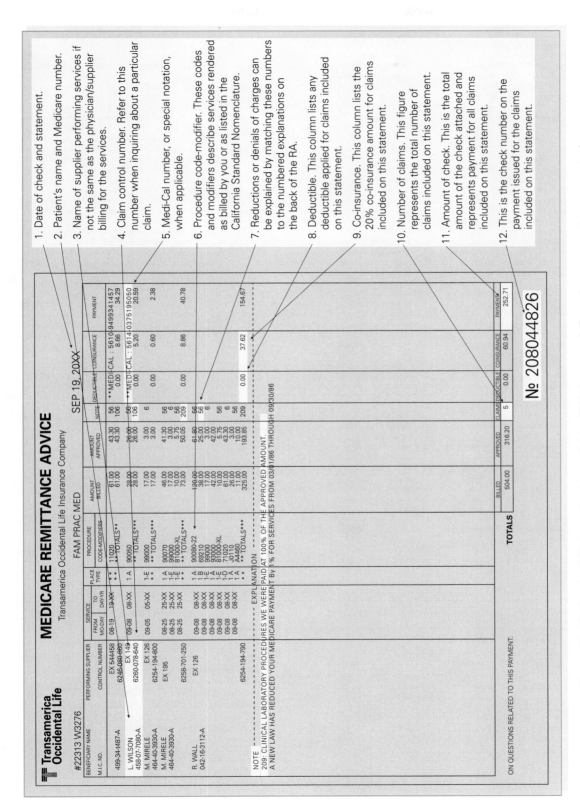

Figure 11-17. Sample of Medicare Remittance Advice (RA) document. A, Front. Insurance carriers are required to use Health Care Financing Administration messages for Medicare RA, but each carrier has its own code numbers to denote the messages.

(Illustration continued on following page)

Content within the figure:

Transamerica Occidental Life

MEDICARE REMITTANCE ADVICE

Transamerica Occidental Life Insurance Company

SEP 19, 20XX

#22313 W3276   FAM PRAC MED

| BENEFICIARY NAME | PERFORMING SUPPLIER | SERVICE | | PLACE TYPE | PROCEDURE | AMOUNT BILLED | AMOUNT APPROVED | NOTE | DEDUCTIBLE | COINSURANCE | PAYMENT |
M.I.C. NO.	CONTROL NUMBER	FROM MO-DAY	TO DAY-YR		CODE-MODIFIERS						
499-34-1487-A	EX 544458	08-19	19-XX	* *	11020	61.00	43.30	56	**MEDICAL :	5610	9499341457
	6246-080-660				***TOTALS**	61.00	43.30	106	0.00	8.66	34.29
L. WILSON	EX 149	09-08	08-XX	1 A	90050	28.00	26.00	56	**MEDICAL :	5614	0375195050
458-07-7080-A	6260-078-640				***TOTALS***	28.00	26.00	106	0.00	5.20	20.59
M. MIRELE	EX 126	09-05	05-XX	1-E	99000	17.00	3.00	6	0.00	0.60	2.38
464-40-3930-A	6254-194-800			* *	***TOTALS***	17.00	3.00				
M. MIRELE	EX 195	08-25	25-XX	1 A	90070	46.00	41.30	56			
464-40-3930-A		08-25	25-XX	1-E	99000	17.00	3.00	6			
	6258-701-250	08-25	25-XX	1-E	81000-XL	10.00	5.75	56			
				* *	***TOTALS***	73.00	50.05	209	0.00	8.86	40.78
R. WALL	EX 126	09-08	08-XX	1 A	90080-22	129.00	61.90	56			
042-16-3112-A		09-08	08-XX	1 B	69210	38.00	25.00	56			
		09-08	08-XX	1-A	99000	17.00	3.00	6			
		09-08	08-XX	1-E	99000	47.00	3.00	56			
		09-08	08-XX	1-D	71020	61.00	5.75	6			
		09-08	08-XX	1 A	J0110	26.00	43.30	56			
	6254-194-790			* *	A4460	11.00	3.00	56			
					TOTALS	325.00	193.85	209	0.00	37.62	154.67

NOTE --------------- EXPLANATION ----------------------------
209: CLINICAL LABORATORY PROCEDURES WE WERE PAID AT 100% OF THE APPROVED AMOUNT.
A NEW LAW HAS REDUCED YOUR MEDICARE PAYMENT By 1% FOR SERVICES FROM 03/01/86 THROUGH 09/30/86

	BILLED	APPROVED	CLAIMS	DEDUCTIBLE	COINSURANCE	PAYMENT
TOTALS	504.00	316.20	5	0.00	60.94	252.71

ON QUESTIONS RELATED TO THIS PAYMENT:

№ 208044826

Callout notes:

1. Date of check and statement.
2. Patient's name and Medicare number.
3. Name of supplier performing services if not the same as the physician/supplier billing for the services.
4. Claim control number. Refer to this number when inquiring about a particular claim.
5. Medi-Cal number, or special notation, when applicable.
6. Procedure code-modifier. These codes and modifiers describe services rendered as billed by you or as listed in the California Standard Nomenclature.
7. Reductions or denials of charges can be explained by matching these numbers to the numbered explanations on the back of the RA.
8. Deductible. This column lists any deductible applied for claims included on this statement.
9. Co-insurance. This column lists the 20% co-insurance amount for claims included on this statement.
10. Number of claims. This figure represents the total number of claims included on this statement.
11. Amount of check. This is the total amount of the check attached and represents payment for all claims included on this statement.
12. This is the check number on the payment issued for the claims included on this statement.

EXPLANATION OF NOTES   Additional notes may be listed on the front of this form.

1 – See enclosed letter.

2 – Claim was filed after the time limit.

4 – These bills are handled by a special intermediary.

5 – This payment is for an adjustment of a previous claim.

6 – Charges over the maximum Medicare allowance are not covered.

7 – Services before Medicare entitlement are not covered.

8 – Services after Medicare entitlement ended are not covered.

10 – Other charges submitted with this claim may be on a separate statement which you have received or will receive soon.

12 – Routine examinations and related services are not covered.

13 – Immunizations or other routine and preventative services are not covered.

16 – We need an itemization of this charge. Please resubmit your claim with this information.

17 – Prescription drugs are not covered.

18 – Charges for this physician/supplier are not covered.

19 – We need a full description of the service or supply to consider this charge. Please resubmit your claim with this information.

23 – We need a written report for this service. Please resubmit your claim with this information.

26 – More than $312.50 annual psychiatric expense is not covered.

27 – We need from the prescribing physician the specific length of time this medical equipment is needed. Please resubmit your claim with this information.

30 – This charge was previously considered.

37 – Claims for these services will be made by a home health agency or hospital.

39 – Equipment that is not medically necessary is not covered. (See Note 89)

42 – These supplies or services are not covered.

45 – Over 62½% of psychiatric expenses is not covered.

46 – Routine foot care is not covered.

47 – Routine eye examinations or eye refractions are not covered.

48 – Partial payment of this claim was made to the beneficiary.

49 – This service cannot be considered until the hospital makes the necessary arrangement with the carrier for its processing.

50 – The beneficiary is not responsible for this reduction/denial under the assignment agreement.

54 – Care before and/or after surgery is included in the surgery benefit. (See Note 50)

56 – This is the full charge allowed based upon the prevailing or usual and customary rate.

62 – Payment has been reduced because this test is commonly part of an automated test group. (See Note 50)

66 – This service is not covered when done by this laboratory.

70 – There were no charges or bills with your claim form. Please resubmit your claim with this information.

72 – We need a signed and dated prescription showing medical necessity and specific length of time needed. Please resubmit your claim with this information.

73 – Before another month's payment can be made, we need a new signed and dated prescription showing further necessity of the medical equipment and specific length of time needed.

80 – We need to know the place of service to consider this charge. Please resubmit your claim with this information.

83 – SSA advises us that they are unable to verify the patient's eligibility for Part B Medical Insurance Plan. For this reason, no payment can be made on this claim.

84 – The patient's HIC number shown on this claim was incorrect. Please use the correct HIC number on all future claims.

85 – The patient's name shown on this claim was incorrect. Please use the correct name on all future claims.

86 – Over 62½% of the allowable charges for psychiatric services is not covered.

89 – If you did not know that Medicare does not pay for this medical service, you may request a review of this decision. See below paragraph entitled "Your right to review of a case."

90 – This service by a chiropractor is not covered.

93 – Over $500.00 annual expense billed by a physical therapist is not covered.

95 – These specific services by this supplier are not covered.

96 – Please verify the date of this service. Resubmit your claim with this information.

99 – We need a complete diagnosis before the claim can be considered. Please resubmit your claim with this information.

106 – The Medicare covered services on this claim have been forwarded for additional processing under Medi-Cal.

107 – This claim was not forwarded for Medi-Cal processing. Please bill Medi-Cal directly and attach a copy of this statement.

108 – The bills for these services have been transferred to Blue Shield of California Medicare Claims, Chico, CA 95976. You will hear from them.

129 – Payment for services prior to July 1 is based on the previous year's payment rate.

131 – Payment for this physician service in a hospital department is reduced since this service is commonly performed in the physician's office. (See Note 50)

138 – This amount is more than Medicare pays for maintenance treatment of renal disease.

147 – This charge is not covered because an allowance for purchase of the same equipment was previously made.

151 – Your claim was transferred to a Health Maintenance Organization for processing.

153 – These are more visits (treatments) for this diagnosis than Medicare covers unless there were unusual circumstances. (See Note 89)

154 – This service is not covered for your patient's reported condition. (See Note 89)

155 – Only one visit per month to a nursing home is covered unless special need is indicated. (See Note 89)

156 – This laboratory test for the reported condition and/or illness is not covered. (See Note 89)

158 – Procedures whose effectiveness has not been proven are not covered. (See Note 89)

161 – The frequency of services for this condition are not covered. (See Note 89)

162 – More than one visit per day for this condition are not covered. (See Note 89)

172 – This type of services billed by a psychologist are not covered.

179 – The amount for this service is included in the approved amount for the consultation/office/hospital visit.

181 – Payment for this service is included in the major surgical fee.

187 – We need the name and address of the individual doctor who performed this service. Please resubmit your claim with this information.

192 – Medicare benefits have been reduced because the patient's employer group health plan has paid some of these expenses.

198 – A claim must be sent to the patient's employer group health plan first. After the claim has been processed by that plan, resubmit this claim with the bills and the notice the other insurance company sent you.

203 – Clinical laboratory services. Blood Gas Studies and Rhythm Strips (1–3 leads) furnished in a hospital setting are reimbursed through the hospital.

205 – The date of this service is after the patient's expiration date provided to us by SSA. If service was rendered to this patient on this date, have the patient's estate contact the local Social Security Office for assistance.

206 – For payment, these services must be billed by the performing laboratory with the assignment accepted.

213 – We did not send this claim to Medicaid. Please send this statement and a copy of the claim to the agency that handles Medicaid in your area.

216 – This service or item cannot be processed until your application for a Medicare provider identification number is received and approved.

218 – Since you are Medicare participating, we have processed this claim as assigned. Future claims must be billed on assignment. If the bill was paid in full, you must immediately refund the amount due to the beneficiary.

219 – We need this charge submitted on your letterhead bill. Please resubmit your claim with this information.

221 – The name and Medicare number submitted on this claim do not match. Please verify for whom these services were rendered and provide the correct name and number on the claim and resubmit.

223 – We did not consider this for payment because you did not send the extra information we asked for. Payment can be requested again by sending us another claim form and all the information.

226 – Medicare will pay rent for the prescribed number of months or until the equipment is no longer needed, whichever occurs first. This is the first monthly rental payment.

227 – You will receive a notice each month when additional rental payments are paid.

231 – Medicare will no longer pay for rental on this item since the purchase price has been paid.

237 – The amount of this payment is the difference between the approved purchase allowance and the rental payments you have received.

YOUR RIGHT TO REVIEW OF A CASE

If you have a problem or question about the way a claim was handled or about the amount paid, please write Transamerica Occidental Life, Box 54905, Terminal Annex, Los Angeles, California 90054, within 6 months of the date of this notice. We will give your request full consideration.

Your Social Security office will help you file a request for review of a claim if it is more convenient for you.

WHERE TO SEND REFUNDS

When refunding a payment you should send a check with a letter of explanation. The letter should include your Transamerica Occidental/Medicare check number, beneficiary name and Medicare identification number (HIC No.), control number to which the payment relates and any other information which may be pertinent to the refund. Send this information to:

Transamerica Occidental Life
C/O Check and Payment Control
Box 54905, Terminal Annex
Los Angeles, CA 90054-0905

KEY TO CODES FOR PLACE AND TYPE OF SERVICE

Place of service	Type of service
1. Office	A. Medical care
2. Home	B. Surgery (includes treatment of fractures)
3. Inpatient hospital	C. Consultation
4. Skilled nursing facility	D. Diagnostic X-ray
5. Outpatient hospital	E. Diagnostic laboratory
6. Independent laboratory	F. Radiation therapy
7. Other	G. Anesthesia
8. Independent kidney disease treatment center	H. Assistance at surgery
	I. Other medical service
	J. Whole blood or packed red cells

Figure 11–17 *Continued. B,* **Back of Medicare Remittance Advice (RA) document.**

to be used as an example, deleting the patient's name to ensure confidentiality. Then use the RA to illustrate to future patients what various terms mean. This will increase patient understanding and save time.

Beneficiary Representative/Representative Payee

Medicare beneficiaries may have memory impairment or may be confined to a wheelchair or bed so they have a legal right to appoint an individual to serve as their representative.

Claims assistance professionals (CAPs) act as a client representative. They have some legal standing and are recognized by Medicare to act on the beneficiary's behalf if the beneficiary completes a Beneficiary Representative Form SSA 1696. This form is available from the Social Security District Office. Copies of the completed form should be sent to the Medicare intermediary or carrier when appropriate.

In contrast, a representative payee is an individual or organization chosen by the SSA to receive and administer SSA benefit funds on behalf of the beneficiary. Other duties consist of assisting the beneficiary with check writing for financial obligations, such as personal care and maintenance, housing, medical service expenses, and investing any surplus monies for the beneficiary's benefit. A representative payee is responsible for using payments received only for the benefit of the beneficiary, accounting for the benefits received on request, and contacting SSA when anything affects eligibility for SSA benefits or prevents the representative payee's ability to perform these responsibilities. Additional information on CAPs is found in Chapters 1 and 17.

Posting Payments

Usually a physician's charge is higher than the charge approved by the Medicare carrier or fiscal agent. This does not mean that his or her charges are unreasonable. As previously mentioned, payments are established using a fee schedule based on an RBRVS, a **volume performance standard (VPS)** for expenditure increases, and a *limiting charge* for nonparticipating physicians.

Because some services may be disallowed or the payments on them may be lower than those charged by the physician, it is important to know how to post payments to the patient's ledger card or computerized account. Figure 11–16 illustrates how

payments and courtesy adjustments are posted. The word "courtesy" implies that Medicare patients are treated well and is preferred to phrases like "not allowed" or "write off."

In regard to the patient's coinsurance payment, Medicare does not allow for the standardized waiving of copayments. Medicare regulations require that a patient be billed for the copayment at least three times before the balance is adjusted off as uncollectible. If the patient is suffering financial hardship, it is important to document this as further justification.

When a remittance advice (RA) is received, it may list many patients (Fig. 11–17). Do not post the entire payment made in a lump sum to the day sheet. Individually post each line item paid to the patient's ledger card or computerized account and to the day sheet (Fig. 11–18). To prevent funds from going astray, some offices prefer to post Medicare payments to a separate day sheet and deposit each multiple reimbursement check separately. This way, the day sheet totals will agree with the deposit slip totals and not get confused with other monies collected.

Figure 11–19A illustrates an example of a Medicare/Medicaid case after payment by Medicare. Medicare applied the patient's full $100 deductible amount to the Medicare allowed amount, reducing payment to $4. The Medicaid RA (see Fig. 11–19B) shows reimbursement of the coinsurance and deductible amounts dual-billed to Medicaid.

Calculations are shown in the following box:

Medicare		Medicaid	
$105	Allowed amount	$105	Medicare allowed amount
−100	Deductible		
5	Balance on which	−32	Medicaid cutback
	payment is	$ 73	Medicaid allowed
× .80	calculated		
$ 4	Medicare paid 80%	−4	Medicare paid
		$ 69	Medicaid payment

When referring to the Medicaid program, a *cutback* means a reduction and would require an adjustment entry on the patient's ledger. Cutbacks are common on Medicaid claims.

Medicare overpayments can occur in the following situations:

▶ Carrier processes the charge more than once.
▶ Physician receives duplicate payments from Medicare and a secondary payer.

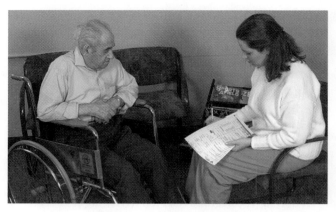

Figure 11–18 Insurance billing specialist explaining a Medicare Remittance Advice document that the physician's office has received.

▶ Physician is paid directly on an unassigned claim.

▶ Item is not covered but is paid.

▶ Payment is made on erroneous information.

If you receive a check and know that it is an overpayment, deposit the check and then write to Medicare notifying them of the overpayment. Include a copy of the check and the RA. This over-

payment will be deducted from your next Medicare payment and be will be shown on the RA. If the physician wishes to repay a Medicare overpayment on the installment plan, form HCFA-379 may be used. This form is sent to the physician when the carrier notifies the physician that money is due back.

For additional information about Explanation of Benefits documents from private insurance carriers, refer to Chapter 7.

Review and Appeal Process

As you have read, Chapter 8 outlines in detail the steps to take for having a claim reviewed and the process of appealing a claim in the Medicare program.

RESOURCES ON THE INTERNET

For current information or to download Medicare publications, visit the Medicare web site: **www.medicare.gov.**

MEDICARE REMITTANCE ADVICE
XYZ Insurance Company

Physician or Supplier Name	Dates of service From To MMDD MMDDYY	See back serv typl	Sub code (alwcode)	Billed amount	Amount allowed	See ** act cde	Beneficiary obligation Deductible Co-ins		Medicare payment to Beneficiary Provider	

BENEFICIARY: BILL HUTCH   HIC NUMBER: 5432-112-34
CONTROL NO.: 92106-30810-00   DE/MI: 2121D52

A	John Doe MD 0310 031094	D 03	120101	145.00	105.00	101	100.00	1.00	0.00	4.00	
	CLAIM TOTALS:			145.00	105.00	101	100.00	1.00	0.00	4.00	

MEDICARE REMITTANCE ADVICE

RECIPIENT NAME	RECIPIENT MEDICAID ID NO.	CLAIM CONTROL NUMBER	SERVICE DATE MO DAY YR	PROCEDURE CODE	PATIENT ACCT. NO.	QTY.	MEDICARE ALLOWED	MEDICAID ALLOWED	PATIENT LIABILITY	COMPUTED MCR AMT.	MEDICAID PAID	EOB MESSAGE
BILL HUTCH	521345678	4006984891200	03 10 94	49555–80		001	105.00	73.00		4.00	.00	
		4006984891200	00 00 00			000	105.00	73.00		4.00	69.00	
B BLOOD DEDUCT 00 DEDUCTIBLE 100.00 COINSUR 1.00 CUTBACK 32.00												CUTBACK 443

Figure 11–19. *A,* Example of a Medicare/Medicaid case after payment by Medicare. *B,* The Medicaid Remittance Advice (RA) shows reimbursement of the coinsurance and deductible amounts dual billed to Medicaid.

STUDENT ASSIGNMENT LIST

✔ Study Chapter 11.

✔ Answer the review questions in the *Workbook* to reinforce the theory learned in this chapter and to help prepare you for a future test.

✔ Complete the assignments in the *Workbook* to give you experience in computing Medicare in mathematic calculations, selecting HCPCS code numbers, abstracting from patients' medical records, preparing ledger cards, and completing forms pertinent to the Medicare program.

✔ Turn to the Glossary at the end of this textbook for a further understanding of the Key Terms used in this chapter.

COMPUTER ASSIGNMENT

Do the exercises for cases 8, 9, and 10 on the computer disk to review concepts you have learned for this chapter.

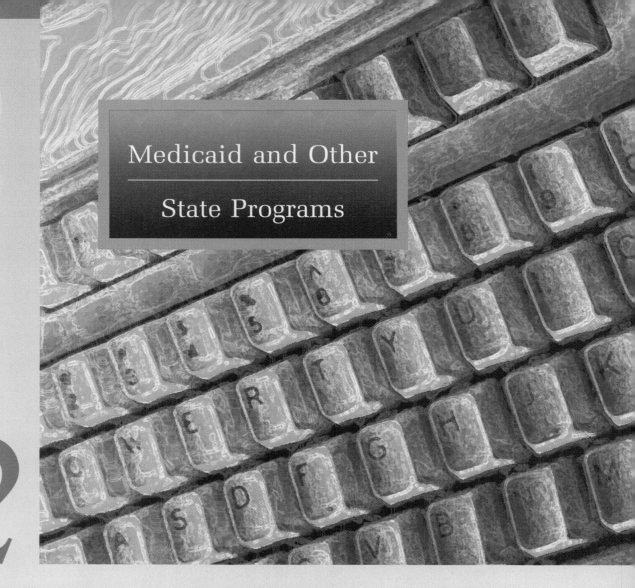

Medicaid and Other
State Programs

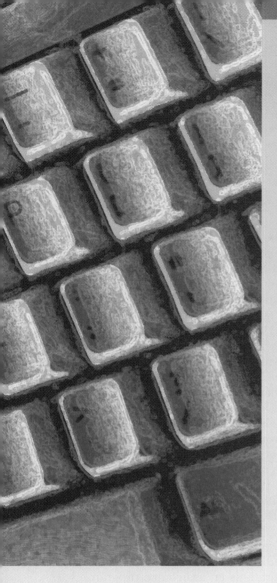

dures for the Maternal and Child Health Program.

■ Identify those eligible for the Medicaid Qualified Medicare Beneficiaries program.

■ Explain basic operations of a Medicaid-managed care system.

■ Describe basic Medicaid claim procedure guidelines.

■ File claims for patients who have Medicaid and other coverage.

■ Minimize the number of insurance forms rejected because of improper completion.

KEY TERMS

categorically needy

covered services

Early and Periodic Screening, Diagnosis, and Treatment (EPSDT)

fiscal agent

Maternal and Child Health Program (MCHP)

Medicaid (MCD)

Medi-Cal

medically needy (MN)

prior approval

recipient

share of cost

Supplemental Security Income (SSI)

OBJECTIVES*

After reading this chapter, you should be able to:

■ Understand the benefits and nonbenefits of Medicaid.

■ Define terminology inherent to Medicaid.

■ Interpret Medicaid abbreviations.

■ Name the two Medicaid eligibility classifications.

■ List important information to abstract from the patient's Medicaid card.

■ State eligibility requirements and claims proce-

*Performance objectives and exercises for hands-on practical experience for this chapter appear in the *Workbook*.

History

Federal participation in providing medical care to needy persons began between 1933 and 1935 when the Federal Emergency Relief Administration made funds available to pay the medical expenses of the needy unemployed. The Social Security Act of 1935 set up the public assistance programs; and although no special provision was made for medical assistance, the federal government paid a share of the monthly assistance payments, which could be used to meet the costs of medical care. However, the payment was made to the assistance recipient rather than to the provider of medical care.

In 1950, Congress passed a law mandating that all states set up a health care program of assistance, which meant that the states had to meet minimum requirements. As a result of this mandate, the states set up **Medicaid (MCD)** programs. Congress authorized *vendor payments* for medical care, that is, payments from the welfare agency directly to physicians, health care institutions, and other providers of medical services. By 1960 four fifths of the states made provisions for medical vendor payments.

A new category of assistance recipient was established for the medically needy aged population. The incomes of these individuals were too high to qualify them for cash assistance payments, but they needed help in meeting the costs of medical care. The federal government financially supports the minimum assistance level, and the states must wholly support any part of the program that goes beyond the federal minimum. This is referred to as *state share.*

In 1965, Title XIX of the Social Security Act became federal law, and Medicaid legally came into being. It was, to a large extent, the result of various attempts over the previous 30 years to provide medical care to the needy. The program has always had somewhat of a split personality. On one hand, it is viewed as an attempt on the part of the government to provide comprehensive quality health care to those unable to afford it. On the other hand, Medicaid has been seen as merely a bill paying mechanism whose purpose is to administer the provision of health care using the most efficient and economic system possible.

Since 1983, the trend in many states has been to expand Medicaid eligibility requirements and services. Changes in Medicaid eligibility allowing more people into the program were made by many states after the passage by the federal government of the Deficit Reduction Act of 1984 (DEFRA) and the Child Health Assurance Program (CHAP).

In 1982, the Tax Equity and Fiscal Responsibility Act (TEFRA) set down laws affecting those under the Medicare program as well as Medicaid medically needy recipients and those in certain other categories. For information about how this act affects Medicare recipients, see Chapter 11.

Medicaid Programs

Title XIX of the Social Security Act provides for a program of medical assistance for certain low-income individuals and families. The program is known as Medicaid in 48 states and **Medi-Cal** in California. Arizona is the only state without a Medicaid program like those existing in other states. Since 1982, it has received federal funds under a demonstration waiver for an alternative medical assistance program (prepaid care) for low-income persons called the Arizona Health Care Cost Containment System (AHCCCS).

Medicaid is administered by state governments with partial federal funding. Coverage and benefits vary widely from state to state because the federal government sets minimum requirements and the states are free to enact more benefits. Thus, each state designs its own Medicaid program within federal guidelines. The Health Care Financing Administration (HCFA) of the Bureau of Program Operations of the United States Department of Health and Human Services is responsible for the federal aspects of Medicaid. Medicaid is not so much an insurance program as an assistance program.

Maternal and Child Health Program

Each state and certain other jurisdictions, including territories and the District of Columbia (56 programs total), operate a **Maternal and Child Health Program (MCHP)** with federal grant support under Title V of the Social Security Act. Although Title V has been amended on a number of occasions, notably between 1981 and 1987, no changes have been as sweeping as those in the Omnibus Budget Reconciliation Act (OBRA) of 1989. Federal funds are granted to states, enabling them to:

▶ Provide low-income mothers and children access to quality maternal and child health services.

▶ Reduce infant mortality and the incidence of preventable diseases and handicapping conditions among children.

▶ Increase the number of children immunized against disease and the number of low-income children receiving health assessments and follow-up diagnostic and treatment services.

▶ Promote the health of mothers and infants by providing prenatal, delivery, and postpartum care for low-income, at-risk pregnant women.

▶ Provide preventive and primary care services for low-income children.

▶ Provide rehabilitation services for the blind and disabled younger than age 16 years.

▶ Provide, promote, and develop family-centered, community-based, coordinated care for children with special health care needs.

The state agency tries to locate mothers, infants, and children younger than age 21 years who may have conditions eligible for treatment under the MCHP. The conditions are diagnosed, and the necessary medical and other health-related care, any hospitalization, and any continuing follow-up care are given.

After a child is examined at an MCHP clinic and a diagnosis is made, the parents are advised about the treatment that will benefit the child. The state agency then helps them locate this care. If the parents cannot afford this care, the agency assists them with financial planning and may assume part or all of the cost of treatment, depending on the child's condition and the family's resources.

Low-Income Medicare Recipients

There are three aid programs for Medicare patients who have low incomes and have difficulty paying Medicare premiums, copayments, and deductibles. Each program addresses a different financial category, and the monthly income figures are adjusted each year. They are:

▶ Medicaid Qualified Medicare Beneficiary Program

▶ Specified Low-Income Medicare Beneficiary Program

▶ Qualifying Individuals Program

The programs are usually administered through county social services departments, the same ones that administer Medicaid. One application is completed that pertains to all three programs, and an individual is placed in one of the programs depending on how he or she qualifies financially.

Medicaid Qualified Medicare Beneficiary Program

The Medicaid Qualified Medicare Beneficiary (MQMB) program was introduced in the Medicare Catastrophic Act of 1988 as an amendment to the Social Security Act. Then, in 1990, the Omnibus Budget Reconciliation Act allowed for assistance to qualified Medicare beneficiaries (QMBs pro-

nounced "kwim-bees") who are aged and disabled and are receiving Medicare and have annual incomes *below the federal poverty level*. Eligibility also depends on what other financial resources an individual might have.

Under this act, states must provide limited Medicaid coverage for QMBs. They must pay Medicare Part B premiums (and, if applicable, Part A premiums), along with required Medicare deductibles and coinsurance amounts. Coverage is restricted to Medicare cost sharing unless the beneficiary qualifies for Medicaid in some other way. Medicaid will not pay for the service if Medicare does not cover the service to the patient.

States are also required to pay Part A premiums, but no other expenses, for qualified disabled and working individuals. It is optional for states to provide full Medicaid benefits to QMBs who meet a state-established income standard.

Specified Low-Income Medicare Beneficiary Program

The Specified Low-Income Medicare Beneficiary (SLMB pronounced "slim-bee") program was established in 1993 for elderly individuals that are *20% above the federal poverty level*. It pays the entire Medicare Part B premium. The patient must pay the deductible, copay, and for noncovered items.

Qualifying Individuals Program

The Qualifying Individuals (QI) program was created in 1997 for qualifying individuals who are *135% above the poverty standard*. It also pays for the Medicare Part B premium.

Medicaid Eligibility

Medicaid is available to certain needy and low-income people, such as the aged (65 years or older), the blind, the disabled, and members of families with dependent children deprived of the support of at least one parent and financially eligible on the basis of income and resources. If a person is eligible for Medicaid, he or she goes to the local welfare office and applies for benefits. After acceptance into the program, the patient brings a form or card to the physician's office that verifies acceptance into the program (Fig. 12–1). Each state decides what services are covered and what the payments are for each service. There are two classifications that contain several basic groups of needy and low-income individuals.

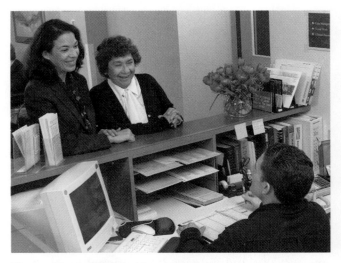

Figure 12–1. A Medicaid patient checking in at the receptionist's desk.

Categorically Needy

The first classification, the **categorically needy** group, includes all cash recipients of the Aid to Families with Dependent Children (AFDC) program, certain other AFDC-related groups, most cash recipients of the **Supplemental Security Income (SSI)** program, other SSI-related groups, Qualified Medicare Beneficiaries (QMBs), and institutional and long-term care and intermediate-care facility patients (Fig. 12–2).

Medically Needy

The second classification involves state general assistance programs for low-income people, medically indigent, and individuals losing employer health insurance. This classification is sometimes referred to as the **medically needy** class. A Medicaid **recipient** in this category may or may not pay coinsurance and/or a deductible, which must be met within the eligibility month or other specified time frame before he or she can receive state benefits (also known as **share of cost**). Emergency care and pregnancy services are exempt by law from copayment requirements. This may be a component of a state's general assistance program for low-income people. For those individuals who may become *medically indigent* as a result of high medical care expenses and inadequate health insurance coverage, a number of states have adopted a State Program of Assistance for the Medically Indigent. For a clear, simple understanding of the classes and basic groups for Medicaid eligibility, see Figure 12–2.

Maternal and Child Health Program Eligibility

Under the Maternal and Child Health Program (MCHP) specific conditions qualify a child for benefits. The state law under which each agency operates either defines the conditions to be included or directs the children's agency to define them. All state laws include children who have some kind of handicap that needs

GROUPS ELIGIBLE FOR MEDICAID BENEFITS	
CLASSIFICATIONS	**GROUPS**

CATEGORICALLY NEEDY	I. Families, pregnant women and children
	    a) Aid to Families with Dependent Children (AFDC)-related groups
	    b) Non-ADFC pregnant women and children
	
	II. Aged and disabled persons
	    a) Supplemental Security Income (SSI)-related groups
	    b) Qualified Medicare Beneficiaries (QMBs)
	
	III. Persons receiving institutional or other long-term care
	     in nursing facilities (NFs) and intermediate care facilities (ICFs)

MEDICALLY NEEDY	IV. Medically indigent low-income individuals and families V. Low-income persons losing employer health insurance coverage (Medicaid purchase of COBRA coverage)

Figure 12–2. Classifications and basic groups eligible for Medicaid benefits.

orthopedic treatment or plastic surgery; a few states add other conditions. A list of both types of conditions that qualify children for MCHP follows:

Cerebral palsy
Chronic conditions affecting bones and joints
Cleft lip
Cleft palate
Clubfoot
Cystic fibrosis*
Epilepsy*
Hearing problems*
Mental retardation*
Multiple handicaps*
Paralyzed muscles
Rheumatic and congenital heart disease*
Vision problems requiring surgery*

Accepting Medicaid Patients

Individual physicians have their own office procedures for handling Medicaid patients. A patient can be on Medicaid 1 month and off the following month or on the program for several months or years; therefore, each case is different. The physician may accept or refuse to treat Medicaid patients but must make the decision on the basis of the entire Medicaid program, not an individual patient's personality, medical situation, or other discriminating factor. It is important that the patient receive quality care and be treated the same as the paying patient. If the physician decides to take Medicaid patients, he or she must accept the Medicaid allowance as payment in full (Fig. 12–13).

When obtaining personal information from the patient at the time of the first visit or a follow-up visit, check the patient's name, address, and telephone number in a reverse address directory to verify that it is correct. Another type of directory available is one that lists everyone on a given block or even in an apartment building who has a telephone. These easy reference guides cut verification time in half. Some Medicaid individuals are homeless and may list fake addresses, which makes locating them difficult.

Identification Card

A plastic or paper Medicaid identification card (or, in some states, coupons) is usually issued monthly. Under certain classifications of eligibility, identification cards are issued in some states on the 1st and 15th of each month, every 2 months, every 3 months, or every 6 months. Sometimes an unborn child can be issued an identification card that is used for services promoting the life and health of the fetus.

Obtain a photocopy of the front and back of the card. Carefully check the expiration date of the card each time the patient visits the physician's office to see whether eligibility is indicated for the month of service. Note whether the patient has other insurance, copayment requirements, or restrictions, such as being eligible for only certain types of medical services.

When professional services are rendered, eligibility for that month must be verified, which may be done in a number of ways. For some states, the Potomac Group, Inc., in Nashville, Tennessee, has developed MediFAX. This is a machine that allows the user to verify coverage in seconds and is available for several states. There are some states that provide their own electronic system for Medicaid verification via touch-tone telephone, modem, or specialized Medicaid terminal equipment. Some states issue cards that contain adhesive labels listing the month of eligibility that must be used on the billing claim form.

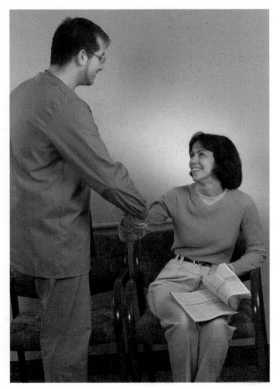

Figure 12–3. A disabled patient being welcomed by an insurance biller and asking for her Medicaid card.

---

*Only some states include this item in their Maternal and Child Health Program.

Retroactive Eligibility

In some cases, retroactive eligibility may be granted to a patient. When patients are seeking medical care who are in hope of qualifying for Medicaid but have not done so at the time of service, the account must be set up as a cash account until retroactive eligibility has been established. If the patient has documentation or a retroactive card confirming this and has paid for any services during the retroactive period, then a refund must be made and Medicaid billed. As described and shown in the previous chapter, a waiver of liability agreement rewritten to the Medicaid program and signed by the patient might be used in such cases.

Medicaid Benefits

Covered Services

Under Federal guidelines, the state Medicaid basic benefits offered to eligible recipients include the types of **covered services** shown in Table 12–1.

Early and Periodic Screening, Diagnosis, and Treatment

Another benefit of the Medicaid program is the **Early and Periodic Screening, Diagnosis, and Treatment (EPSDT)** service. This is a program of prevention, early detection, and treatment of welfare children (younger than age 21) (Fig. 12–4). In California (Medi-Cal), it is known as the Child Health and Disability Prevention (CHDP) program.

The EPSDT guidelines include a medical history and physical examination; immunization status assessment; dental, hearing, and vision screening; developmental assessment; and screening for anemia and lead absorption, tuberculosis, bacteriuria, and sickle cell disease and trait. States are required to provide necessary health care, diagnostic services, treatment, and other services to correct physical or mental defects found.

Disallowed Services

If a service is totally disallowed by Medicaid (denied claim), a physician is within legal rights to bill the patient. However, it is wise to have the patient sign a waiver of liability agreement if the service to be provided may be a denied service from known past claim submission experience. An example of a waiver of liability agreement is shown in Chapter 11, Figure 11–10. To obtain up-to-date information and details on the Medicaid program

TABLE 12–1   **Medicaid Basic Benefits**
Family planning
Home health care
Immunizations
Inpatient hospital care
Laboratory and x-ray
Outpatient hospital care
Physicians' care
Screening, diagnosis, and treatment of children younger than 21 years of age
Skilled nursing care
Transportation to and from health care providers
In some states, additional services included might be the following:
Allergy care
Ambulance services
Certain medical cosmetic procedures
Chiropractic care
Clinic care
Dental care
Dermatologic care
Diagnostic, screening, preventive, and rehabilitative services (e.g., physical therapy)
Emergency department care
Eyeglasses and eye refractions
Hospice care
Intermediate care
Occupational therapy
Optometric services
Podiatric care
Prescription drugs
Private duty nursing
Prosthetic devices
Psychiatric care
Respiratory care
Speech therapy

in your state, write or telephone your state agency (see Appendix A).

Medicaid Managed Care

As early as 1967, some states began bringing managed care to their Medicaid programs. In the past decade, many states have adopted pilot projects to see whether a managed care system will work and what benefits might be received. Mainly this has been done as an effort to control escalating health care costs by curbing unnecessary emergency department visits and emphasizing preventive care.

When the last state, Arizona, joined Medicaid, it began with prepaid care rather than the way most states have structured their programs. By then,

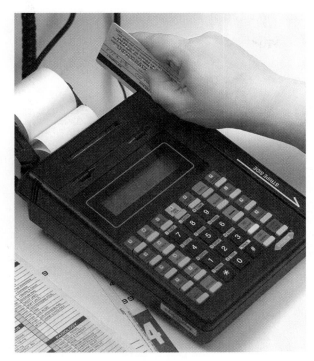

Figure 12–4. An insurance biller using a special machine to check a patient's Medicaid eligibility.

most states had been struggling with Medicaid for nearly 20 years. In these systems the Medicaid recipient enrolls either in an existing or specifically formed plan similar to a health maintenance organization (HMO). Some plans are run by independent commissions appointed by county boards of supervisors. Usually the patient can either choose or be assigned a gatekeeper (primary care physician), who must approve all specialty care and inpatient or outpatient hospital treatment. Patients must use physicians, clinics, and hospitals participating in their assigned plan.

Patients can be cared for side by side with private-paying patients. Some states have adopted capitated (a flat fee per patient) rather than fee-for-service reimbursement. There may be a small copayment for services. In programs run for a number of years, it has been found that if they are well managed, there is better access to primary health care and savings of monies in delivering the care.

Claim Procedure

Medicaid policies and claim procedures regarding identification cards, prior approval regulations, claim forms, and time limits vary from state to state. General guidelines for submitting claims are stated here.

For specific state guidelines, consult your current Medicaid Handbook and/or state fiscal agent. See Appendix A for the name and address in your region.

Claim procedures and information on the Medi-Cal program are presented in Appendix C for those working as an insurance billing specialist for a clinic or physician's practice in California.

Copayment

There are two types of copayment requirements that may apply to your state. Some states require a small fixed copayment paid to the provider at the time services are rendered. This policy was instituted to help pay some of the administrative costs of physicians participating in the Medicaid program.

Another requirement is the *share of cost* copayment. Some Medicaid recipients must meet this copayment requirement each month before Medicaid benefits can be claimed. The amount may change from month to month so be sure and verify it each time it is collected. It is important to obtain this copay amount when the patient comes in for medical care and report on the claim form that it has been collected.

Prior Approval

Many times **prior approval** is required for various services, except in a bona fide emergency. Some of these services might be

- durable medical equipment
- hearing aids
- hemodialysis
- home health care
- inpatient hospital care
- long-term care facility services
- medical supplies
- medications
- prosthetic/orthotic appliances
- surgical procedures
- transportation
- some vision care

Usually, prior authorization forms are completed to obtain permission for a specific service or hospitalization (Fig. 12–5) and mailed or faxed to the Department of Health or a certain office in your region for approval. In some cases, time does not allow for a written request to be sent for prior approval so an immediate authorization can be obtained via a telephone call to the proper department in your locale. Note the date and time the authorization was given, the name of the person who gave authorization, and any verbal number given to you by the field office. Usually a treat-

STATE USE ONLY

SERVICE CATEGORY

CONFIDENTIAL   PATIENT INFORMATION
FOR F.I. USE ONLY

F.I. USE ONLY
40 ☐ 41 ☐
42 ☐ 43 ☐

TYPEWRITER ALIGNMENT Elite Pica

CCN

TREATMENT AUTHORIZATION REQUEST
STATE OF CALIFORNIA DEPARTMENT OF HEALTH SERVICES

TYPEWRITER ALIGNMENT Elite Pica

(PLEASE TYPE)   FOR PROVIDER USE   (PLEASE TYPE)

VERBAL CONTROL NO.

TYPE OF SERVICE REQUESTED
☐ DRUG ☒ OTHER

REQUEST IS RETROACTIVE?
☐ YES ☒ NO

IS PATIENT MEDICARE ELIGIBLE?
☐ YES ☒ NO

PROVIDER PHONE NO.
(013) 555-1111
AREA

PATIENT'S AUTHORIZED REPRESENTATIVE (IF ANY)
ENTER NAME AND ADDRESS
•
•
•
•

PROVIDER NAME AND ADDRESS

PROVIDER NO.
HSC12345F

PLEASE TYPE YOUR NAME AND ADDRESS HERE

SMITH, SUSAN MD
727 ELM BLVD
ANYTOWN, CA 90101

30 83

FOR STATE USE

33   PROVIDER; YOUR REQUEST IS:

1 ☒ APPROVED AS REQUESTED   ☐   ☐ DEFERRED

2 ☐ APPROVED AS MODIFIED (ITEMS MARKED BELOW AS AUTHORIZED MAY BE CLAIMED)   ☐ JACKSON VS RANK PARAGRAPH CODE

BY _John Doe_
MEDICAL CONSULTANT

REVIEW COMMENTS INDICATOR

I.D. #   DATE
34 |0|1| 35 |0|8|2|0|X|X| 44 ☐

NAME AND ADDRESS OF PATIENT

PATIENT NAME (LAST, FIRST, M. I.)
APPLEGATE, NANCY

MEDICAL IDENTIFICATION NO.
253971060   CD CHECK ☐

STREET ADDRESS
1515 RIVER ROAD

SEX AGE DATE OF BIRTH
F   32   06 18 65

CITY, STATE, ZIP CODE
SACRAMENTO, CA 95822

☒ HOME ☐ BOARD AND CARE

PHONE NUMBER
(013) 545-1123

PATIENT STATUS: ☐ SNF/ICF ☐ ACUTE HOSPITAL

COMMENTS/ EXPLANATION
_____
_____
_____
_____
_____
_____

DIAGNOSIS DESCRIPTION:
ENDOMETRIOSIS

ICD-9-CM DIAGNOSIS CODE
617.9

MEDICAL JUSTIFICATION:
VISTA HOSPITAL - 1200 MAPLE ST., ANYTOWN, CA

UNCONTROLLABLE ENDOMETRIOSIS

RETROACTIVE AUTHORIZATION GRANTED IN ACCORDANCE WITH SECTION 51003 (B)
36 ☐1 ☐2 ☐3 ☐4 ☐5 ☐6

	AUTHORIZED YES NO	APPROVED UNITS	SPECIFIC SERVICES REQUESTED	UNITS OF SERVICE	PROCEDURE OR DRUG CODE	QUANTITY	CHARGES
1	9 ☒ ☐	10 _3_	DAYS: 3 HOSPITAL DAYS REQUESTED		11	12	$
2	13 ☒ ☐	14 _1_	HYSTERECTOMY	1	15 5815070	16 1	$ $1300.00
3	17 ☐ ☐	18			19	20	$
4	21 ☐ ☐	22			23	24	$
5	25 ☐ ☐	26			27	28	$
6	29 ☐ ☐	30			31	32	$

TO THE BEST OF MY KNOWLEDGE, THE ABOVE INFORMATION IS TRUE, ACCURATE AND COMPLETE AND THE REQUESTED SERVICES ARE MEDICALLY INDICATED AND NECESSARY TO THE HEALTH OF THE PATIENT.

Susan Smith   _MD_   _8-10-XX_
SIGNATURE OF PHYSICIAN OR PROVIDER   TITLE   DATE

AUTHORIZATION IS VALID FOR SERVICES PROVIDED

37 FROM DATE   38 TO DATE
|0|9|0|1|X|X| |0|9|3|0|X|X|

TAR CONTROL NUMBER

36 OFFICE
12

SEQUENCE NUMBER
61240229

PI
0

NOTE: AUTHORIZATION DOES NOT GUARANTEE PAYMENT. PAYMENT IS SUBJECT TO PATIENT'S ELIGIBILITY. BE SURE THE IDENTIFICATION CARD IS CURRENT BEFORE RENDERING SERVICE.   SEND TO FIELD SERVICES (F.I. COPY)

SEE YOUR PROVIDER MANUAL FOR ASSISTANCE REGARDING THE COMPLETION OF THIS FORM.
50-1 12/87

Figure 12–5. Example of a completed prior authorization form.

ment authorization form indicating that the service was already authorized must be sent in as follow-up to the telephone call.

Time Limit

Each state has its own time limit for the submission of a claim. The time limit can vary from 2 months to 1 year from the date that the service was rendered. If a bill is submitted after the time limit, it can be rejected, unless there is some valid justification that the state recognizes. Some states have separate procedures for billing Over One Year (OOY) claims. A percent of the claim may be reduced according to the date of a delinquent submission. Prescription drugs and dental services are often billed to a different intermediary than services performed by a physician, depending on the state guidelines.

Reciprocity

Most states have reciprocity for Medicaid payments if a patient requires medical care while out of state. Contact the Medicaid intermediary in the patient's home state and ask for the appropriate forms. If the case was an emergency, state this on the form. File the papers with Medicaid in the patient's home state. Reimbursement will be at that state's rate.

Claim Form

As of October 1, 1986, federal law mandates that the HCFA-1500 Insurance Claim Form be adopted for the processing of Medicaid claims in all states that do not optically scan their claims for payment. States that use optical scanners must adopt a form that is as close as possible to the format of Form HCFA-1500.

Physicians either submit a claim form to a **fiscal agent,** which might be an insurance company, or the bill is sent directly to the local Department of Social Services (Fig. 12–6). Refer to Appendix A for the Medicaid fiscal agent's address for your state.

In Chapter 6, there are general instructions for block by block entries on how to complete the HCFA-1500 claim form for the Medicaid program. Because guidelines for completing the form vary among all Medicaid intermediaries, refer to your local Medicaid intermediary for their directions. Figure 6–77 is a template emphasizing placement of basic elements on the claim form and shaded blocks that do not require completion.

To keep up-to-date, always read the current bulletins or newsletters on the Medicaid or Medi-Cal program published by the fiscal agent in your state. Obtain your state published handbook with updates

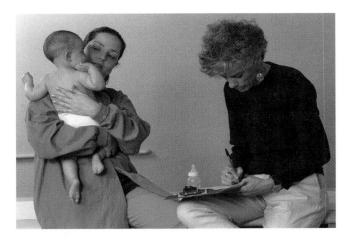

Figure 12–6. A physician with a child interacting with an insurance biller.

of its Medicaid rules. Read and implement the rule changes and updates to avoid rejected claims.

Medicaid Managed Care

When filing a claim for a Medicaid managed care patient, send the bill to the managed care organization (MCO) and not the Medicaid fiscal agent. The MCO receives payment for services rendered to eligible members via the capitation method.

Maternal and Child Health Program

Each jurisdiction operates its own MCHP with its own unique administrative characteristics. Thus, each has its own system and forms for billing and related procedures. The official plans and documents are retained in the individual state offices and are not available on either a regional or national office basis. For specific information about your state's policies, write to the MCHP state agency listed in Appendix A.

Medicaid and Other Plans

When Medicaid and a third party payer cover the patient, Medicaid is always considered the payer of last resort. The third party payer is billed first.

Government Programs and Medicaid

When a Medicaid patient has Medicare (referred to as a Medi-Medi case), TRICARE, or CHAMPVA, always send the insurance claim first to the federal program fiscal agent servicing your region. Then bill Medicaid second and attach to the claim form the remittance advice/explanation of benefits

(RA/EOB) that has been received from the federal program. Only send in a claim if the other coverage denies payment, pays less than the Medicaid fee schedule, or if Medicaid covers services not covered by the other policy.

Electronic claims may be automatically crossed over from primary government programs. Chapter 11 gives additional information on Medi-Medi claim submission. In Chapter 6, Figure 6–10 is a template emphasizing placement of basic elements on the claim form and shaded blocks that do not require completion for a Medi-Medi claim. Chapter 13 gives further information on patients who receive benefits from TRICARE and CHAMPVA.

Group Health Insurance and Medicaid

It is possible that a person can be eligible for Medicaid and also have group health insurance coverage through an employer. If any entity is liable to pay all or part of the medical cost of injury, disease, or disability, this is called third party liability. In these cases, the primary carrier is the other program or insurance carrier and they are sent the claim first. After receiving an RA/EOB from the primary carrier, Medicaid, being the secondary carrier, is billed enclosing a copy of the RA/EOB.

Medicaid and Aliens

Some aliens may have Medicare Part A or Part B or both (see Chapter 11, Aliens). If an alien is older than 65 years and on Medicaid (Medi-Cal in California) and not eligible for Medicare benefits, bill the Medicaid processing agent and use the proper Medicaid claim form for your region. On the HCFA-1500 claim form in Block 19 indicate, "Alien is older than 65 years and not eligible for Medicare benefits."

After Claim Submission

Remittance Advice

A remittance advice (RA), formerly known as an explanation of benefits (EOB) form, accompanies all Medicaid payment checks sent to the physician. Sometimes five categories of adjudicated claims appear on an RA—adjustments, approvals, denials, suspends, and audit/refund (A/R) transactions—although this terminology may vary from one fiscal agent to another (Fig. 12–7).

Adjustments occur from overpayments or underpayments. Approval is when an original claim or a previously denied claim is approved for payment. Denied claims are listed with a reason code on the RA. Claims in suspense for a certain period

of time may be listed on the RA. A/R transactions are miscellaneous transactions as a result of cost settlements, state audits, or refund checks received. An RA for a Medicare/Medicaid case may be found in Chapter 11, Figure 11–19A and B.

Appeals

The time limit to appeal a claim varies from state to state, but it is usually 30 to 60 days. Most Medicaid offices consider an appeal filed when they receive it, not when you send it. Usually appeals are sent on a special form or with a cover letter along with photocopies of documents applicable to the appeal (i.e., claim form, remittance advice, preauthorization forms). Appeals go first to the regional fiscal agent or Medicaid bureau, next to the Department of Welfare, and then to an appellate court that evaluates decisions by local and government agencies. At each level, an examiner looks at the case and makes a decision. If not satisfied, the physician may ask for further review at the next level.

Medicaid Fraud Control

Each state has a Medicaid Fraud Control Unit (MFCU), which is a federally funded state law enforcement entity usually located in the state Attorney General's office. The MFCU investigates and prosecutes cases of fraud and other violations, including complaints of mistreatment in long-term care facilities. The state Medicaid agency must cooperate and ensure access to records by the MFCU and agree to refer suspected cases of provider fraud to this division of the Attorney General's office for investigation.

RESOURCES ON THE INTERNET

 Many states have Medicaid web sites. Get the Internet address for your state by contacting your local Medicaid office. To compare state-to-state Medicaid programs and to obtain general data, contact the Health Care Financing Administration's web site at **http://www.hcfa.gov/Medicaid/medicaid.htm.**

STUDENT ASSIGNMENT LIST

✔ Study Chapter 12.
✔ Answer the review questions in the *Workbook* to reinforce the theory learned in this chapter and to help prepare you for a future test.

MEDICAID REMITTANCE ADVICE

TO: ANYBODY, FERNANDO G.
1000 ELM STREET
ANYTOWN, XY 12345-0001

REFER TO PROVIDER MANUAL FOR DEFINITION OF RAD CODES

PROVIDER NUMBER 00AX65800	CLAIM TYPE MEDICAL	WARRANT NO 39248026	EDS SEQ NO 20000617	DATE 06/01/20XX	PAGE 1 of 1 pages

RECIPIENT NAME	RECIPIENT MEDICAID I.D. NO.	CLAIM CONTROL NUMBER	SERVICE DATES FROM MMDDYY	TO MMDDYY	PROCED CODE MODIFIER	PATIENT ACCOUNT NUMBER	QTY	BILLED AMT	PAYABLE AMT		PAID AMT	RAD CODE
APPROVES (RECONCILE TO FINANCIAL SUMMARY)												
TORRES R	559978557	5079350917901	030720XX	030720XX	Z4802		0001	20.00	16.22		16.22	0401
		5079350917901	030720XX	030720XX	Z4802		0001	20.00	16.22		16.22	0401
						TOTAL		40.00	32.44		32.44	
CHAN B	561198435	5044351314501	020320XX	020320XX	Z4800		0001	30.00	27.03		27.03	0401
		5044351314501	020320XX	020320XX	Z4800		0001	20.00	16.22		16.22	0401
						TOTAL		50.00	43.25		43.25	
		TOTALS FOR APPROVES						90.00	75.69		75.69	
											75.69	AMT PAID
DENIES (DO NOT RECONCILE TO FINANCIAL SUMMARY)												
GOMEZ M	624163192	501134031900	122720XX	122720XX	Z4800		0001	30.00				0036
		TOTAL NUMBER OF DENIES					0001					
SUSPENDS (DO NOT RECONCILE TO FINANCIAL SUMMARY)												
HERN D	562416373	5034270703001	010520XX	010520XX	Z4800		0001	20.00				0602
MART E	623105478	5034270712305	010520XX	010520XX	Z4800		0001	20.00				0602
		5034270712305	010520XX	010520XX	Z4800		0001	20.00				0602
						TOTAL		40.00				0602
LOPEZ C	560291467	5034270712502	012420XX	012420XX	Z4800		0001	20.00				0602
		PAT LIAB 932.00 OTH COVG			0.00	SALES TX		0.00				
		TOTAL NUMBER OF SUSPENDS					0004	80.00				

EXPLANATION OF DENIAL/ADJUSTMENT CODES

0401 PAYMENT ADJUSTED TO MAXIMUM ALLOWABLE
0036 RESUBMISSION TURNAROUND DOCUMENT WAS EITHER NOT RETURNED OR WAS RETURNED UNCORRECTED, THEREFOR YOUR CLAIM IS FORMALLY DENIED
0602 PENDING ADJUDICATION
        OHC CARRIER NAME AND ADDRESS
N049 NORTHWESTERN NATIONAL LIFE   111 WASHINGTON AVE. FL 3   MINNEAPOLIS MN 55401

Figure 12–7. Example of a Medicaid Remittance Advice form showing adjustments, cutbacks, denied claims, and claims in suspense.

✔ Complete the assignments in the *Workbook* to give you hands-on experience in abstracting from case histories, posting to ledger cards, and completing forms pertinent to the Medicaid program in your state. Note: For students in California, study Appendix C, Medi-Cal. Complete the assignments in the *Workbook* for Chapter 12 and apply the knowledge learned from Appendix C.

✔ Turn to the Glossary at the end of this textbook for a further understanding of the Key Terms used in this chapter

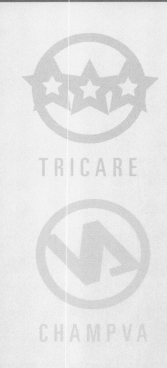

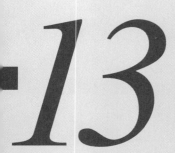

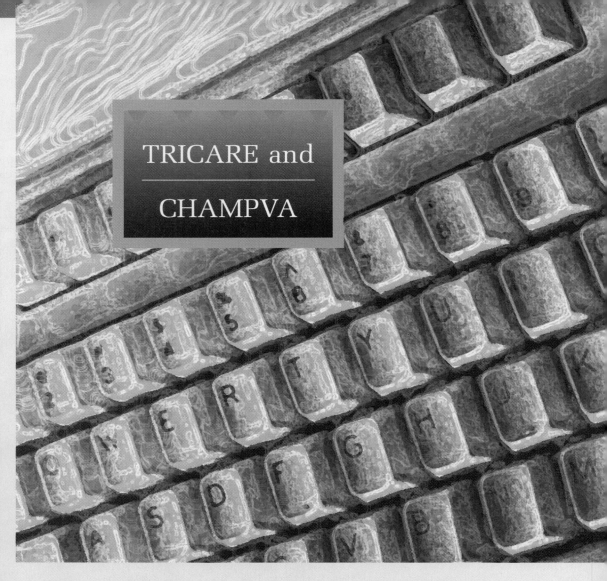

TRICARE and CHAMPVA

13

CHAPTER OUTLINE

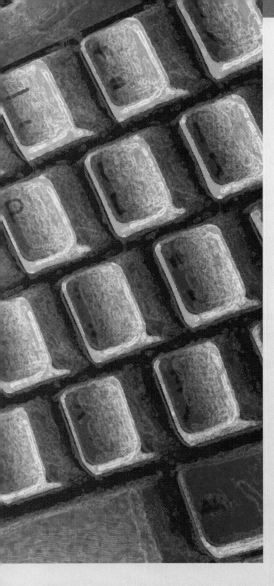

OBJECTIVES*

After reading this chapter you
should be able to:

■ State who is eligible for
TRICARE and CHAMPVA.
■ Define pertinent TRICARE
and CHAMPVA terminol-
ogy and abbreviations.
■ Enumerate the differences
between TRICARE prime
and extra and the TRICARE
standard program.
■ Identify the difference between the TRICARE pro-
gram and CHAMPVA.
■ Explain the benefits and
nonbenefits of these government programs.
■ Name various forms used
with these federal health
care programs.
■ List the circumstances
when a nonavailability
statement is required.
■ Describe how to process
claims for individuals who
are covered by TRICARE
and CHAMPVA.

KEY TERMS

**active duty service
member (ADSM)**

allowable charge

authorized provider

beneficiaries

catastrophic cap

CHAMPVA

cooperative care

coordination of benefits

cost-share

**Defense Enrollment
Eligibility Reporting
System (DEERS)**

emergency

fiscal intermediary (FI)

**health benefits advisor
(HBA)**

**Health Care Finder
(HCF)**

**medically (or
psychologically) necessary**

**military treatment facility
(MTF)**

**Nonavailability Statement
(NAS)**

**nonparticipating provider
(nonpar)**

**other health insurance
(OHI)**

participating provider (par)

partnership program

**point-of-service (POS)
option**

preauthorization

**primary care manager
(PCM)**

continued

---

*Performance objectives and exercises for hands-on practical experience for this chapter
appear in the *Workbook*.

History of TRICARE

The U.S. Congress created CHAMPUS in 1966 under Public Law 89-614 because individuals in the military were finding it increasingly more difficult to pay for the medical care required by their families. CHAMPUS was the acronym for *Civilian Health and Medical Program of the Uniformed Services*, which was a congressionally funded comprehensive health benefits program. Beginning in 1988, to control escalating medical costs and to standardize benefits for active duty families, military retirees, and their dependents, CHAMPUS beneficiaries had a choice of either retaining their benefits under CHAMPUS or enrolling in a managed care plan called CHAMPUS Prime. Then in January 1994, TRICARE became the new title for CHAMPUS. Under TRICARE, individuals have three choices to obtain health care:

▶ TRICARE Standard (fee-for-service cost-sharing type of option)
▶ TRICARE Extra (preferred provider organization type of option)
▶ TRICARE Prime (health maintenance organization type of option)

TRICARE Programs

Eligibility

Those who are entitled to medical benefits under TRICARE are
▶ Eligible family members of active duty service members
▶ Military retirees and their eligible family members
▶ Surviving eligible family members of deceased active or retired service members
▶ Wards and preadoptive children
▶ Former spouses of active or retired service members who meet certain length-of-marriage rules and other requirements
▶ Family members of active duty service members who were court-martialed and separated for spouse or child abuse
▶ Abused spouses, former spouses, or dependent children of service members who were retirement-eligible but lost that eligibility as a result of abuse of the spouse or child
▶ Spouses and children of North Atlantic Treaty Organization (NATO) nation representatives, under certain circumstances
▶ Families of activated reservists and National Guard members if military sponsor's active duty orders are for 30 consecutive days or an indefinite period
▶ Disabled beneficiaries younger than 65 years of age who have Medicare parts A and B and qualify under one of the aforementioned categories

Those *not* eligible for TRICARE are

▶ Medicare-eligible beneficiaries (except active duty dependents older than age 65 and those with end-stage renal disease)
▶ CHAMPVA beneficiaries

Individuals who qualify for TRICARE are known as **beneficiaries,** and the active duty service member is called the **sponsor.**

A person who is retired from a career in the armed forces is known as a **service retiree** or **military retiree** and remains in a TRICARE program until age 65, at which time the individual becomes eligible for the Medicare program. In the event that an active duty military person served from 4 to 6 years and then chose to leave the armed services, thereby giving up a military career, no further family benefits are provided.

Defense Enrollment Eligibility Reporting System

All TRICARE-eligible persons must be enrolled in the **Defense Enrollment Eligibility Reporting System (DEERS)** computerized database. TRICARE claims processors check DEERS before processing claims to verify beneficiary eligibility. A TRICARE beneficiary may check his or her status by contacting the nearest personnel office of any branch of the service or by calling the toll-free number of the DEERS center.

Nonavailability Statement

A **Nonavailability Statement (NAS)** is a certification from a military hospital stating that it cannot provide the care needed (Fig. 13–1). This type of certification is required for all TRICARE and CHAMPVA beneficiaries who wish to receive treatment as *inpatients* at a civilian hospital and who live within a catchment area surrounding a **military treatment facility (MTF)**. An MTF is a uniformed services hospital sometimes referred to as military hospital, formerly called a U.S. Public Health Service (USPHS) hospital. If this certification is not obtained, TRICARE may not pay. An NAS is no longer required for an outpatient procedure.

An NAS is not needed for inpatient care in the following situations:

1. In a medical emergency when delay could cause death or serious threat to health.
2. When the patient has other non-TRICARE major medical insurance that pays first on the bills for TRICARE covered care (i.e., when TRICARE is second pay).
3. When the person is a TRICARE beneficiary and lives within the service area of a uniformed hospital.
4. When maternity care and birthing services are at a TRICARE Standard-authorized birthing center or a hospital-based birthing room.
5. When inpatient services are needed in substance use disorder rehabilitation facilities, skilled nursing facilities, student infirmaries, and residential treatment centers.

Catchment Area

The catchment area is defined by ZIP codes and is based on an area of approximately 40 miles in radius surrounding each U.S. MTF. Individuals whose home address ZIP code falls outside the local military hospital's service area do not need an NAS before they seek civilian health care under TRICARE.

Automated NAS System

Since October 1, 1991, the NAS system has been automated. This means that instead of a paper copy of the NAS being sent in with the TRICARE or CHAMPVA claim, the uniformed service medical facility enters the NAS electronically into the DEERS (Defense Enrollment Eligibility Reporting System) computer files. Always ask the patient if he or she is enrolled in DEERS. Electronically filed statements are the only ones accepted for processing claims. A hard (paper) copy of DD Form 1251 may be printed if the patient needs one to show the hospital or physician.

TRICARE Standard

Enrollment

Those entitled to medical benefits under TRICARE are automatically enrolled in the TRICARE Standard program.

Identification Card

All dependents 10 years of age or older are required to have a Uniformed Services (military) identification and privilege card for TRICARE Standard. Dependents and survivors of active duty personnel and retirees carry a military identification card DD Form 1173 (Fig. 13–2). Dependents younger than 10 years of age are not normally issued Uniformed Services identification cards; information for their claims should be provided from either parent's card. Refer to the back of the card under "medical" to ensure that the card authorizes civilian medical benefits. Essential information must be abstracted from the front and back of the card, so photocopy both sides to retain in the patient's medical record.

Benefits

In the TRICARE Standard program, beneficiaries may receive a wide range of civilian health care services, with a significant portion of the cost paid

NONAVAILABILITY STATEMENT DEPENDENTS MEDICAL CARE PROGRAM

(AR 40-121, SECNAV INST 6320.8A, AFR 160-41, PHS GEN CIR NO 6)

(This Statement is Issued for your Immediate use)

THE ISSUANCE OF THIS STATEMENT MEANS:

1. The medical care requested is not available to you at a Uniformed Services facility in this area.
2. If you receive medical care from civilian sources and such care is determined to be authorized care under the Medicare Program, it will be paid for by the Government to the extent that the program permits.
3. If you receive medical care from civilian sources and it is determined that all or part of the care is not authorized under the Medicare Program, THE GOVERNMENT WILL NOT PAY for the unauthorized care.

The determination of whether medical care you may receive from civilian sources is authorized for payment cannot be made at this time because this determination depends, among other things, upon the care you actually receive, Further, no statement regarding your condition or diagnosis made hereon will be considered in any way determinative as to whether care rendered for such condition is payable under the Medicare Program.

The use of this statement is subject to the conditions and limitations set forth in the regulation issued under the Dependents' Medical Care Act as codified in 10 U.S.C. 1071-1085.

This form must be presented with your Uniformed Services Identification and Privilege Card (DD Form 1173), identified below, when you obtain civilian medical care.

DEPENDENT, SPOUSE OR CHILD, RESIDING WITH SPONSOR

DEPENDENT'S LAST NAME - FIRST NAME - MIDDLE INITIAL	UNIFORMED SERVICES IDENTIFICATION AND PRIVILEGE CARD (DD FORM II73)			
	CARD NUMBER			EXPIRATION DATE
	PREFIX	NUMERICAL	SUFFIX	
DOE, MARY B.	EU	18352	A	20XX JUNE 15

DEPENDENT'S ADDRESS (Complete mailing address)

503 CORN DRIVE, WOODLAND HILLS, XY 12345-0002

SPONSOR MEMBER OF UNIFORMED SERVICES ON ACTIVE DUTY

SPONSOR'S LAST NAME - FIRST NAME - MIDDLE INITIAL	BRANCH OF SERVICE
DOE, JOHN B.	☐ ARMY ☒ NAVY ☐ AIR FORCE

SERVICE NUMBER	GRADE OR RANK	
000-00-0001	LT/03	☐ MARINE CORPS ☐ PUBLIC HEALTH
		☐ COAST GUARD ☐ COAST & GEODETIC SURVEY

ORGANIZATION AND OFFICIAL DUTY STATION

POINT MUGU NAVAL STATION, POINT MUGU, CALIFORNIA

REMARKS

STATION AT WHICH PERMIT ISSUED	DATE ISSUED
POINT MUGU NAVAL STATION, POINT MUGU, CALIFORNIA	20XX MAY 12

GRADE OR RANK AND POSITION OF ISSUING OFFICER	SIGNATURE OF ISSUING OFFICER
COMMANDING OFFICER LT CMDR	*George M. Plates*

DISTRIBUTION *(Three signed copies of this statement will be furnished the dependent for distribution as follows):*

DEPENDENT *(Original Copy)*   ATTENDING PHYSICIAN *(Duplicate copy)*   CIVILIAN MEDICAL FACILITY *(Triplicate copy)*

Figure 13–1. TRICARE Nonavailability Statement DD Form 1251 for inpatient care rendered in a nonmilitary hospital.

Front of card

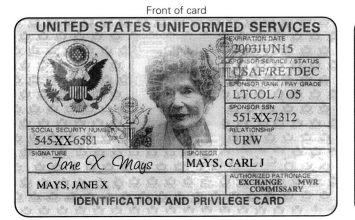

Back of card

Figure 13-2. Sample TRICARE Standard family member dependent's identification card, DD Form 1173, from which essential information must be abstracted. Dependents younger than 10 years of age are not normally issued identification cards; information on their claims should reflect information from either parent's card. This type of card has been issued since 1994.

by the federal government. Patients are not limited to using network providers, and benefits include medical or psychological services or supplies that are considered appropriate care. Such services are generally accepted by qualified professionals to be reasonable and adequate for the diagnosis and treatment of illness, injury, pregnancy, and mental disorders, or that are reasonable and adequate for well-baby care. These services are referred to as **medically (or psychologically) necessary.**

Beneficiaries may also receive urgent care and emergency care services. The differences between these two types of care are as follows. **Urgent care** is medically necessary treatment that is required for an immediate illness or injury that would not result in further disability or death if not treated *immediately.* Treatment should not be delayed but should occur within 24 hours to avoid development of further complications. An **emergency** is a sudden and unexpected medical condition, or the worsening of a condition, which poses a threat to life, losing a limb, or sight and requires immediate treatment to alleviate suffering (e.g., shortness of breath, chest pain, drug overdose). It is usually obtained at a hospital emergency department.

Ordinarily TRICARE Standard patients seek care from a military hospital near their home. If the service hospital that is managing the TRICARE Standard patient cannot provide a particular service or medical supplies, the military physician may refer the patient to a civilian source. These services or supplies may be cost-shared by TRICARE Standard under certain conditions, and this is known as **cooperative care.**

Another option that lets TRICARE Standard-eligible persons receive inpatient or outpatient treatment from civilian providers of care in a military hospital, or from uniformed services providers of care in civilian facilities, is called a **partnership program.** Whether a partnership program is instituted at a particular military hospital is up to the facility's commander, who makes the decision based on economics.

In addition, there are times when there is no service hospital in the area and a TRICARE Standard beneficiary may seek care through a private physician's office or hospital. Delivery of care through the private physician will be emphasized in this chapter.

To see the overall picture of TRICARE benefits, which includes cost-sharing (deductibles and copayments), read carefully through Figures 13-3 and 13-4.

Fiscal Year

The TRICARE fiscal year begins October 1 and ends September 30. It is different from most programs so office staff need to be alert when collecting deductibles.

Authorized Providers of Health Care

An **authorized provider** may treat a TRICARE Standard patient; these include:

Doctor of Medicine (MD)
Doctor of Osteopathy (DO or MD)
Doctor of Dental Surgery (DDS)
Doctor of Dental Medicine (DDM)
Doctor of Podiatric Medicine or Surgical Chiropody (DPM or DSC)
Doctor of Optometry (DO)
Psychologist (PhD)

BENEFITS AND COVERAGE CHART

Inpatient Services   **Beneficiary Cost**

SERVICES	TRICARE PRIME	TRICARE EXTRA	TRICARE STANDARD
HOSPITALIZATION++ Semiprivate room (and when medically necessary, special care units), general nursing, and hospital service. Includes inpatient physician and their surgical services, meals including special diets, drugs and medications while an inpatient, operating and recovery room, anesthesia, laboratory tests, x-rays and other radiology services, necessary medical supplies and appliances, blood and blood products.	+ Active Duty Family Members: No copayment. + Retirees and their Family Members and Survivors: No copayment for professional services. $75 per day to $750 maximum per admission.	+ Active Duty Family Members: No copayment. + Retirees and their Family Members and Survivors: copayment of $250 per day or 25% of plan allowable, whichever is less, plus 20% of separately billed professional charge at Plan allowable rate.	Active Duty Family Members: $25 copayment or $11.45*** per day whichever is higher. + Retirees and their Family Members and Survivors: copayment of $401*** per day or 25% of billed charges, whichever is less, plus 25% of TRICARE allowable for separately billed professional charges.
MATERNITY++ Hospital and professional services (prenatal, postnatal).			Active Duty Family Members: $25 copayment or $11.45*** per day, whichever is higher.
SKILLED NURSING FACILITY CARE Semiprivate room, regular nursing services, meals including special diets, physical, occupational and speech therapy, drugs furnished by the facility, necessary medical supplies, and appliances.			Retirees and their Family Members and Survivors: 25% of billed charges, plus 25% of TRICARE allowable for separately billed professional charges.
HOSPITALIZATION FOR MENTAL ILLNESS++ 18 and under, 45 days per year, 19 and older, 30 days per year as medically necessary. Up to 150 days for treatment in a Residential Treatment Center. The number of days may be subject to change pending new legislation.	+++ Active Duty Family Members: $20 copayment for civilian hospital. +++ Retirees and their Family Members and Survivors: copayment of $40 per day or 25% of Plan allowable, whichever is less.	+++ Active Duty Family Members: $20 copayment for civilian hospital. +++ Retirees and their Family Members and Survivors: copayment of $40 per day or 25% of Plan allowable, whichever is less, plus 20% of separately billed professional charge at Plan allowable rate.	Active Duty Family Members: $25 copayment or $11.45*** per day, whichever is higher. Retirees and their Family Members and Survivors: 25% of TRICARE allowable billed charges, plus 25% of TRICARE allowable for separately billed professional charges.
ALCOHOLISM++ 7 days for detoxification and 21 days for rehabilitation per 365 days. Maximum of one rehabilitation program per year and three per lifetime. Detoxification and rehabilitation days count toward 30-day limit for mental health benefits.			

*** This figure is for Fiscal Year 2001 and is subject to change each **October 1 at the beginning of each Fiscal Year.**
This is only a summary description of the coverage. See the TRICARE Standard Handbook and a TRICARE Prime Member Handbook for more complete description of all terms and conditions. In addition, TRICARE rregulations and the interpretations under those regulations are the final authority on covered services.
+   Unlimited, with authorization, as medically necessary.
++ NAS Note: The patient must obtain a Non-availability Statement if you live within a designated service area around a military hospital. This may be a restricted NAS requiring the patient to use TRICARE network providers.
+++ With authorization.
For Active Duty Family members, the maximum family liability (Catastrophic Cap Benefit) is $1000 for deductibles and cost-shares based on allowable charges for the Basic Program services and supplies recieved in a Fiscal Year. For all other beneficiary families, the Fiscal Year cap is $7,500. After a Fiscal Year cap is met, the TRICARE determined allowable amount shall be paid in full for all covered services and supplies under the Basic Program received through the end of that Fiscal Year. In order to get credit for all family expenditures allowed toward the Catstrophic Cap Benefit, the beneficiary may be required to submit appropriate documentation (e.g. TRICARE Explanation of Benefits).

Figure 13–3. TRICARE Prime, Extra, and Standard Inpatient Services Benefits and Coverage Chart.

BENEFITS AND COVERAGE CHART

Outpatient Services　　　　**Beneficiary Cost**

SERVICES	TRICARE PRIME*	TRICARE EXTRA**	TRICARE STANDARD**
ANNUAL DEDUCTIBLE** (10–1 to 9–30) (Applied to Outpatient Services)	None	$150/person or $300/ family per fiscal year.***	$150/person or $300/ family per fiscal year.***
PHYSICIAN SERVICES*+ Office visits; outpatient office-based medical and surgical care; consultation, diagnosis, and treatment by a specialist; allergy tests and treatment; osteopathic manipulation; medical supplies used within the office including casts, dressings and splints.	No copayment per visit.*	Active Duty Family Members: 15% of Plan allowable after deductible has been satisfied. Retirees and their Family Members and Survivors: 20% of Plan allowable after deductible has been satisfied.	Active Duty Family Members : 20% of TRI-CARE allowable after deductible has been satisfied. Retirees and their Family Members and Survivors: 25% of TRICARE allowable after deductible has been satisfied.
LABORATORY and X-RAY SERVICES (Including Mammograms)	$6 copayment. (No copayment if included in the office visit.)		
ROUTINE PAP SMEARS Frequency depends on physician recommendations based on the published guidelines of the American Academy of Obstetrics and Gynecology.	$6 copayment per visit. (No copayment if included in the office visit.)		
AMBULANCE SERVICES When medically necessary as currently defined and covered by OCHAMPUS.	$10, $15, or $20 copayment per occurrence, depending on pay grade.		
EMERGENCY SERVICES Outpatient, both in and out of service area for emergency and urgently needed care.	$10, $20, or $30 copayment, depending on pay grade use. $15 copayment for urgent care center use.		
DURABLE MEDICAL EQUIPMENT, PROSTHETIC DEVICES, AND MEDICAL SUPPLIES PRESCRIBED BY YOUR PHYSICIAN AND WHEN A CHAMPUS BENEFIT (If dispensed for use outside of the office or after the home visit.)	10%, 15%, or 20%, depending on pay grade.		
HOME HEALTH CARE Part-time skilled nursing care, physical, speech and occupational therapy as currently defined by OCHAMPUS (when medically necessary).	$6 or $12 copayment per visit, depending on pay grade.		
FAMILY HEALTH SERVICES Family planning and well-baby care (up to 24 months of age). Certain exclusions apply as currently defined by OCHAMPUS.	$6 or $12 copayment per visit, depending on pay grade.		
OUTPATIENT MENTAL HEALTH One hour of therapy no more than two times each week (when medically necessary). Outpatient Medication Management	$10 copayment for individual visits. $5 copayment for group visits. $5 copayment per visit		

*　No copayment for primary care or preventive services for family members of sponsors with pay grades of E-5 and below (both active duty and retired). The Fiscal Intermediary has the responsibility for defining primary care; some office visits are subject to copayment(s).

**　Please note that TRICARE Extra and TRICARE Standard annual deductibles and cost shares are subject to change.

***　Except for families whose Active Duty sponsor's pay grade is E-4 and below, for whom the annual deductible is $50/person or $100/family.

This is only a summary description of the coverage. See the TRICARE Standard Handbook and a TRICARE Prime Member Handbook for a more complete description of all terms and conditions. In addition, TRICARE regulations and interpretations under those regulations are the final authority on covered services.

\+　Certain outpatient procedures require a Nonavailability Statement (NAS). The patient must obtain an NAS when residing within a designated service area near a military treatment facility if the care is not available at the facility. This may be a restricted NAS requiring the patient to use TRICARE network providers.

Figure 13–4. TRICARE Prime, Extra, and Standard Outpatient Services Benefits and Coverage Chart.

(Illustration continued on following page)

BENEFITS AND COVERAGE CHART

Outpatient Services   **Beneficiary Cost**

SERVICES	TRICARE PRIME*	TRICARE EXTRA**	TRICARE STANDARD**
ANNUAL DEDUCTIBLE** (10–1 to 9–30) (Applied to Outpatient Services)	None	$150/person or $300/family per fiscal year.***	$150/person or $300/family per fiscal year.***
PARTIAL HOSPITALIZATION FOR ALCOHOLISM TREATMENT Up to 21 days for rehabilitative treatment on a limited hour-per-day basis. Does not count toward the mental health inpatient limit, but does count toward 60-day partial hospitalization limit.	Subject to inpatient mental health copayment.	Subject to inpatient mental health copayment.	Subject to inpatient mental health copayment.
PARTIAL HOSPITALIZATION FOR PSYCHIATRIC TREATMENT Limited to 60 treatment days (whether a full day or a partial day program) in a fiscal year or in an admission. Not counted toward the 30/45 day inpatient limit.	Subject to inpatient mental health copayment.	Subject to inpatient mental health copayment.	Subject to inpatient mental health copayment.
PERIODIC PHYSICAL EXAMINATIONS Conducted by Primary Care Managers for ages over 24 months. For well-baby care up to 24 months of age, see "Family Health Services."	Free	Not covered.	Not covered.
PHYSICAL, OCCUPATIONAL, SPEECH AND RADIATION THERAPY.	$5 copayment per visit.	Active Duty Family Members: 15% of Plan allowable after deductible has been satisfied. Retirees and their Family Members and Survivors: 20% of Plan allowable after deductible has been satisfied.	Active Duty Family Members: 20% of TRICARE allowable after deductible has been satisfied. Retirees and their Family Members and Survivors: 25% of TRICARE allowable after deductible has been satisfied.
WELLNESS CLASSES, COMMUNITY, HEALTH SERVICES AND COMMUNITY RESOURCE COORDINATION	No charge or minimal cost.	Not covered.	Not covered.

*   No copayment for primary care or preventive services for family members of sponsors with pay grades of E-4 and below (both active duty and retired). The Fiscal Intermediary has the responsibility for defining primary care; some office visits are subject to copayment(s).

**   Please note that TRICARE Extra and TRICARE Standard annual deductibles and cost shares are subject to change.

*** Except for families whose Active Duty sponsor's pay grade is E-4 and below, for whom the annual deductible is $50/person or $100/family.

This is only a summary description of the coverage. See the TRICARE Standard Handbook and a TRICARE Prime Member Handbook for a more complete description of all terms and conditions. In addition, TRICARE regulations and interpretations under those regulations are the final authority on covered services.

++   An outpatient Nonavailability Statement (NAS) may be required. Consult the Health Care Finder. This may be a restricted NAS requiring the patient to use TRICARE network providers.

+++ With authorization.

For Active Duty Family Members, the maximum family liability (Catastrophic Cap Benefit) is $1000 for deductibles and cost-shares based on allowable charges for the Basic Program services and supplies received in a Fiscal Year. For all other beneficiary families, the Fiscal Year cap is $7,500. After a Fiscal Year cap is met, the TRICARE-determined allowable amount shall be paid in full for all covered services and supplies under the Basic Program received through the end of that Fiscal Year. In order to get credit for all family expenditures allowed toward the catastrophic cap benefit, the beneficiary may be required to submit appropriate documentation (e.g., TRICARE Explanation of Benefits).

Figure 13–4. *Continued.* TRICARE, Prime, Extra, and Standard Outpatient Services Benefits and Coverage Chart.

BENEFITS AND COVERAGE CHART

Outpatient Services **Beneficiary Cost**

SERVICES	TRICARE PRIME*	TRICARE EXTRA**	TRICARE STANDARD**
ANNUAL DEDUCTIBLE** (10–1 to 9–30) (Applied to Outpatient Services)	None	$150/person or $300/ family per fiscal year.***	$150/person or $300/ family per fiscal year.***
PRESCRIPTION DRUGS No charge for prescriptions at the military treatment facility.	$5 copayment per Rx up to a 30-day supply for Active Duty Family Members. $9 copayment per Rx up to a 30-day supply for Retirees, their Family Members, and Survivors.	Active Duty Family Members: 15% of Plan allowable. Retirees and their Family Members and Survivors: 20% of Plan allowable. The deduction is waived for prescriptions at a network pharmacy.	Active Duty Family Members: 20% of TRICARE allowable after deductible has been satisfied. Retirees and their Family Members and Survivors: 25% of TRICARE allowable after deductible has been satisfied.
EYE EXAMS One routine examination per year.	Active Duty Family Members: $6 copayment E4 and below; $12 copayment, E5 and above. Retirees and their Family Members, and Survivors 18 years of age and over: Not covered.	Active Duty Family Members: 15% of Plan allowable after deductible has been satisfied. Retirees and their Family Members and Survivors: Not covered.	Active Duty Family Members: 20% of TRICARE allowable after deductible has been satisfied. Retirees and their Family Members and Survivors: Not covered.
AMBULATORY SURGERY (same day)++ Authorized hospital-based or freestanding ambulatory surgical center that is TRICARE Certified.	+++ Active Duty Family Members: $25 copayment. +++ Retirees and their Family Members and Survivors: $5 copayment for primary surgeon only.	+++ Active Duty Family Members: $25 copayment. +++ Retirees and their Family Members and Survivors: 20% of Plan allowable after deductible has been satisfied.	Active Duty Family Members: $25 copayment for hospital charges. Retirees and their Family Members and Survivors: 25% of billed charges after deductible has been satisfied.
IMMUNIZATIONS Pediatric and adult immunizations as recommended by the American Academy of Pediatrics for children and by the U.S. Public Health Service for adults. If immunizations are needed for overseas travel, it is recommended you contact the military hospital or clinic and/or Public Health Department.	$5 copayment per visit up to 24 months of age. (See Family Health Services.) $5 copayment per immunization for over 2 years old.	For official travel, PCS orders outside the U.S. only. Active Duty Family Members: 15% of Plan allowable after deductible has been satisfied. Retirees and their Family Members and Survivors: Not covered.	For official travel, PCS orders outside the U.S. only. Active Duty Family Members: 20% of TRICARE allowable after deductible has been satisfied. Retirees and their Family Members and Survivors: Not covered.

*   No copayment for primary care or preventive services for family members of sponsors with pay grades of E-4 and below (both active duty and retired). The Fiscal Intermediary has the responsibility for defining primary care; some office visits are subject to copayment(s).

** Please note that TRICARE Extra and TRICARE Standard annual deductibles and cost shares are subject to change.

*** Except for families whose Active Duty sponsor's pay grade is E-4 and below, for whom the annual deductible is $50/person or $100/family.

This is only a summary description of the coverage. See the TRICARE Standard Handbook and a TRICARE Prime Member Handbook for a more complete description of all terms and conditions. In addition, TRICARE regulations and interpretations under those regulations are the final authority on covered services.

++ An outpatient Nonavailability Statement (NAS) may be required. Consult the Health Care Finder. This may be a restricted NAS requiring the patient to use TRICARE network providers.

+++ With authorization.

For Active Duty Family Members, the maximum family liability (Catastrophic Cap Benefit) is $1000 for deductibles and cost-shares based on allowable charges for the Basic Program services and supplies received in a Fiscal Year. For all other beneficiary families, the Fiscal Year cap is $7,500. After a Fiscal Year cap is met, the TRICARE-determined allowable amount shall be paid in full for all covered services and supplies under the Basic Program received through the end of that Fiscal Year. In order to get credit for all family expenditures allowed toward the catastrophic cap benefit, the beneficiary may be required to submit appropriate documentation (e.g., TRICARE Explanation of Benefits).

Figure 13–4. *Continued*

Other authorized nonphysician providers include audiologists, certified nurse midwives, clinical social workers, licensed practical nurses, licensed vocational nurses, psychiatric social workers, registered nurses, registered physical therapists, and speech therapists.

Preauthorization

There are certain referral and **preauthorization** requirements for TRICARE Standard patients. When specialty care or hospitalization is required, the military treatment facility must be used if services are available. If services are not available, the **Health Care Finder (HCF)** will assist with the referral or preauthorization process. An HCF is a health care professional, usually a registered nurse, who helps the patient work with his or her primary care physician to locate a specialist or obtain a preauthorization for care. HCFs are found at a **TRICARE Service Center (TSC),** which is an office staffed by HCFs and beneficiary service representatives. All admissions, ambulatory surgical procedures, and other selected procedures require preauthorization. Certain types of health care services requiring prior approval from the TRICARE health contractor are:

▶ Arthroscopy
▶ Breast mass or tumor removal
▶ Cardiac catheterization
▶ Cataract removal
▶ Cystoscopy
▶ Dental care
▶ Dilatation and curettage
▶ Durable medical equipment purchases
▶ Gastrointestinal endoscopy
▶ Gynecologic laparoscopy
▶ Hernia repairs
▶ Laparoscopic cholecystectomy
▶ Ligation or transection of fallopian tubes
▶ Magnetic resonance imaging (MRI)
▶ Mental health care
▶ Myringotomy or tympanostomy
▶ Nose repair (rhinoplasty and septoplasty)
▶ Neuroplasty
▶ Strabismus repair
▶ Tonsillectomy or adenoidectomy

Payment

Deductible and Copayment

Deductibles and copayments are determined according to two groups: (1) active duty family members and (2) retirees, their family members, and survivors.

Spouses and Children of Active Duty Members

For inpatient (hospitalized) care, the beneficiary pays the first $25 of the hospital charge or a small fee for each day, whichever is greater, and TRICARE pays the remainder of the allowable charges for authorized care.

For outpatient (nonhospitalized) care, the beneficiary pays the first $150 (deductible) plus 20% of the charges over the $150 deductible. A family with two or more eligible beneficiaries pays a maximum of $300 (deductible) plus 20% of the charges in excess of $300. TRICARE pays the remainder of the allowable charges, which is 80%.

All Other Eligible Beneficiaries

This category includes retired members, dependents of retired members, dependents of deceased members who died in active duty, and so forth.

For inpatient (hospitalized) care, the beneficiary pays 25% of the hospital charges and fees of professional personnel. TRICARE pays the remaining allowable charges for authorized care, or 75%.

For outpatient (nonhospitalized) care, the beneficiary pays $150 (deductible) plus 25% of the charges over the $150 deductible. A family with two or more eligible beneficiaries pays a maximum of $300 plus 25% of the charges in excess of $300. TRICARE pays the remainder of the allowable charges for authorized care, which is 75%.

Refer to Figures 13–3 and 13–4 for further clarification and to see the differences in benefits between the three TRICARE program options.

Participating Provider

For a TRICARE Standard case, if the physician agrees to *accept assignment*, then the **participating provider (par)** agrees to accept the TRICARE-determined **allowable charge** as payment in full. Providers may choose to accept TRICARE assignment on a case-by-case basis. Always accept assignment in cases when the service member is transferring within 6 months because this will avoid collection problems. The provider may bill the patient for his or her **cost-share** or coinsurance (20% to 25% of the allowable charge after the deductible has been met) and for any noncovered services or supplies. The provider may not bill for the difference between the provider's usual charge and the allowable charge.

Beneficiaries pay only a certain amount each year for the cost-share and annual deductible. This amount is known as the **catastrophic cap.** After this cap is reached, TRICARE pays 100% of the allowable charges for the rest of the year. Attach a note to the claim when the patient has met the catastrophic cap, and this may help expedite claims processing and payment. After completing the claim and sending it to the fiscal intermediary, the payment will go directly to the physician.

Nonparticipating Provider

A health care provider who chooses not to participate in TRICARE is called a **nonparticipating provider (nonpar)** and, as of November 1, 1993, may not bill the patient more than 115% of the TRICARE allowable charge. For example, if the TRICARE allowable charge for a procedure is $100, providers who decide not to participate in

TRICARE may charge TRICARE patients no more than $115 for that procedure. When the physician does not accept assignment, the patient pays the deductible, 20% or 25% of the charges determined to be allowable, and any amount over the allowable charge up to 115%.

TRICARE Extra

Enrollment

TRICARE Extra is a preferred provider organization type of option in which the individual does not have to enroll or pay an annual fee. On a visit-by-visit basis, the individual may seek care from an authorized network provider and receive a discount on services and reduced cost-share (copayment). A nonenrolled beneficiary automatically becomes a TRICARE Extra beneficiary when care is rendered by a network provider. If a nonenrolled beneficiary receives care from a non-network provider, the services received are covered under TRICARE Standard. Providers receive a contract rate for giving care.

Identification Card

A TRICARE Extra beneficiary must present the military identification card when receiving care as proof of eligibility. The military identification card will indicate a "Yes" in Box 15B (back of card) if the beneficiary is eligible. Children younger than 10 years of age may use the sponsor's identification card (attach a copy of the child's card to the claim). Individuals older than age 10 years must have their own identification card. To verify eligibility, contact the local HCF. Active duty and retiree dependents and survivors carry an orange or brown military identification card (see Fig. 13–2). Retirees carry a blue-gray military identification card.

Benefits

See Figures 13–3 and 13–4 for outpatient and inpatient benefits and deductible and copayment amounts.

Network Provider

The network provider is the physician who provides medical care to TRICARE beneficiaries under the TRICARE Extra program at contracted rates.

Preauthorization

Referrals from other network providers are coordinated through the HCF. The network provider refers the beneficiary for additional services, when necessary, following precertification requirements and completing a referral form.

Payments

Deductible and Copayment

Deductibles and copayments are determined according to two groups: (1) active duty family members and (2) retirees, their family members, and survivors.

Spouses and Children of Active Duty Members

For inpatient (hospitalized) care, there is no copayment required.

For outpatient (nonhospitalized) care, the beneficiary pays the first $150 (deductible) plus 15% of the charges over the $150 deductible. A family with two or more eligible beneficiaries pays a maximum of $300 (deductible) plus 15% of the charges in excess of $300. TRICARE pays the remainder of the allowable charges, which is 85%.

All Other Eligible Beneficiaries

For inpatient (hospitalized) care, the copayment is $250 per day or 25% of the plan's allowable charges, whichever is less, plus 20% of separately billed professional charges at the plan's allowable rate.

For outpatient (nonhospitalized) care, the beneficiary pays $150 (deductible) plus 20% of the charges over the $150 deductible. A family with two or more eligible beneficiaries pays a maximum of $300 plus 20% of the charges in excess of $300. TRICARE pays the remainder of the allowable charges for authorized care, which is 80%.

See Figures 13–3 and 13–4 for further clarification of deductibles and copayments.

TRICARE Prime

TRICARE Prime is a voluntary health maintenance organization-type (HMO) option. Participation in TRICARE Prime is optional. Beneficiaries who are *not* enrolled as members in TRICARE Prime may continue to receive services through TRICARE Extra from network providers or through TRICARE Standard using non-network providers. Once enrolled in TRICARE Prime, the beneficiary may no longer use the TRICARE Standard program.

Enrollment

To become a TRICARE Prime member, an individual must complete an application and enroll for a minimum of 12 months. There is an annual enrollment fee charged per person or per family except for active duty families, who may enroll free. Active duty service members are enrolled automatically in TRICARE Prime and are not eligible for benefits under TRICARE Standard or TRICARE Extra. These members are able to use the local military and civilian provider network with necessary authorization.

Enrollees normally receive care from within the Prime network of civilian and military providers. The beneficiary has the option of choosing or being assigned a primary care manager (PCM) for each family member. The PCM manages all aspects of the patient's health care (except emergencies) including referrals to specialists. Enrolled beneficiaries may not use a non-network provider, except in emergencies or for pharmaceuticals, without a specific referral from an HCF.

Identification Card

Individuals who enroll are issued a TRICARE Prime identification card, as shown in Figure 13−5. This card does not guarantee TRICARE eligibility, so providers *must* check the TRICARE Uniformed Services military identification card for the effective and expiration dates or call the local HCF. Always make copies of the military identification card and the TRICARE Prime card and retain them in the patient's file. For TRICARE Prime patients, check both cards at *every* visit.

Benefits

Covered services are the same as those for TRICARE Standard patients plus additional preventive and primary care services. For example, periodic physical examinations are covered at no charge under TRICARE Prime but are not covered under TRICARE Extra or TRICARE Standard. Prime also covers certain immunizations and annual eye examinations for dependent children of retirees that are not a benefit under Extra or Standard. A dental plan is available for an additional monthly premium. An NAS is required for certain inpatient services if the beneficiary resides within the designated military treatment facility catchment area. See Figures 13−3 and 13−4 for outpatient and inpatient benefits and deductible and copayment amounts.

Primary Care Manager

The **primary care manager (PCM)** is a physician who is responsible for coordinating and managing all the beneficiary's health care unless there is an emergency. A provider who decides to participate in a managed care program goes through a credentialing process. This is done approximately every 2 years for all physicians who participate as providers. The PCM may refer the beneficiary for additional services, when necessary, but specific referral and preauthorization requirements must be carried out. Referral patterns are evaluated to determine excessive or inappropriate referrals to specialists. A pattern of such referrals could result in termination of participation in TRICARE Prime.

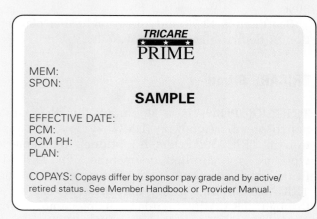

Figure 13−5. Sample TRICARE Prime Identification card (red, white, and blue in color).

Preauthorization

All admissions, ambulatory surgical procedures, and other selected procedures require preauthorization. Outpatient or ambulatory surgery must be on the approved procedure list before it is performed. The list is in the TRICARE Policy Manual available on the web site: *www.tricare-on@csdmail.med com.amedd.army.mil.*

An NAS may be needed for some types of surgery performed in approved ambulatory surgery centers or hospitals.

Call the **health benefits advisor (HBA)** at the nearest military medical facility to find out if an NAS statement is needed for the procedure before scheduling the surgery in the approved facility. An HBA is a person at a military hospital or clinic who is there to help beneficiaries obtain medical care needed through the military and through TRICARE. If no authorization is obtained, a **point-of-service (POS) option** is available. This means that the individual can choose to get TRICARE-covered nonemergency services outside the Prime network of providers without a referral from the PCM and without authorization from the HCF. If the POS option is used, there is an annual deductible and 50% cost-share.

Payments

Copayment

TRICARE Prime copayments vary for active duty family members and retirees and their family members and survivors for inpatient hospital services. For outpatient services, copayments are the same for active duty family members and retirees and their family members and survivors but vary in amounts depending on the type of service received. They should always be collected at the time services are rendered. Refer to Figures 13−3 and 13−4 for further clarification of copayments.

TRICARE Prime Remote Program

Enrollment

TRICARE Prime Remote (TPR) is a program designed for **active duty service members (ADSMs)** who work and live more than 50 miles or 1 hour from military treatment facilities (military hospitals and clinics). ADSMs must enroll for this program, which enables them to receive care from any civilian provider.

Family members of active duty service members in the TPR program are *not eligible* for TPR. They may enroll in TRICARE Prime or receive care through the TRICARE Standard and TRICARE Extra options.

Identification Card

Active duty service members must present their military identification card to receive care from providers (Fig. 13−6). Photocopy front and reverse sides of the card so information will be available for reference when completing the insurance claim form.

Benefits

TPR program benefits are similar to TRICARE Prime. Services may be received from an MTF

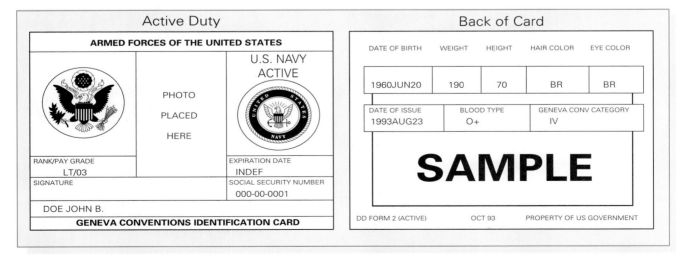

Figure 13−6. Sample military identification card for an active duty individual in the Armed Forces. It is used as the identification card for the TRICARE Remote Program and is considered a sponsor identification card.

when available or from any civilian provider. Primary routine care does not require prior authorization (e.g., office visits and preventive health care). The HCF must be contacted to receive authorization for referrals, inpatient admissions, maternity, physical therapy, orthotics, hearing appliances, family planning (tubal ligation/vasectomy), outpatient and inpatient behavioral health services, and transplants. See Figure 13−7 for a summary of the unique aspects of TPR.

Payments

Those covered and receiving benefits under TPR are not responsible for any out-of-pocket costs. Active duty service member claims for services

provided by a TRICARE network provider are paid at the same contracted rate as other TRICARE beneficiary claims.

Supplemental Health Care Program

Enrollment

The Supplemental Health Care Program (SHCP) covers both military treatment facility referred care as well as civilian health care provided to active duty service members. The military treatment facility always administers routine care (e.g., routine office visits and preventive health care).

	TRICARE Prime Remote (TPR)	Supplemental Health Care Program (SHCP)
Plan description	TPR is a program for Active Duty Service Members (ADSMs) who live and work more than 50 miles or one hour from a military treatment facility. ADSMs must enroll.	SHCP is a program for • Active Duty Service Members (ADSMs) • Inpatients at military treatment facilities who are not TRICARE eligible (e.g., eligible parents, parents-in-law) referred by an MTF to a civilian provider for care (usually for a specific test, procedure or consultation). • Non-MTF referred ADSMs (e.g., ROTC students, cadets/midshipmen, eligible foreign military).
Provider type	Any civilian provider.	Any civilian provider.
Beneficiary access to care	TPR ADSMs recieves services from any civilian provider, or from a military treatment facility when available. Under TPR, ADSMs will have the same priority to care as other ADSMs at the MTF.	The beneficiary may receive services from any civilian provider, in accordance with referral and preauthorization requirements, below.
Beneficiary responsibility	TPR ADSMs have no annual deductible, cost-shares or copayment. The TPR ADSM must present his/her Military ID card at the time care is received.	ADSMs and others, eligible for SHCP referred to civilian providers have no copayment, deductible, or cost share. Beneficiary must present his/her Military ID card at the time care is recieved.
Point-of-Service (POS)	Point-of-Service does not apply. If the ADSM receives care without a referral or preauthorization, the claim will be processed if it meets all other TRICARE requirements on a case-by-case basis.	The Point-of-Service option does not apply.
Program benefits	Offers benefits similar to TRICARE Prime. Some benefits (including all behavioral health care) require preauthorization.	Offers benefits similar to TRICARE Prime. Some benefits (including all behavioral health care) require preauthorization.
Referrals and preauthorizations	Primary care − ADSMs can receive primary care from a provider without a referral or preauthorization. ADSMs with an assigned PCM will receive primary care from their PCM. ADSMs with no PCM can use any TRICARE-certified provider. Or, he/she can contact a HCF for assistance in locating a provider. Specialty and inpatient care − The SPOC will review requests for specialty and inpatient care.	Specialty and inpatient care − The MTF will review all requests for specialty and inpatient care for ADSMs. **The MTF Commander or designee signature on a DD Form 2161** is required for designated patients **referred** for civilian care. Preauthorization for **non-referred** Active Duty Service Members for specialty, inpatient, and behavioral health care must be **obtained from the SPOC or the Health Care Finder.**

Figure 13−7. Summary of unique aspects of TRICARE Remote Program and Supplemental Health Care Program.

Identification Card

Active duty service members must present their military identification card to receive care from providers (see Fig. 13–6). Photocopy front and reverse sides of the card so information will be available for reference when completing the insurance claim form.

Benefits

See Figure 13–7 for a summary of the unique aspects of SHCP.

SHCP enables beneficiaries to be referred to a civilian provider for care. The military treatment facility must initiate all referrals to civilian providers using DD Form 2161 signed by the facility commander. There is no deductible, copayment, or cost-share for services provided by a civilian provider.

Payments

Those covered and receiving benefits under SHCP are not responsible for any out-of-pocket costs. Active duty service member claims for services provided by a TRICARE network provider are paid at the same contracted rate as other TRICARE beneficiary claims.

TRICARE Hospice Program

The TRICARE hospice program is based on Medicare's hospice program. It is designed to provide care and comfort to patients who are expected to live less than 6 months if the terminal illness runs its normal course. Those persons who receive care under the hospice program cannot receive other services under the TRICARE basic programs (treatments aimed at a cure) unless the hospice care has been formally revoked. There are a number of additional rules and limits to the hospice program, so call the HBA at the nearest military medical facility and ask for a copy of the guidelines.

TRICARE and HMO Coverage

TRICARE considers HMO coverage to be the same as any other primary health insurance coverage. TRICARE shares the cost of covered care received from an HMO (including the HMO's user fees), after the HMO has paid all it is going to pay, under the following conditions:

◗ Provider must meet TRICARE provider certification standards
◗ Type of care must be a TRICARE benefit and medically necessary

TRICARE will not pay for emergency services received outside the HMO's normal service area.

TRICARE will not cost-share services an individual obtains outside the HMO, if the services are available through the HMO. For example, if an HMO provides psychiatric services but the patient does not like the HMO's psychiatrist and obtains services outside the HMO, then TRICARE will not pay anything on the claim.

CHAMPVA Program

The Veterans Health Care Expansion Act of 1973 (PL93-82) authorized a CHAMPUS-like program, **CHAMPVA,** which became effective on September 1, 1973. The acronym stands for *Civilian Health and Medical Program of the Veterans Administration* (now known as the Department of Veterans Affairs). CHAMPVA *is not an insurance program* in that it does not involve a contract guaranteeing the indemnification of an insured party against a specified loss in return for a premium paid. It is considered a **service benefit program;** therefore, there are no premiums.

This program is for the spouse and children of a veteran with a **total, permanent service-connected disability** or for the surviving spouse and children of a veteran who died as a result of a service-connected disability. A **veteran** is any person who has served in the armed forces of the United States, is no longer in the service, and has received an honorable discharge. Just as in the TRICARE program, individuals who qualify for CHAMPVA are known as beneficiaries and the active duty service member is called the sponsor.

Examples of service-connected total, permanent disability are when an individual suffers an injury with paraplegic results, receives a bullet wound with neurologic damage, loses a limb, and so on. This contrasts to a chronic or temporary service-connected disability, which might exist if an individual, while in the Navy, improperly lifts a heavy object, suffers a back injury with ongoing sporadic symptoms, and requires continuing medical care after leaving the service. Both scenarios present service-connected disabilities, but the first example illustrates a person permanently disabled whereas the second example illustrates what may be a chronic or temporary disability.

Eligibility

The following persons are eligible for CHAMPVA benefits as long as they *are not eligible* for TRI-CARE Standard and not eligible for Medicare Part A as a result of reaching age 65:

▶ The husband, wife, or unmarried child of a veteran with a total disability, permanent in nature, resulting from a service-connected injury.

▶ The husband, wife, or unmarried child of a veteran who died as the result of a service-connected disability or who, at the time of death, had a total disability, permanent in nature, resulting from a **service-connected injury.**

▶ The husband, wife, or unmarried child of an individual who died in the line of duty while on active service.

Children are those unmarried and younger than the age of 18 regardless of whether dependent or not, or up to the age of 23 if enrolled in a course of instruction at an approved educational institution.

Determination of eligibility is the responsibility of the Department of Veterans Affairs. The prospective beneficiary goes to the nearest VA medical center and, if eligible, receives a VA identification card.

Enrollment

Dependents of veterans must have a Social Security number and have established dependency to the veteran sponsor by contacting the local VA regional office. The individual obtains and completes an application by phone, fax, or downloading from the VA's web site (see Internet section at the end of this chapter).

Identification Card

The issuing station's number appears on the identification card to identify the home station where the beneficiary's case file is kept. The identification card number is the veteran's VA file number with an alpha suffix. The suffix is different for each beneficiary of a sponsor. All dependents 10 years of age or older are required to have a Uniformed Services (military) identification and privilege card for CHAMPVA as shown in Figure 13–8.

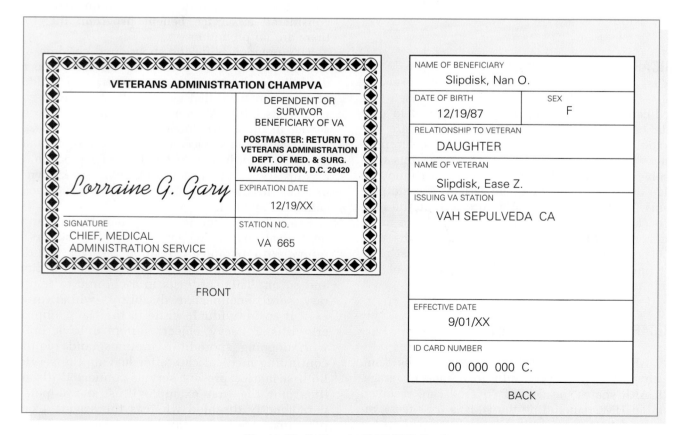

Figure 13–8. Sample CHAMPVA Card.

Benefits

The Department of Veterans Affairs (VA) elected to provide these beneficiaries with benefits and cost-sharing plans similar to those received by dependents of retired and deceased uniformed services personnel under TRICARE Standard. To see the overall picture of CHAMPVA benefits, which includes cost-sharing (deductibles and copayments), study Figure 13–9.

Provider

The beneficiaries of the CHAMPVA program have complete freedom of choice in selecting their civilian health care providers.

Benefit [2]	Beneficiary Pays [3, 4]			CHAMPVA Pays
	Deductible ($50/individual or $100/family per calendar year)	Cost Share [5]	Additional Costs (costs above CHAMPVA allowable)	
Outpatient services	Yes	25% of allowable	No	75% of allowable
Ambulatory surgery *Family services*	No	25% of allowable	No	75% of allowable
Professional services	Yes	25% of allowable	No	75% of allowable
Pharmacy services	Yes	25% of allowable	No	75% of allowable
Durable Medical Equipment (DME)				
Non–VA source	Yes	25% of allowable	No	75% of allowable
VA source	No	NONE	No	100% of VA cost
Inpatient services *Facility services* DRG based	No	Lesser of: 1) per day amt x number of inpatient days; 2) 25% of billed amount; or 3) DRG rate	No	DRG rate less beneficiary cost share
Non–DRG based	No	25% of allowable	No	75% of allowable
Mental health High volume/RTC	No	25% of allowable	No	75% of allowable
Low volume	No	Lesser of: 1) per day amt x number of inpatient days; 2) 25% of billed amount.	No	Balance of allowable AFTER beneficiary cost share
Professional services	No	25% of allowable	No	75% of allowable

CHAMPVA Cost Share Summary [1]

[1]Except for Medicaid, policies that are purchased exclusively for the purpose of supplementing CHAMPVA benefits, and State Victims of Crime Compensation Programs, CHAMPVA is always the *secondary* payer.
[2]Covered services only.
[3]Services received at VA healthcare facilities under the CITI (CHAMPVA Inhouse Treatment Initiative) program are exempt from beneficiary cost sharing.
[4]Under catastrophic protection plan (Cat Cap), annual beneficiary cost sharing is limited to $7,500.
[5]Claims involving a payment from another health insurance (OHI) plan may result in a reduced beneficiary cost share or, depending on the combined OHI and CHAMPVA payment, no cost share at all.

Figure 13–9. CHAMPVA Service Benefits and Cost Share Summary Chart.

Preauthorization

Preauthorization is required for organ and bone marrow transplants, hospice services, most mental health/substance abuse services, all dental care, and all durable medical equipment with a purchase price or total rental cost of $300 or more. Preauthorization for mental health and substance abuse care must be requested from Health Management Strategies (HMS) International, Inc., at 800-240-4068 or mailed to CVAC-MHP, P.O. Box 26128, Alexandria, VA 22313. All other preauthorization requests are made directly to CHAMPVA at 303-331-7599, by fax at 303-331-7804, or by mail to VA Health Administration Center, CHAMPVA, Attn: Preauthorization, P.O. Box 65023, Denver, CO 80206-9023.

Medical Record Access

Privacy Act of 1974

The Privacy Act of 1974 became effective on September 27, 1975, and establishes an individual's right to review his or her medical records maintained by a federal medical care facility, such as a VA medical center or U.S. Public Health Service facility, and to contest inaccuracies in such records. The Act directs each agency to make its own rules establishing access procedures. Agencies are allowed to adopt special procedures when it is believed that direct access could be harmful to a person. The Act requires that an individual from whom personal information is requested be informed of (1) the authority for the request, (2) the principal purpose of the information requested, (3) routine use of the information, and (4) the effect on an individual who does not provide the information.

Computer Matching and Privacy Protection Act of 1988

Another act, the Computer Matching and Privacy Protection Act of 1988, was established and permits the government to verify information by way of computer matches.

Both of these acts are mentioned on the back of the HCFA-1500 claim form. It is important that TRICARE patients be made aware of this information by physicians who treat them, so that they are knowledgeable about routine use and disclosure of medical data.

Patients may make a Privacy Protection Act request in writing, in person, or by telephone. Individuals should call the facility to determine the required procedures to obtain access to the records and what to include in making a written request.

Claims Procedure

Fiscal Intermediary

TRICARE Standard is governed by the Department of Defense (DOD). As such, it is not subject to those state regulatory bodies or agencies that control the insurance business. The DOD and the VA have agreed to use the Office of the Assistant Secretary of Defense and the TRICARE Standard system of fiscal intermediaries and hospital contractors to receive, process, and pay CHAMPVA claims, following the same procedures currently used for TRICARE Standard.

A **fiscal intermediary (FI)** (also known as a contractor or claims processor) is an organization under contract to the government that handles insurance claims for care received under the TRICARE Standard or CHAMPVA program.

TRICARE Standard and CHAMPVA

TRICARE Standard and CHAMPVA claims must be billed on the HCFA-1500 claim form and submitted to the claims processor (fiscal intermediary). Remember to abstract the correct information from front and back sides of the patient's identification card. Refer to Chapter 6 and follow the TRICARE or CHAMPVA instructions for completing the HCFA-1500 claim form. Refer to Figure 6–82 for an example of a completed TRICARE case with no other insurance and Figure 6–83 for an example of a completed CHAMPVA case. If electing to complete the VA Form 10-1759A for a CHAMPVA case, refer to the instructions presented later in this chapter.

If the physician is nonparticipating and *does not accept assignment,* the patient completes the top portion of the HCFA-1500 claim form, attaches the physician's itemized statement, and submits the claim. Alternatively, the patient may submit on the white TRICARE claim DD Form 2642 Patient's Request for Medical Payment. Patients and providers of care for health services in foreign countries must use DD Form 2520. The Uniform Bill, UB-92, form is used for inpatient hospital billing.

Time Limit

Effective January 1, 1993, claims must be filed within 1 year from the date a service is provided or (for inpatient care) within 1 year from the patient's date of discharge from the inpatient facility.

Claims Office

The TRICARE program is administered by the Department of Defense, TRICARE Management Activity, 16401 East Centretech Parkway, Aurora, CO 80011-9043, but claims are not processed in Colorado. Refer to Appendix A for the address for submitting a TRICARE Standard claim in your state. Write to the TRICARE Support Office or contact the health benefits advisor (HBA) at the nearest MTF to obtain a current TRICARE *Standard Handbook* or to answer any questions about the name of the regional claims processor, benefits, nonbenefits, when an NAS is required, and so on.

The CHAMPVA program is administered by the Department of Veterans Affairs, Health Administration Center, P.O. Box 65023, Denver, CO 80206-9023.

TRICARE Extra and TRICARE Prime

The beneficiary does not file any claim forms under TRICARE Extra or TRICARE Prime programs when using network providers. Providers must submit claims on HCFA-1500 claim forms to TRICARE subcontractors listed in Appendix A for services given to beneficiaries. Referral and preauthorization numbers are required claims information when applicable.

Time Limit

For *outpatient* care, a claim must be *received by* the state's or region's TRICARE contractor within 1 year of the date the provider rendered the service to the patient. For *inpatient* care, a claim must be *received by* the contractor within 1 year from the date the patient was discharged from the facility. If a claim covers several different medical services or supplies that were provided at different times, the 1-year deadline applies to each item on the claim.

When a claim is submitted on time but the contractor returns it for more information, resubmit the claim with the requested information so it is received by the contractor no later than 1 year after the medical services or supplies were provided or 90 days from the date the claim was returned to you, whichever is later.

A contractor may grant exemptions from the filing deadlines for several reasons. Submit a request to the contractor including a complete explanation of the circumstances of the late filing, all available documentation supporting the request, and the claim denied for late filing.

Claims Office

See Appendix A for the name and address to which to submit claims and to obtain further information about this program.

TRICARE Prime Remote and Supplemental Health Care Program

Outpatient professional services are submitted using an HCFA-1500 claim form. Primary care service claims are processed and paid without a referral or preauthorization from a network or non-network provider. For specialty medical/surgical care and for behavioral health counseling and therapy sessions, a referral number provided by the HCF must be included on the claim form. The POS option and NAS requirements do not apply to TPR and SHCP claims.

Time Limit

A claim must be filed within 1 year from the date a service is provided or (for inpatient care) within 1 year from the patient's date of discharge from the inpatient facility.

Claims Office

Do not file claims of active duty armed service patients to TRICARE. Claims for patients on active duty must be sent to the specific branch of service (e.g., Army, Navy, Air Force, Marines). Claims are submitted to Palmetto Government Benefits Administrators (PGBAs) for processing and payment (see Appendix A for the address).

TRICARE/CHAMPVA and Other Insurance

By law, TRICARE/CHAMPVA is usually second payer when a beneficiary is enrolled in **other health insurance (OHI),** a civilian health plan, or belongs to a health maintenance organization (HMO) or preferred provider organization (PPO). However, there are two exceptions:

▶ When a plan is administered under Title XIX of the Social Security Act (Medicaid)
▶ When coverage is specifically designed to supplement TRICARE benefits (e.g., Medigap health plan)

When the patient has other health insurance that is primary (meaning that it pays before TRICARE Standard or CHAMPVA does), submit the claim using the HCFA-1500 insurance claim form. Attach the explanation of benefits from the primary carrier. If the patient is submitting his or her claim to the other insurance, take these steps.

1. Bill the other insurance carrier with the form it has supplied.
2. Bill TRICARE or CHAMPVA by completing the top section of the HCFA-1500 after receiving payment and an explanation of benefits from the other insurance company. Submit the physician's itemized statement, which must contain the following:
   a. Provider's name
   b. Date the services/supplies were provided
   c. Description of each service/supply
   d. Place of treatment
   e. Number/frequency of each service
   f. Fee for each item of service or supply
   g. Procedure code numbers
   h. Diagnostic code number or description of condition for which treatment is being received

   Billing statements showing only total charges, canceled checks, or cash register receipts (or similar type receipts) are not acceptable as itemized statements.
3. Attach a photocopy of the explanation of benefits from the other insurance company.
4. Send the TRICARE or CHAMPVA claim to the local claims processor (fiscal intermediary).

Medicaid and TRICARE/CHAMPVA

File TRICARE or CHAMPVA claims first if the beneficiary is a recipient of the Medicaid program.

Medicare and TRICARE

TRICARE is considered secondary to Medicare for persons younger than age 65 who have Medicare Part A as a result of a disability and who have enrolled in Medicare Part B. Those eligible for Medicare Part A are *not* covered by TRICARE unless disabled. Claims should be submitted to Medicare, then to TRICARE with a copy of the Medicare remittance advice. Services covered by TRICARE but not covered by Medicare (e.g., prescriptions) will be paid by TRICARE. Participating providers may obtain a TRICARE fee schedule by contacting their fiscal intermediary.

Medicare and CHAMPVA

Effective December 5, 1991, CHAMPVA became secondary payer to Medicare for persons younger than age 65 who are enrolled in Medicare Parts A and B and who are otherwise eligible for CHAMPVA. Because CHAMPVA is secondary payer, claims must first be submitted to Medicare.

Dual or Double Coverage

If a patient has additional insurance that provides double coverage, a claim must be filed. Refusal by the beneficiary to claim benefits from other health insurance coverages will result in a denial of TRICARE benefits. In double coverage situations, TRICARE will pay the lower of:

1. The amount of TRICARE allowable charges remaining after the double coverage plan has paid its benefits *or*
2. The amount TRICARE would have paid as primary payer

So that there is no duplication of benefits paid between the double coverage plan and TRICARE, there must be **coordination of benefits.**

Third Party Liability

If the patient is in an automobile accident or receives an injury that may have third party involvement, the following two options are available for reimbursement:

Option 1: TRICARE Form DD 2527 (Statement of Personal Injury—Possible Third Party Liability) must be sent in with the regular claim form for cost-sharing of the civilian medical care. All five sections of the form should be completed by the patient. This form allows TRICARE to evaluate the circumstances of the accident and the possibility that the government may recover money for the medical care from the person who injured the patient. If an HCFA-1500 claim form is submitted without TRICARE Form DD 2527, a request will be made to complete it. This form must be returned within 35 days of the request, or the claims processor will deny the original and all related claims. Then the fiscal intermediary submits a claim to the third party for reimbursement or files a lien for reimbursement with the liability insurance carrier, the liable party, or the attorneys or court involved.

Option 2: The provider can submit claims exclusively to the third party liability carrier for reimbursement. Claims submitted with ICD-9-CM diagnostic codes between 800 and 999 (Injury and Poisoning) trigger the fact that there might be third party litigation, and the claims processor may request the completion of DD Form 2527.

Workers' Compensation

If a TRICARE or CHAMPVA beneficiary is injured on the job or becomes ill because of his or her work, this becomes a workers' compensation case, and the claim must be filed with the compensation insurance carrier. When all workers' compensation benefits have been exhausted, then TRICARE or CHAMPVA can be billed.

In some cases it can happen that the case is in the state of determining whether it is a work-related accident or illness and the claim might be sent to the TRICARE or CHAMPVA claims processor. In those instances, the claims processor files a lien with the workers' compensation carrier for recovery when the case is settled.

PROCEDURE: Completing a CHAMPVA Claim Form

An example of a completed CHAMPVA claim form is provided in Figure 13−10.

1: Enter the patient's last name, first name, and middle initial (do not use nicknames or abbreviations).

2: Enter the patient's Social Security number exactly as it appears on the Social Security card. If the patient does not have a Social Security number, print "None."

3: Enter the patient's complete address. If the patient's address has changed, place an "X" in the box.

4: Enter the patient's home telephone number. Include area code.

5A: Enter the number from Item 6 of the patient's current CHAMPVA Authorization Card.

5B: Enter the date from Item 4 of the patient's current CHAMPVA Authorization Card.

5C: Enter the date from Item 5 of the patient's current CHAMPVA Authorization Card.

6: Enter the patient's date of birth.

7: Enter the patient's relationship to sponsor.

8: Enter the patient's gender.

9: Enter the sponsor's last name, first name, and middle initial (do not use nicknames or abbreviations).

10: Enter sponsor's VA Claim/File Number.

11: Enter the sponsor's complete address (if different from the patient's).

12A: Place an "X" in the appropriate box if the patient is covered under any other medical benefits plan or health insurance coverage. *CHAMPVA will not duplicate benefits of any other health insurance plan or program.*

12B: Place an "X" beside all applicable types of medical plans or other health insurance to which the patient is entitled.

12C: Enter the name and address of the other insurance carrier.

12D: Enter the name and address of the employer if other health insurance is provided by the patient's employer.

12E: Enter the policy identification number of the other health insurance carrier.

12F: Enter the insurance agent's name. If this information is not known, enter "Unknown."

12G: Enter the insurance agent's telephone number. If this information is not known, enter "Unknown."

13: Check the appropriate box according to the type of medical care the patient received.

 ▶ Inpatient: For admission to a civilian hospital, check the Inpatient box.
 ▶ Outpatient: Check the Outpatient box for all eligible CHAMPVA beneficiaries provided medical care from civilian facilities unless otherwise authorized by the VA.
 ▶ Pharmacy: Check the Pharmacy box for claims for payment of drugs and medicines requiring a prescription by law.
 ▶ Travel: Check Travel box for claims for ambulance travel to, from, or between hospitals for Inpatient care.
 ▶ Dental: Check the Dental box for dental care for which the patient has an approved preauthorization.
 ▶ DME: Check the DME box for payment of durable medical equipment costing more than $100.
 ▶ College Infirmary: Check the Other box for College Infirmary.
 ▶ Other Inpatient Care: Check the Inpatient box for admissions to an approved nursing facility (including a Christian Science sanatorium).

14: If the patient needs treatment for any kind of an injury (e.g., broken toe, sprained knee, lacerated forehead, back injury), check "YES" and briefly describe the injury and circumstances of how the patient was injured.

15: Be sure to read the release of medical record information contained in this item and complete the blanks, if appropriate.

16: CHAMPVA is a benefit program. As such the patient (or sponsor) MUST assign the benefit to the provider of care if he or she wishes the payment to be made to the provider. Otherwise, payment will be made to the patient.

17A: Every CHAMPVA claim must be signed by a patient 18 years of age or older. If the beneficiary is unable to sign on his or her own behalf, the sponsor (or other parent) may sign. In the absence of either parent, a guardian or

OMB NC: 2900-
Estimated burden: 30 min

VA Department of Veterans Affairs	CHAMPVA CLAIM FORM

CHAMPVA CENTER, 4500 Cherry Creek Drive South, Box 300, Denver CO 80222

WARNING: IF YOU KNOWINGLY MAKE A FALSE STATEMENT OF ANY MATERIAL FACT IN OR IN CONNECTION WITH THIS CLAIM, YOU ARE SUBJECT TO PROSECUTION IN A U.S. COURT

PART 1 - PATIENT INFORMATION (To be completed by the beneficiary, patient or sponsor)

1. PATIENT'S NAME
CHIEU, MARION W.

2. PATIENT'S SOCIAL SECURITY NUMBER
742-11-0491

3. PATIENT'S ADDRESS (Street, City, State, ZIP)   (Check if new address)
321 OAK STREET,   WOODLAND HILLS, XY 12345

4. TELEPHONE NUMBER (Include area code)
(013) 492-7800

5A. CHAMPVA IDENTIFICATION CARD/AUTHORIZATION NUMBER
49-467-081C

	5B. EFFECTIVE DATE			5C. EXPIRATION DATE		
	MONTH	DAY	YEAR	MONTH	DAY	YEAR
	09	01	XX	12	19	XX

6. PATIENT'S DATE OF BIRTH (Month, day, year)
12-01-77

7. PATIENT'S RELATIONSHIP TO SPONSOR (Check one)
☒ SPOUSE   ☐ CHILD

8. PATIENT'S SEX (Check one)
☐ MALE ☒ FEMALE

PART II - SPONSOR INFORMATION (To be completed by the beneficiary, patient or sponsor)

9. SPONSOR'S NAME (Last, first, middle initial)
CHIEU, FRANK T.

10. VA CLAIM/FILE NUMBER
421-05-0129

11. SPONSOR'S ADDRESS IF DIFFERENT FROM PATIENT'S (Street, City, State, Zip)

PART III - PATIENT INSURANCE INFORMATION (To be completed by the beneficiary, patient or sponsor)

12A. IS PATIENT'S TREATMENT COVERED BY OTHER HEALTH INSURANCE
☐ YES   ☒ NO   IF YES, PLEASE COMPLETE ITEMS 12B THROUGH 12G BELOW

12B. TYPE OF COVERAGE
☐ GROUP HEALTH   ☐ PRIVATE (NON–GROUP)
☐ MEDICARE   ☐ CHAMPVA SUPPLEMENTAL
☐ MEDICAID   ☐ WORKERS COMPENSATION
☐ OTHER   ☐ NONE

12C. NAME AND ADDRESS OF INSURANCE CARRIER

12D. IF COVERAGE IS THROUGH WORK, NAME AND ADDRESS OF EMPLOYER

12E. POLICY IDENTIFICATION NUMBER

12F. INSURANCE AGENT'S NAME

12G. AGENT'S TELEPHONE NUMBER

PART IV - TREATMENT INFORMATION (To be completed by the beneficiary, patient or sponsor)

13. TYPE OF CLAIM (Check one)
☐ INPATIENT   ☐ DENTAL
☒ OUTPATIENT   ☐ DME
☐ PHARMACY   ☐ OTHER
☐ TRAVEL

14. WAS NEED OF TREATMENT DUE TO A PHYSICAL INJURY?   YES ☐   NO ☒
(If "Yes", briefly describe injuries and give a statement of circumstances)

15. I authorize the identified provider of service to disclose to CHAMPVA medical record information that pertains to the medical services described on this form. Unless limitations are shown below, this consent pertains to all of my medical records, including records related to treatment for medical or dental conditions, psychological or psychiatric impairments, drug or alcohol abuse, acquired immune deficiency syndrome (AIDS) or infection with the human immunodeficiency virus (HIV), and sickle cell disease.

The information will be used to process my CHAMPVA claim and determine my (or the patient identified above) eligibility for medical benefits. I also authorize the release of or obtaining of medical and/or other coverage information to and from another organization with which I have other medical benefits plan or health insurance coverage. I understand that I may revoke this authorization at any time, except to the extent that action has already been taken to comply with it. Without my express revocation, this consent will automatically expire: (1) upon satisfaction of the need for disclosure; (2) on February 2, 20XX (date supplied by the beneficiary); or (3) under the following conditions:

LIMITATIONS:

16. I assign payment to the provider(s) of these claim services   ☐ YES   ☒ NO

17. I CERTIFY THAT THE ABOVE STATEMENTS AND ATTACHMENTS ARE CORRECT AND REPRESENT ACTUAL SERVICES, DATES AND FEES CHARGED TO ME OR MY ELIGIBLE DEPENDENTS.

17A. CLAIMANT'S SIGNATURE

17B. DATE
2–2–XX

17C. RELATIONSHIP TO SPONSOR
WIFE

Figure 13–10. Example of a completed CHAMPVA Claim Form VA Form 10-7959A, used when billing for professional services. (A)

PATIENT'S NAME (Last, first, middle initial)	SPONSOR'S NAME (Last, first, middle initial)
CHIEU, MARION W.	CHIEU, FRANK T.

PART V - PHYSICIAN/OTHER PROVIDER (To be completed by physician or other provider)

18. PROVIDER'S NAME	19. PROVIDER'S TAX I.D. NUMBER	20. NAME OF REFERRING PHYSICIAN OR OTHER SOURCE (e.g. public health agency)
DOE, JOHN M.D.	93-4267890	

21. WHEN SERVICES ARE RELATED TO A PERIOD OF HOSPITALIZATION, GIVE DATES		22. NAME AND ADDRESS OF FACILITY WHERE SERVICES RENDERED (if other than home office)
ADMITTED	DISCHARGED	

23. DIAGNOSIS OR NATURE OF ILLNESS OR INJURY. RELATE DIAGNOSIS TO PROCEDURE BY USING PROCEDURE NUMBER IN COLUMN 24E BELOW.

A. Dysfunctional uterine bleeding.

B.

C.

24A DATE OF SERVICE	24B * PLACE OF SERVICE	24C PROCEDURE CODE	24D DESCRIBE UNUSUAL SERVICE OR CIRCUMSTANCES	24E DIAGNOSIS CODE	24F CHARGES	24G DAYS OR UNITS	24H TYPE OF SERVICE
02-02-XX	0	99213	Ofc visit Eval & Mgmt Level 3	626.8	45 00	1	1

25. I certify that the statements on the reverse of this bill apply and are made a part hereto.	26. PROVIDER'S SOCIAL SECURITY NO 272-49-5731	27. TOTAL CHARGES	45.00	
John Doe, MD 02-02-XX SIGNATURE OF PROVIDER DATE	28. PROVIDER'S ADDRESS, ZIP CODE AND TELEPHONE NUMBER 123 MAIN STREET, WOODLAND HILLS, XY 12345 013/486-9002			

```
* PLACE OF SERVICE CODE FOR ITEM 24B
    IN -INPATIENT HOSPITAL          NCF -NIGHT CARE FACILITY (PSY)        IL -INDEPENDENT LABORATORY
    OH -OUTPATIENT HOSPITAL         NH -NURSING HOME                      OF -OTHER MEDICAL/SURGICAL FACILITY
    O -DOCTOR'S OFFICE              SNF -SKILLD NURSING FACILITY          RTC -RESIDENTIAL TREATMENT CENTER
    H -PATIENT'S HOME               AMB -AMBULANCE                        STF - SPECIALIZED TREATMENT FACILITY
    DCF -DAY CARE FACILITY (PSY)    OL -OTHER LOCATIONS
```

PART VI- PHARMACY INFORMATION (To be completed by pharmacist)				PATIENT'S NAME	
29A. NATIONAL DRUG CODE	29B. RX NUMBER	29C. PHARMACY NAME	29D. FILL DATE (Month, day, year)	29E. PHYSICIAN NAME	29F. CHARGES

30. TOTAL CHARGES – $

VA FORM 10-7959A
DEC 1990   Pg II

reference initials

Figure 13–10. *Continued*

fiduciary may sign. (*Note:* For privacy reasons, a patient younger than 18 years of age may sign his or her own claim form.)

17B: Insert date of signature.

17C: Enter the claimant's relationship to sponsor.
Part V: To be completed by physician or other provider.
Top of page II: Enter patient and sponsor's last name, first name, and middle initial.

18: Enter provider's (physician's) name and title.

19: Enter provider's tax identification number.

20: Enter the name of the referring physician or agency.

21: Enter the admission and discharge dates if the patient is hospitalized.

22: Enter the name and address of the facility where services were rendered if other than home or office.

23: Enter diagnostic description or nature of illness or injury.

24A: Enter the date of service.

24B: Enter the place of service using one of the codes shown midway down on this page of the form.

24C: Enter the CPT procedure code number with modifier.

24D: Insert a description of the service or procedure.

24E: Enter the ICD-9-CM diagnostic code number for each diagnosis as described in Item 23.

24F: Enter the fee for each service, procedure, or test described in 24D.

24G: Enter the number of days or units. This block is commonly used for multiple visits, number of miles, units of supplies including drugs, anesthesia minutes, or oxygen volume.

24H: Enter the type of service code from the following list:

1 Medical care
2 Surgery
3 Consultation
4 Diagnostic x-ray
5 Diagnostic laboratory dialysis
6 Radiation therapy
7 Anesthesia
8 Assistance at surgery
9 Other medical service
0 Blood or packed red cells
A Used DME
F Ambulatory surgical center
H Hospice
L Renal supply in home
M Alternate payment for maintenance
N Kidney donor
V Pneumococcal vaccine
Y Second opinion on elective surgery
Z Third opinion on elective surgery

25: Show the signature of the physician, or his or her representative, and the date the form was signed.

26: Enter the provider's Social Security number.

27: Enter the total of all charges.

28: Enter the provider's street address, city, state, ZIP code, and telephone number, including area code.

Items 29A through 30 may be completed if the patient is receiving prescription drugs.

After Claim Submission

TRICARE Summary Payment Voucher

For each TRICARE claim, the claims processor issues a **summary payment voucher** (Fig. 13–11) detailing the payment of the claim. When the provider participates (accepts assignment), the voucher is sent to him or her with the check. The patient always receives a copy of the voucher, even if the provider receives payment directly from the fiscal intermediary.

CHAMPVA Explanation of Benefits Document

Upon completion of the processing of a claim, a payment check is generated and an explanation of benefits document is sent to the beneficiary (including the provider if the claim is filed by the provider). The explanation of benefits summarizes the action taken on the claim and contains information as graphically illustrated and explained in Figure 13–12. Beneficiaries who receive durable medical equipment or VA services from a CHAMPVA Inhouse Treatment Initiative (CITI, pronounced "city") do not receive an explanation of benefits.

Quality Assurance

A **quality assurance program** continually assesses the effectiveness of inpatient and outpatient care. The quality assurance department reviews providers' outpatient records on a random basis for clinical and administrative quality. Grievance procedures have been established for members and providers if any complaint arises from an administrative process, a service provided by a physician, or an issue involving quality of care.

TRICARE-managed care programs have a quality assurance program to continually assess the effectiveness of care and services rendered by providers. This includes inpatient and outpatient hospital care,

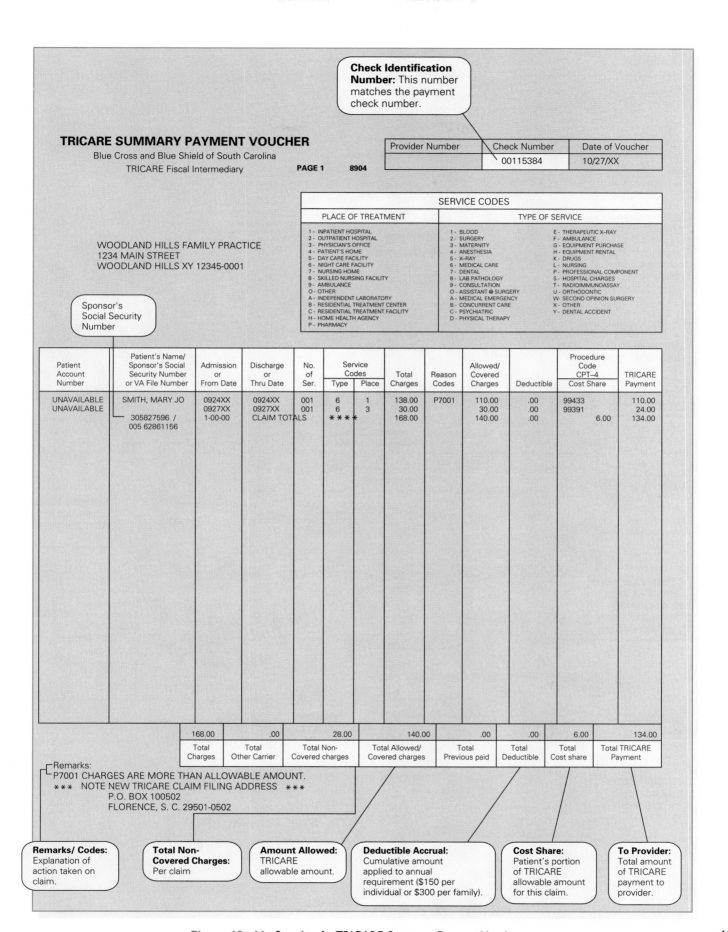

Figure 13–11. Sample of a TRICARE Summary Payment Voucher.

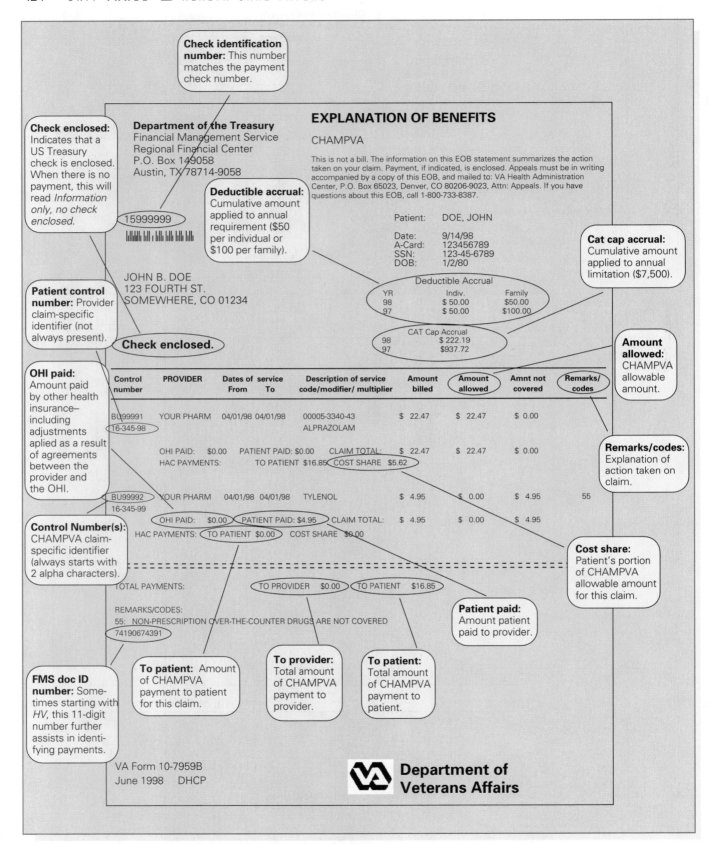

Check identification number: This number matches the payment check number.

Check enclosed: Indicates that a US Treasury check is enclosed. When there is no payment, this will read *Information only, no check enclosed.*

Deductible accrual: Cumulative amount applied to annual requirement ($50 per individual or $100 per family).

Patient control number: Provider claim-specific identifier (not always present).

OHI paid: Amount paid by other health insurance—including adjustments applied as a result of agreements between the provider and the OHI.

Control Number(s): CHAMPVA claim-specific identifier (always starts with 2 alpha characters).

FMS doc ID number: Sometimes starting with *HV*, this 11-digit number further assists in identifying payments.

Cat cap accrual: Cumulative amount applied to annual limitation ($7,500).

Amount allowed: CHAMPVA allowable amount.

Remarks/codes: Explanation of action taken on claim.

Cost share: Patient's portion of CHAMPVA allowable amount for this claim.

Patient paid: Amount patient paid to provider.

To patient: Amount of CHAMPVA payment to patient for this claim.

To provider: Total amount of CHAMPVA payment to provider.

To patient: Total amount of CHAMPVA payment to patient.

Department of the Treasury
Financial Management Service
Regional Financial Center
P.O. Box 149058
Austin, TX 78714-9058

15999999

JOHN B. DOE
123 FOURTH ST.
SOMEWHERE, CO 01234

Check enclosed.

EXPLANATION OF BENEFITS

CHAMPVA

This is not a bill. The information on this EOB statement summarizes the action taken on your claim. Payment, if indicated, is enclosed. Appeals must be in writing accompanied by a copy of this EOB, and mailed to: VA Health Administration Center, P.O. Box 65023, Denver, CO 80206-9023, Attn: Appeals. If you have questions about this EOB, call 1-800-733-8387.

Patient: DOE, JOHN

Date: 9/14/98
A-Card: 123456789
SSN: 123-45-6789
DOB: 1/2/80

Deductible Accrual

YR	Indiv.	Family
98	$ 50.00	$50.00
97	$ 50.00	$100.00

CAT Cap Accrual

| 98 | $ 222.19 |
| 97 | $937.72 |

Control number	PROVIDER	Dates of service From	To	Description of service code/modifier/ multiplier	Amount billed	Amount allowed	Amnt not covered	Remarks/ codes
BU99991 16-345-98	YOUR PHARM	04/01/98	04/01/98	00005-3340-43 ALPRAZOLAM	$ 22.47	$ 22.47	$ 0.00	

OHI PAID: $0.00   PATIENT PAID: $0.00   CLAIM TOTAL: $ 22.47 $ 22.47 $ 0.00
HAC PAYMENTS: TO PATIENT $16.85   COST SHARE $5.62

| BU99992 16-345-99 | YOUR PHARM | 04/01/98 | 04/01/98 | TYLENOL | $ 4.95 | $ 0.00 | $ 4.95 | 55 |

OHI PAID: $0.00   PATIENT PAID: $4.95   CLAIM TOTAL: $ 4.95 $ 0.00 $ 4.95
HAC PAYMENTS: TO PATIENT $0.00   COST SHARE $0.00

TOTAL PAYMENTS: TO PROVIDER $0.00   TO PATIENT $16.85

REMARKS/CODES:
55: NON-PRESCRIPTION OVER-THE-COUNTER DRUGS ARE NOT COVERED
74190674391

VA Form 10-7959B
June 1998   DHCP

Department of Veterans Affairs

Figure 13–12. CHAMPVA Explanation of Benefits document.

mental health services, long-term care, home health care, and programs for the handicapped. Providers are notified in writing when a potential quality issue has been confirmed as a breach of quality standards. Recommended corrective action plans are given, and noncompliance may lead to suspension or termination of a provider.

Claims Inquiries and Appeals

Through the appeal process, providers may request reconsideration of a denial of certification for coverage or of the amount paid for a submitted claim. See Chapter 8 for inquiring about the status of a claim and to learn the procedures on how to file reviews and appeals.

RESOURCES ON THE INTERNET

To download a TRICARE manual, visit the TRICARE web site:

> **http://www.tricare.osd.mil/tricare-manuals/**

For information on CHAMPVA, visit the CHAMPVA web site:

> **www.va.gov/hac/champva/champva.html**

For VA government forms, visit the VA web site:

> **www.va.gov/forms/medical.htm**

STUDENT ASSIGNMENT LIST

✔ Study Chapter 13.
✔ Answer the review questions in the *Workbook* to reinforce the theory learned in this chapter and to help prepare you for a future test.
✔ Complete the assignments in the *Workbook* for computing mathematical calculations and giving you hands-on experience in completing TRICARE and CHAMPVA insurance claim forms and proficiency in procedural and diagnostic coding.
✔ Turn to the Glossary at the end of this textbook for a further understanding of the Key Terms used in this chapter.

COMPUTER ASSIGNMENT

Complete Case 7 on the computer disk to review concepts you have learned for this chapter.

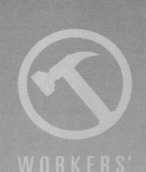

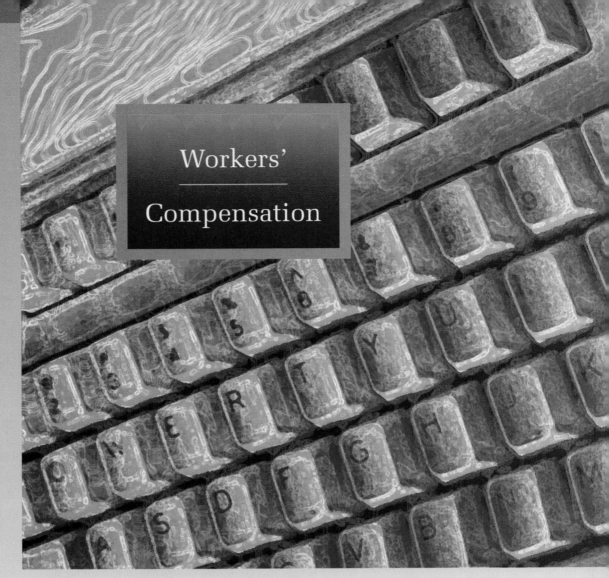

Workers'
Compensation

14

CHAPTER OUTLINE

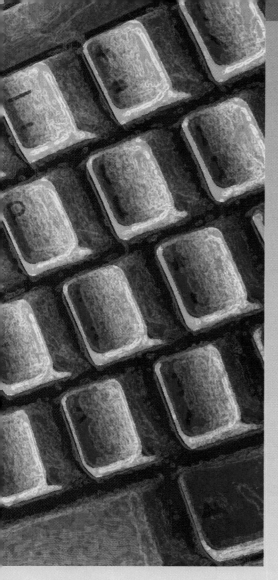

OBJECTIVES*

After reading this chapter you should be able to:

- State the purpose of workers' compensation laws.
- Enumerate who is covered under federal workers' compensation laws.
- Name who is covered under state workers' compensation laws.
- Differentiate between workers' compensation insurance and employers' liability insurance.
- Determine the waiting period in each state before benefits begin.
- Describe the types of compensation benefits.
- Define nondisability, temporary disability, and permanent disability claims.
- Explain OSHA's role in protecting employees.
- Define third party subrogation.
- Define second-injury fund.
- Name the contents of a medical report.
- Complete workers' compensation forms properly.
- Explain how to handle out-of-state claims.
- Define terminology and abbreviations pertinent to workers' compensation cases.
- Explain the advantages of filing a lien.
- List signs of fraud and abuse involving employees, employers, insurers, medical providers, and lawyers.
- State when to report fraud or abuse involving a workers' compensation claim.
- Describe workers' compensation record keeping methods.
- Explain two ways in which depositions are used.
- Describe actions to take in following up on delinquent workers' compensation claims.

KEY TERMS

accident

adjudication

by report (BR)

claims examiner

compromise and release (C and R)

deposition

ergonomic

extraterritorial

Federal Employees' Compensation Act (FECA)

fee schedule

independent medical evaluator (IME)

injury

insurance adjuster

lien

medical service order

nondisability (ND) claim

occupational illness (or disease)

Occupational Safety and Health Administration (OSHA)

permanent and stationary (P and S)

permanent disability (PD)

petition

second injury fund

sequelae

sub rosa films

continued

---

*Performance objectives and exercises for hands-on practical experience for this chapter appear in the *Workbook*.

History

Before the establishment of a workers' compensation program in the United States, the employer was responsible for any injury or death to his or her employees resulting from administrative negligence. *Employees* are individuals employed by another, generally for wages, in exchange for labor or services. A physician who is incorporated is also considered an employee under workers' compensation laws.

Originally, the worker had to legally prove that injury was due to negligence on the part of the employer. By the close of the 19th century, the number of accidents had increased and legal processes were uncertain; therefore, federal and state legal provisions were required. As an outcome, in the early 1900s employers' liability laws were adopted by many states, but there was still a great need for improvement. In 1911, the first workers' compensation laws were enacted allowing injured employees to receive medical care without first taking employers to court. Today, all states have workers' compensation laws.

Workers' compensation insurance is the most important coverage written to insure industrial accidents. Previously, this form of insurance was known as workmen's compensation. The term *workmen* was changed to *workers* for a more generic title and to avoid sexual bias in language. Employers will use employers' liability coverage occasionally to protect themselves when their employees do not come within the scope of a compensation law.

Workers' Compensation Statutes

There are two kinds of statutes under workers' compensation: federal compensation laws and state compensation laws. Federal laws apply to miners, maritime workers, and those who work for the government; they do not apply to state and private business employees. State compensation laws apply to employers and employees within each state, but the laws vary for each state.

The workers' compensation statutes relieve the employer of liability for injury received or illness contracted by an employee in a work situation except in gross negligence cases. They also enable the employee to be more easily and quickly compensated for loss of wages, medical expenses, and permanent disability. Before these statutes were passed, the employer could be found legally responsible for his or her employees' injuries or illnesses, and frequently there were delays in the employee's attempt to recover damages.

Workers' Compensation Reform

By 1994 in many U.S. cities, dysfunctional workers' compensation systems were costing companies more than $65 billion annually, driving insurers to deny insurance to businesses and causing companies to close their doors. Some employers began moving their businesses to states requiring lower premiums. Widespread legal and medical corruption and abuse had evolved throughout the system in the form of record high medical treatment and legal expenses. Because of these problems, reforms of the compensation of health care workers became necessary. Reform laws have been introduced in a number of states. They deal with the following:

▶ Antifraud legislation and increased penalties for workers' compensation fraud
▶ Antireferral provisions (i.e., restrictions of physicians referring patients for diagnostic studies to sites where the physician has a financial interest)
▶ Proof of the medical necessity for treatment (or tests), as well as appropriate documentation. If not adhered to, the carrier may refuse to pay the entire fee (i.e., utilization review of inpatient and outpatient claims and treatment plans)
▶ Preauthorization for major operations and expensive tests (e.g., computed tomography and magnetic resonance imaging)
▶ Caps on vocational rehabilitation
▶ Utilization of a disabled worker in another division of the company he or she was employed in so that the person may be gainfully employed while not using the injured part of the body
▶ Increase in occupational safety measures
▶ Employers offering a variety of managed care plans from which employees can choose, with some of these restricting their choice of provider (i.e., HMOs, PPOs)
▶ Development of fee schedules
▶ Medical bill review (mandatory review by law or payers' voluntary review identifying duplicate claims and billing errors)
▶ Use of mediators instead of lawyers to reach agreement between employers and the injured employee
▶ Prosecuting physicians, lawyers, and employees who abuse the system

Although far from perfect or complete, much progress has been made toward reducing high costs by trimming reimbursement for medical services and minimizing abuses of the system.

Workers' Compensation Laws and Insurance

Purposes of Workers' Compensation Laws

There are a variety of reasons for workers' compensation laws. They have been developed to accomplish the following:

1. Provide the best available medical care necessary to ensure a prompt return to work of any injured or ill employee, as well as the achievement of maximum recovery.

2. Provide income to the injured or ill worker or to his or her dependents, regardless of fault.
3. Provide a single remedy and reduce court delays, costs, and workloads arising out of personal injury litigation.
4. Relieve public and private charities of financial drains resulting from uncompensated industrial accidents.
5. Eliminate payment of fees to attorneys and witnesses as well as time-consuming trials and appeals.
6. Encourage maximum employer interest in safety and rehabilitation through an appropriate experience-rating mechanism.
7. Promote the study of causes of accidents and reduce preventable accidents and human suffering rather than concealing fault.

Self-Insurance

Another way that employers can fight high medical costs after an accident is self-insurance. A very large employer can save money by self-insuring employees for a predetermined amount of money and then purchasing policies with large deductibles to cover catastrophic problems. A self-insuring company pays for medical expenses instead of insurance premiums. Benefits are variable from plan to plan, and precertification for certain services may be required. Generally, the state insurance commissioner does not have jurisdiction over such plans. Some states may have laws that regulate self-insurers. Physicians who care for individuals under such plans may wish to negotiate payment terms to be 60 days or less.

A form of self-insurance designed to serve a small manufacturing company is known as *captive insurance.* This is best for companies that have good safety records and those willing to implement worker safety programs to keep claims to a minimum. Members of captive self-insurance programs hire an outside firm to process claims and purchase extra insurance for major claims. They share overhead expenses and investment income if any remains after paying expenses and claims. Most captive programs are based in Bermuda or the Cayman Islands to take advantage of favorable tax benefits.

Managed Care

Increasing numbers of employers are seeking managed care contracts with preferred provider organizations (PPOs) and health maintenance organizations (HMOs). Some states have adopted laws authorizing managed care programs, and other states are conducting pilot programs to test the effectiveness of managed care networks. Managed care contracts are not uniform and may limit the choice of providers, use fee schedule-based payments, require precertification for certain procedures, implement hospital and medical bill review, and incorporate utilization review of medical services.

Eligibility

Individuals entitled to workers' compensation insurance coverage are private business employees, state employees, and federal employees (e.g., postal workers, IRS employees, coal miners, maritime workers). **Workers' compensation (WC) insurance** coverage provides benefits to employees and their dependents if employees suffer work-related injury, illness, or death.

Industrial Accident

An **accident** is an unplanned and unexpected happening traceable to a definite time and place and causing **injury** (damage or loss).

Workers' compensation (industrial) accidents do not necessarily occur at the work site. For example, an individual may be asked to obtain and cash for the petty cash reserve during the lunch hour; while walking to the bank, he or she missteps off the curb, suffering a fractured ankle. This person is considered to be working, although not at the work site, and the injury is covered under workers' compensation insurance.

Occupational Illness

Occupational illness is any abnormal condition or disorder caused by exposure to environmental factors associated with employment, including acute and chronic illnesses or diseases that may be caused by inhalation, absorption, ingestion, or direct contact. Occupational diseases usually become apparent soon after exposure. However, some diseases may be latent for a considerable amount of time. Some states, therefore, have extended periods during which claims may be filed for certain slowly developing occupational diseases. These diseases might be silicosis, asbestosis, pneumoconiosis, berylliosis, anthracosilicosis, radiation disability, loss of hearing, cumulative trauma, or repetitive motion illnesses (e.g., carpal tunnel syndrome).

Coverage

Federal Laws

Employees who work for federal agencies are covered by a number of federal workers' compensation laws:

▶ *Workmen's Compensation Law of the District of Columbia.* This law became effective on May 17, 1928, and provides benefits for those working in Washington, DC.
▶ *Federal Coal Mine Health and Safety Act.* This act, also referred to as the Black Lung Benefits Act, became effective on May 7, 1941. The act provides benefits to coal miners and is administered through the national headquarters in Washington, DC.
▶ *Federal Employees' Compensation Act.* The **Federal Employees' Compensation Act (FECA)** was instituted on May 30, 1908, to provide benefits for on-the-job injuries to all federal employees. The insurance is provided through an exclusive fund system. Many different claim forms are used, depending on the type of injury. Payment is based on a schedule of maximum allowable charges. The time limit for submitting a bill is by December 31 of the year after the year in which services were rendered (or by December 31 of the year after the year the condition was accepted as work compensable, whichever is later). For further information, contact the Office of the Federal Employees' Compensation Act (FECA) by writing to the nearest office as listed in Appendix A.
▶ *Longshoremen's and Harbor Workers' Compensation Act (LHWCA).* This act became effective on March 4, 1927, and provides benefits for private or public employees engaged in maritime work nationwide. It is administered through regional offices in Boston, Chicago, Cleveland, Denver, Honolulu, Jacksonville, Kansas City, New Orleans, New York City, Philadelphia, San Francisco, Seattle, and Washington, DC. This type of insurance corresponds to that available through the private insurance system. For further information contact the nearest district office, as listed in Appendix A.

State Laws

State compensation laws cover those workers not protected by the previously mentioned federal statutes. Federal law mandates that states set up laws to meet minimum requirements. If an employer does not purchase workers' compensation insurance from a private insurance company, the employer must self-insure and have enough cash in reserve to cover the cost of medical care for all workers who suffer work-related injuries. In some instances, an employer may be reluctant to file a workers' compensation report with the state, preferring to pay medical expenses out of pocket because of not wanting premium rates to increase. It is illegal for an employer to fail to report a work-related accident when it is required by state law, and some states consider it a misdemeanor. Different penalties can be imposed, depending on state law, such as imprisonment or assessment of fines of from $50 to $2,500 or more.

In addition to workers' compensation protection, statutes also require that employers have employers' liability insurance. The difference between workers' compensation insurance and employers' liability insurance is that the latter is coverage that protects for claims arising out of bodily injury to others or damage to their property when someone is on business premises. It is not considered insurance coverage for someone who is working at a business site.

State compensation laws are either compulsory or elective, and this may be defined as follows:

1. *Compulsory law.* Each employer is required to accept its provisions and provide for specified benefits.
2. *Elective law.* The employer may accept or reject the law. If the statute of the law is rejected, the employer loses the three common-law defenses, which are
   a. Assumption of risk
   b. Negligence of fellow employees
   c. Contributory negligence

However, coverage is only elective in two states, New Jersey and Texas. Practically, this means that all laws, in effect, are "compulsory."

Minors

Minors are covered by workers' compensation, and in some states double compensation or added penalties are provided. In many states, minors also receive special legal benefit provisions.

Interstate Laws

If a worker's occupation takes him or her into another state, questions may arise as to which state's law determines payment of compensation benefits. Most compensation laws are **extraterritorial** (effective outside of the state) by either specific provisions or court decision.

Volunteer Workers

Several states have laws to compensate civil defense and other volunteer workers, such as firemen, who are injured in the line of duty.

Funding

Six states (Nevada, North Dakota, Ohio, Washington, West Virginia, Wyoming), two U.S. territories, and most provinces require employers to insure through a *monopolistic state* or *provincial fund.* Puerto Rico and the Virgin Islands require employers to insure through a *territorial fund.* In 48 states and territories, employers may qualify as self-insurers. A number of states permit employers to purchase insurance from either a competitive state fund or a private insurance company.

The employer pays the premiums for workers' compensation insurance, the amount depending on the employee's job and the risk involved in job performance. The physician usually must supply comprehensive information, and the reporting requirements vary from state to state (Table 14–1). To obtain instructions and proper forms, contact your state bureau or individual insurance carriers. State bureaus are listed in Appendix A.

Second-Injury Fund (Subsequent Injury Fund)

The **second injury fund,** also known as the **subsequent injury fund (SIF),** was established to meet problems arising when an employee has a preexisting injury or condition and is subsequently injured at work. The preexisting injury combines with the second injury to produce disability that is greater than that caused by the latter alone.

Two functions of the fund are (1) to encourage hiring of the physically handicapped and (2) to allocate more equitably the costs of providing benefits to such employees. Second-injury employers pay compensation related primarily to the disability caused by the second injury, even though the employee receives benefits relating to the combined disability; the difference is made up from the subsequent injury fund.

Scenario

Bob Evans loses his left thumb while working a lathe. Then, 2 years later, Bob loses his left index finger in a second work-related accident. A question could arise of whether the second injury added to a preexisting condition or was related to the prior injury. This case illustrates that the existence of the former injury or disability substantially increased (added to) the disability caused by the latter injury.

TABLE 14–1   **Employers' and/or Physicians' Report of Accident[1]**

Jurisdiction	Time Limit	Injuries Covered
Alabama	Within 15 days	Death or disability exceeding 3 days
Alaska	Within 10 days	Death, injury, disease, or infection
Arizona	Within 10 days	All injuries
Arkansas	10 days from notice of injury	Indemnity, injuries, or death. Medical claims reported monthly[2]
California	Immediately[3] (employer)	Death or serious injuries
	As prescribed	1-day disability or more than first aid
	Within 5 days	Occupational diseases or pesticide poisoning
Colorado	Immediately[4]	Death
	Within 10 days[4]	Injuries causing lost time of 3 days or more[4b]
	Immediately	Any accident in which three or more employees are injured
	10 days[4]	Occupational disease cases
	10 days[4]	Cases of permanent physical impairment
Connecticut	7 days or as directed	Disability of 1 day or more
Delaware	Within 48 hours[5]	Death or injuries requiring hospitalization
	Within 10 days	Other injuries
District of Columbia	Within 10 days	All injuries
Florida	Within 24 hours[6]	Death
	Within 7 days of carrier receipt of notice	All injuries
Georgia	Within 21 days[7]	All injuries requiring medical or surgical treatment or causing over 7 days of absence
Guam	Within 10 days[8]	Injury, illness, or death
Hawaii	Within 48 hours	Death
	Within 7 working days	All injuries
Idaho	As soon as practicable but not later than 10 days after the accident[9]	All injuries requiring medical treatment or causing 1 day's absence
Illinois	Within 2 working days	Death or serious injuries
	Between 15th and 25th of month	Disability of over 3 days
	As soon as determinable	Permanent disability
Indiana	Within 7 working days[10]	Disability of more than 1 day
Iowa	Within 4 days	Disability of more than 3 days, permanent partial disability, death
Kansas	Within 28 days[11]	Death
	Within 28 days	Disability of more than remainder of day or shift
Kentucky	Within 7 days[12]	Disability of more than 1 day
Louisiana	Within 10 days of employer's actual knowledge of injury[13]	Lost time over 1 week or death
Maine	Within 7 days[14]	Only injuries causing 1 day or more of lost time[14]
Maryland	Within 10 days	Disability of more than 3 days
Massachusetts	Within 7 days, except Sundays and holidays	Disability of 5 or more calendar days
Michigan	Immediately	Death disability of 7 days or more, and specific losses
Minnesota	Within 48 hours	Death or serious injury
	Within 14 days	Disability of 3 days or more
Mississippi	Within 10 days	Death or disability of more than 5 days[15]
Missouri	Within 10 days[16]	Death or injury
Montana	Within 6 days	All injuries
Nebraska	Within 48 hours[17]	Death
	Within 7 days	All injuries
Nevada	Within 6 working days after report from physician[18]	All injuries requiring medical treatment
New Hampshire	Within 5 calendar days	All injuries involving lost time or medical expenses
New Jersey	Immediately[19]	All injuries
New Mexico	Within 10 days of employer notification	Any injury or illness resulting in 7 or more days of lost time

TABLE 14–1   *continued*

Jurisdiction	Time Limit	Injuries Covered
New York	Within 10 days	Disability of 1 day beyond working day or shift on which accident occurred or requiring medical care beyond 2 first aid treatments
North Carolina	Within 5 days[20]	Disability of more than 1 day
North Dakota	Within 7 days	All injuries
Ohio	Within 1 week	Injuries causing total disability of 7 days or more
Oklahoma	Within 10 days or a reasonable time	All injuries causing lost time or requiring treatment away from worksite
Oregon	Within 5 days[21]	All injuries requiring medical treatment[21]
Pennsylvania	Within 48 hours	Death
	After 7 days but not later than 10 days	Disability of 1 day or more
Puerto Rico	Within 5 days	All injuries
Rhode Island	Within 48 hours	Death
	Within 10 days	Disability of 3 days of more and all injuries requiring medical treatment
	Within 2 years of injury	Any claim resulting in medical expense to be reported within 10 days
South Carolina	Within 10 days[22]	All injuries requiring medical attention costing more than $500, more than 1 day disability or permanency
South Dakota	Within 7 days	All injuries[23]
Tennessee	Within 14 days	All injuries requiring medical attention
Texas	Within 8 days[22]	Disability of more than 1 day, or occupational disease
Utah	Within 7 days	All injuries requiring medical attention
Vermont	Within 72 hours[22]	Disability of 1 day or more requiring medical care
Virgin Islands	Within 8 days	Injury or disease
Virginia	Within 10 days[22]	All injuries
Washington	Within 8 hours	Death and accidents resulting in workers' hospitalizations or inability to work
West Virginia	Within 5 days	All injuries
Wisconsin	Within 14 days	Disability beyond 3-day waiting period
Wyoming	Within 10 days	Compensable injuries
FECA	Immediately	All injuries involving medical expenses, disability, or death
LHWCA	10 days	Injuries that cause loss of 1 or more shifts of work or death

[1]Federal Occupational Safety and Health Act of 1970 established uniform requirements and forms to meet its criteria for all businesses affecting interstate commerce to be used for statistical purposes and compliance with the Act. 12 U.S.C. §651.

[2]Arkansas—Medical only claims reported monthly.

[3]California. To Division of Occupational Safety and Health. Within 5 days of employer's notice or knowledge of employee death, employer must report death to the Department of Industrial Relations.

[4]Colorado. (a) Failure to report tolls time limit for claims. (b) Disability of less than 3 days must be reported to insurer.

[5]Delaware. Supplemental report upon termination of disability.

[6]Florida. Report to carrier within 7 days, if injury caused employee to lose 7 or more work days. Supplemental report within 30 days after final payment.

[7]Georgia. Supplemental report on first payment and suspension of payment and within 30 days after final payment.

[8]Guam. Failure to report tolls limits for claims.

[9]Supplemental report required after 60 days (for Rhode Island and South Carolina every 6 months), or upon termination of disability.

[10]Indiana. Supplemental report within 10 days after termination of compensation period.

[11]Kansas. Failure to report tolls time limit for claims. Childress v. Childress Painting Co., 1979.

[12]Kentucky. Supplemental report required after 80 days or upon termination of disability

[13]Louisiana. Employers with more than 10 employees must also report, within 90 days, death, any nonfatal occupational illness or injury causing loss of consciousness, restriction of work or motion, job transfer, or medical treatment other than first aid. Violation of confidentiality of any record, subject to $500 fine.

[14]Maine. Must report asbestosis, mesothelioma, silicosis, and exposure to heavy metals no later than 30 days from date of diagnosis.

[15]Mississippi—Permanent disability, serious head or facial disfigurement also covered. $100 may be added to any award and $100 may be ordered payable to the Commission.

continued

TABLE 14-1	*continued*

[16]Missouri. Supplemental report within 1 month after original notice to Division.

[17]Nebraska. Report may be made by insurance carrier or employer. Failure to report tolls time limits.

[18]Nevada. For minor injuries not requiring medical treatment, the employee may file a "Notice of Injury," which must be retained by the employer for 3 years.

[19]New Jersey. Uninsured employers are required to report compensable injuries only. If insured, carrier is also required to make report.

[20]North Carolina. Supplemental report required after 60 days or upon termination of disability.

[21]Oregon. Insurers to send disabling claims to Workers' Compensation Department within 21 days of employer knowledge.

[22]South Carolina, Texas, Vermont, and Virginia. Supplemental report required after 60 days or upon termination of disability.

[23]South Dakota. Any injury that requires treatment other than first aid or that incapacitates employee for at least 7 calendar days.

Minimum Number of Employees

Table 14–2 shows the minimum number of employees required by each state before the state workers' compensation law comes into effect. There are exemptions in many states for certain occupations such as domestic or casual employees, laborers, babysitters, newspaper vendors or distributors, charity workers, and gardeners. Some states do not require compensation insurance for farm laborers or may need a larger number of farm employees than the number shown in the table.

Waiting Periods

The laws state that a **waiting period (WP)** must elapse before income benefits are payable. This waiting period affects only wage compensation because medical and hospital care are provided immediately. To find the waiting period of your state, see Table 14–3.

State Disability and Workers' Compensation

Five states and one U.S. territory have state disability insurance (also known as unemployment

TABLE 14–2	**Minimum Number of Employees for State Workers' Compensation Laws**

No. of Employees				
1		*3*	*4*	*5*
Alaska	Nebraska	American Samoa	Florida	Alabama
Arizona	Nevada	Arkansas	South Carolina	Mississippi
California	New Hampshire	Georgia		Missouri
Colorado	New Jersey	Michigan		Tennessee
Connecticut	New York	New Mexico		
Delaware	North Dakota	North Carolina		
District of Columbia	Ohio	Virginia		
Guam	Oklahoma			
Hawaii	Oregon			
Idaho	Pennsylvania			
Illinois	Puerto Rico			
Indiana	Rhode Island			
Iowa	South Dakota			
Kansas	Texas			
Kentucky	Utah			
Louisiana	Vermont			
Maine	Virgin Islands			
Maryland	Washington			
Massachusetts	West Virginia			
Minnesota	Wisconsin			
Montana	Wyoming			

| TABLE 14–3 | Waiting Period for Income Benefits; Medical Benefits* | | |

Jurisdiction	Waiting Period (Days)	Jurisdiction	Waiting Period (Days)
Alabama	3	Nebraska	7
Alaska	3	Nevada	5
Arizona	7	New Hampshire	3
Arkansas	7	New Jersey	7
California	3	New Mexico	7
Colorado	3	New York	7
Connecticut	3	North Carolina	7
Delaware	3	North Dakota	5
District of Columbia	3	Ohio	7
Florida	7	Oklahoma	3
Georgia	7	Oregon	3
Guam	3	Pennsylvania	7
Hawaii	3	Puerto Rico	3
Idaho	5	Rhode Island	3
Illinois	3	South Carolina	7
Indiana	7	South Dakota	7
Iowa	3	Tennessee	7
Kansas	0	Texas	7
Kentucky	7	Utah	3
Louisiana	7	Vermont	3
Maine	7	Virgin Islands	0
Maryland	3	Virginia	7
Massachusetts	5	Washington	3
Michigan	7	West Virginia	3
Minnesota	3	Wisconsin	3
Mississippi	5	Wyoming	3
Missouri	3	FECA	3
Montana	6	LHWCA	3

*These are statutory provisions for waiting periods. Statutes provide that a waiting period must elapse during which income benefits are not payable. This waiting period affects only compensation, because medical and hospital care are provided immediately.

FECA. Federal Employees Compensation Act. LHWCA. Longshoremen's and Harbor Workers' Compensation Act.

compensation disability insurance): California, Hawaii, New Jersey, New York, and Rhode Island, along with Puerto Rico. If a recipient is collecting benefits from a workers' compensation insurance carrier and the amount that the compensation carrier pays is less than that allowed by the state disability insurance program, then the latter will pay the balance. See Chapter 15 for further information on state disability insurance.

Benefits

Five principal types of state compensation benefits that may apply in ordinary cases are

1. *Medical treatment.* This includes hospital, medical, and surgical services, medications, and prosthetic devices. Treatment may be rendered by a licensed physician, osteopath, dentist, or chiropractor.
2. *Temporary disability indemnity.* This is in the form of weekly cash payments made directly to the injured or ill person.
3. *Permanent disability indemnity.* This may consist of either weekly or monthly cash payments based on a rating system that determines the percentage of permanent disability or a lump sum award. California has a unique system of permanent disability evaluation that requires a separate determination by the disability rating bureau in San Francisco. No other state has this system.
4. *Death benefits for survivors.* This consists of cash payments to dependents of employees who

are fatally injured. In some states, a burial allowance is also given.

5. *Rehabilitation benefits.* In cases of severe disabilities, this can be either medical or vocational rehabilitation.

Types of State Claims

There are three types of state workers' compensation claims: nondisability claims, temporary disability claims, and permanent disability claims. Each type will be discussed in detail for a clear definition and an understanding of the determination process.

Nondisability Claim

This is the simplest type of claim. Generally, a **nondisability (ND) claim** involves a minor injury in which the patient is seen by the doctor but is able to continue working (Fig. 14–1). This type of case would not require weekly temporary disability payments.

Temporary Disability Claim

Temporary disability (TD) occurs when a worker has a work-related injury or illness and is unable to perform the duties of his or her occupation. The time period of temporary disability can extend from the date of injury until the worker either returns to full duty without residual rateable disability (discussed later), returns to modified work, or has rateable residual disability that the physician states is permanent and stationary.

An **insurance adjuster** is the person at the workers' compensation insurance carrier overseeing the industrial case. He or she is responsible for keeping in contact with the physician's office regarding the patient's ongoing progress. The insurance adjuster's most important function is to *adjust an industrial claim.* This means that the insurance adjuster must evaluate the injury or illness, predict in advance the amount of money reserves needed to cover medical expenses, and calculate as accurate a reserve as possible for weekly TD payments to the injured. This is frequently a difficult task, because a seemingly minor back strain may ultimately require fusion or a small cut may become gangrenous and lead to an amputation. The insurance carrier wants to provide the best possible medical care for the patient. If a specialist is required on a case, the patient will be immediately referred to the specialist.

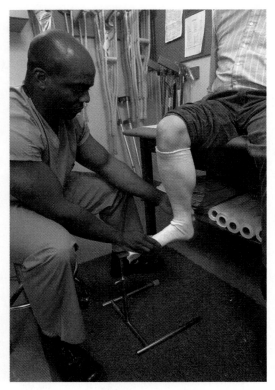

Figure 14–1. Physician interacting with an injured worker in the examination room.

Usually workers' compensation weekly TD payments are based on the employee's earnings at the time of the injury. Compensation benefits are not subject to income tax.

Sometimes a patient is released to modified work to effect a transition between the period of inactivity due to disability and a return to full duty, especially when heavy work is involved. Other times an employee is returned to the company and placed in a different department or division so he or she is gainfully employed while not using the injured body part. This topic is further detailed in the next section.

Vocational Rehabilitation

Many states provide rehabilitation in the form of retraining, education, job guidance, and placement, to assist an injured individual in finding work before temporary disability compensation benefits expire. In any successful rehabilitation program, insurance carrier, physician, physical therapist, employer supervisor, and personnel department must act as a team with the common goal of getting an injured employee back to light duty or regular work as soon as possible. It is believed that the longer a person remains out of work, the less chance there is that he or she will return to the workplace. The employer and insurance adjuster must keep in communication with rehabilitation center therapists to determine when the injured person will be able to resume some form of work. The physician may suggest a rehabilitation center that provides good care, or the employer may have an in-house program.

Work Hardening

Sports medicine therapy and physical medicine rehabilitation are often used to strengthen the injured worker. Physical medicine/therapy CPT codes 97001 to 97542 are used to report these services. Another type of therapy, called **work hardening,** is an individualized program using simulated or real work tasks to build up strength and improve the worker's endurance toward a full day's work. CPT codes 97545 and 97546 are used to report work hardening conditioning.

Ergonomics

In some cases, an **ergonomic** evaluation of the work site is performed and modifications may be instituted to the job or work site to lessen the possibility of future injury and to get the employee back to gainful employment. CPT code 97537 may be used to report a work site modification analysis. Injured individuals may also be retrained into another career field if their disability prevents them from returning to their former occupation.

Permanent Disability Claim

In this type of claim the patient or injured party is usually on TD benefits for a time and then concludes that he or she is unable to return to his or her former occupation. The physician states in the report that the patient has residual disability that will hamper his or her opportunity to compete in the open job market. Examples of residual disability include loss of a hand, an eye, or a leg or neurologic problems. Each patient who has **permanent disability (PD)** is rated according to the severity of the injury, the age of the injured person, and the patient's occupation at the time of the injury. The older the person, the greater the PD benefit. One might think that a younger person deserves higher compensation because he or she will be disabled for a longer portion of his or her working career. However, the workers' compensation laws assume that a young person has a better chance of being rehabilitated into another occupation.

In a PD claim, the physician's final report must include the words **"permanent and stationary" (P and S).** This phrase means that damage from the injury or illness is permanent, the patient has recovered to the fullest extent possible, the physician is unable to do anything more for the patient, and the patient will be hampered by the disability to some extent for the rest of his or her life. The P and S examination is usually a comprehensive examination, and a level 5 CPT code may be appropriate. Depending on the fee schedule, a modifier indicating that the Evaluation and Management service is a P and S examination may also be used. The case is rated for PD, and a settlement is made called a **compromise and release (C and R).** This is an agreement between the injured party and the insurance company on a total sum. The case can then be closed.

Reasons that may delay closing a workers' compensation case include the following:

1. Unanswered questions or incomplete answers to data required on workers' compensation forms by either the employee, employer, or physician
2. Vague terminology used by the physician in medical reports
3. Omitted signatures on forms or written reports by the employee, employer, or physician
4. Incorrect billing by the physician's office
5. Inadequate progress reports (e.g., the physician fails to send in a medical report routinely to update the insurance carrier when the injured employee is seen in subsequent visits)

Rating

Final determination of the issues involving settlement of an industrial accident is known as **adjudication,** or the rating of a case. A physician does not rate disability but renders a professional opinion on whether the injured individual has temporary or permanent disability that prevents him or her from gainful employment. Rating itself is carried out by the state's industrial accident commission or workers' compensation board. Wage loss, earning capacity, and physical impairment are three categories that may be taken into consideration to rate temporary partial, permanent partial, or total disabilities.

In addition, permanent partial disabilities may be rated by using a scheduled or nonscheduled injury award system. This system is based on a set number of weeks of compensation for a specific loss, such as 288 weeks for the loss of a leg. Scheduled injuries may include loss of a body part, disfigurement, permanent hearing loss, and so on. Nonscheduled injuries are more general, such as disability due to injury to the back or neck.

If an injured person is dissatisfied with the rating after the case has been declared P and S, he or she may appeal the case (by **petition**—formal written request) to the **Workers' Compensation Appeals Board (WCAB)** or the Industrial Accident Commission.

Surveillance

In rating a case, **sub rosa films** are sometimes provided to document the extent of a patient's permanent disability. Sub rosa means "under the rose." In ancient times, the rose was a symbol of silence or secrecy. Videotapes are made over a period of 2 to 3 days without the patient's knowledge. This surveillance is expensive and is used as a last resort, especially in cases where a person receiving workers' compensation benefits is suspected of making exaggerated complaints. It is also used in cases when a worker has been off work for a long period of time and is supposedly unable to perform any work activity, not even light duty.

Investigators have been known to carry a camera in a gym bag and videotape a supposedly disabled claimant bench pressing at the gym. Patients have also been videotaped going into the physician's office for an appointment wearing a neck brace and removing the brace on returning to their car.

Fraud and Abuse

In the 1990s, increases for fraudulent workers' compensation claims were noted throughout many large metropolitan cities. These problems involved employers, employees, insurers, medical providers, and lawyers. An increasing number of states have enacted some kind of antifraud legislation and stiffened penalties for workers' compensation fraud, making it a felony. Some states require reporting suspected insurance fraud and have forms to incorporate wording in regard to fraudulent statements. An example is shown in Figure 14–2.

Physicians are responsible for determining the legitimacy of work injuries and reporting findings accurately. If a report is prepared with the intent to use it in support of a fraudulent claim, or if a fraudulent claim is knowingly submitted for payment under an insurance contract, the physician may be subject to fines and/or imprisonment and the revocation or suspension of a medical license. Some physicians sign and send a disclosure statement with the medical report certifying that they personally performed an evaluation. The physician may list the total time spent in reviewing records, face-to-face time with the patient, preparation of a report, and other relevant activities.

It is the responsibility of all individuals who deal with workers' compensation cases to notify the insurance carrier of any suspicious situation. By doing so, action can be taken to have the case investigated further by personnel from the fraud divisions or referred to the district attorney's office. Perpetrators and signs of workers' compensation fraud and abuse are listed in Table 14–4.

For further information on fraud and abuse in the medical setting, see Chapters 1, 11, and 12.

Occupational Safety and Health Administration (OSHA) Act of 1970

Background

Congress has established an office known as the **Occupational Safety and Health Administration (OSHA)** to protect employees against on-the-job health and safety hazards. This program includes strict health and safety standards and a sensible complaint procedure enabling individual workers to trigger enforcement measures.

Work standards are designed to minimize exposure to on-the-job hazards such as faulty machinery, noise, dust, and toxic chemical fumes. Employers are required by law to meet these health and safety standards. Failure to do so can result in fines against the employer that could run into thousands of dollars.

Coverage

The Act provides that if a state submits an OSHA plan and it is approved by the government, then the state may assume responsibility for carrying out OSHA policies and procedures and is excluded from federal jurisdiction.

The Act applies to almost all businesses, large or small. It applies to heavy, light, and service industries, nonprofit and charitable institutions, churches' secular activities in hospitals, farmers, and retailers. Employees of state and local governments are also covered. Federal employees, a farmer's immediate family, church employees engaged in religious activities, independent contractors, and household domestic workers are *not* covered.

Regulations

Specific regulations that affect the medical setting are those aimed at minimizing exposure to hepatitis B virus (HBV), human immunodeficiency virus (HIV), and other bloodborne pathogens. Any worker who comes in contact with human blood

State of California
Department of Industrial Relations
DIVISION OF WORKERS' COMPENSATION

Estado de California
Departmento de Relaciones Industriales
DIVISION DE COMPENSACIÓN AL TRABAJADOR

EMPLOYEE'S CLAIM FOR WORKERS' COMPENSATION BENEFITS

PETICION DEL EMPLEADO PARA BENEFICIOS DE COMPENSACIÓN DEL TRABAJADOR

If you are injured or become ill because of your job, you may be entitled to workers' compensation benefits.

Complete the **"Employee"** section and give the form to your employer. Keep the copy marked **"Employee's Temporary Receipt"** until you receive the dated copy from your employer. You may call the Division of Workers' Compensation at **1-800-736-7401** if you need help in filling out this form or in obtaining your benefits. An explanation of workers' compensation benefits is included on the back of this form.

You should also have received a pamphlet from your employer describing workers' compensation benefits and the procedures to obtain them.

Si Ud. se ha lesionado o se ha enfermado a causa de su trabajo, Ud. tiene derecho a recibir beneficios de compensación al trabajador.
Complete la sección "Empleado" y entregue la forma a su empleador. Quédese con la copia designada "Recibo Temporal del Empleado" hasta que Ud. reciba la copia fechada de su empleador. Si Ud. necesita ayuda para completar esta forma o para obtener sus beneficios, Ud. puede hablar con la Division de Compensación al Trabajador llamando al 1-800-736-7401. En la parte de atrás de esta forma se encuentra una explicación de los beneficios de la compensación al trabajador.

Ud. también debería haber recibido de su empleador un folleto describiendo los beneficios de compensación al trabajador lesionado y los procedimientos para obtenerlos.

Any person who makes or causes to be made any knowingly false or fraudulent material statement or material representation for the purpose of obtaining or denying workers' compensation benefits or payments is guilty of a felony.

Toda aquella persona que a propósito haga o cause que se produzca cualquier declaración o representación material falsa o fraudulenta con el fin de obtener o negar beneficios o pagos de compensación a trabajadores lesionados es culpable de un crimen mayor "felonía".

Employee: *Empleado*

1. Name. *Nombre.* Ima B. Hurt   Today's date. *Fecha de hoy.* 4-3-20XX
2. Home address. *Dirección residencial.* 300 East Central Avenue
3. City. *Ciudad.* Woodland Hills   State. *Estado.* XY   Zip. *Código postal* 12345-0001
4. Date of injury. *Fecha de la lesión (accidente).* 4-3-XX   Time of injury. *Hora en que ocurrió.* ___ a.m. 2:00 p.m.
5. Address and description of where injury happened. *Dirección/lugar dónde occurió el accidente.* The Conk Out Company
   45 South Gorman Street, Woodland Hills, XY 12345   injured in stock room
6. Describe injury and part of body affected. *Describa la lesión y parte dél cuerpo afectada.* Fell off ladder in stock room.
   Injured left ankle.
7. Social Security Number. *Número de Seguro Social del Empleado.* 120 23 6542
8. Signature of employees. *Firma del empleado.* *Ima B. Hurt*

Employer—complete this section and give the employee a copy immediately as a receipt.
Empleador–complete esta sección y déle inmediatamente una copia al empleado como recibo.

9. Name of employer. *Nombre del empleador.* The Conk Out Company
10. Address. *Dirección.* 45 South Gorman Street, Woodland Hills, XY 12345
11. Date employer first knew of injury. *Fecha en que el empleador supo por primera vez de la lesión o accidente.* 4-3-20XX
12. Date claim form was provided to employee. *Fecha en que se le entregó al empleado la petición.* 4-3-20XX
13. Date employer received claim form. *Fecha en que el empleado devolvió la petición al empleador.* 4-3-20XX
14. Name and address of insurance carrier or adjusting agency. *Nombre y dirección de la compañía de seguros o agencia administradora de seguros.* XYZ Insurance Company, P.O. Box 5, Woodland Hills, XY 12345
15. Insurance policy number. *El número de la poliza del Seguro.* B 12345
16. Signature of employer representative. *Firma del representante del empleador.* *J. D. Hawkins*
17. Title. *Título.* Owner   18. Telephone. *Teléfono.* 013-430-3488

Employer: You are required to date this form and provide copies to your insurer or claims administrator and to the employee, dependent or representative who filed the claim within **one working day** of receipt of the form from the employee.

SIGNING THIS FORM IS NOT AN ADMISSION OF LIABILITY

Empleador: Se requiere que Ud. feche esta forma y que provéa copias a su compañía de seguros, administrador de reclamos, o dependiente/répresentante de reclamos y al empleado que hayan presentado esta petición dentro del plazo de **un día hábil** desde el momento de haber sido recibida la forma del empleado.

EL FIRMAR ESTA FORMA NO SIGNIFICA ADMISION DE RESPONSABILIDAD

Original (Employer's Copy)
DWC Form 1 (REV. 1/94)

ORIGINAL (Copia del Empleador)
DWC Forma 1 (REV. 1/94)

Figure 14–2. Employee's Claim for Workers' Compensation Benefits. Notice the insert regarding fraudulent material.

TABLE 14–4	Perpetrators and Signs of Workers' Compensation Fraud and Abuse

Employee

■ Misses the first physician's visit
■ Cannot describe the pain or is overly dramatic, such as an employee who comes into the physician's office limping on the left leg, suddenly starts limping on the right leg, and then goes back to limping on the left leg
■ Delays in reporting the injury
■ Does not report Friday's injury until Monday morning
■ First reports an injury to a legal or regulatory agency
■ Reports an injury after missing several days of work
■ Changes physicians frequently
■ Is a short-term worker
■ Has a curious claim history
■ Fabricates an injury
■ Exaggerates a work-related injury to obtain larger benefits, such as an injured employee who has a back pain and claims inability to bend over or lift. Surveillance cameras capture the individual at work on weekends repairing cars in the driveway at home—a task he is supposedly unable to perform
■ Blames an injury that occurred off the job on the employer

Employer

■ Misrepresents the annual payroll to get lower premium rates
■ Misrepresents the number of workers employed
■ Gives a false address with the least expensive premium rates
■ Falsely classifies the job duties of workers (as not hazardous), such as stating the job title as a clerical worker when, in fact, the employee is using a lathe every day

Insurer

■ Refuses to pay valid medical claims
■ Forces the injured worker to settle by using unethical tactics. An insurance agent told an employee that he had a back sprain. Relying on that information, the worker settled the case. Later, a myelogram revealed a herniated intervertebral disk. The patient was left with a permanent partial disability.

Medical Provider

■ Orders or performs unnecessary tests
■ Renders unnecessary treatment
■ Charges the insurance carrier for services never rendered
■ Participates in a provider mill scheme (see explanation under "lawyer")
■ Makes multiple referrals from a clinic practice regardless of type of injury
■ Sends medical reports that look photocopied with the same information typed in (e.g., employer's address, description of injury) or that read almost identical to other reports
■ Sends in many claims in which injuries are of a subjective nature, such as stress, emotional distress, headaches, inability to sleep
■ Sends in claims from one employer showing several employees with similar injuries, using the same physicians and/or attorneys

Lawyer

■ Overbills clients
■ Participates in a medical provider mill scheme. An individual is solicited while in the unemployment line by a recruiter known as a "capper." The capper tells the worker it is possible to obtain more money on disability than through unemployment. The worker is referred to an attorney and a "provider mill" clinic, which help the individual fabricate a claim by claiming stress or an on-the-job injury. In some states, such acts may be considered a public offense and punishable as a misdemeanor or felony.

and infectious materials must receive proper information and training and use universal precautions to avoid infection. Vaccinations must be provided for those who are at risk for exposure to hepatitis B, and comprehensive records must be maintained. For fact sheets, booklets, and guidelines on bloodborne pathogens, contact the nearest OSHA office or write to OSHA Publications Office, 200 Constitution Avenue, NW, Room N3101, Washington, DC 20210.

In many work settings, chemicals and hazardous substances are used that impose dangers. Businesses are required to obtain material safety data sheets (MSDS) for each hazardous chemical used on site. Employers that produce a hazardous chemical must develop material safety data sheets. A compliance kit is available from the Superintendent of Documents, U.S. Government Printing Office, Washington, DC 20402.

Filing a Complaint

To file a complaint, the proper form is obtained from the federal Division of Industrial Safety or a state OSHA office and completed by the employee.

It is against the law for an employer to take any adverse action against an employee who files such a complaint.

Inspection

A compliance officer (inspector) may call for an appointment or may be sent unannounced to the place of employment. If an officer arrives unannounced, the office manager must be notified so an appointment may be arranged for the inspection to take place. A court warrant may be required to search a company's premises if the employer does not consent to OSHA entry. A business may be cited and, depending on the violation, fines and/or criminal penalties may be imposed.

Record Keeping and Reporting

Employers must keep records of their employees' work-related injuries and illnesses on OSHA Form No. 200. Forms may be obtained from the OSHA office or from any office of the U.S. Department of Labor. This document must be on file at the workplace and available to employees and OSHA compliance officers on request. Form 200 must be retained in the file for 5 years. After 6 days, a case recorded on Form 200 must have a supplementary record, OSHA Form 101, completed and kept in the files. Some states have modified their workers' compensation forms so they may be used as substitutes for Form 101. Certain low-hazard industries are exempt from having to complete and retain Forms 200 and 101.

Companies with under 11 employees must complete safety survey OSHA Form 200-S. Companies are also required to display OSHA posters to inform employees of their job safety rights. Federal law states that an accident that results in the death or hospitalization of five or more employees must be reported to OSHA.

Legal Situations

Medical Evaluator

Physicians who conduct medicolegal evaluations of injured workers must pass a complex medical examination. They are then certified by the Industrial Medical Council (IMC) and may be referred to under one of the following titles:

▶ Agreed Medical Evaluator (AME)
▶ Independent Medical Evaluator (IME)
▶ Qualified Medical Evaluator (QME)

The medical evaluator is hired by the insurance company or appointed by the referee or appeals board to examine an individual, independent from the attending physician, and render an unbiased opinion regarding the degree of disability of an injured worker. When the physician performs an evaluation on an injured worker, the workers' compensation fee schedule may have specific procedure codes to bill for the examination. Evaluation and Management consultation codes or the CPT code for work-related evaluation by "other" physician, 99456, may be used. Some state fee schedules may have specific medical legal (ML) procedure codes to bill for various levels of examination. When a case involves a medical evaluation, a deposition may be taken of his or her testimony.

Depositions

A **deposition** is a proceeding in which an attorney asks a witness questions regarding a case, and the witness answers under oath but not in open court. It may take place in the attorney's office or often in the physician's office. In permanent disability workers' compensation cases, depositions are usually taken from the physician and the injured party by the attorney representing the workers' compensation insurance company. If the witness is the defendant, his or her attorney is also present. Direct and cross examination may be done by both attorneys.

The session may be recorded on a stenotype machine, in shorthand, or by audio or videotape. Video depositions are used in several instances. For example, if a plaintiff in a case is terminally ill and the plaintiff's attorney wishes to preserve the plaintiff's testimony, a video deposition may be used as substantive (essential) evidence. Or, if a witness cannot be present at the trial, a video deposition may be taken. In a case in which a witness may be in Arizona and cannot appear in Pennsylvania, the attorney takes the deposition in Arizona and proves to the court that the witness is beyond its jurisdiction. The same is true for a physician defendant who is not available for some reason.

Exhibits may be entered into evidence. The witness is allowed to read the transcript and make corrections or changes. The witness may be asked to sign the transcript but can waive signature if his or her attorney does not wish this to be done. The deposition is used when the case comes to trial.

Depositions may be taken to find out additional information, the physician's version of the facts, the patient's version of the facts, what kind of witnesses the physician and the patient will be, and so on. Another use for a deposition is to impeach (challenge the credibility or validity of) a witness on cross examination. If the witness takes the stand and the testimony is inconsistent with the deposition, the attorney will make this known to the jury.

Medical Testimony

In the instance of an accident case with third party liability, the physician may have to testify as an expert witness, take time to give a deposition, or attend a pretrial conference. It is important that there be a clear understanding of the terms of testimony and payment to eliminate any future misunderstandings. A written agreement from the patient's lawyer should be obtained stating exactly what compensation the physician will receive for research (preparation), time spent waiting to testify (if appointments must be canceled), and actual testimony time (Fig. 14–3). In some cases, the physician may want to ask for partial payment in advance. If the physician is subpoenaed, he or she must appear in court regardless of whether an agreement exists. The correct CPT code for medical testimony is 99075. This agreement should be signed by the physician and sent to the attorney. The attorney should return the original to the physician, retaining a copy for his or her files.

Liens

The word **lien** derives from the same origin as the word *liable*, and the right of lien expresses legal claim on the property of another for the payment of a debt (Fig. 14–4). Liens are sometimes called encumbrances and may be filed for a number of reasons.

MEDICAL TESTIMONY AGREEMENT

AGREEMENT made this _____ day of _____ 20xx, between _____
herein referred to as attorney, and _____ ,
of _____ , _____ , _____ _____ , a licensed _____ .
 (street address)   (city)   (state)   (ZIP code)

In consideration of their mutual covenants set forth herein, the parties agree as follows:

1. The doctor will give medical testimony in the case of:
_____
as a treating physician or as an expert witness (delete the unwanted phrase).

2. The doctor agrees to appear promptly when called and to present his medical testimony in a well-prepared professional manner.

3. The doctor will be compensated for time away from the practice of his or her medical duties in accordance with the following:
  (a) $_____ per hour for reports and preparation of medical testimony.
  (b) $_____ per hour for pre-trial conferences.
  (c) $_____ per hour for court appearance, including travel time to and from the office.
  (d) $_____ per hour for deposition.
  (e) $_____ per hour for being on call with cancellation of appointments but not appearing in court.

4. The doctor will appear in court on_____ hour's notice from the attorney, unless prior arrangements have been made for the exact time of appearance.

5. The doctor will be compensated on completion of his or her medical testimony and payment will not be contingent upon the outcome of the case. However, if the case is settled before reaching the court, the doctor will be compensated for being on call as noted above.

This contract shall be binding upon the parties.

IN WITNESS WHEREOF, the said parties hereto have subscribed their respective signatures.

_____
 (physician)

_____
 (attorney)

Date:_____

Figure 14–3. Example of a medical testimony agreement between physician and attorney. This is signed by the physician and sent to the attorney for signature. A copy is retained by the attorney, and the original is kept by the physician.

The advantages of filing a lien are as follows:

▶ It is a written agreement and will be recognized in court.

▶ It is a source of protection in the event of litigation.

▶ It ensures that payment for previously rendered medical services will be received when the attorney and patient have reached a settlement with the insurance company in an accident case.

▶ It is an inexpensive method of collecting the fee. The physician can file suit and try to get a judgment against the patient, but this is relatively expensive in comparison with filing a lien.

▶ The physician will collect the full fee. If the physician assigns such a delinquent account to a collection agency, he or she may lose as much as 50% of the fee when it is collected.

▶ If the physician wishes to bill more than what is allowed for a given service or services, a lien can be filed and the judge will determine whether it is reasonable.

▶ It avoids harassment in trying to collect the bill.

The chief disadvantage of not filing a lien is that there is no legal documentation should the case go to court as far as collecting monies owed to the physician. A case could be settled, the attorney would get his or her fee, and the physician's fee may be placed last on the list for payment or remain unpaid.

Scenarios

Problem 1. Suppose Attorney Blake advises a client Roger Reed not to pay the physician until after the trial. Or, what happens if payment is not made for Dr. Practon's courtroom testimony and the case is lost? Suppose medical reports are ordered and Attorney Blake neglects to pay for them. What happens if Roger Reed forgets about the physician's bill?

Solution. If a lien had been signed, then once the case has been settled, the money would be paid to the physician; otherwise, the settlement would belong to the patient, Roger Reed, and he could take any action with the money that he wanted.

Problem 2. Suppose Dr. Practon had an oral agreement covering his fee. The patient, Katie Crest, was unable to pay for medical treatment except on legal monetary recovery. When Katie Crest settled her case, the proceeds went almost entirely to welfare agencies because she received retroactive Medicaid. Dr. Practon sued the patient's attorney and lost.

Solution. If Dr. Practon had gotten a written assignment of the proceeds, the lawyer could have been held liable for the fee.

When you fill out a lien form, specify a time limit, because litigation may take several years before settlement is reached. Some patients may be persuaded to pay before a legal settlement is made or at least to make payments until a settlement is reached. At the end of the time limit, the lien becomes null and void. If the patient's financial status has changed, you might be able to collect because you can now bill the patient. If not, file an amended or subsequent lien stating the actual balance of the patient's account. Type the word "amended" on the new lien below the Workers' Compensation Appeals Board case number.

Protect the physician's fee by asking the attorney to sign the lien, thereby indicating that he or she will pay the physician directly from any money received in a settlement. This makes the attorney responsible for the fee. The patient's file must be placed in a Hold for Settlement category until the case comes up in court. In some states, the physician's fee owed by the patient constitutes a first lien against any such money settlement, and the attorney must first satisfy the lien of the physician before the patient or attorney receives any money from the settlement. Check the laws of your state. Call the office of the patient's attorney at least quarterly for an update.

If there is a third party litigation involved in an industrial case or a decision has not been reached as to whether an accident is due to industrial or nonindustrial causes, file both a regular lien and a workers' compensation lien. In most states, a special lien form for workers' compensation filing is available and should be used. A copy of the lien should be completed and sent to all concerned parties:

▶ Appeals board
▶ Employer of the patient
▶ Employee (the patient)
▶ Insurance carrier
▶ Physician's files (lien claimant or one who is filing for the lien)

The patient/employee consents to the lien by his or her signature. Do not accept a lien form unless it is also signed by the patient's attorney. Check with your local Division of Industrial Accidents for forms pertinent to filing a lien and instructions on the formalities, number of copies required, and where they are to be sent.

Third Party Subrogation

The legal term **third party subrogation** means "to substitute" one person for another. When applied to workers' compensation cases, it means a transfer of the claims and rights from the original creditor (workers' compensation insurance carrier) to the third party liability carrier. In a compensation case involving third party subrogation, the participants are the patient, the insurance carrier, and a third party responsible for the injury sometimes referred to as **third party liability.**

Scenario

Problem. Monica Valdez, a secretary, goes to the bank to deposit some money for her employer. While on the errand, Monica's car is rear-ended by another automobile and she is injured.

Solution. In such a case there is no question of fault and no question of cause. Monica was hurt during the performance of her work, and the workers' compensation insurance carrier is liable. The carrier must adjust the claim, provide all medical treatment, and pay all TD and PD benefits.

However, the insurance carrier does have legal recourse. It may send a representative to visit with Monica, explain to her that she has a good subrogation case, encourage her to seek the advice of an attorney, and sue the third party (other automobile driver) in civil court. This is sometimes referred to as litigation, which is the process of carrying on a lawsuit. If Monica agrees to sue, the insurance carrier files a demand with the court for repayment of all the money that it has paid out. This is called a lien, which was discussed earlier in the chapter. When the case is settled, if an award is made to Monica, the insurance carrier is reimbursed for all that it has paid and Monica receives the balance. In some states, such as California, the patient is legally prevented from collecting twice.

If the patient's attorney should call the physician's office for information, it is only ethical and legal to get a signed authorization from the patient and also to ask permission from the insurance carrier before giving out any medical information. Remember that the contract exists between the physician and the insurance carrier, not the physician and the patient.

Medical Reports

Confidentiality

There is a difference in the treatment of confidentiality for certain records in industrial cases. In most states, insurance claims adjusters have unlimited access to the injured employee's medical records that pertain only to the industrial case. Some states allow employers similar access. However, check with your state laws to see if both employer and insurance company must sign an authorization to release records before giving them to a third party.

Documentation

Documentation must always show the necessity for the procedures performed. If there is not an accurate diagnostic code to explain the patient's condition, a report should be sent describing the details of the diagnosis. CPT code 99080 may be used to bill for workers' compensation reports. The monetary value assigned to the code is usually determined by the number of pages in the report. If medical records are reviewed before consulting or treating a workers' compensation patient, submit a bill for this service. Refer to Chapter 3, Documentation, for comprehensive information on this topic.

Medical Record Keeping

If a private patient comes to the office with an industrial injury, set up a separate medical record (chart) and financial record (ledger) for the work-related injury. Never mix a private medical record with an industrial case because there are separate disclosure laws for each and because the workers' compensation case may go to court. Some medical practices use a colored file folder or colored tabs for the industrial medical record, making filing of all private and workers' compensation documents easier for the insurance billing specialist. If two charts are maintained, it is easy to pull the industrial medical record and ledger quickly without having to dig through the patients' previously unrelated private medical records.

It is preferable never to schedule a patient to see the physician for a workers' compensation follow-up examination and an unrelated complaint during the same appointment time. Separate appointments (back to back, if necessary) need to be arranged. This allows for separate dictation without intermixing the required documentation for each chart.

Terminology

A majority of workers' compensation cases involve accidents causing bodily injuries. Therefore, it is important to become familiar with anatomic terms, directional and range of motion words, types of fractures, body activity terms, and words that describe pain and symptoms. This terminology appears in progress chart notes and industrial injury

**REQUEST FOR ALLOWANCE OF LIEN
ASSIGNMENT AND AUTHORIZATION**

WHEREAS, I have a right or cause of action arising out of personal injury, to wit:

I,_____ hereby authorize _____ ,
  patient's name   physician's name

to furnish, upon request, to my attorney_____ ,
any and all medical records, or reports of examination, diagnosis, treatment, or prognosis but not necessarily limited to those items as set forth herein, in addition to an itemized statement of account for services rendered therefore or in connection therewith, which my attorney may from time to time request in connection with the injuries described above and sustained by me on the _____ day of_____ , 20XX.

   I, hereby irrevocably authorize and direct my said attorney set forth herein to pay to_____ all charges for attendance in court,
                       physician's name

if required as an expert witness whether he testifies or not; reports or other data supplied by him; depositions given by said doctor; medical services rendered or drugs supplied; and any other reasonable and customary charges incurred by my attorney as submitted by_____ and in
                                       physician's name

connection with said injury. Said payment or payments are to be made from any money or monies received by my attorney whether by judgment, decree, or settlement of this case, prior to disbursement to me and payment of the amount as herein directed shall be the same as if paid by me. This authorization to pay the aforementioned doctor shall constitute and be deemed as assignment of so much of my recovery I receive. It is agreed that nothing herein relieves me of the primary responsibility and obligation of paying my doctor for services rendered, and I shall at all times remain personally liable for such indebtedness unless released by the aforementioned doctor or by payment disbursed by my attorney.
I accept the above assignment:
Dated: _____ Patient:_____

As the attorney of record for the above-named patient, I hereby agree to observe the terms of this agreement, and to withhold from any award in this case such sums as are required for the adequate protection of Dr._____
_____ .

Date: _____ Attorney:_____

Figure 14–4. Patient's authorization to release information to an attorney and to grant lien to the physician against proceeds of settlement in connection with accident, industrial, or third party litigation cases.

reports. The more knowledgeable you become about the meaning of the documentation the more proficient you are in knowing if the procedure and diagnostic codes assigned are substantiated or if code selection is deficient and needs to be enhanced for better payment. Carefully study each illustration in this chapter, Figures 14–5 through 14–9 and Tables 14–5 and 14–6. Look up the definitions of the words in the dictionary and learn how to spell them.

Directional Terms

Directional terms are commonly used in workers' compensation reports. Figure 14–5 illustrates positional and directional terms referring to movements and planes of the body. The subject is standing upright, facing forward, arms at the sides with palms forward, and feet parallel. Imaginary lines divide the body in half, forming body planes (e.g., frontal plane dividing right and left sides, coronal plane dividing front and back).

The positional and directional terms indicate the location or direction of the body part with respect to each other (e.g., medial, toward the midline of the body, and lateral, toward the sides of the body).

Range of Motion of Upper and Lower Extremities

Figure 14–6 shows commonly dictated terms for range of motion (ROM) of upper and lower extremities. ROM tests determine if the body part is able to move to the full extent possible. Often after an injury to an extremity or joint there is restriction of motion and loss of strength (e.g., grip). This can be improved with activity and therapy and is measured and documented each time a patient is examined using special measurement devices.

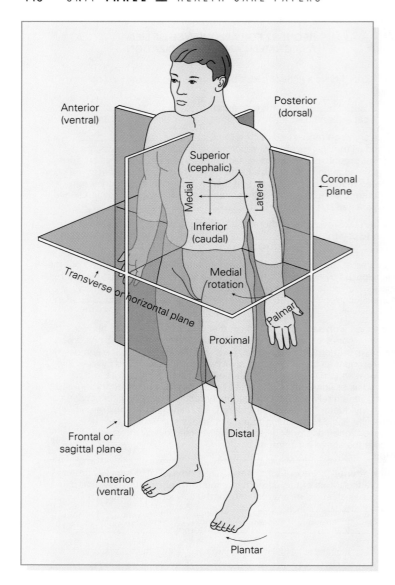

Anterior
(ventral)

Posterior
(dorsal)

Superior
(cephalic)

Medial

Lateral

Coronal
plane

Inferior
(caudal)

Transverse or horizontal plane

Medial
rotation

Palmar

Proximal

Frontal or
sagittal plane

Distal

Anterior
(ventral)

Plantar

Figure 14–5. Directional terminology. (Modified from Chabner DE: Medical Terminology: A Short Course. Philadelphia, WB Saunders, 1999, p 47.)

Types of Fractures

A fracture is a break in the continuity of a bone. Figure 14–9 explains each type of fracture. Such injuries can occur from falling, blows, impact hits, a disease process, or direct violence, such as in an automobile accident. Healing may take months and depends on the location and severity of the injured part, associated injury, and complications or infections.

Reporting Requirements

Employer's Report

The laws clearly state that the injured person must promptly report the industrial injury or illness to his or her employer or immediate supervisor. In most states, the first report of an industrial injury submitted by the employer and the physician is required by law. The employer sends in an Employer's Report of Occupational Injury or Illness Form (Fig. 14–10) to the insurance company. In different states, the time limit on submission of this form varies from immediately to as long as 30 days (see Table 14–1. Many states have adopted the form shown in Figure 14–10 to meet the requirements of the Federal Occupational Safety and Health Act of 1970 and for state statistical purposes.

Medical Service Order

In addition to the employer's report, the employer may complete and sign a **medical service order,** giving this to the injured employee to take

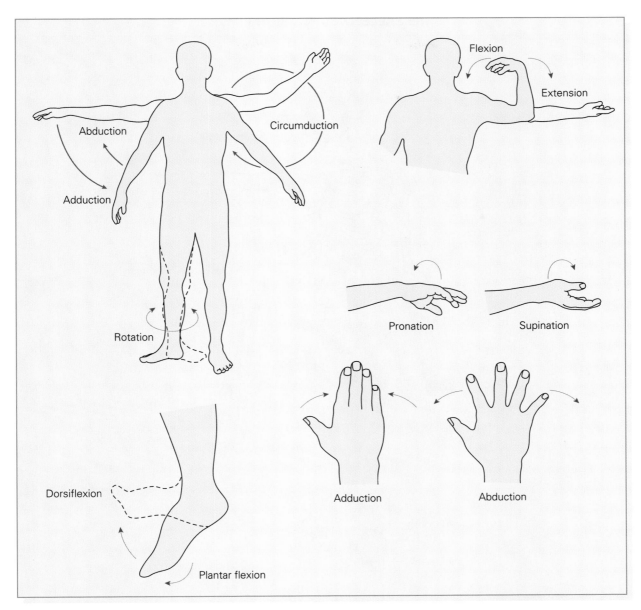

Figure 14–6. Range of motion for upper and lower extremities. (Modified from Sloane S, Fordney MT: Saunders Manual of Medical Transcription. Philadelphia, WB Saunders, 1994.)

to the physician's office (Fig. 14–11). This authorizes the physician to treat the injured employee. Photocopy the form, retaining the copy for the physician's files, and attach the original to the Doctor's First Report of Occupational Injury or Illness (preliminary report). An employer may prefer to write the service order on his or her business letterhead, billhead, or a piece of scratch paper.

Authorizations may also be obtained over the telephone. However, some offices prefer that, if a patient arrives for an appointment without written authorization, the employer be telephoned and asked that the authorized person fax the permission for treatment. Subsequently, if payment is not received or the claim is disputed, it may be easier to collect if a copy of the written authorization is included when sending collection follow-up correspondence.

In a situation where the patient has a managed care plan and neglects to bring in an authorization, collect the copayment. It is the patient's responsibility to get the authorization if injured on the job (Fig. 14–12).

If an appointment was arranged by the employer or insurance company for a workers' compensation patient and was not canceled 72 hours

THE SKELETON (ANTERIOR VIEW)

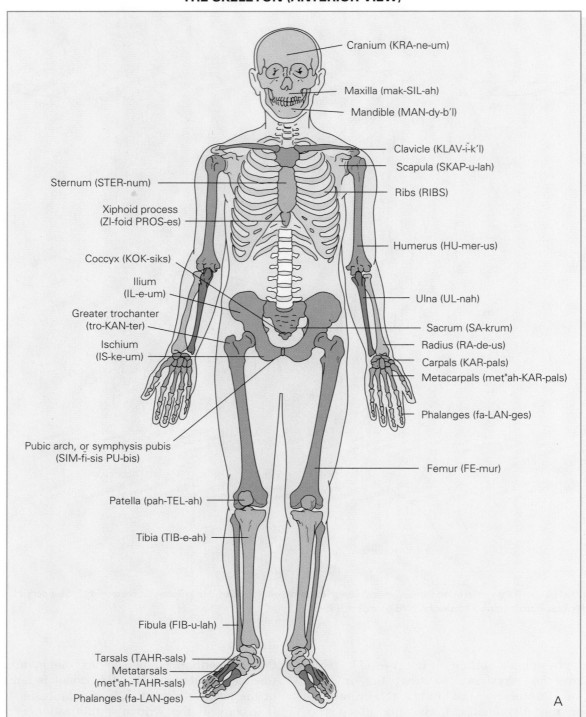

Cranium (KRA-ne-um)

Maxilla (mak-SIL-ah)

Mandible (MAN-dy-b'l)

Clavicle (KLAV-i-k'l)

Scapula (SKAP-u-lah)

Sternum (STER-num)

Ribs (RIBS)

Xiphoid process (ZI-foid PROS-es)

Humerus (HU-mer-us)

Coccyx (KOK-siks)

Ilium (IL-e-um)

Ulna (UL-nah)

Greater trochanter (tro-KAN-ter)

Sacrum (SA-krum)

Radius (RA-de-us)

Ischium (IS-ke-um)

Carpals (KAR-pals)

Metacarpals (met"ah-KAR-pals)

Phalanges (fa-LAN-ges)

Pubic arch, or symphysis pubis (SIM-fi-sis PU-bis)

Femur (FE-mur)

Patella (pah-TEL-ah)

Tibia (TIB-e-ah)

Fibula (FIB-u-lah)

Tarsals (TAHR-sals)

Metatarsals (met"ah-TAHR-sals)

Phalanges (fa-LAN-ges)

A

Figure 14–7. A and B, Terminology pertinent to the skeletal anatomy commonly used in reports on injury cases. (Modified from Chabner DE: The Language of Medicine, 6th ed. Philadelphia, WB Saunders, 1999, p 545.)

before the appointment time, a charge can be made. This policy may vary depending on state laws, so check with the insurance company.

If outside testing or treatment is necessary, obtain authorization from the employer or the adjuster for the insurance company. When this is done by telephone, state the name of the procedure or test and the medical necessity for it. Obtain the name and title of the person giving authorization and write this in the patient's chart

THE SKELETON (POSTERIOR VIEW)

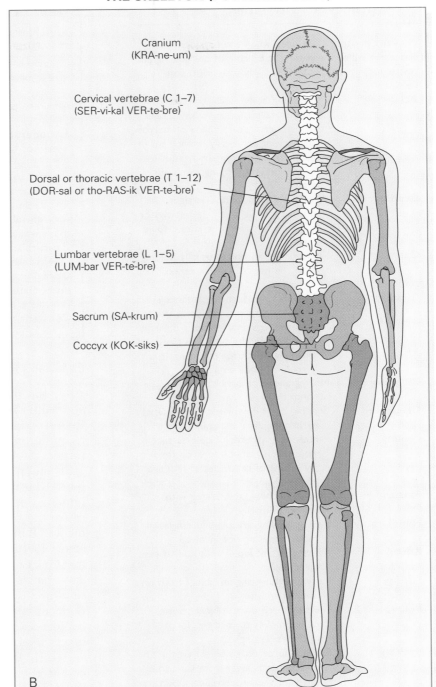

Cranium
(KRA-ne-um)

Cervical vertebrae (C 1–7)
(SER-vi-kal VER-te-bre)

Dorsal or thoracic vertebrae (T 1–12)
(DOR-sal or tho-RAS-ik VER-te-bre)

Lumbar vertebrae (L 1–5)
(LUM-bar VER-te-bre)

Sacrum (SA-krum)

Coccyx (KOK-siks)

B

Figure 14–7 *Continued.* B

and on the order form as well as the date. No authorization numbers are issued in workers' compensation cases.

If a translator is needed for a workers' compensation patient, contact the insurance adjuster handling the case. He or she will make arrangements for an official translator to be present for all appointments. Do not allow a member of the patient's family or the patient's friend to serve as a translator because if information is miscommunicated leading to a bad outcome, there may be no legal recourse for the physician.

TABLE 14-5	Body Activity Terms

Body activity terms are used when the physician describes activities the patient is capable of performing and restrictions when a patient returns to work before full recovery.

Balancing	Maintaining body equilibrium to prevent falling when walking, standing, crouching, or running on narrow, slippery, or erratically moving surfaces, or maintaining body equilibrium when performing gymnastic feats.
Bending	Angulation from neutral-straight position about joint (e.g., elbow) or spine (e.g., forward or lateral spine flexion).
Carrying	Transporting an object usually holding it in the hands or arms or on the shoulder.
Climbing	Ascending or descending ladders, stairs, scaffolding, ramps, and poles using feet and legs and/or hands or arms. For climbing, the emphasis is placed on body agility; for balancing, it is placed on body equilibrium.
Crawling	Moving about on hands and knees or hands and feet.
Crouching	Bending body downward and forward by bending legs and spine.
Feeling	Perceiving attributes of objects such as size, shape, temperature, or texture by means of receptors in skin like those of fingertips.
Fingering	Picking, pinching, or working with fingers primarily.
Handling	Seizing, holding, grasping, turning with hands, fingering not involved.
Kneeling	Bending legs at knees to come to rest on knees.
Lifting	Raising or lowering an object from one level to another.
Pulling	Exerting force on an object so the object moves toward the force (includes jerking).
Pushing	Exerting force on an object so the object moves away from the force (includes slapping, striking, kicking, and treadle action).
Reaching	Extending the arm(s) in any direction.
Sitting	Remaining in the normal seated position.
Standing	Remaining on one's feet in the upright position at a work station without moving about.
Stooping	Bending body downward and forward by bending spine and waist.

TABLE 14-6	Terms That Describe Intensity of Pain and Frequency of Occurrence of Symptoms

Definitions that describe intensity of pain and frequency of symptoms were developed to assist the physician when documenting subjective complaints.

A **severe** pain would preclude the activity causing the pain.

A **moderate** pain could be tolerated but would cause marked handicap in the performance of the activity precipitating the pain.

A **slight** pain could be tolerated but would cause some handicap in the performance of the activity precipitating the pain.

A **minimal** (mild) pain would constitute an annoyance but would cause no handicap in the performance of the particular activity. It would be considered a nonrateable permanent disability.

Occasional means approximately 25% of the time.

Intermittent means approximately 50% of the time.

Frequent means approximately 75% of the time.

Constant means 90% to 100% of the time.

Physician's First Report

After the physician sees the injured person, he or she sends in a completed First Treatment Medical Report (Fig. 14–13) or a Doctor's First Report of Occupational Injury or Illness form (used in California; see Fig. 14–14) as soon as possible.

If the physician prefers to submit a narrative letter, the medical report should include the components, if relevant, shown in Table 14–7. Because the time limit for filing this report varies, refer to Table 14–1 for the requirements of your state. Failure to file the report can be a misdemeanor. Copies of the report form go to the insurance carrier and the state. Some physicians also send a copy to the employer.

Because the report is a legal document, each copy *must be signed in ink* by the physician. The insurance company waits for the physician's report and bill, then issues payment to the physician; and if there is no further treatment or disability, the case can be closed.

PROCEDURE: Completing the Doctor's First Report of Occupational Injury or Illness

---

The submission of this form (Fig. 14–14) has a deadline, from immediately to within 5 days after the patient has been seen by the physician, de-

BONES OF THE HAND AND FOOT

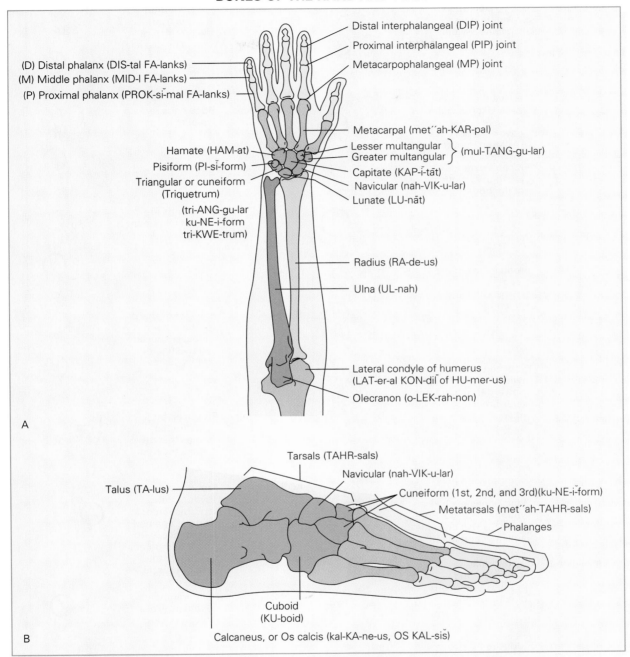

Figure 14–8. Terminology pertinent to the hand (A) and the foot (B), indicating the common medical terms seen in reports on injury cases. (A, Redrawn from Marble HC: The Hand: A Manual and Atlas for the General Surgeon. Philadelphia, WB Saunders, 1960; B, redrawn from Chabner DE: The Language of Medicine, 4th ed. Philadelphia, WB Saunders, 1991.)

pending on each state's law. Distribute an original and three or four copies as follows:

▶ Original to the insurance carrier (unless more copies are required)
▶ One copy to the state agency
▶ One copy to the patient's employer

▶ One copy retained for the physician's files in the patient's workers' compensation file folder

In some states, attending physicians may file a single report directly to the insurer or self-insured employer within a specified number of days from initial treatment. The insurer or self-insured em-

Fracture	Definition		Fracture	Definition	
Closed or simple	Broken bone is contained within intact skin.		Pathologic	Results from weakening of bone by disease	
Open or compound	Skin is broken above the fracture, which is thus open to the external environment, resulting in potential for infection.		Nondisplaced	Bone ends remain in alignment	
Longitudinal	Fracture extends along the length of the bone.		Displaced	Bone ends are out of alignment	
Transverse	Produced by direct force applied perpendicularly to a bone		Spiral	Have long, sharp, pointed bone ends; produced by twisting or rotary forces	
Oblique	Produced by a twisting force with an upward thrust; fracture ends are short and run at an oblique angle across the bone		Compression	Produced by transmitted forces that drive bones together	
Greenstick	Produced by compression or angulation forces in long bones of children younger than 10. Bone is cracked on one side and intact on the other due to softness.		Avulsion	Produced by forceful contraction of a muscle against resistance, with a bone fragment tearing at the site of muscle insertion	
Comminuted	Has multiple fragments and is produced by severe direct violence		Depression	Bone fragments of the skull are driven inward	
Impacted	Produced by strong forces that drive bone fragments firmly together				

Figure 14–9. Terminology and illustration of different types of fractures. (From Chester GA: Modern Medical Assisting. Philadelphia, WB Saunders, 1998.)

State of California	Please complete in triplicate (type, if possible). Mail two copies to:	OSHA Case No.
EMPLOYER'S REPORT OF OCCUPATIONAL INJURY OR ILLNESS	Insurance Carrier Name and Address	# 18 ☐ Fatality

Any person who makes or causes to be made any knowingly false or fraudulent material statement or material representation for the purpose of obtaining or denying workers' compensation benefits or payments is guilty of a felony.

NOTICE: California law requires employers to report within **five days** of knowledge every occupational injury or illness which results in lost time beyond the date of the incident **OR** requires medical treatment beyond first aid. If an employee subsequently dies as a result of a previously reported injury or illness, the employer must file within **five days** of knowledge an amended report indicating death. In addition, every serious injury/illness, or death must be reported **immediately** by telephone or telegraph to the nearest office of the California Division of Occupational Safety and Health.

EMPLOYER

1. FIRM NAME *The Conk Out Company*
1A. POLICY NUMBER *B12345*
DO NOT USE THIS COLUMN — Case No.

2. MAILING ADDRESS (Number and Street, City, ZIP) *45 South Gorman St. Woodland Hills, XY 12345*
2A. PHONE NUMBER *013-430-3488*

3. LOCATION, IF DIFFERENT FROM MAILING ADDRESS (Number and Street, City, ZIP)
3A. LOCATION CODE — Ownership

4. NATURE OF BUSINESS, e.g., painting contractor, wholesale grocer, sawmill, hotel, etc. *Plumbing Repair*
5. STATE UNEMPLOYMENT INSURANCE ACCT. NO. — Industry

6. TYPE OF EMPLOYER ☒ PRIVATE ☐ STATE ☐ CITY ☐ COUNTY ☐ SCHOOL DIST. ☐ OTHER GOVERNMENT - SPECIFY _____ — Occupation

EMPLOYEE

7. EMPLOYEE NAME *Ima B. Hurt*
8. SOCIAL SECURITY NUMBER *120-23-6542*
9. DATE OF BIRTH (mm/dd/yy) *3-4-66* — Sex

10. HOME ADDRESS (Number and Street, City, ZIP) *300 E. Central Ave. Woodland Hills, XY 12345*
10A. PHONE NUMBER *476-9899* — Age

11. SEX ☐ MALE ☒ FEMALE
12. OCCUPATION (Regular job title — NO initials, abbreviations or numbers) *Clerk Typist*
13. DATE OF HIRE (mm/dd/yy) *1-20-86* — Daily Hours

14. EMPLOYEE USUALLY WORKS *8* hours per day *5* hours per week *40* total weekly hours
14A. EMPLOYMENT STATUS (check applicable status at time of injury) ☒ regular full-time ☐ part-time ☐ temporary ☐ seasonal
14B. Under what class code of your policy were wages assigned? *7219* — Days per week

15. GROSS WAGES/SALARY $ *700.00* per *week*
16. OTHER PAYMENTS NOT REPORTED AS WAGES/SALARY (e.g. tips, meals, lodging, overtime, bonuses, etc.)? ☐ YES $ _____ PER _____ ☒ NO — Weekly hours

INJURY OR ILLNESS

17. DATE OF INJURY OR ONSET OF ILLNESS (mm/dd/yy) *4-3-XX*
18. TIME INJURY/ILLNESS OCCURRED ☐ A.M. *2:00* ☒ P.M.
19. TIME EMPLOYEE BEGAN WORK *8:00* ☒ A.M. ☐ P.M.
20. IF EMPLOYEE DIED, DATE OF DEATH (mm/dd/yy) — Weekly wage

21. UNABLE TO WORK AT LEAST ONE FULL DAY AFTER DATE OF INJURY? ☒ YES ☐ NO
22. DATE LAST WORKED (mm/dd/yy) *4-3-XX*
23. DATE RETURNED TO WORK (mm/dd/yy)
24. IF STILL OFF WORK, CHECK THIS BOX ☒ — County

25. PAID FULL WAGES FOR DAY OF INJURY OR LAST DAY WORKED? ☒ YES ☐ NO
26. SALARY BEING CONTINUED? ☐ YES ☒ NO
27. DATE OF EMPLOYER'S KNOWLEDGE/NOTICE OF INJURY/ILLNESS (mm/dd/yy) *4-3-XX*
28. DATE EMPLOYEE WAS PROVIDED *4-3-XX* — Nature of injury

29. SPECIFIC INJURY/ILLNESS AND PART OF BODY AFFECTED, MEEDICAL DIAGNOSIS, if available, e.g. second degree burns on right arm, tendonitis of left elbow, lead poisoning. *ankle injury swelling, possible fracture* — Part of body

30. LOCATION WHERE EVENT OR EXPOSURE OCCURED (Number, Street, City) *45 South Gorman St. Woodland Hills, XY 12345*
30B. ON EMPLOYERS PREMISES? ☐ YES ☒ NO — Source

31. DEPARTMENT WHERE EVENT OR EXPOSURE OCCURED, e.g., shipping department, machine shop. *stock room*
32. OTHER WORKERS INJURED/ILL IN THIS EVENT? ☐ YES ☒ NO — Event

33. EQUIPMENT, MATERIALS AND CHEMICALS THE EMPLOYEE WAS USING WHEN EVENT OR EXPOSURE OCCURRED, e.g., acetylene, welding torch, farm tractor, scaffold. *6 foot ladder* — Sec. Source

34. SPECIFY ACTIVITY THE EMPLOYEE WAS PERFORMING WHEN EVENT OR EXPOSURE OCCURRED, e.g., welding seams of metal forms, loading boxes onto truck. *climbed ladder to remove pipe fittings from shelf; fell* — Extent of injury

35. HOW INJURY/ILLNESS OCCURRED. DESCRIBE SEQUENCE OF EVENTS. SPECIFY OBJECT OR EXPOSURE WHICH DIRECTLY PRODUCED THE INJURY/ILLNESS, e.g., worker stepped back to inspect work and slipped on scrap material. As he fell, he brushed against fresh weld, and burned right hand. USE SEPERATE SHEET IF NECESSARY.
worker climbed ladder to remove pipe fittings from top shelf in stock room. She was descending and mis-stepped falling to the floor. She tried to land upright, and her left leg took the brunt of the fall.

36. NAME AND ADDRESS OF PHYSICIAN (Number and Street, City, ZIP) *Martin Feelgood, MD 4567 Broad Ave., Woodland Hills, XY 12345*
36A. PHONE NUMBER *013-486-9002*

37. IF HOSPITALIZED AS AN INPATIENT, NAME AND ADDRESS OF HOSPITAL (Number and Street, City, ZIP)
37A. PHONE NUMBER

| Completed by (type or print) *J.D. Hawkins* | Signature *J.D. Hawkins* | Title *owner* | Date *4-3-XX* |

FILING THIS REPORT IS NOT AN ADDMISSION OF LIABILITY

Figure 14–10. Employer's Report of Occupational Injury or Illness. This form complies with OSHA requirements as well as California State Workers' Compensation laws.

WORKERS' COMPENSATION MEDICAL SERVICE ORDER

To: Dr./Clinic _____ Martin Feelgood, MD _____

Address   _____ 4567 Broad Avenue, Woodland Hills, XY 12345 _____

We are sending _____ Mrs. Ima Hurt _____

Address   _____ 300 East Central Ave. Woodland Hills, XY 12345 _____

Social Security No. _____ 120-23-6542 _____ Date of birth 3-4-1966 _____
        to you for treatment in accordance with the terms of the Worker's
        Compensation Laws. Please submit your report to the
        _____ XYZ Insurance Company _____
        at once. Compensation cannot be paid without complete medical
        information.

Insurance carrier _____ XYZ Insurance Company _____

Address P.O. Box 5, Woodland Hills, XY 12345 Telephone 013-271-0562

Employer   _____ The Conk Out Company _____

Address 45 S. Gorman St. Woodland Hills, XY 12345 Telephone 013-430-3488

Signature _____ *J.A.HAWKINS* _____ Date _____ 4-3-20XX _____
        If patient is able to return to work today or tomorrow, please
        show date and time below — sign and give to patient to return to
        employer. If there are any work restrictions indicate on the back
        of this form. Please submit your usual first report in any case.

Date/Time _____ By _____

Figure 14–11. Medical Service Order.

ployer, in turn, is required to send a report to the state agency. This cuts down on paperwork and postage. Refer to Table 14–1 to find out the time limit in your state during which the physician must submit the initial report.

1. Enter the insurance carrier's complete name, street address, city, state, and ZIP code.
2. Enter the employer's full name and policy number if known. Some insurance carriers file by employer and then by policy number. Sometimes the employer's telephone number is required on this line.
3. Enter the employer's street address, city, state, and ZIP code.
4. Enter the type of business the company is involved in (e.g., repairing shoes, building construction, retailing men's clothes).
5. Enter the patient's complete first name, middle initial, and last name.
6. Enter a check mark in the appropriate box to indicate the patient's gender.
7. Enter the patient's birth date and list the year as four digits.
8. Enter the patient's street address, city, state, and ZIP code.
9. Enter the patient's home telephone number.
10. Enter the patient's specific job title. It is important to be accurate in listing the occupation with the job title so that the insurance carrier may be certain the patient was doing the job for which he or she was insured.

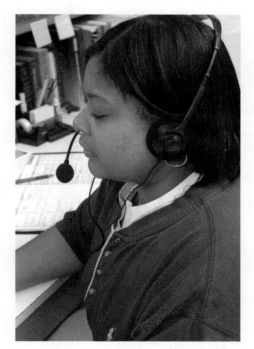

Figure 14–12. Receptionist receiving a Medical Service Order via telephone for the worker to receive medical services.

NEBRASKA WORKERS' COMPENSATION COURT
First Treatment Medical Report
(Must be filed with Compensation Court & Employer within 14 days of first treatment)
(Shaded sections are not required)

TYPE OR PRINT

PATIENT & INSURED (SUBSCRIBER) INFORMATION

1. PATIENT'S NAME (First, name, middle initial, last name)	2. PATIENT'S DATE OF BIRTH	3. INSURED'S NAME (Employer)
Lester M. Task	05 | 06 | 60	Jonas Construction Company

4. PATIENT'S ADDRESS (Street, City, State, ZIP Code)	5. PATIENT'S SEX	6. INSURED'S I.D. NO. (Include any letters)
5400 Holly Street Woodland Hills, XY 12345	[x] MALE [ ] FEMALE	B 785700

	7. PATIENT'S RELATIONSHIP TO INSURED	8 INSURED'S GROUP NO. (Or Group Name)
	[ ] SELF [ ] SPOUSE [ ] CHILD [x] OTHER	5601

9. OTHER HEALTH INSURANCE COVERAGE - Enter Name of Policyholder and Plan Name and Address and Policy or Medical Assistance Number	10. WAS CONDITION RELATED TO:
	
	A. PATIENT'S EMPLOYMENT
	   [x] YES [ ] NO
	
	B. AN AUTO ACCIDENT
	   [ ] YES [ ] NO
		11. INSURED'S ADDRESS (Street, City State, ZIP Code)
		
		300 Main Street
		Woodland Hills, XY 12345

12. PATIENT'S OR AUTHORIZED PERSON'S SIGNATURE I Authorize the Release of any Medical Information Necessary to Process this Claim SIGNED	12A. PATIENT'S SOCIAL SECURITY NO 578 | 03 | 1921 DATE 11-8-XX	13. I AUTHORIZE PAYMENT OF MEDICAL BENEFITS TO UNDERSIGNED PHYSICIAN OR SUPPLIER FOR SERVICE DESCRIBED BELOW SIGNED (Insured or Authorized Person)

PHYSICIAN OR SUPPLIER INFORMATION

14. DATE OF:	ILLNESS (FIRST SYMPTOM OR INJURY (ACCIDENT)	15. DATE FIRST CONSULTED YOU FOR THIS CONDITION	16. HAS PATIENT EVER HAD SAME OR SIMILAR SYMPTOMS?
11-8-XX	◄	11-8-XX	[ ] YES [x] NO

17. DATE PATIENT ABLE TO RETURN TO WORK	18. DATES OF TOTAL DISABILITY		DATES OF PARTIAL DISABILITY
	FROM 11-8-XX	THROUGH 12-8-XX	FROM THROUGH

19. NAME OF REFERRING PHYSICIAN	20. FOR SERVICES RELATED TO HOSPITALIZATION GIVE HOSPITALIZATION DATES
	ADMITTED 11-8-XX | DISCHARGED 11-10-XX

21. NAME & ADDRESS OF FACILITY WHERE SERVICES RENDERED (If other than home or office)	22. WAS LABORATORY WORK PERFORMED OUTSIDE YOUR OFFICE?
Community Hospital, 400 Oak St., Woodland Hills, XY 12345	[ ] YES [x] NO CHARGES:

23. DIAGNOSIS OR NATURE OF ILLNESS OR INJURY, RELATE DIAGNOSIS TO PROCEDURE IN COLUMN D BY REFERENCE TO NUMBERS 1,2,3, ETC. OR DX CODE

1. fracture of right patella   822.1
2.
3.
4.

24. A DATE OF SERVICE	B* PLACE OF SERVICE	C FULLY DESCRIBE PROCEDURES, MEDICAL SERVICE OR SUPPLIES FURNISHED FOR EACH DATE GIVEN PROCEDURE CODE (IDENTIFY:)	(EXPLAIN UNUSUAL SERVICES OR CIRCUMSTANCES)	D DIAGNOSIS CODE	E CHARGES	F
11-8-XX	1	99222	Initial hospital care	1	125 00	
11-8-XX	1	27524	Open TX patellar fracture with internal fixation	1	600 00	

24A. HISTORY. GIVE BRIEF DESCRIPTION OF WHAT OCCURRED. PATIENT'S ACCOUNT OF ACCIDENT.

Patient was up on a scaffold at a construction site and fell off of it about

8 feet hitting the ground with his right knee.

25. SIGNATURE OF PHYSICIAN OR SUPPLIER SIGNED *Gregory T. Getwell, MD* DATE 11-8-XX	26. ACCEPT ASSIGNMENT (GOVERNMENT CLAIMS ONLY) [ ] YES [ ] NO PHYSICIAN'S SOCIAL SECURITY NO.	27. TOTAL CHARGE 725.00	28. AMOUNT PAID	29. BALANCE DUE 725 | 00

32. YOUR PATIENT'S ACCOUNT NO.	33. YOUR EMPLOYER I.D. NO. 95-3208976	31 PHYSICIAN'S OR SUPPLIER'S NAME, ADDRESS, ZIP CODE & TELEPHONE NO Gregory T. Getwell, MD 60 North State Street Woodland Hills, XY 12345 I.D. NO. A123456 013-459-0087

*PLACE OF SERVICE CODES

1—(IH) - INPATIENT HOSPITAL	4—(H) PATIENT'S HOME	7—(NH) NURSING HOME	O—(OL) OTHER LOCATIONS
2—(OH) - OUTPATIENT HOSPITAL	5— DAY CARE FACILITY (PSY)	8—(SNF) SKILLED NURSING FACILITY	A—(IL) INDEPENDENT LABORATORY
3—(O) - DOCTOR'S OFFICE	6— NIGHT CARE FACILITY(PSY)	9— AMBULANCE	B— OTHER MEDICAL/SURGICAL FACILITY

NWCC FORM 45 (Rev. 86)

reference initials

Figure 14–13. First Treatment Medical Report form used in Nebraska. This form follows the format of the Health Insurance Claim Form HCFA-1500 developed by the American Medical Association Council on Medical Service (see Chapter 6).

STATE OF CALIFORNIA

DOCTOR'S FIRST REPORT OF OCCUPATIONAL INJURY OR ILLNESS

Within 5 days of your initial examination, for every occupational injury or illness, send two copies of this report to the **employer's workers' compensation insurance carrier** or the **self-insured employer.** Failure to file a timely doctor's report may result in assessment of a civil penalty. **In the case of diagnosed or suspected pesticide poisoning,** send a copy of this report to Division of Labor Statistics and Research, P.O. Box 420603, San Francisco, CA 94142-0603, and notify your local health officer by telephone within 24 hours.

	PLEASE DO NOT USE THIS COLUMN
1. **INSURER NAME AND ADDRESS** XYZ Insurance Company, P.O. Box 5, Woodland Hills, XY 12345	
2. **EMPLOYER NAME** The Conk Out Company Policy# B12345	Case No.
3. Address No. and Street City Zip 45 So. Gorman St. Woodland Hills, XY 12345	Industry
4. Nature of business (e.g., food manufacturing, building construction, retailer of women's clothes) plumbing repair	County
5. **PATIENT NAME** (first name, middle initial, last name) Ima B. Hurt 6. Sex ☐ Male ☒ Female 7. Date of Mo. Day Yr. birth 3-4-1966	Age
8. Address: No. and Street City Zip 300 East Central Ave., Woodland Hills, XY 12345 9. Telephone number (013) 476-9899	Hazard
10. Occupation (Specific job title) clerk typist 11. Social Security Number 120-23-6542	Disease
12. Injured at: No. and street City County 45 So. Gorman St., Woodland Hills, XY 12345 Humboldt	Hospitalization
13. Date and hour of injury Mo. Day Yr. Hour or onset of illness 4-3-20XX ____ a.m. 2:00 p.m. 14. Date last worked Mo. Day Yr. 4-3-20XX	Occupation
15. Date and hour of first Mo. Day Yr. Hour examination or treatment 4-3-20XX ____ a.m. 4:00 p.m. 16. Have you (or your office) previously treated patient? ☐ Yes ☒ NO	Return date/Code

Patient please complete this portion, if able to do so. Otherwise, doctor please complete immediately. Inability or failure of a patient to complete this portion shall not affect his/her rights to workers' compensation under the California Labor Code.

17. **DESCRIBE HOW THE ACCIDENT OR EXPOSURE HAPPENED** (Give specific object, machinery or chemical. Use reverse side if more space is required.)

I climbed a ladder in the stock room and while I was coming
down I missed a step, lost my balance, and fell hurting my left ankle.

18. **SUBJECTIVE COMPLAINTS** (Describe fully. Use reverse side if more space is required.)

Pain in left ankle.

19. **OBJECTIVE FINDINGS** (Use reverse side if more space is required.)

A. Physical examination

Pain, swelling and discoloration of l. ankle.

B. X-ray and laboratory results (state if none or pending.) Ankle x-ray (left) 3 views

20. **DIAGNOSIS** (if occupational illness specify etiologic agent and duration of exposure.) Chemical or toxic compounds involved? ☐ Yes ☒ No

Trimalleolar ankle fracture (left)

ICD-9 Code ___824.6___

21. Are your findings and diagnosis consistent with patient's account of injury or onset of illness?   ☒ Yes   ☐ No if "no", please explain.

22. Is there any other current condition that will impede or delay the patient's recovery?   ☐ Yes   ☒ No if "yes", please explain.

23. **TREATMENT RENDERED** (Use reverse side if more space is required.)

Examination, x-rays, closed treatment of trimalleolor ankle fracture (left) without manipulation. Return in one week for recheck.

24. If further treatment required, specify treatment plan/estimated duration.

25. If hospitalized as inpatient, give hospital name and location   Date admitted   Mo. Day Yr.   Estimated stay

26. WORK STATUS–Is patient able to perform usual work?   ☐ Yes ☒ No
If "no", date when patient can return to: Regular work _5_ / _17_ /20XX
                                         Modified work ___ /___ /___   Specify restrictions _____

Doctor's signature __*Martin Feelgood, MD*__   4-3-20XX   CA license number __A 12345__
Doctor name and degree (please type) __Martin Feelgood, MD__   IRS number __95-3664021__
Address _____4567 Broad Avenue, Woodland Hills, XY 12345__   Telephone number __(013) 486-9002__

FORM 5021 (REV. 4)
1992

Any person who makes or causes to be made any knowingly false or fraudulent material statement or material representation for the purpose of obtaining or denying workers' compensation benefits or payments is guilty of a felony.

reference initials

Figure 14–14. Doctor's First Report of Occupational Injury or Illness form, used in California.

TABLE 14–7	**Narrative Medical Report Issues, if Relevant**
History	Outline all specific details of accident, injury, or illness. Physician should state whether there is a causal connection between the accident and conditions that may appear subsequently but are not obvious **sequelae** (diseased conditions following, and usually resulting from, a previous disease). If facts were obtained by reviewing prior records or x-ray films, the source should be mentioned. When a history is obtained through an interpreter, include that person's name.
Present Complaints	Usually given as subjective complaints. *Subjective* refers to statements made by the patient about symptoms and how he or she feels. Subjective disability is evaluated by ▶ A description of the activity that produces the disability. ▶ The duration of the disability. ▶ The activities that are precluded by, and those that can be performed with, the disability. ▶ The means necessary for relief.
Past History	Description of any previous, current, subsequent medical information relevant to this injury or illness and state whether there is a preexisting defect that might entitle the injured person to benefits from the subsequent injury fund or represent the actual cause of the present condition.
Examination Findings	Usually given as *objective findings*. State all significant physical or psychiatric examination, testing, laboratory, or imaging findings.
Diagnostic Impression	State all diagnostic findings and opinion as to *relationship,* if any, between the injury or disease and the condition diagnosed. Use diagnostic terminology that corresponds to the diagnostic code book.
Disability/Prognosis	A) Period during which the patient has been unable to work because of the injury or illness. B) Opinion as to probable further temporary disability and a statement as to when the patient will be able to return to work or has returned to work. C) Statement indicating whether the condition is currently permanent and stationary, as well as the probability of future permanent disability. D) Statement indicating "All objective tests for organic pathology are negative. There is obviously a strong functional or emotional overlay," when a patient has multiple complaints but no clinical objective findings.
Work Limitations	Description of any limitations to all activities.
Causation	Description of how the permanent disability is related to the patient's occupation and the specific injury or cumulative events causing the illness.

11. Enter the patient's Social Security number. Some insurance carriers use the Social Security number as the industrial case number.

12. Enter the exact location where the patient was injured. Many times the injury may occur off the premises of the company or factory, depending on the type of job on which the employee was working. List the county where the patient was injured.

13. Enter the date the patient was injured and time of the injury. List the year as four digits.

14. Enter the date the patient last worked. This date should coincide with the date the patient reported to work and worked any portion of

his or her shift (workday). This may be the same date of injury. This item is important because it informs the insurance carrier of the working status of the patient or whether the patient has been disabled and cannot return to work. List the year as four digits.

15. Enter the date and hour of the physician's first examination. It is important for the insurance carrier to know how soon after the accident the patient sought medical attention. List the year as four digits.

16. Enter a check mark in the appropriate box indicating whether the physician or an associate has previously treated the patient.

17. Have the patient complete this section if possible in his or her own words stating how the illness or injury occurred. Or the physician may dictate this information after obtaining it from the patient.

18. Enter the answers to these questions regarding the patient's complaints and medical findings, which may be found in the patient's medical record. List all of the patient's subjective complaints.

19. A. Enter all objective findings from physical examination. B. Enter all x-ray and laboratory results; or if none, state "none" or "pending."

20. Enter a check mark in "yes" or "no" to indicate if chemical or toxic compounds are involved. Enter the diagnosis and diagnostic code number. Specify etiologic agent and duration of exposure if occupational illness.

21. Enter a check mark in "yes" or "no" to indicate if the findings and diagnosis are consistent with the history of injury or onset of illness. If "yes," insert an explanation.

22. Enter a check mark in "yes" or "no" to indicate if there is any other current condition that will impede or delay the patient's recovery. If "yes," insert an explanation.

23. Enter a full description of what treatment was rendered.

24. Enter an explanation if further treatment is required and, if so, specify the treatment plan. Indicate if physical therapy is required and its frequency and duration.

25. Enter the name and location of the hospital, admission date, and estimated stay if the patient is to be hospitalized.

26. Enter a check mark in "yes" or "no" to indicate whether the patient is able to work as usual. If the answer is "no," give the date when it is estimated that the patient will be able to return to regular or modified work. List the year as four digits. Specify any work restrictions. It is very important for the insur-

ance company to anticipate how long the patient will be off work so that money may be set aside for temporary disability benefits, medical benefits, and, if necessary, permanent disability benefits. If the estimated date of return to work should change after the form is submitted, a supplemental report or progress note should be sent to the insurance carrier to change the date of the disability.

Bottom of Form: If not preprinted, enter the physician's name and degree (e.g., MD, DC), complete address, state license number, federal tax identification number, and telephone number. Indicate the date the report is submitted. The insurance billing specialist should type reference initials in the lower left-hand corner of the form. This form *must be signed in ink* by the physician. Any carbon copies or photocopies must also be signed in ink. A stamped signature will *not* be accepted because sometimes these cases may go into litigation or may be presented for a permanent disability rating. Only those documents considered as original medical records are acceptable, and this means a handwritten signature by the attending physician.

Progress or Supplemental Report

In a TD case, a *supplemental report* is sent to the insurance carrier after 2 to 4 weeks of treatment to give information on the current status of the patient. If there is a significant change in the prognosis, a detailed progress report (sometimes called a *reexamination report)* is sent to the insurance carrier. Subsequent progress or supplemental reports should be sent to the insurance carrier after each hospitalization and office visit to update the progress of a case and may be narrative and are not necessarily completed on the special forms available in most states (Fig. 14–15). If the disability is ongoing over a period of time, monthly progress reports should be submitted. A follow-up report must contain the following information:

1. Date of most recent examination
2. Present condition and progress since last report
3. Measurements of function
4. X-ray or laboratory report since last examination
5. Treatment (give type and duration)
6. Work status (patient working or estimated date of return to work)
7. Permanent disability to be anticipated

The insurance carrier authorizing the examination should be furnished with the report in triplicate or quadruplicate, depending on its needs. A copy should always be retained for the physician's files.

ATTENDING PHYSICIAN'S REPORT

Employee: Mrs. Ima B. Hurt   Claim number: 120 23 6542
Employer: The Conk Out Company   Date of injury(ies): 4-3-20XX   Date of next exam: 4-24-20XX
Date of this exam: 4-10-XX   Patient Social Security No: 120 23 6542
Current diagnosis: 824.6 closed fracture; L. trimalleolar ankle
(include ICD•9 code)

PATIENT STATUS

Since the last exam, this patient's condition has:

☒ improved as expected.   ☐ improved, but slower than expected.   ☐ not improved significantly.

☐ worsened.   ☐ plateaued, no further improvement is expected.   ☐ has been determined to be non-work related.

Briefly, describe any change in objective or subjective complaint:

TREATMENT

Treatment plan: (only list changes from prior status)   ☐ No change   ☐ Patient is/was discharged from care on
Est. discharge date: 5-18-20XX   Medications: Tylenol for pain
Therapy: Type   Times per week   Estimated date of completion
Diagnostic studies: X-ray, L. ankle 3 views
Hospitalization/surgery:
Consult/other service:

WORK STATUS

The patient has been instructed to:

☐ return to full duty with no limitations or restrictions.

☐ remain off the rest of the day and return to work tomorrow:

_____ with no limits or restrictions._____ with limits listed below.

☐ return to work on
   work limitations:

☒ remain off work until 5-17-20XX — discharge exam scheduled

Estimated date patient can return full duty: 5-18-20XX

DISABILITY STATUS

☐ Patient discharged as cured.

Please supply a brief narrative report if any of the below apply:

☐ Patient will be permanently precluded from engaging in his/her usual and customary occupation.

☐ Patient's condition is permanent and stationary.

☐ Patient will have permanent residuals   ☐ Patient will require future medical care.

Physician name: Martin Feelgood, MD   Address: 4567 Broad Avenue, Woodland Hills, XY 12345
Date: April 10, 20XX   Telephone: (013) 482-9002
Signature: Martin Feelgood, MD

reference initials

Figure 14–15. Physician's Supplemental Report form.

Final Report

TD ends when the physician tells the insurance carrier that the patient is able to return to work. Sometimes a physician submits a final report at the time of discharge. When the patient resumes work, the insurance carrier closes the case, and the TD benefits cease.

A physician's final report should be sent indicating any impairment or permanent disability and accompanied by a statement listing total expenses incurred (Fig. 14–16).

Claim Submission

Financial Responsibility

As discussed in Chapter 2, the contract for treatment in a personal illness or injury case is between the physician and the patient, who is responsible for the entire bill. However, when a business is self-insured, a person is under a state program for care, or an individual is being treated as a workers' compensation case, the financial responsibility exists between the physician and insurance company or state program. As long as treatment is authorized by the insurance carrier, the insurance company is responsible for payment. A physician who agrees to treat a workers' compensation case must agree to accept payment in full according to the workers' compensation fee schedule. You cannot collect a copayment amount or balance bill the patient for any amount not covered.

If an injured worker refuses to accept the physician retained by the insurance company for the employer, then the patient may be responsible for the cost of medical treatment. The employee should contact the employer first, and the insurance company second to find out if there are any provisions for a change of physicians.

Some states have a medical program where employers can reduce their workers' compensation rates by paying the first $1,000 in medical bills. This is similar to a deductible for the employer's policy. In this situation, send the statement to the employer for payment.

Always obtain health insurance information in case you need to bill for services provided that are not work related or if the injury or illness is declared nonindustrial. To assist in informing patients of financial responsibility for nonrelated illness, have the worker sign an agreement for nonrelated medical expenses, as shown in Figure 14–17.

Sometimes while examining an injured worker the physician may discover a problem unrelated to the industrial injury or illness, such as high blood pressure. The physician may bill the workers' compensation carrier for the examination but needs to code the claim carefully with regard to the treatment of the injury. If treatment is initiated for the patient's high blood pressure, then that portion of the examination becomes the financial obligation of the patient and not the workers' compensation carrier.

Fee Schedules

Some states have developed and adopted a workers' compensation **fee schedule,** whereas other states pay medical claims based on the Medicare fee schedule plus a certain percentage. Fee schedules assist with the following:

1. They limit the fees providers can charge for standard medical procedures paid by workers' compensation companies.
2. They limit the amount that providers will be paid.
3. They make the allowable charges and procedures more consistent.
4. They provide follow-up procedures in case of a fee dispute.

Some workers' compensation fee schedules list maximum reimbursement levels for physicians and other nonhospital providers. Generally, however, the physician is expected to accept payment by the insurance company as payment in full when based on a fee schedule. If the fee charged is more than the amount listed, the following factors may be considered:

▶ Provider's medical training, qualifications, and time in practice
▶ Nature of services provided
▶ Fees usually charged by the provider
▶ Fees usually charged by others in the region where services were given
▶ Other economic factors of the provider's practice that are relevant
▶ Any unusual circumstances in the case

If documentation is sent validating the fee and noting these aforementioned facts, sometimes the insurance carrier will pay the additional amount.

Types of Fee Schedules

Types of fee schedules include the following:

▶ *Percentile of charge schedule*, which is designed to set fees at a percentile of the providers' usual and customary fee.
▶ *Relative value scale schedule*, which takes into account the time, skills, and extent of the ser-

XYZ INSURANCE COMPANY

DOCTOR'S FINAL (OR MONTHLY) REPORT AND BILL

Monthly itemized bills required on all cases under continuing treatment.
Services beginning late in month and extending into succeeding month may be itemized on one statement.

CASE No. __120 23 6542__

EMPLOYEE __Mrs. Ima B. Hurt__
DATE OF INJURY __April 3, 20XX__
EMPLOYER __The Conk Out Company__

SERVICES FOR MONTH OF __May__ 20 __XX__

Patient refused treatment _____ 20 ___
Patient stopped treatment
    without orders _____ 20 ___
Patient entered hospital _____ 20 ___
Further treatment anticipated? __X__
        (Yes)   (No)

Patient able to return to work __May 18,__ 20 __XX__
Patient discharged as cured _____ 20 ___
Condition at time of last visit __fracture healed__

__P.T. L. Ankle 2 x wk 3 wks__
Any other charges authorized such as Drugs? _____ Hospital? _____
               (Check)   (Check)

Code: O—Office: V—Home Visit: H—Hospital Visit: N—Night Visit: S—Operation: X—X-ray.

Month	1	2	3	4	5	6	7	8	9	10	11	12	13	14	15	16	17	18	19	20	21	22	23	24	25	26	27	28	29	30	31
May							O										O														

	RVS CODE	TOTALS
First aid treatment *(describe)* _____ # _____		$ _____
Office Visits __5/7/XX and 5/17/XX__ #	99213	$ 40.20
Home Visits _____ #	99213	$ 40.20
Hospital Visits _____ #		$ _____
Operations _____ #		$ _____
MATERIAL *(Itemize at cost)* __Left ankle films; complete 5/7/xx__ #	73610	$ 34.26
__5/17/xx__ #	73610	$ 34.26
_____ #		$ _____

Any charges shown above which are in excess of the scheduled fee must
be explained regarding nature of such services, indicating the date rendered. TOTAL $ __148.92__

Make check payable to:

Doctor __Martin Feelgood, MD__

Address __4567 Broad Avenue__
            (Street)
__Woodland Hills, XY 12345__
   (City)   (Zip)

Internal Revenue Code Section 6109
requires you to furnish your Internal
Revenue Service Employer Identification
Number or Social Security Number.
Please enter the Identification Number
here __95-3664021__

Signature __*Martin Feelgood, MD*__

Date __May 18, 20XX__

LEAVE BLANK	
	APPROVED
	BY _____
(Dollars) (Cents)	DATE _____

IMPORTANT—
Bills Must Be Submitted in Duplicate
MAIL ADDRESS: P.O. BOX S, WOODLAND HILLS, XY 12345

SCIF FORM 60 REV 5 78

Figure 14–16. Doctor's Final (or Monthly) Report and Bill form.

vice provided by the physician. Each procedure is rated on how difficult it is, how long it takes, the training a physician must have to perform it, and expenses the physician incurs, including the cost of malpractice insurance. Many of the fee schedules are similar to the CPT format in regard to sections (i.e., Evaluation and Management; Anesthesia; Surgery; Radiology, Nuclear Medicine, and Diagnostic Ultrasound; Pathology and Laboratory; and Medicine).

A *conversion factor* that uses a specific dollar amount is used for each of the sections of the fee schedule. Conversion factors may be adjusted to reflect regional differences and in some states are recalculated on an annual basis.

1999 Conversion Factors for Workers' Compensation in California

$8.50/unit	Evaluation and Management section
$6.15/unit	Medicine section
$34.50/unit	Anesthesia section
$153.00/unit	Surgery section
$12.50/unit	Radiology section (total unit value column)
$1.95/unit	Professional component
$1.50/unit	Technical component
$1.50/unit	Pathology section technical component

Actual covered procedures, descriptions, modifiers, global periods, and other elements of a fee guideline may significantly differ from those used for other plans or programs. Sometimes a schedule may include modifiers and code numbers not listed in the CPT code book. Use the workers' compensation codes regardless of what you do for other insurance plans.

With regard to enforcement of fee schedules, reviews or audits may be performed by the following entities:

▶ The state agency or state fund responsible for overseeing workers' compensation (bill review)
▶ The payer, employer, or insurance carrier (bill review)
▶ The payer (bill review) and state agency (compliance audit)

Helpful Billing Tips

The following are helpful hints for billing workers' compensation claims.

1. Ask whether the injury occurred within the scope of employment and verify insurance in-
formation with the benefits coordinator at the employer. This will promote filing initial claims with the correct insurance carrier.
2. Request that the patient obtain the claim number of his or her case when he or she comes in for the initial visit.
3. Educate the patient with regard to the medical practice's billing policies for workers' compensation cases by having him or her complete the patient agreement form shown in Figure 14–17.
4. Verify if prior authorization is required before a surgical procedure is performed.
5. Document in a telephone log or patient's record all data for authorization of examination, diagnostic studies, or surgery (e.g., date, name of individual who authorizes, response).
6. Obtain the workers' compensation fee schedule for your state.
7. Use appropriate five-digit code numbers and modifiers to ensure prompt and accurate payment for services rendered.
8. Complete the Doctor's First Report of Occupational Injury or Illness form for your state and submit it within the time limit shown in Table 14–1.
9. Submit a monthly itemized statement or bill on the termination of treatment for nondisability claims.
10. Clearly define any charges in excess of the fee schedule. Attach any x-ray reports, operative reports, discharge summaries, pathology reports, and so forth to clarify such excess charges or when **by report (BR)** is shown for a code selected from the workers' compensation procedure code book.
11. Itemize in detail and send invoices for drugs and dressings furnished by the physician. Bill medical supplies on a separate claim or statement and do not bill with services because this may be routed to a different claims processing department.
12. Call the insurance carrier and talk with the **claims examiner** who is familiar with the patient's case, if you have a question regarding the fee.
13. Search the Internet for a web site or write to the workers' compensation state plan office in your state for booklets, bulletins, forms, and legislation information. See Appendix A for the workers' compensation address in your state.

Billing Claims

For efficiency in processing industrial claims, many insurance carriers have developed their own forms for workers' compensation cases whereas others al-

PATIENT AGREEMENT

Patient's Name _____ James Doland _____ Soc. Sec. # _431-07-1942_

Address _67 Blyth Dr., Woodland Hills, XY 12345_ Tel. No. _013-372-0101_

WC Insurance Carrier _____ Industrial Indemnity Company _____

Address _30 North Dr., Woodland Hills_ Telephone No. _013-731-7707_

Date of illness _2-13-20XX_ Date of first visit _2-13-20XX_

Emergency Yes _X_ No _____

Is this condition related to employment Yes _X_ No _____

If accident: Auto _____ Other _____

Where did injury occur? _Construction site_

How did injury happen? _fell 8 ft from scaffold suffering fractured right tibia_

Employee/employer who verified this information _Scott McPherson_

Employer's name and address _Willow Construction Company_

Employer's telephone No. _013-526-0611_

In the event the claim for worker's compensation is declared fraudulent for this illness or condition or it is determined by the Workers' Compensation Board that the illness or injury is not a compensable workers' compensation case, I _James Doland_ , hereby agree to pay the physician's fee for services rendered.

I have been informed that I am responsible to pay any services rendered by Dr. _Raymond Skeleton_ with regard to the discovery and treatment of any condition not related to the workers' compensation injury or illness. I agree to pay for all services not covered by workers' compensation and all charges for treatment and personal items unrelated to my workers' compensation illness or injury.

Signed _James Doland_ Date _2-13-20XX_

Figure 14–17. Patient agreement to pay the physician's fees if the case is declared not work related or if an illness is discovered and treated that is not work related.

low use of the HCFA-1500 claim form. Some carriers have made slight modifications to the HCFA-1500 claim form as depicted in Figure 14–13, First Treatment Medical Report form used in Nebraska.

Figure 6–15 in Chapter 6 is an illustration of a completed workers' compensation case on a nonmodified HCFA-1500 claim form.

Electronic Claims Submission and Reports

Uniform data processing codes and universal electronic injury report forms have been developed by the American National Standards Institute (ANSI) and the International Association of Industrial Accident Boards and Commissions (IAIABC). ANSI is a national organization founded in 1918 to coordinate the development of voluntary business standards in the United States. Texas is one of the first states to establish an insurance regulation requiring workers' compensation carriers to use universal electronic transmission for first report of injury forms and subsequent reports developed by IAIABC.

Electronic Data Systems, Inc. (EDS) in Dallas, Texas, and Insurance Value-Added Network Services (IVANS) in Greenwich, Connecticut, introduced the nation's first coast-to-coast electronic claims processing and report-filing network, called Workers' Compensation Reporting Service. EDS processes all claims and follow-up reports. IVANS provides the network service and marketing of software to employers. This system is operational in many states.

Some workers' compensation insurance companies are using telephone reporting of claims. Employers report injuries occurring on the job by calling a toll-free number. Calls go to a regional center where service representatives document the first report of injury and electronically transmit it to the local claim office handling workers' compensation insurance. Employers avoid tardiness of reporting when using this system. Employers neglecting prompt report of injuries could delay payments to physicians.

Because workers' compensation is operated under state laws, each state is required to report financial data, statistics on injuries and illnesses, and other information to state insurance regulators. In the states that use telephone reporting service, workers' compensation payers use the system to reduce the paper processing costs that have escalated out of proportion and to improve administrative efficiency.

Out-of-State Claims

When billing for an out-of-state claim, insurance billing specialists must follow all workers' compensation regulations from the jurisdiction (state) in which the injured was hired and not the state where the injury occurred.

Companies that have employees who travel to other states are required to obtain workers' compensation insurance in those states. Sometimes a patient may seek care from a physician in an adjacent state because he or she feels the physician provides a higher quality of care or the patient needs a specialized type of surgery, expensive diagnostic tests, or treatment. It is important that referral requirements be met before the patient is seen (e.g., letter of referral or preauthorization from the managing doctor with a copy to the workers' compensation carrier). Nine states hold the injured employee responsible for unauthorized care (Alabama, Alaska, Arkansas, New Jersey, North Dakota, Ohio, Washington, West Virginia, and Wisconsin). When a patient crosses a state line for treatment, he or she may be liable for some balance billing, and the patient should be informed of this fact.

Obtain the out-of-state fee schedule to determine the proper procedure codes, modifiers, and amounts for billing the claim. Ask whether the claimant's jurisdiction accepts electronic submission of the HCFA-1500 claim form or another form. Determine whether other documents (e.g., the operative report) are required to be submitted with the bill.

Delinquent Claims

If a workers' compensation claim becomes 45 days delinquent, the insurance billing specialist should send a letter to the insurance carrier (Fig. 14–18). For problem claims it may be wise to obtain and complete a *Certificate of Mailing* form from the U.S. Postal Service. The form is initialed and postmarked at the post office and returned to the insurance biller for the office file. Because the post office does not keep a record of the mailing, this certificate costs less than certified mail. It shows proof that a special communication was mailed or sent on a certain date if a deadline is in question.

After receiving a response from the insurance carrier, it may be necessary to send subsequent letters to the employer. For example, if the insurance company notifies the physician's office that the employer's preliminary report of injury has not been received, then send a letter to the employer (Fig. 14–19).

If 30 days have elapsed from the date the letter was sent requesting the Employer's Report of Work Injury and the employer has not responded, send a letter to the Workers' Compensation Board or Industrial Accidents Commission in your state (Fig. 14–20).

Refer to Chapter 8 for additional information and helpful suggestions on following up on delinquent claims.

Martin Feelgood, MD
4567 Broad Avenue
Woodland Hills, XY 12345
013-486-9002

June 20, 20XX

XYZ Insurance Company
P. O. Box S
Woodland Hills, XY 12345

Dear Madam or Sir:

Re: Case No.:   120 23 6542
       Injured: Mrs. Ima B. Hurt
       Date of Injury: April 3, 20XX
       Employer: The Conk Out Company
       Amount: $148.92

Our records indicate that our final statement for the above case dated ___5/18/20XX___ remains unpaid.

Your cooperation in furnishing us the present status of this statement will be appreciated. A notation on the bottom of this letter will be sufficient.

Very truly yours,

Martin Feelgood ,MD

ref initials

- -

_____No Employer's Report on file
_____No Doctor's First Report on file
_____Did not receive itemized billing statement
_____Payment was made. Check No.____Date_____
_____Other reason(s) _____

Figure 14–18. If a workers' compensation claim becomes 45 days delinquent, the insurance billing specialist should send this letter to the insurance carrier.

Martin Feelgood, MD
4567 Broad Avenue
Woodland Hills, XY 12345
013-486-9002

June 20, 20XX

The Conk Out Company
45 South Gorman Street
Woodland Hills, XY 12345

Dear Madam or Sir:

Re: Case No.:   120 23 6542
       Injured: Mrs. Ima B. Hurt
       Date of Injury: April 3, 20XX

I have been informed by your workers' compensation
insurance carrier that they have not as yet received the
employer's report in regard to the above injured person.

Unless you have already done so, may I ask your cooperation
in completing and sending this report so that the case may be
closed.

Should you have any questions or if I can be of assistance to
you in any way, please do not hesitate to call on me.

Very truly yours,

Martin Feelgood , MD

ref initials

Figure 14–19. If the insurance company notifies the physician's office that the employer's preliminary report of injury has not been received, send this letter to the employer.

Martin Feelgood, MD
4567 Broad Avenue
Woodland Hills, XY 12345
013-486-9002

July 15, 20XX

Division of Industrial Accidents
State Office Building
107 South Broadway, Room 4107
Woodland Hills, XY 12345

Dear Madam or Sir:

Re: Failure of employer to follow Section No. 3760

Your office is being solicited to help secure an Employer's
Report of Work Injury from the employer listed below.

       Case No.:   120 23 6542
       Name of Employer: The Conk Out Company
          Address: 45 South Gorman Street
                                   Woodland Hills, XY 12345
       Name of Injured: Mrs. Ima B. Hurt
          Address: 300 East Central Avenue
                                   Woodland Hills, XY 12345
       Date of Injury: April 3, 20XX
       Name of Insurance Carrier: XYZ Insurance Company
       Amount of Unpaid Bill: $148.92

Your cooperation in this matter will be greatly appreciated. If you
need further information, please feel free to contact my office.

Sincerely yours,

Martin Feelgood , MD

ref initials

Figure 14–20. If the employer does not respond to your letter requesting the Employer's Report of Work Injury after 30 days have elapsed from the date of the letter, send this letter to the Workers' Compensation Board or Industrial Accident Commission in your state.

RESOURCES ON THE INTERNET

Contact the following for information about federal benefits:
Department of Labor, Employment Standards Administration, Washington, DC 20210

www.dol.gov/dol/esa/

Inquiry can be directed to one of these departments:

Division of Coal Mine Workers' Compensation

www.dol.gov/dol/esa/public/regs/compliance/ owcp/bltable.htm

Division of Federal Employees' Compensation

www.dol.gov/dol/esa/public/regs/compliance/ owc

Division of Longshoremen's and Harbor Workers' Compensation

www.dol.gov/dol/esa/public/regs/compliance/ owc

STUDENT ASSIGNMENT LIST

✔ Study Chapter 14.
✔ Answer the review questions in the *Workbook* to reinforce the theory learned in this chapter and to help prepare you for a future test.
✔ Complete the assignments in the *Workbook* for hands-on experience in completing workers' compensation insurance claim forms and reports, as well as enhanced proficiency in procedural and diagnostic coding.
✔ Turn to the Glossary at the end of this textbook for a further understanding of the Key Terms used in this chapter.

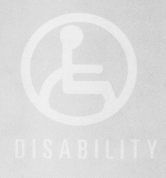

DISABILITY

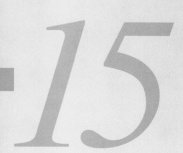

15

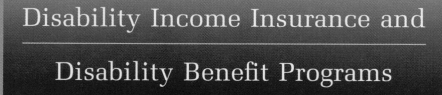

Disability Income Insurance and Disability Benefit Programs

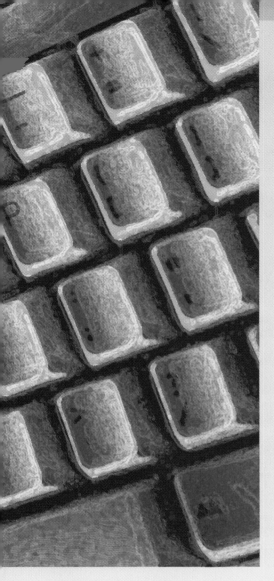

- Name federal disability benefit programs.
- Differentiate between SSDI and SSI.
- State eligibility requirements, benefits, and limitations of SSDI and SSI.
- Explain disability benefit programs for disabled active military personnel, veterans, and their dependents.
- Name states that have state disability insurance plans.
- State eligibility requirements, benefits, and limitations of state disability plans.
- Explain voluntary disability insurance plans.
- Recognize forms used for processing state disability plans.
- Describe topics and contents of a medical history report.
- List guidelines for federal, state, individual, and group disability claim procedures.

OBJECTIVES*

After reading this chapter you should be able to:

- Define terminology and abbreviations pertinent to disability insurance and disability benefit programs.
- Describe benefits and exclusions contained in individual and group disability income insurance.
- Define the words *temporary disability* and *permanent disability,* as related to each type of disability program.

*Performance objectives and exercises for hands-on practical experience for this chapter appear in the *Workbook.*

KEY TERMS*

accidental death and dismemberment

Armed Services Disability

benefit period*

Civil Service Retirement System (CSRS)

consultative examiner (CE)

cost-of-living adjustment

Disability Determination Services (DDS)

disability income insurance

double indemnity

exclusions*

Federal Employees Retirement System (FERS)

future purchase option

guaranteed renewable*

hearing

long-term disability insurance

noncancelable clause*

partial disability*

reconsideration

regional office (RO)

residual benefits*

short-term disability insurance

Social Security Administration (SSA)

Social Security Disability Insurance (SSDI) program

continued

---

*Some of the insurance terms presented in this chapter are shown marked with an asterisk and may seem familiar from previous chapters. However, their meanings may or may not have a slightly different connotation when referring to disability income insurance.

Disability Claims

Not everyone has disability insurance, but when working with patients who have it, you may encounter some interesting and unique accidents, injuries, or illnesses. After reading these extracts or direct quotations from disability insurance claim applications, you may ask: "How in the world could something like this happen?" The following gems show just how funny some situations can appear:

Describe How Your Disability Occurred

"A hernia from pulling cork out of bottle."

"Put tire patch on Playtex girdle and it caused infection on right thigh."

"While waving goodnight to friends, fell out a two-story window."

"Back injury received from jumping off a ladder to escape being hit by a train."

One victim graphically described an experience most of us have had: "Getting on a bus, the driver started before I was all on." Can you hear them asking at the hospital, "Was this your assigned seat?"

Another victim stated, "I dislocated my shoulder swatting a fly." When asked, "Have you ever dislocated a shoulder at this sport?" He stated, "I have—I knocked over two table lamps, several high-balls, and skinned an elbow."

Because you have come to the end of your course on insurance billing and have learned a great deal, you may feel a bit bogged down by the many rules and regulations and their ever-changing nature. It is hoped that the introduction to this chapter added a bit of levity to your perspective on the world of disability insurance.

This chapter introduces various types of disability income insurance plans as well as a number of disability benefit programs. The first topic, **disability income insurance,** is a form of health insurance providing periodic payments under certain conditions when the insured is unable to work because of illness, disease, or injury—not as a result of a work-related accident or condition.

A second section describes major programs administered by the U.S. government related to industrial accidents and other disability benefit programs unrelated to work injuries.

The third part of the chapter deals with nonindustrial state disability programs administered in five states and Puerto Rico, as well as voluntary disability insurance plans.

Guidelines for federal, state, individual, and group disability claim procedures are presented at the end of the chapter.

History

Before the late 1800s disability income insurance provided only accident protection. Some life insurance contracts had disability income riders attached to them offering limited benefits. In the early 1880s, insurance companies began selling disability income policies that offered coverage for accident and illness. Then in the early 1900s, the Paul Revere Life Insurance Company introduced the first noncancelable disability income policy. This meant that the contract would be in force for a certain period of time and guaranteed that the premium would not be increased. By 1956, Congress had enacted legislation providing for disability income protection under the Social Security program for disabled individuals older than the age of 50 years. This program was expanded in 1965 to cover workers without regard to age as long as certain eligibility standards were met.

Today, disability income insurance is available from private insurance companies (individual policies) and employer-sponsored plans (group policies). Government-funded and state benefit programs are also available for disabled persons. In this chapter all of these plans and programs are discussed, along with the role of the insurance billing specialist in dealing with this type of insurance.

Disability Income Insurance

Individual

Individual disability income insurance is coverage that provides a specific monthly or weekly income when a person becomes unable to work, temporarily or totally, because of an illness or injury. Disability income policies *do not* provide medical expense benefits. The disability *cannot be* work related. As learned in the previous chapter, with workers' compensation insurance the illness or accident *must be* work related.

For individuals who are self-employed, this insurance is particularly important because a business could not meet its financial obligations if the owner became injured or too ill to work. For example, if an individual is self-employed with a home-based business, repetitive stress injuries (RSIs) would not allow that individual to use the computer for several months. The main purpose of these policies is to provide some benefits while the person is not able to work. To collect benefits, the individual must meet the policy's criteria of what constitutes partial, temporary, or total disability.

These policies terminate when the individual retires or reaches a certain age, usually 65 years.

Waiting Period

The time period from the beginning of disability to receiving the first payment of benefits is called an *elimination period* or **waiting period.** During this initial period, a disabled individual is not eligible to receive benefits even though he or she is unable to work.

Benefit Period

A **benefit period** is the maximum amount of time that benefits will be paid to the injured or ill person for the disability (e.g., 2-year, 5-year, to age 65, or lifetime).

Benefits

Benefits paid to the insured disabled person are called *indemnity* and can be received daily, weekly, monthly, or semiannually depending on the policy. Premiums and benefits hinge on several risk factors, such as age, gender, health history and physical state, income, and occupational duties. Some policies include residual or partial disability income benefits. Benefits are not taxable if premiums are paid by the individual.

Residual benefits pay a partial benefit when the insured is not totally disabled. If one becomes partially disabled or can work only part-time or in a limited capacity, the residual benefits make up the difference between what an individual can earn at present and what he or she would have earned working full-time.

Supplemental benefits may consist of insurance provisions that will increase monthly indemnity, such as a **future purchase option** or a **cost-of-living adjustment.** Provisions also distribute a percentage of the policy premiums if an individual keeps a policy in force for 5 or 10 years or does not file any claims.

An **accidental death and dismemberment** benefit is written into some contracts. This offers the insured person protection when loss of sight or loss of limb(s) occurs. In some policies, such as life insurance, if an unintended, unexpected, and unforeseeable accident occurs resulting in death, a special provision known as **double indemnity** applies. This feature provides for twice the face amount of the policy to be paid if death results from accidental causes.

Types of Disability

A disability may be partial, temporary, or total. The definition of **total disability** that is stated in each disability income policy varies from one to the other because there is no standard definition. An example of a liberal definition might read: "The insured must be unable to perform the major duties of his or her specific occupation." Social Security has a restrictive definition that you will read later in this chapter.

The terms *residual disability* and **partial disability** are defined as "when an illness or injury prevents an insured person from performing *one or more* of the functions of his or her regular job"—in other words, when a person cannot perform all of his or her job duties.

Temporary disability exists when a person cannot perform all the functions of his or her regular job for a limited period of time.

Clauses

When a policy is **guaranteed renewable,** this means that the insurer is required to renew the policy as long as premium payments are made for a specified number of years or to a specified age, such as 60, 65, 70, or for life. However, the premium may be increased when it is renewed. When the policy has a **noncancelable clause,** this means the premium cannot be increased.

A **waiver of premium,** if included in the insurance contract, means that while disabled, the policy pays all premiums and the employee does not have to pay. Usually this provision is used as a total and permanent disability benefit and may be available in certain other cases.

Exclusions

Exclusions are provisions written into the insurance contract denying coverage or limiting the scope of coverage. Examples are preexisting conditions; disability due to war, riot, self-inflicted injury, or attempted suicide; mental or nervous conditions; disability while legally intoxicated or under the influence of narcotics unless prescribed by a licensed physician; conditions arising from normal pregnancy or during the act of committing a felony; or if benefits are being received under workers' compensation or a government program. The phrase *legally intoxicated* means intoxication in an individual who has a certain amount of alcohol in the blood when tested that exceeds limits set by state law.

Acquired Immunodeficiency Syndrome and Human Immunodeficiency Virus Infection

States have statutes governing questions that can and cannot be asked on insurance application forms regarding AIDS and HIV testing; therefore, *each* state has developed its own forms. If a private insurance company wishes to test an applicant, a consent/notice form including acceptance of pretest and post-test counseling must be signed.

Group

Some employers elect to offer group disability income insurance as a fringe benefit. These contracts are drawn up between the insurer and the employer. Premiums may be paid by the employer with or without contributions from the employee. Employees hold certificates of insurance and are covered under the employer's policy, so they are not called policyholders. When the employee leaves the company, the insurance terminates unless the employee is disabled. A few group policies allow conversion to a limited benefit individual policy.

Benefits

Benefits vary from one plan to another but are usually for **short-term disability insurance** (13 weeks to 24 months) or **long-term disability insurance** (to age 65). To qualify for benefits, an individual must be unable to perform the major duties of his or her occupation during the initial period of disability (i.e., the first 2 years). Benefits cease when the employee returns to work, even part-time. These policies offer the worker partial disability income benefits to motivate a disabled individual to return to work on a part-time basis. Monthly benefits are usually paid directly to the employee and are taxable if the employee is not making any contribution toward the premiums.

Exclusions

Disabilities commonly excluded from coverage include those seen in individual disability income insurance policies as previously described.

Federal Disability Programs

Workers' Compensation

The federal government has a number of programs that cover workers from loss of income because of work-related disability. These programs were mentioned in Chapter 14 because work-related disabilities fall under workers' compensation laws. When an individual is eligible under more than one program, coordination of benefits is used so that a worker cannot receive benefits that result in an amount greater than what the person receives when working. *Coordination of benefits* is a provision preventing double payment for expenses by making one of the programs the primary payer and ensuring that no more than 100% of the costs are covered.

Disability Benefit Programs

The government's major disability programs are:
▸ **Social Security Disability Insurance (SSDI) program**
▸ Supplemental Security Income (SSI)
▸ **Civil Service Retirement System (CSRS)**
▸ **Federal Employees Retirement System (FERS)**
▸ **Armed Services Disability**
▸ **Veterans Affairs (VA) disability program**

The **Social Security Administration (SSA)** manages two programs that pay monthly disability benefits to people younger than age 65 who cannot work for at least a year because of a severe disability: SSDI and SSI. Medical requirements are the same for both programs.

Social Security Disability Insurance Program

Background

In 1935, the Social Security Act, the Old-Age, Survivors, Disability, and Health Insurance Program (OASDHI), was enacted, providing benefits for death, retirement, disability, and medical care. Then in 1956, Congress decided to establish a program for long-term disability known as Social Security Disability Insurance (SSDI) under Title II of the Social Security Act. This is an entitlement, not welfare, program providing monthly benefits to workers and those self-employed who meet certain conditions.

Disability Definition

Disability under Social Security has a strict definition: "Inability to engage in any substantial gainful activity by reason of any medically determinable physical or mental impairment which can be expected to result in death or which has lasted or can be expected to last for a continuous period of not less than 12 months."

Eligibility

The following is a list of individuals who meet eligibility requirements for SSDI:
▸ Disabled workers younger than age 65 years and their families
▸ Individuals who become disabled before age 22 years, if a parent (or, in certain cases, a grandparent) who is covered under Social Security retires, becomes disabled, or dies
▸ Disabled widows or widowers, age 50 years or older, if the deceased spouse worked at least 10 years under Social Security
▸ Disabled surviving divorced spouses older than age 50 years, if the ex-spouse was married to the disabled person for at least 10 years
▸ Blind workers whose vision in the better eye cannot be corrected to better than 20/200 or whose visual field in the better eye, even with corrective lenses, is 20 degrees or less

Workers must be fully insured in accordance with standards set by the Social Security Administration in terms of age, number of quarters worked, and amount of wages earned per quarter. The processing of eligibility application forms may take up to 2 months.

Benefits

Monthly benefits are paid to qualified individuals. After 24 months of disability payments, the disabled individual also becomes eligible for Medicare. When an individual reaches age 65, the benefits convert to retirement benefits.

Supplemental Security Income

Eligibility

The Supplemental Security Income (SSI) program is under Title XVI of the Social Security Act and provides disability payments to needy people (adults and children) with limited income and few resources. No prior employment is needed. Many SSI recipients also qualify for Medicaid, a state assistance program. The following individuals may qualify for SSI disability payments:
▸ Disabled persons younger than age 65 years who have very limited income and resources
▸ Disabled children younger than age 18 years, if the disability compares in severity with one that would keep an adult from working and has lasted or is expected to last at least 12 months or result in death
▸ Blind adults or children who, in the better eye, with the use of corrective lenses, have a visual

acuity no better than 20/100 or have a visual field of 20 degrees or less

Disability Determination Process

To establish disability under SSDI or SSI, an individual calls or visits any Social Security office and completes application forms with the help of a social worker. Then, a determination process is set into action. A physician may be involved in the determination process in one of three ways: (1) as a treating source who provides medical evidence on behalf of his or her patient, (2) as a **consultative examiner (CE)** who is paid a fee and examines and/or tests the applicant, or (3) as a full- or part-time medical or psychologic consultant reviewing claims for a state or **regional office (RO).**

In addition to a medical report from one of these sources, other criteria taken into consideration are the individual's age and vocational and educational factors that may contribute to the person's ability to work. It is possible that a person may be eligible for disability payments under one government program and not eligible under Social Security because the rules differ. If the applicant has reports from another agency, they may be used to determine whether a person is disabled for Social Security purposes. Many SSA state agencies have a division known as **Disability Determination Services (DDS).** The physician does not make the disability determination. Determination of disability is made by a DDS team composed of a physician/psychologist and disability examiner (DE).

Appeals Evaluation Process

If a claimant does not agree with the determination of disability, a four-level appeals process is available.

1. A **reconsideration,** which is a complete review of the claim by a medical or psychologic consultant/disability examiner team that did not take part in the original disability determination.
2. A **hearing** before an administrative law judge who had no part in the initial or reconsideration determinations of the claim. The hearing is held within 75 miles of the claimant's home. The claimant and his or her representative are permitted to present their case in person and to present a written statement. They also are permitted to review information the judge will use to make a decision and to question any witnesses.
3. A *review by the Appeals Council,* which considers all requests for review, but it may deny a request if it believes the decision by the administrative law judge was correct. If the Appeals Council decides the case should be reviewed, it will either make a decision on the case or return it to an administrative law judge for further review.
4. A *review by the federal court,* for which the claimant may file an action where he or she resides.

From time to time, disability cases are reviewed to be sure the individuals are still disabled. The frequency depends on the nature and severity of the impairment, the likelihood of improvement, rehabilitation, ability to work, and so on.

Benefits

Social Security disability programs are designed to give long-term protection and benefits to individuals totally disabled who are unable to do any type of work in the national economy. In contrast, short-term disability may be provided through workers' compensation, insurance, savings, and investments.

Work Incentives

Special rules allow disabled or blind people presently receiving Social Security or SSI to work and still receive monthly benefits as well as Medicare or Medicaid. There is a limit on how much the person can earn in a calendar year. These encouragements are referred to as "work incentives," and the rules are different for Social Security beneficiaries and SSI recipients.

Civil Service and Federal Employees Retirement System Disability

Eligibility

Federal employees who work in civil service fall under the Civil Service Retirement System (CSRS). This system has provisions for those who become totally disabled. This program is a combination of federal disability and Social Security disability. Both portions of the program must be applied for by the worker. The disability cannot be work related, and 5 years of service are required before benefits are payable. Eighteen months of service are required under the Federal Employees Retirement System (FERS).

Benefits

Those who qualify are entitled to benefits that are payable for life.

An example is an individual who works for the Internal Revenue Service performing clerical and filing job duties and has an automobile accident on the weekend. The head injuries are so severe that the person is unable to return to gainful employment at any job. He or she could apply for benefits either under the CSRS or FERS depending on their eligibility status.

Armed Services Disability

Eligibility

Individuals covered under this program must be members of the armed services on active duty.

Benefits

If a disability occurs or is aggravated while serving in the military service, monthly benefits are payable for life. Benefit amounts are based on years of service, base pay, and severity of disability. This, too, is subject to review.

Veterans Affairs Disability

Eligibility

The Veterans Affairs (VA) is authorized by law to provide a wide range of benefits to those who have served their country in the armed forces and to their dependents. If a veteran who is honorably discharged files a claim for a *service-connected disability* within 1 year of sustaining that injury, he or she is eligible for outpatient treatment. Veterans with *non–service-connected disabilities* who are in receipt of housebound or aid-in-attendance benefits are eligible for treatment by a private physician if they are unable to travel to a VA facility owing to geographic inaccessibility. Their identification card, benefits, and claims procedures are identical to those of veterans with service-connected disabilities receiving outpatient medical care.

Benefits

The following is a general list of veterans' medical benefits. Each benefit requires that certain criteria be met. These criteria are ever-changing and will not be mentioned here. A complete up-to-date booklet listing all the benefits is available.*

▶ Hospital care in a VA hospital
▶ Nursing home care in a VA facility

---

*Federal Benefits for Veterans and Dependents. Department of Veterans Affairs, Washington, DC 20420. The booklet is published annually and is available for a small fee from the Superintendent of Documents, U.S. Government Printing Office, Mail Stop: SSOP, Washington, DC 20402-9328.

▶ Domiciliary care
▶ Outpatient medical treatment at a VA facility or by a private physician
▶ Emergency treatment in a hospital for a service-connected condition
▶ Prescription drugs and medication issued by a VA pharmacy or other participating pharmacy. Only bona fide emergency prescriptions can be filled by a private pharmacy
▶ Certain medical equipment, such as oxygen, prosthetics, and so on
▶ Travel expenses when receiving VA medical care
▶ Outpatient dental treatment (if the veteran files a claim within 90 days from the date that he or she was discharged from the service)
▶ Treatment for Agent Orange or nuclear radiation exposure
▶ Alcohol and drug dependence outpatient care
▶ Readjustment counseling services

In regard to a service-connected disability, any professional service that is not related to the service disability must be paid by the veteran out of his or her own pocket. The physician must accept what the VA pays as payment in full and cannot bill the patient for any additional charges, even if there is a balance after the VA pays the claim. If the treatment is likely to cost more than $40 per month, the physician must obtain prior authorization from the nearest VA facility. A separate ledger card must be prepared for VA benefits if the physician is also treating the patient for ailments other than a service-connected disability.

Veterans with non–service-connected disabilities may have copayments when seeking treatment. For example, individuals on Medicare may be responsible for the deductible for the first 90 days of care during any 365-day period. For each additional 90 days of hospital care, the patient is charged one-half the Medicare deductible, $10 a day of hospital care, and $5 a day for VA nursing home care. For outpatient care, the copayment is 20% of the cost of an average outpatient visit.

Outpatient Treatment

Veterans eligible for outpatient treatment may obtain outpatient medical care only for the disability as listed on the **Veterans Affairs (VA) outpatient clinic** card (Fig. 15–1). Usually a veteran seeks care at the nearest VA outpatient clinic. However, when a VA facility is not within reasonable distance, when the veteran is too ill to travel to the nearest location, or when the condition needs prompt attention, the veteran can apply for and be granted medical care by a private physician through the Home Town Care Program. The VA outpatient

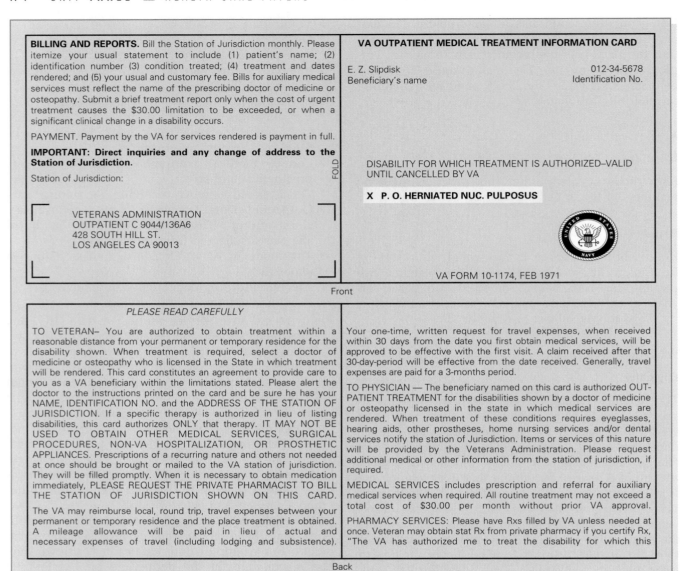

BILLING AND REPORTS. Bill the Station of Jurisdiction monthly. Please itemize your usual statement to include (1) patient's name; (2) identification number (3) condition treated; (4) treatment and dates rendered; and (5) your usual and customary fee. Bills for auxiliary medical services must reflect the name of the prescribing doctor of medicine or osteopathy. Submit a brief treatment report only when the cost of urgent treatment causes the $30.00 limitation to be exceeded, or when a significant clinical change in a disability occurs.

PAYMENT. Payment by the VA for services rendered is payment in full.

IMPORTANT: Direct inquiries and any change of address to the Station of Jurisdiction.

Station of Jurisdiction:

FOLD

VETERANS ADMINISTRATION
OUTPATIENT C 9044/136A6
428 SOUTH HILL ST.
LOS ANGELES CA 90013

VA OUTPATIENT MEDICAL TREATMENT INFORMATION CARD

E. Z. Slipdisk   012-34-5678
Beneficiary's name   Identification No.

DISABILITY FOR WHICH TREATMENT IS AUTHORIZED–VALID UNTIL CANCELLED BY VA

X   P. O. HERNIATED NUC. PULPOSUS

VA FORM 10-1174, FEB 1971

Front

PLEASE READ CAREFULLY

TO VETERAN– You are authorized to obtain treatment within a reasonable distance from your permanent or temporary residence for the disability shown. When treatment is required, select a doctor of medicine or osteopathy who is licensed in the State in which treatment will be rendered. This card constitutes an agreement to provide care to you as a VA beneficiary within the limitations stated. Please alert the doctor to the instructions printed on the card and be sure he has your NAME, IDENTIFICATION NO. and the ADDRESS OF THE STATION OF JURISDICTION. If a specific therapy is authorized in lieu of listing disabilities, this card authorizes ONLY that therapy. IT MAY NOT BE USED TO OBTAIN OTHER MEDICAL SERVICES, SURGICAL PROCEDURES, NON-VA HOSPITALIZATION, OR PROSTHETIC APPLIANCES. Prescriptions of a recurring nature and others not needed at once should be brought or mailed to the VA station of jurisdiction. They will be filled promptly. When it is necessary to obtain medication immediately, PLEASE REQUEST THE PRIVATE PHARMACIST TO BILL THE STATION OF JURISDICTION SHOWN ON THIS CARD.

The VA may reimburse local, round trip, travel expenses between your permanent or temporary residence and the place treatment is obtained. A mileage allowance will be paid in lieu of actual and necessary expenses of travel (including lodging and subsistence).

Your one-time, written request for travel expenses, when received within 30 days from the date you first obtain medical services, will be approved to be effective with the first visit. A claim received after that 30-day-period will be effective from the date received. Generally, travel expenses are paid for a 3-months period.

TO PHYSICIAN — The beneficiary named on this card is authorized OUT-PATIENT TREATMENT for the disabilities shown by a doctor of medicine or osteopathy licensed in the state in which medical services are rendered. When treatment of these conditions requires eyeglasses, hearing aids, other prostheses, home nursing services and/or dental services notify the station of Jurisdiction. Items or services of this nature will be provided by the Veterans Administration. Please request additional medical or other information from the station of jurisdiction, if required.

MEDICAL SERVICES includes prescription and referral for auxiliary medical services when required. All routine treatment may not exceed a total cost of $30.00 per month without prior VA approval.

PHARMACY SERVICES: Please have Rxs filled by VA unless needed at once. Veteran may obtain stat Rx from private pharmacy if you certify Rx, "The VA has authorized me to treat the disability for which this

Back

Figure 15–1. Sample Veterans Affairs outpatient clinic card.

clinic must be notified within 15 days of the treatment rendered. In such cases, the treating physician must submit evidence of medical necessity (i.e., detailed justification on the invoice) to the VA outpatient clinic. Form 10-583, Claim for Payment of Cost of Unauthorized Medical Services (Fig. 15–2), generally used for hospital emergency care, can also be used for professional care if the doctor is billing after the 15-day period has elapsed.

Veterans Affairs Installations

For information on veterans' benefits or assistance in locating Veterans Affairs Installations, write or call one of the regional offices listed in Appendix A. Many states have toll-free telephone services to the

Department of Veterans Affairs from communities in the state. Consult the local telephone directory or information assistance operator for the latest listing of these numbers.

State Disability Insurance

Background

In 1944, Rhode Island began a **State Disability Insurance (SDI)** program that proved successful. This form of insurance is part of an employment security program that provides temporary cash benefits for workers suffering a wage loss due to off-the-job illness or injury. It can be referred to as

Form Approved
Budget Bureau No. 76-H0325

VETERANS ADMINISTRATION
CLAIM FOR PAYMENT OF COST OF
UNAUTHORIZED MEDICAL SERVICES

Each person, firm or institution claiming payments or reimbursements must complete this form. No carbon paper is necessary. Please use typewriter or ball point pen, and submit both copies.

1A. VETERAN'S LAST NAME – FIRST – MIDDLE INITIAL	1B. CLAIM NO.	1C. SOCIAL SECURITY NO.
Thornberg, Joey T.	c–	421-00-4182

1D. PRESENT ADDRESS (*include zip code*)

4628 Image Street, Woodland Hills, XY 12345-1290

2. NAME AND ADDRESS OF PERSON, FIRM OR INSTITUTION MAKING CLAIM (*Leave blank if same as above*)

Gerald Practon, MD 4567 Broad Ave., Woodland Hills, XY 12345-0001

3. STATEMENT OF CIRCUMSTANCES UNDER WHICH THE SERVICES WERE RENDERED (Include diagnosis, symptoms, whether emergency existed, and reason VA facilities were not used)

Patient fell on sidewalk in front of home and suffered traumatic injury of right arm.
Symptoms: Localized pain, swelling, and bruising of right arm near elbow.
AP and lateral x-rays of right elbow show anterior dislocation right radius. Negative for fracture.
Medical care rendered in Emergency Dept. at College Hospital (99282).
Patient unable to go to VA facility as this is 60 miles away.
Treatment of closed elbow dislocation without anesthesia (23400).
Diagnosis: Anterior closed dislocation right radius (Dx code No. 832.01).

4. AMOUNT CLAIMED	*Attach bills or receipts showing services furnished, dates, and charges*
$ 237.02	attached

5. COMPLETE A OR B, AS APPROPRIATE

A. Amount claimed does not exceed that charged the general public for similar services, and payment has not been received.	B. I certify that the amount claimed has been paid and reimbursement has not been made.
Gerald Practon, MD 5/11/XX	*Joey T. Thornberg* 5/11/XX
SIGNATURE AND TITLE OF PROVIDER OF SERVICE, AND DATE	SIGNATURE OF VETERAN OR REPRESENTATIVE, AND DATE

FOR VETERANS ADMINISTRATION USE ONLY

6. ACTION ☐ APPROVED $ _____ ☐ DISAPPROVED	Treatment was provided in an emergency for a service-connected or adjunct disability, any disability of a veteran who has a total disability permanent in nature from a service-connected disability, or for any illness, injury, dental condition in the case of a veteran eligible under Chapter 31 (Vocational Rehabilitation) Title 38, U. S. Code. VA facilities were not feasibly available and delay would have been hazardous.

7. SIGNATURE, CHIEF, MEDICAL ADMINISTRATION SERVICE	8. DATE	9. ADMINISTRATION VOUCHER NO.

VA FORM
MAY 1974   10-583   SUPERSEDES VA FORM 10-583 FEB 1966 AND WHICH WILL NOT BE USED.

Figure 15–2. Veterans Affairs Form 10-583, Claim for Payment of Cost of Unauthorized Medical Services.

unemployment compensation disability (UCD) or **temporary disability insurance (TDI).** California became the second state to add nonindustrial disability coverage to the Social Security protection afforded to its citizens by appending Article 10 to the Unemployment Insurance Act. This became law on May 21, 1946; and when the legislation took effect on December 1, 1946, this article diverted the 1% tax formerly paid by workers for unemployment insurance to a disability insurance fund. New York and New Jersey soon followed with similar programs. Two decades later, in 1969,

Puerto Rico and Hawaii passed nonindustrial disability insurance laws.

Some accidents that occur are quite serious at the time but upon reviewing them can appear rather humorous.

Unique Accident

The patient was under the kitchen sink repairing a leak when the family cat came along, watched for awhile, then playfully—but painfully—reached up and clawed him. Startled, the man threw his head back, cracked it on the bottom of the sink, and was knocked out cold. He came to as he was being carried out on a stretcher and explained to the attendants what had happened. One stretcher bearer laughed so hard, he relaxed his hold and the patient fell to the ground and broke his arm.

State Programs

As of 2000, nonindustrial disability insurance programs exist in only five states and Puerto Rico. In each area, the law is known by a different name:

State	Name of Law	Web Site
California	California Unemployment Insurance Code.	www.edd.ca.gov
Hawaii	Temporary Disability Insurance Law	
New Jersey	Temporary Disability Benefits Law	www.state.nj.us
New York	Disability Benefits Law	www.web.state.ny.us
Puerto Rico	Disability Benefits Law	
Rhode Island	Temporary Disability Insurance Act	www.state.ri.us

Web sites for most of these programs can also be found at the end of this chapter.

Funding

To fund state disability insurance, a small percentage of the wage is deducted from employees' paychecks each month, or the employer may elect to pay all or part of the cost of the plan as a fringe benefit for employees. The money is then sent in quarterly installments to the state and put into a special fund.

Eligibility

To receive state disability insurance benefits, an employee must be:

- Employed full or part time or actively looking for work when disability begins
- Suffering a loss of wages because of disability
- Eligible for benefits depending on the amount withheld during a previous period before disability began
- Under the care and treatment of a physician who certifies the employee is disabled
- Disabled at least 7 or 8 calendar days or hospitalized as an inpatient
- Filing a claim within the time limit

If the worker was employed at the time of disability, benefits are not subject to federal income tax. An employee who retires is no longer eligible for the insurance. A worker may file a claim with the state seeking exemption from program participation on religious grounds.

Types of workers not covered are employees of school districts, community college districts, and churches; state workers; federal employees; interstate railroad workers; nonprofit organization employees; and domestic workers.

Benefits

Weekly benefits are determined by the wages earned in a base period or based on a percentage of average weekly wages (Table 15–1). Benefits begin after the seventh consecutive day of disability. There is no provision under the law for hospital or other medical benefits except in Hawaii and Puerto Rico, where hospital benefits are payable under a prepaid health care program if the employee meets certain eligibility requirements.

Limited Benefits

In some states, a patient may qualify for benefits if he or she is a resident of an approved alcoholic recovery facility or an approved drug-free residential facility.

Reduced Benefits

An individual may be entitled to partial benefits if receiving certain types of income, such as

- Sick leave
- Vacation
- Wages paid by employer
- Insurance settlement for the disability
- Workers' compensation benefits
- Unemployment benefits

TABLE 15–1	**State Disability Information Summary**				
State	**Name of State Law**	**Maximum Benefit Period (Wk)**	**Time Limit for Filing Claims**	**2000 Deductions From Salary (%)**	**Benefits**
California	California Unemployment Insurance Code	52	49 days from disability	0.7	Based on earnings in a 12-mo base period, which begins approximately 18 mo before disability
Hawaii	Temporary Disability Insurance Law	26	90 days from disability	0.5	Based on 58% of average weekly wage
New Jersey	Temporary Disability Benefits Law	26	30 days from disability	0.5	Based on average weekly wage
New York	Disability Benefits Law	26	30 days from disability	0.5 (max. 60 cents/wk)	Based on 50% of average weekly wage (max. $170/wk)
Puerto Rico	Disability Benefits Act	26	3 months from disability	0.3 employee; 0.3 employer	Based on wages earned during base year
Rhode Island	Temporary Disability Insurance Act	30	1 year from disability	1.2	Based on 4.62% of wages in the base period quarter in which wages were the highest

Time Limits

A claim for state disability insurance should be filed within the time limit of the state laws (see Table 15–1). There is usually a grace period of 7 or 8 days after the deadline. After the claim is approved, basic benefits become payable on the eighth day of disability or the first day of hospital confinement, whichever comes first. In California, benefits are paid from day 1 if the disability extends to 22 calendar days or more. A person may continue to draw disability insurance for a maximum of 26 weeks in Hawaii, New Jersey, New York, Puerto Rico, and Rhode Island and 52 weeks in California on the same illness or injury or overlapping disabilities. An employee is also entitled to disability benefits 15 days after recovery from a previous disability or illness. In other words, if a patient is discharged by the physician to return to work and is on the job 15 calendar days and then becomes ill with the same ailment, he or she may file a new claim.

Medical Examinations

The claimant may be required to submit to an examination or examinations by an independent medical examiner to determine any mental or physical disability. Fees for such examinations are paid by the state department handling disability insurance. Code 99450 for billing these medical examinations may be found in the Special Evaluation and Management Services section of *Current Procedural Terminology.*

Restrictions

There are many restrictions on disability insurance. A few of the major situations in which a claim could possibly be denied are listed here.

1. *Conditions covered by workers' compensation,* unless the rate is less than the disability insurance rate. In that case, the state pays the difference between the two rates.
2. Applicants receiving *unemployment insurance benefits over a certain specified amount.* Exception: If the applicant is on unemployment insurance and then becomes ill or injured, he or she is put on temporary disability insurance until able to go for a job interview.
3. *Disabilities beginning during a trade dispute.* If an employee is on strike and is injured while

walking a picket line, he or she is not eligible for benefits. However, if the union is on strike and an individual member remains at home and then becomes ill or injured, he or she can claim disability and will receive benefits.

4. *Confinement by court order or certification in a public or private institution* as an alcoholic, drug addict, or sexual psychopath.
5. *When legal custody is the cause of unemployment.*
6. *When the employing company has a voluntary disability plan and is not paying into a state fund.*
7. *Religious exemption certificate* on file by employee or company and no payment is made into a state fund.
8. *Pregnancy-related disability,* unless the pregnancy is complicated (e.g., cases in which the patient has diabetes, varicose veins, ectopic pregnancy, or cesarean section). *Exceptions:* California, Hawaii, New Jersey, and Rhode Island have maternity benefits that may be applied for at the time the physician tells the patient to stop working.

Voluntary Disability Insurance

Persons residing and working in states that do not have state disability insurance programs may elect to contact a local private insurance carrier to arrange for coverage under a **voluntary disability insurance** plan. If these persons become ill or disabled, they receive a fixed weekly or monthly income, usually for approximately 6 months. If the disability or illness is permanent and the individual is unable to return to work, there is sometimes a small monthly income for the duration of the person's life. Some of the state laws provide that a "voluntary plan" may be adopted instead of the "state plan" if a majority of company employees consent to private coverage.

PROCEDURE: Claims Submission

Disability Income Claims

When the insurance billing specialist is handling disability income claim forms, he or she should note that the insured (claimant) is responsible to notify the insurance company of the disability. A proof of loss form is completed to establish disability.

The facts required are
▶ Date the disability occurred
▶ Date the disabled is expected to be well enough to return to work
▶ Description of how the disability occurred
▶ Name of treating physician
▶ Explanation of how the disability prevents the insured from work

The report must show that the patient's disability meets the policy's definition of disability, or benefits will be denied. Because the definition of disability varies among policies, the critical issues are the content and wording on the claim form.

A portion of this form is usually completed by the attending physician. The following data are required:
▶ Medical history
▶ Dates patient became disabled
▶ Subjective symptoms (patient's own words about his or her chief complaints)
▶ Objective findings on physical examination (e.g., rashes, lacerations, abrasions, contusions)
▶ Severity of the illness or injury (range of motion tests)
▶ Photocopies of laboratory tests, x-ray studies, hospital discharge report
▶ Medication
▶ Treatment dates
▶ Diagnosis
▶ Prognosis (outcome of the disease or injury)
▶ Names of any other treating physician
▶ Date patient expected to return to work
▶ Description of job duties and patient's ability to perform work

This information helps verify the disability. In some cases, the physician may wish to dictate a medical report and attach it to the claim form instead of completing a portion of the form. The insurance billing specialist must be prepared to extract data from source documents, such as medical and financial records, to complete the claim form. In such situations, ask the physician to read the information carefully before signing the document. Always ask the patient to sign an authorization form to release medical information. Reasons for denial of benefits are often improper choice of words or inadequate medical information.

The insurance company may request information from other places to justify payment of benefits, such as employer's records, employee's wage statements and/or tax forms, or the attending physician's medical records. A company representative may interview the insured if conflicting information exists.

If disability continues, additional claim forms may need to be completed monthly, or more frequently, by the insured and attending physician. Other sources of information may be requested, for example, records from medical specialists or Social Security records.

If the validity of the case is in question, an independent medical examiner may be asked by the insurance company to examine the disabled individual. If the claimant neglects to return claim forms, refuses telephone calls, misses appointments, or engages in questionable activities, then the insurance company will discreetly engage in surveillance of the insured through the services of a professional investigation firm.

Federal Disability Claims

The Social Security Administration division called Disability Determination Services (DDS) has a teledictation service so the physician or psychologist can dictate the medical report over the telephone instead of completing a medical report form. The service is available at any time, including nights and weekends. A typed transcript is sent to the physician to review, sign, and return to the SSA state agency, or a report may be typed on the physicians' stationery. The physician may photocopy relevant portions of the patient's chart and submit that information, but it should be legible. Be sure the patient has signed an authorization to release information. Copies of consultation reports and hospital summaries are also helpful. By law only recent data no more than 1 year old are allowed.

A medical report must include

▶ Relevant medical history, past history, social history, and family history
▶ Subjective complaints (patient's symptoms)
▶ Objective findings on physical examination (e.g., results of physical or mental status examination, blood pressure)
▶ Laboratory and x-ray findings
▶ Diagnostic studies (e.g., treadmill tests, pulmonary function tests, electrocardiographic tracings)
▶ Diagnosis (statement of disease or injury based on signs and symptoms)
▶ Treatment prescribed, with patient's response and prognosis
▶ Medical prognosis regarding disability based on medical findings. A description is required of the individual's ability to perform work-related activities, such as standing, sitting, lifting, carrying, walking, handling objects, hearing, speaking, and traveling. For cases of mental impairment, the statement should present the individual's capacity for understanding and memory, sustained concentration and persistence, social interaction, and adaptation.

Veterans Affairs Disability Outpatient Clinic Claims

The processing of invoices from private physicians is a somewhat lengthy procedure as required by VA regulations and involves several steps. To keep the delay in payment to a minimum, private physicians are urged to bill the VA on a monthly basis. To ensure prompt processing, invoices should contain the following information:

1. Patient's name as shown on the I.D. card, VA Form 10-1174 (see Fig. 15–1).
2. Patient's Social Security number.
3. Condition treated, shown on every invoice, because this is the basis for approval of payment.
4. Diagnosis being treated must be listed on the I.D. card or authorized by the statement "for any condition." Abstract the diagnosis exactly as it is stated on the I.D. card.
5. Treatment given and dates rendered
6. Physician's usual and customary fee for services rendered
7. Name and address of private physician and his or her Social Security or Federal Taxpayer I.D. number. If the I.D. number is assigned to a group and the physician desires to be paid individually, the VA outpatient clinic must be so advised.

Private physicians, as well as veterans, are urged to read the instructions on the I.D. card carefully. This is sometimes neglected and can lead to misunderstanding.

If the physician does not wish to bill the VA outpatient clinic, the patient can pay the physician and then be reimbursed, but the veteran must carefully follow the instructions on the back of the VA outpatient clinic card.

State Disability Claims

Residents of a state that provides state disability benefits may call or write to the nearest office that handles state disability insurance to obtain a claim form and insurance pamphlet. A list of offices and addresses for each state is provided in Appendix A.

In some states, the claim form is in three parts and must be completed by the claimant, employer, and physician. In other states, the form is in two parts and is completed by the claimant and physician (Figs. 15–3 and 15–4). In either instance, the case must be substantiated by a physician before the applicant may begin receiving benefits. Carefully read all information from the state disability insurance office and follow the directions. Provide the data requested and have the physician and pa-

CLAIM STATEMENT OF EMPLOYEE *Please read instructions on back before completing this form.*
COMPLETE *ALL* ITEMS. IF INCOMPLETE, THIS FORM WILL BE RETURNED, CAUSING A DELAY IN BENEFIT PAYMENTS

1. Print your full name: FIRST   INITIAL   LAST

    MARCIA   M.   MONROE

Other Names (including maiden, married and ethnic surnames) Used:

Your Mailing Address:

STREET ADDRESS, P.O. BOX OR RFD   APT. NO.   CITY OR TOWN   STATE AND ZIP CODE

3501 Maple Street, Woodland Hills,   XY 12345

Your Home Address: (Required if different from mailing address)
IF YOU HAVE NO STREET ADDRESS, YOU **MUST** PROVIDE SPECIFIC DIRECTIONS TO YOUR HOME

Male ☐   Female ☒   Birthdate MONTH 03 DAY 04 YEAR 1952

Do you need assistance in a language other than English? ☒ No   ☐ Yes
If yes, write that language here:_____
¿Prefiere Ud. formularios escritos en español? No ☐   Sí ☐

2. **IMPORTANT:** Enter your Social Security Account Number

    5 4 0   2 1   9 8 8 1

2A. If you have used another Social Security number, enter that number here

    _ _ _   _ _   _ _ _ _

3. What was the first day you were too sick to perform all the duties of your regular or customary work, even if it was a Saturday, Sunday, holiday, or a normal day off?:

    MONTH 10   DAY 10   YEAR 20xx

4. What was the last day you worked prior to your disability?

    MONTH 10   DAY 09   YEAR 20xx

5. Current or Last Employer's Business Name: Telephone Number

    A and B Company   (013) 487-9980

Current or Last Employer's Business Address   NUMBER AND STREET   CITY   STATE AND ZIP CODE

    401 State Street   Woodland Hills,   XY   12345

6. Your occupation with this employer. secretary   Your Badge or Payroll number: 4399

7. a. What is your usual occupation? secretary

   b. Have you been retrained for a new occupation? If yes, please give name of that occupation: Yes ☐   No ☒

8. Are you self-employed?   Yes ☐   No ☒

9. Did you lose any time from work because of this illness or injury during the two weeks before the last day you worked as shown in item (4) above?   Yes ☐   No ☒

10. Did you stop work because of sickness, injury or pregnancy?
    If "No," please give reason: Yes ☒   No

11. Have you filed for or received UNEMPLOYMENT INSURANCE benefits between the last day you worked and the first day you became disabled?   Yes ☐   No ☒

12. a. Has, or will your employer continue your pay by means of sick leave, pension, gift or other means?   Yes ☐   No ☒

    b. Do you authorize the Employment Development Department to disclose benefit eligibility information to your employer to be used only for the purpose of integrating your employer's wage continuation/sick leave program with your benefits? (This information is limited to the claim effective date; the weekly and maximum benefit amounts; and the periods covered by benefit payments.) Yes ☒   No

13. Was this disability or any other disability during this claim period caused by your work?   Yes ☐   No ☒
    If "Yes," please provide: (a) The date of your work-caused injury: _____ and (b) The name and address of any insurance carrier from whom you are claiming or receiving Workers' Compensation benefits.

14. Have you recovered from your disability?
    If "Yes," enter date of recovery: Yes ☐   No ☒

15. Have you returned to work for any day, part-time or full-time, after the beginning date of your disability as shown in item (3) above?
    If "Yes," please enter such dates: Yes ☐   No ☒

16. At any time during your disability, were you, as a result of an arrest, confined to a jail, detention center, prison medical center or other correctional institution or any other place: If "Yes," give dates: Yes ☐   No ☒

I hereby claim benefits and certify that for the period covered by this claim I was unemployed and disabled, that the foregoing statements, including any accompanying statements, are to the best of my knowledge and belief true, correct and complete. I hereby authorize my attending physician, practitioner, hospital, vocational rehabilitation counselor, employer, and California Department of Industrial Relations to furnish and disclose all facts concerning my disability and wages or earnings that are within their knowledge and to allow inspection of and provide copies of any medical, vocational rehabilitation, and billing records concerning my disability that are under their control. I understand that authorizaitons contained in this claim statement are granted for a period of five years from the date of my signature or the effective date of the claim, whichever is later. I agree that a photocopy of this authorization shall be as valid as the original.

Claim signed on: ▶   MONTH 10 DAY 12 YEAR 20xx   Claimant's signature: ▶   (DO NOT PRINT)   Telephone Number (013) 487-9980

Under Section 2101 of the California Unemployment Insurance Code, it is a violation to willfully make a false statement or knowingly conceal a material fact in order to obtain the payment of any benefits, such violation being punishable by imprisonment and/or by a fine not exceeding $20,000 or both.

If your signature is made by mark (X) it must be attested by two witnesses with their addresses.
SIGNATURE-WITNESS   SIGNATURE-WITNESS

ADDRESS   ADDRESS

If an authorized agent is filing for benefits for an INCAPACITATED or DECEASED claimant, or a spouse is filing for a MENTALLY INCAPACITATED individual, contact the office below for the required forms and instructions.

480

Figure 15–3. Form DE 2501, Claim Statement of Employee. This is a two-part form, and this side is completed by the claimant.

DOCTOR'S CERTIFICATE

Certification may be made by a licensed medical or osteopathic physician and surgeon, chiropractor, dentist, podiatrist, optometrist, designated psychologist or an authorized medical officer of a United States Government facility. Certification may also be made by a licensed nurse-midwife or nurse practitioner for the purposes of disability related to normal pregnancy or childbirth. All items on this sheet must be completed legibly.

Patient File No.	Name MARCIA M. MONROE	Social Security Number 540-21-9881

17. I attended the patient for the present medical problem

	MONTH DAY YEAR		MONTH DAY YEAR
from:	10-12-20XX	To present	At intervals of: two visits to date

18. Are you completing this form for the sole purpose of referral or recommendation to an alcoholic recovery home or drug-free facility?
Yes ☐ No ☒ If yes, please enter facility name and address in item #28.

19. History:
cough of 2 wks duration, chest pain, 100°F

Objective Findings/Detailed Statement of Symptoms

Diagnosis:
(REQUIRED)
bilateral pneumonitis

bilateral pneumonitis

ICD-9 Disease Code, Primary:
(REQUIRED)   486

ICD-9 Disease Code, Secondary:

Type of treatment and/or medication rendered to patient:
Bed rest   Rx   antibiotic

20. Diagnosis confirmed by: **(Specify type of test or X-ray)**
AP and lateral chest x-rays

21. Is this patient now pregnant or has she been pregnant since the date of treatment as reported above?
Yes ☐ No ☒
If "Yes," date pregnancy terminated or future EDC.

Is the pregnancy normal?
Yes ☐ No ☐
If "No," state the abnormal and involuntary complication causing maternal disability:

22. Operation: Date performed or to be performed   DNA

Type of Operation:

ICD-9 Procedutre Code:
(REQUIRED)

23. Was or is patient confined as a registered bed patient in a hospital? Yes ☐ No ☒
If "Yes," please provide dates:
Entered hospital on _____, 20____
Discharged from hospital on _____, 20____

24. Has the patient at any time during your attendance for this medical problem, been incapable of performing his or her regular work as a _____? Yes ☒ No ☐ If "Yes" the disability commenced on: 10-10-20XX

25. APPROXIMATE date, based on your examination of patient, disability (if any) should end or has ended sufficiently to permit the patient to resume regular or customary work. Even if considerable question exists, make SOME "estimate." This is a requirement of the Code, and the claim will be delayed if such date is not entered. Such answers as "Indefinite" or "don't know" will not suffice.
(ENTER DATE)
10-30-20XX

26. Based on your examination of patient, is this disability the result of "occupation" either as an "industrial accident" or as an "occupational disease"?
Yes ☐ No ☒
This should include aggravation of pre-existing conditions by occupation.

27. Have you reported this OR A CONCURRENT DISABILITY to any insurance carrier as a Workers' Compensation Claim?
Yes ☐ No ☒ If "yes" to whom? _____
(Name of carrier or firm)

28. Was or is patient a resident in an alcoholic recovery home or drug-free residential facility? Yes ☐ No ☒
If "Yes," please provide name and address:

29. Would the disclosure of this information to your patient be medically or psychologically detrimental to the patient?
Yes ☐ No ☒

I hereby certify that, based on my examination, the above statements truly describe the patient's disability (if any) and the estimated duration thereof, and that I am a ___MD___ | ___GP___ licensed to practice by the State of ___California___
(TYPE OF DOCTOR)   (SPECIALTY, IF ANY)

▶ David W. Smith, MD
PRINT OR TYPE DOCTOR'S NAME AS SHOWN ON LICENSE

▶
ORIGINAL SIGNATURE OF ATTENDING DOCTOR
- RUBBER STAMP IS NOT ACCEPTABLE -

▶ 4567 Broad Ave., Woodland Hills, XY 12345
NO. AND STREET   CITY   ZIP CODE

▶ C 14020   (013) 486-9002   10-19-20XX
STATE LICENSE NUMBER   TELEPHONE   DATE OF SIGNING THIS FORM

Under Section 2116 of the California Unemployment Insurance Code, it is a violation for any individual who, with the intent to defraud, falsely certifies the medical condition of any person in order to obtain disability insurance benefits, whether for the maker or for any other person, and is punishable by imprisonment and/or a fine not exceeding twenty thousand dollars. Section 1143 requires additional administrative penalties.

Figure 15–4. Form DE 2501, Doctor's Certificate. This side is completed by the attending physician and submitted within a set period of time from the beginning date of disability to initiate benefits. If the patient is seen by a second physician, this form is mailed to the claimant to secure the certification of a new physician or to clarify a specific claimed period of disability.

tient sign the forms. Send in the form within the stated time limits.

After the claim has been completed by all parties concerned, it is submitted to the nearest local office for processing. The most important items on the claim form are

1. The claimant's Social Security number; without it the claim cannot be researched properly to establish wages earned in the base period.
2. The first day the patient was too sick to perform all of his or her regular work duties (item 3); this cannot be the same day the patient worked, even if the patient went home sick.
3. The last day the patient worked (item 4); list the last day the patient worked even if for only part of the day.

Note: The two dates listed in items 2 and 3 cannot be the same; for example, if the patient went home sick on October 4, that would be considered the last day worked and October 5 becomes the first day the patient was unable to go to work.

For examples of the different forms used in the processing of disability insurance, California has been selected as the model state. To establish a claim, the First Claim for Disability Insurance Form DE 2501 must be completed by both the patient (see Fig. 15−3) and the attending physician (see Fig. 15−4). If an extension of disability is required, the Physician's Supplementary Certificate Form DE 2525XX must be completed by the physician (Fig. 15−5). This accompanies the last check issued to the patient. For additional medical information that might be required, Forms DE 2547 and DE 2547A are sometimes sent to the attending physician for completion (Figs. 15−6 and 15−7).

Remember that all follow-up correspondence should include the patient's name and Social Security number. The insurance billing specialist should promptly report any change of address, telephone number, or return to work date to the state disability insurance office. Patients must report any income received to the state disability insurance office, because this may affect benefits.

Conclusion

As a finale to this subject, I wish to take you behind the scenes to the desk of a claims adjuster. Many disability insurance application forms completed by employees came across this desk. These gems were taken from actual cases.

Spelled as:	Should have been:
yellow "jonders"	yellow jaundice
"goalstones"	gallstones
"limp glands"	lymph glands
"falls teeth"	false teeth
"high pretension"	hypertension
"Pabst smear"	Pap smear
"wrecktum"	rectum

RESOURCES ON THE INTERNET

Websites pertaining to the law for non-industrial disability insurance programs: California Unemployment Insurance Code

www.edd.ca.gov
Temporary Disability Benefits Law (New Jersey)
www.state.nj.us
Disability Benefits Law (New York)
www.web.state.ny.us
Temporary Disability Insurance Act (Rhode Island)
www.state.ri.us
(Hawaii and Puerto Rico do not have websites.)

STUDENT ASSIGNMENT LIST

✔ Study Chapter 15.
✔ Answer the review questions in the *Workbook* to reinforce the theory learned in this chapter and to help prepare you for a future test.
✔ Complete the assignments in the *Workbook*. These assignments will provide you with hands-on experience in working with patient histories and completing disability insurance claim forms described in this chapter.
✔ Turn to the Glossary at the end of this textbook for a further understanding of the Key Terms used in this chapter.

NOTICE OF FINAL PAYMENT

The information contained in your claim for Disability Insurance indicates that you are now able to work, therefore, this is the final check that you will receive on this claim.

IF YOU ARE **STILL** DISABLED: You should complete the Claimant's Certification portion of this form and contact your doctor immediately to have him/her complete the Physician's Supplementary Certificate below.

IF YOU BECOME DISABLED **AGAIN:** File a new Disability Insurance claim form.

IF YOU ARE UNEMPLOYED AND AVAILABLE FOR WORK: Report to the nearest Unemployment Insurance office of the Department for assistance in finding work and to determine your entitlement to Unemployment Insurance Benefits.

This determination is final unless you file an appeal within twenty (20) days from the date of mailing of this notification. You may appeal by giving a detailed statement as to why you believe the determination is in error. All communications regarding this Disability Insurance claim should include your Social Security Account Number and be addressed to the office shown.

CLAIMANT'S CERTIFICATION

I certify that I continue to be disabled and incapable of doing my regular work, and that I have reported all wages, Workers' Compensation benefits and other monies received during the claim period to the Employment Development Department.

ENTER YOUR SOCIAL SECURITY NUMBER *540 21 9881*

Sign Your Name *Marcia M. Monroe*   Date signed *October 29* 20 *xx*

PHYSICIAN'S SUPPLEMENTARY CERTIFICATE   Department Use Only

1. Are you still treating patient? *Yes* Date of last treatment *October 29* 20 *xx*

2. What present condition continues to make the patient disabled?

bilateral pneumonitis; infiltrate still present

3. Date patient recovered, or will recover sufficiently (even if under treatment) to be able to perform his/her regular and customary work *November 7* 20 *xx*   Please enter a specific or estimated recovery date.

4. Would the disclosure of this information to your patient be medically or psychologically detrimental to the patient?

Yes ☐   No ☒

I hereby certify that the above statements in my opinion truly describe the claimant's condition and the estimated duration thereof.

Date *October 29* 20 *xx*   Doctor's Signature *David W. Smith M.D.*

                                            Phone Number *013-486-9002*

DE 2525XX Rev. 13 (3-86)   —Version en español el dorso—

Figure 15–5. Notice of Final Payment/Physician's Supplementary Certificate Form DE 2525XX. This form indicates that the period of disability is "closed" or terminated with the accompanying check, based on information in the claim records. Benefits will cease unless the reverse side of the form is completed by the claimant's physician, extending the duration of disability. This form is pink. One side of the form is in English, and the other is in Spanish.

STATE OF CALIFORNIA
EMPLOYMENT DEVELOPMENT DEPARTMENT

FOR DEPT. USE ONLY

REFER TO

4920   – Our File No.
Marcia M. Monroe   – Your Patient
Secretary   – Regular or Customary Work

REQUEST FOR ADDITIONAL
MEDICAL INFORMATION

David W. Smith, MD
4567 Broad Avenue
Woodland Hills, XY 12345

The original basic information and estimate of duration of your patient's disability have been carefully evaluated. At the present time, the following additional information based upon the progress and present condition of this patient is requested. This will assist the Department in determining eligibility for further disability insurance benefits. Return of the completed form as soon as possible will be appreciated.

WM. C. SCHMIDT, M.D., MEDICAL DIRECTOR

CLAIMS EXAMINER   **DOCTOR: Please complete either Part A or B, date and sign.**

PART A   IF YOUR PATIENT HAS RECOVERED SUFFICIENTLY TO BE ABLE TO RETURN TO HIS/HER REGULAR OR CUSTOMARY WORK LISTED ABOVE, PLEASE GIVE THE DATE, _____ 20_____.

PART B   THIS PART REFERS TO PATIENT WHO IS STILL DISABLED.

Are you still treating the patient?   YES ☒   NO ☐   ___November___ __15__, 20 __xx__
                                                                                        DATE OF LAST TREATMENT

What are the medical circumstances which continue to make your patient disabled?

Bilateral pneumonitis. Patient has had continual fever 100° F to 102° F,

productive cough, chest pains, and lethargy

What is your present estimate of the date your patient will be able to perform his/her regular or customary work listed above? Date __November   30__ 20__xx__ .

Further Comments: _____

Would the disclosure of this information to your patient be medically or psychologically detrimental to the patient?   YES ☐   NO ☒

Date __November   17__ 20__xx__

David W. Smith M.D.
DOCTOR'S SIGNATURE

SE   David W. Smith, MD
ENCLOSED IS A STAMPED PREADDRESSED ENVELOPE FOR YOUR CONVENIENCE.

DE 2547 R v. 18 (8-84)

Figure 15–6. Request for Additional Medical Information Form DE 2547. This form is mailed to the physician when the normal expectancy date of the disability is reached, provided that the physician has requested a longer-than-normal duration without complications as indicated.

Figure 15-7. Medical Inquiry Form DE 2547A. This form is mailed to the physician at any time during the life of the claim if any questions need to be answered or if the physician has failed to enter a prognosis date.

STATE OF CALIFORNIA

EMPLOYMENT DEVELOPMENT DEPARTMENT
P.O. Box 1529, Santa Barbara, CA 93102
(805) 963-9611

For Dept. Use Only

REFER TO

MEDICAL INQUIRY

4920
Marcia M. Monroe
Secretary

- Our File No.
- Your Patient
- Regular Work

David W. Smith, MD
4567 Broad Avenue
Woodland Hills, XY 12345

A review of the medical certificate received in conjunction with a claim for disability insurance benefits filed by your patient, named above, reveals that some additional information is needed in order to evaluate the claim properly. Your cooperation in answering the question or questions below and returning the form in the enclosed stamped and addressed envelope will be appreciated.

WM. C. SCHMIDT, MD, MEDICAL DIRECTOR

CLAIMS EXAMINER

What is the name and address of the facility that took the x-rays on this patient?

Speedy Radiology Service
4598 Main Street
Woodland Hills, XY 12345

Would the disclosure of this information to your patient be medically or psychologically detrimental to the patient: Yes ☐   No ☒

October 24   20xx   *David W. Smith MD*
Date   Doctor's Signature
SE   David W. Smith, MD

DE 2547A Rev. 10 (9-84)

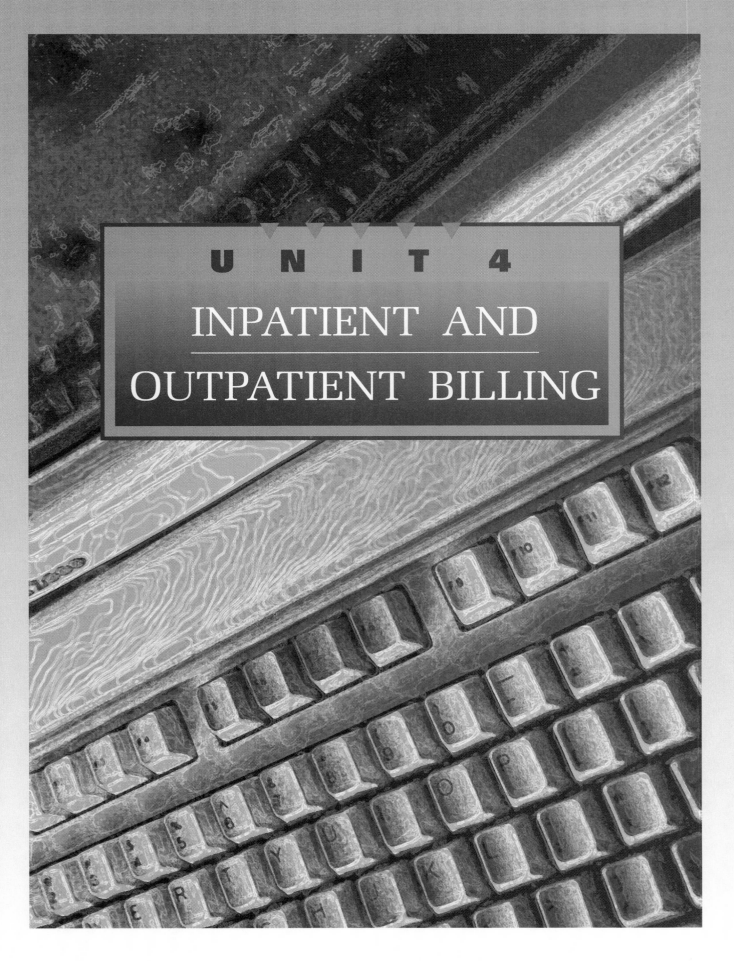

U N I T 4

INPATIENT AND
OUTPATIENT BILLING

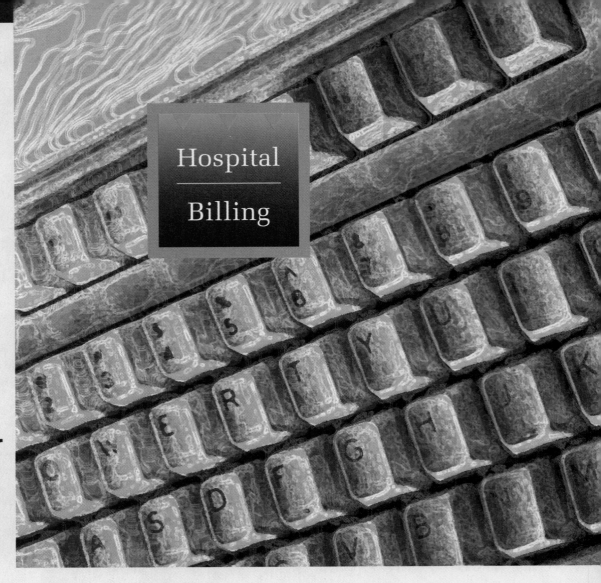

Hospital
Billing

16

CHAPTER OUTLINE

plan administrator tries to obtain discount rates for participation by a hospital in the plan in exchange for an increased volume of patients. These programs use any one or a combination of various payment methods. Refer to Chapter 10, Managed Care Systems, for definitions on types of managed care plans. A brief description of some reimbursement methods follows:

Ambulatory Payment Classifications. An outpatient classification scheme developed by Health Systems International is **ambulatory payment classifications (APCs).** This method is based on procedures rather than on diagnoses. Services associated with a specific procedure or visit are bundled into the APC reimbursement. More than one APC may be billed if more than one procedure is performed, but discounts may be applied to any additional APCs. This topic is discussed in detail at the end of this chapter.

Bed Leasing. A managed care plan leases beds from a facility (e.g., payment to the hospital of $300 per bed for 20 beds regardless of whether those beds are used).

Capitation or Percentage of Revenue. Capitation means reimbursement to the hospital on a per-member per-month basis regardless of whether the patient is hospitalized. **Percentage of revenue** means a fixed percentage paid to the hospital to cover charges.

Case Rate. Case rate is an averaging after a *flat* rate (set amount paid for a service) has been given to certain categories of procedures (e.g., normal vaginal delivery is $1,800 and cesarean section is $2,300). Utilization is expected to be 80% vaginal deliveries and 20% cesarean section; therefore, the case rate is $1,900 for all deliveries. Specialty procedures may also be given a case rate (e.g., coronary artery bypass graft surgery or heart transplantation). *Bundled case rate* means an all-inclusive rate is paid for both institutional and professional services; for example, for coronary artery bypass graft surgery, a rate is used to pay all who provide services connected with that procedure. Bundled case rates are seen in teaching facilities in which a faculty practice plan works closely with the hospital.

Diagnosis-Related Groups (DRGs). A classification system called **diagnosis-related groups (DRGs)** categorizes patients who are medically related with respect to diagnosis and treatment and are statistically similar in length of hospital stay. Medicare and some private hospital insurance payments are based on fixed dollar amounts determined by DRGs. DRGs are discussed in detail later in the chapter.

Differential by Day in Hospital. The first day of the hospital stay is paid at a higher rate (e.g., the first day may be paid at $1,000 and each subsequent day at $500). Most hospitalizations are more expensive on the first day. This type of reimbursement method may be combined with a per diem arrangement.

Differential by Service Type. The hospital receives a flat per-admission reimbursement for the service to which the patient is admitted. If services are mixed, a prorated payment may be made (e.g., 50% for intensive care and 50% medicine). Service types are defined in the contract (e.g., medicine, surgery, intensive care, neonatal intensive care, psychiatry, obstetrics).

Fee Schedule. A comprehensive listing of charges based on procedure codes, under a fee-for-service (FFS) arrangement, or discounted FFS, states fee maximums paid by the health plan within the period of the managed care contract. Usually the fee schedule is based on CPT codes. For industrial cases, whether managed care or not, this may be called a workers' compensation fee schedule. This document may also be known as a *fee maximum schedule* or *fee allowance schedule.*

Flat Rate. A set amount (single charge) per hospital admission is paid by the managed care plan regardless of the cost of the actual services the patient receives.

Per Diem. Per diem is a single charge for a day in the hospital regardless of actual charges or costs incurred (e.g., a plan that pays $800 for each day regardless of the actual cost of service).

Periodic Interim Payments (PIPs) and Cash Advances. These are methods in which the plan advances cash to cover expected claims to the hospital. The fund is replenished periodically. Insurance claims may be applied to the cash advance or may be paid outside it. This is generally done by Medicare.

Withhold. In this method part of the plan's payment to the hospital may be withheld or set aside in a bonus pool. If the hospital meets or exceeds the criteria set down, then the hospital receives its withhold or bonus; also called *bonus pools, capitation, risk pools, or withhold pools.*

Managed Care Stop Loss Outliers. Stop loss is a form of guarantee that may be written into a contract using one of a variety of methods. The purpose is to limit the exposure of cost to a reasonable level to prevent excessive loss. Stop loss is the least understood of reimbursement issues and can leave many thousands of dollars uncollected. There are a number of different ways stop loss can be applied; each contract is different. Familarize yourself with each contract and the stop loss provisions in it. Following are some methods that you may encounter.

1. Case-based stop loss: This is the most common stop loss and can apply to the physician, on a smaller case basis, as well as to the individual hospital claim. For example, in cases of premature infants of extremely low birth weight, the hospital bill may run over $1 million. The contract may pay $2,000 to $3,000 per day, which may reimburse the hospital several hundred thousand dollars, but the hospital must absorb the excess. Stop loss provisions may pay 65% of the excess over $100,000. Thus, the hospital and the insurance carrier share the loss.

2. Reinsurance stop loss: The hospital buys insurance to protect against lost revenue and receives less of a capitation fee and the amount they do not get helps pay for the insurance. For example, after a case reaches $100,000, the plan may receive 80% of expenses in excess of $100,000 from the reinsurance company for the remainder of the year.

3. Percentage stop loss: Some managed care contracts pay a percentage of charges when the total charge exceeds $65,000.

4. Medicare stop loss: Medicare provides stop loss called *outliers* in its regulations. There are *day outliers* for patients who remain in the hospital for long spells of illness. Medicare provides *cost outliers* for those cases in which charges exceed the DRG or $30,000. DRGs are discussed at the end of this chapter.

Some reimbursement methods not used very much are:

Charges. In a managed care plan, **charges** are the dollar amount owed to a participating provider for health care services rendered to a plan member, according to a fee schedule set by the managed care plan. This is the most expensive and least desirable type of reimbursement contract, so not many of these contracts exist.

Discounts in the Form of Sliding Scale. For example, a 10% reduction in charges for 0 to 500 total bed days per year with incremental increases in the discount up to a maximum percentage.

Sliding Scales for Discounts and Per Diems. Based on total volume of business generated, this is a reimbursement method in which an interim per diem is paid for each day in the hospital. For example, a lump sum is either added to or withheld from the payment due at the end of each year to adjust for actual hospital usage. Because this can be done either monthly or annually, it is difficult to administer.

Electronic Data Interchange

As early as 1980s, large hospitals began submitting electronic claims for payment to third party payers instead of printing out the UB-92 claim form; this is called electronic data interchange (EDI). The claim arrives at the insurance company the same day and receives priority for payment. This method of claim submission reduces the cost to the hospital and expedites payment. Confirmation of claim transmission/receipt is received the following day. Use of computer software assists the insurance billing editor in checking for errors before forwarding the claim to the proper claims office. This is called *cleaning the bill*. Medicare, Medicaid, group health carriers, many managed care plans, and some workers' compensation carriers mandate use of EDI. All hospital electronic billing goes through a clearinghouse where additional edits are made and claims are batched and sent electronically to insurance companies. Billing can be set up according to days or dollar amounts, typically every 30 days. If a Medicare patient remains in an acute hospital, you may bill on the 60th day and not again until discharge. For detailed information on this topic refer to Chapter 7, Electronic Data Interchange.

Hard Copy Billing

When a printed paper copy of the UB-92 is generated from the computer system, it is referred to as a hard copy. The same edits are made and the claim is cleaned before it is sent. Some insurance companies do not have the capability of receiving electronic claims so billing by hard copy is mandatory. All secondary insurance companies and all claims that require attachments also fit into this category.

Receiving Payment

Timeliness of payment may be included in a contract to encourage a hospital to join a plan (e.g., an additional 4% discount for paying a clean claim within 14 days of receipt), or a hospital may demand a penalty for clean claims not processed within 30 days. Some states require this payment by law.

After receipt of payment from insurance and managed care plans, the patient is sent a net bill that lists any owing deductible, coinsurance amount, and charges for services not covered under the insurance policy. Standard bookkeeping procedures are used to post entries showing payments and adjustments. Financial management for managed care programs is discussed and shown in figures in Chapter 10, Managed Care Systems.

Outpatient Insurance Claims

The term **outpatient** is used when an individual receives medical service from the hospital and goes home the same day. If an individual has an accident, injury, or acute illness, he or she may seek the services of medical personnel in the emergency department of the hospital. When seen in this department, a patient is considered an outpatient unless he or she is admitted for overnight hospital stay. Many elective surgeries are done on an outpatient surgery basis. **Elective surgery** indicates a surgical procedure that can be scheduled in advance, is not an emergency, and is discretionary on the part of the physician and patient. Elective procedures are those that are deferrable, which means that the patient will not experience serious consequences if the operation is postponed or there is failure to undergo the operation. Some insurance policies require a second opinion for elective surgery. If the patient does not seek a second opinion and chooses to undergo surgery, the insurance company may not pay. See Chapter 11 for elective surgery in regard to the Medicare program. Patients may also receive certain types of therapy and diagnostic testing services on an outpatient basis.

Hospital Professional Services

Although physicians make daily hospital visits to their patients, perform surgeries, discharge patients from the hospital, and are called to the hospital to provide consultations and emergency department treatment, their professional services are submitted on the HCFA-1500 insurance claim form by the physician and not by the hospital billing department. Only services provided by the hospital should be submitted by the hospital unless the hospital is billing for physicians. Such hospital services include:

- Emergency department (ED) facility fee (supplies)
- Laboratory (technical component)
- Radiology (technical component)
- Physical and occupational therapy facility fee

Personnel who work in these departments (e.g., ED physician, pathologist, radiologist, and physical therapist) might be employees of the hospital. In that situation, the hospital would submit bills for professional services. If not an employee, the professional would bill independently.

Avoid using the hospital for surgical or medical consultations that could be done in a specialist's office unless the patient physically requires admission. This necessity should be documented. If a patient is admitted for consultation only, the entire payment for hospital admission will be denied as well as any physician fees involved.

Billing Problems

Many times, patients receive hospital bills, are stunned by the total balance due, and are unable to make sense of specific items, abbreviations, or codes on the statement. A bill should never show unexplained codes or items without descriptions. A brief hospital stay may translate into hundreds of individual charges. A patient has the right to request, examine, and question a detailed statement, as mentioned in the Patient's Bill of Rights—a nationally recognized code of conduct published by the American Hospital Association. If the bill lumps charges together under broad categories such as pharmacy, surgical supplies, and radiology and the patient requests an itemized invoice, then it should be provided at no cost to the patient. In fact, consumer advocates and policies governing the Medicare program encourage consumers to scrutinize their hospital bills for mistakes. If the charges seem exorbitant, the hospital may receive a call or letter from the patient asking for an explanation of the charges. Sometimes hospital billing personnel, a hospital patient representative or advocate, the attending physician, and his or her staff may be able to satisfactorily explain a confusing charge.

Some common billing errors are:

- Incorrect name—Use of maiden name instead of married name
- Wrong subscriber—Patient's name listed in error
- Covered days versus noncovered days

Duplicate Statements

Duplicate billings, which may confuse the patient, can occur when a patient receives both inpatient and outpatient preadmission tests or services. Perhaps a test was canceled and rescheduled, and a charge is shown for the canceled test. Or several physicians may have consulted on a case and each ordered the same test or therapy. Possibly, a technician took the incorrect amount of blood or produced an unclear radiograph, submitting a charge for the service performed in error as well as for the correct service and thereby generating two charges for one test. These examples are hospital personnel errors, and patients should not have to pay for such mistakes.

Double Billing

Another example involving a violation of Medicare policy is double billing, which results when a patient undergoes routine outpatient testing for a specific diagnosis and then develops unanticipated problems related to that diagnosis, requiring hospital admission. Outpatient personnel may not be aware that the patient was later admitted, and inpatient personnel may not know that the patient had undergone outpatient testing within the previous 72 hours. A hospital billing for such services may be fined because it would be in violation of the Medicare 72-Hour Rule. Such charges must be bundled into the inpatient DRG payment. Therefore, it is imperative that the hospital billing department develops procedures to check for potential double-billing problems.

Phantom Charges

Physicians order admission procedures for each patient who enters the hospital. If a patient has refused some of these tests, make sure that the charges were deleted from the financial records before the bill is sent out. Similarly, if, for example, a patient refuses to take sleeping pills or takes only a few aspirin, he or she should not be charged for refused medication or a bottle of aspirin. The hospital may offer a standard kit of supplies on admission or, when appropriate, a new-mother packet. If the patient does not accept some of these supplies, he or she should not have to pay for them. If a patient requests a semiprivate room but is sent to a private room because all semiprivate rooms are occupied, the patient should not be billed at the higher rate. Phantom charges may appear if a scheduled test is canceled by a physician or if the patient is re-

leased early, making it imperative to check the dates and times of admission and discharge. Charges that should appear on a patient's itemized statement may be missing because the charges were transferred to the wrong patient's bill. This requires a review of the patient's medical records. When a charge cannot be accounted for by a review of the patient's medical record or by talking to the attending physician, the charge should be deleted from the bill.

Hospital Billing Claim Form

Uniform Bill Inpatient and Outpatient Claim Form

In 1982, the UB-82 claim form was developed for hospital claims and was printed in green ink. A need was seen to update this form, so a revision was issued in 1992. The **Uniform Bill (UB-92) claim form** is also known as the HCFA-1450. This form is considered a summary document supported by an itemized or detailed bill. It is used by institutional facilities (e.g., inpatient and outpatient departments, rural health clinics, chronic dialysis services, and adult day health care) to submit claims for inpatient and outpatient services. This claim form is printed in red ink on white paper for processing with optical scanning equipment. Figure 16–5 illustrates a completed UB-92 claim form. Dates of service and monetary values are entered without spaces or decimal points (e.g., $200.00 should be shown as 20000, and June 23, 1995 should be shown as 062395). Dates of birth are entered using two sets of two-digit numbers for the month and day and a four-digit number for the year (e.g., June 23, 1995 should be shown as 06231995). (For information on how to complete the HCFA-1500 Claim Form for professional services, see Chapter 6, The Health Insurance Claim Form).

Instructions for Completing the UB-92 Claim Form

Only general guidelines for completing the UB-92 claim form are mentioned here. Always refer to the medical hospital manual and, if available, your local UB-92 manual to determine whether there are billing guidelines that pertain to your region. At the time of this edition, no guidelines have been published in regard to insertion of the ambulatory payment classification (APC) group number for outpatient claims. Some facilities are grouping claims in-house that relate to APCs before submitting them to the fiscal intermediaries. The following color screens, item numbers, and descriptions correspond to Figure 16–5, which shows a completed UB-92 claim form for inpatient claims.

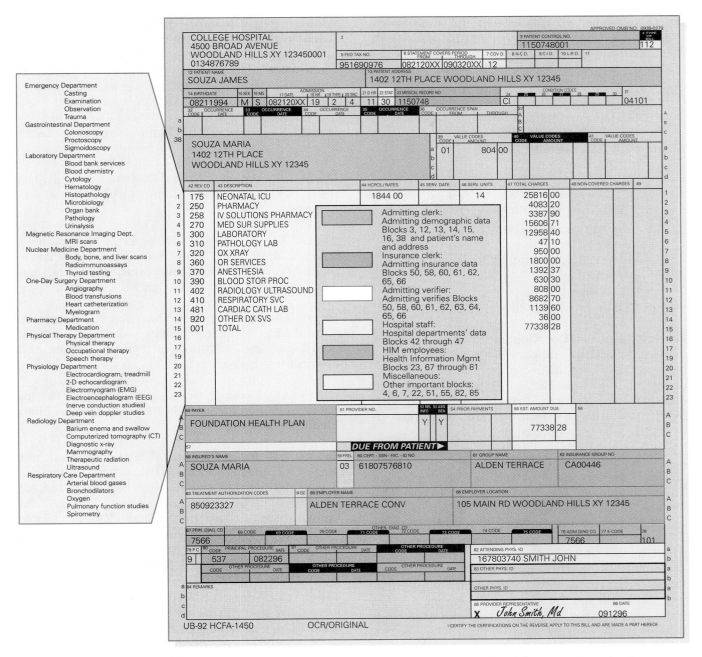

Figure 16–5. Scannable (red ink) Uniform Bill (UB-92) insurance claim form completed for an inpatient showing hospital departments that input data for hospital services. Colored blocks indicate data obtained by various hospital personnel. Job titles and the exact data each one obtains may vary from facility to facility. Block-by-block guidelines vary and may not always follow the visual guide presented here.

Block 1. Field Name/Description. Enter the provider name, address, city, state, and zip code on the first three lines. Enter telephone number, fax number, or county code applicable to the provider on the fourth line. **Medicaid, Medi-Cal, and Medicare:** The fourth line is optional. **TRI-CARE:** The fourth line is required.

Block 2. Untitled. Leave blank.

Block 3. Patient Control Number. This is an optional block that can be used to identify an individual patient account. In some facilities, it is the patient's medical record number or account number. **Medicare:** Required.

Block 4. Type of Bill. Enter the appropriate three-digit bill code as specified in the UB-92 Manual Billing Procedures. The digits indicate the following:

First digit (type of facility)
    1 = Hospital (acute)
    2 = Skilled nursing facility
    3 = Home health
Second digit (bill classification)
    1 = Inpatient
    3 = Outpatient
Third digit (frequency) Use of this digit may change according to facility
    1 = Admit to discharge
    2 = Interim—First claim
    3 = Interim—Continuing claim
    4 = Interim—Last claim
    5 = Late charge bill
Medi-Cal: Optional. **Medicare:** Required.

Block 5. Federal Tax Number. Enter the facility's provider federal tax number. This number is also called a tax identification number (TIN) or employer identification number (EIN). **Medi-Cal** and **Medicare:** Not required. **Private payers** and **TRICARE:** Required. **Some Medicaid programs:** A number in this field may be required.

Block 6. Statement Covers Period. Enter beginning and ending dates of service for the period shown on the bill (e.g., 011820XX to 012020XX). The electronic version requires an eight-character date listing year, month, and day: 20XX0118 to 20XX0120. **Medicare** and **Private payers:** Required. **Medi-Cal:** Not required.

Block 7. Covered Days. Enter number of inpatient days covered by primary insurance carrier. **Medicare:** Required. **Private payers** and **Medicaid:** Depending on plan or state policies, may be required. **Medi-Cal** and **TRICARE:** Not required.

Block 8. Noncovered Days. Enter the days of care not covered by the primary insurance carrier. **Medicare:** Required. **Private payers** and **Medicaid:** Depending on plan or state policies, may be required. **Medi-Cal** and **TRICARE:** Not required.

Block 9. Coinsurance Days. Medicare: Enter inpatient days occurring after the 60th day and before the 91st day of one illness. **Medicare/Medicaid** and **Medicare/supplemental insurance:** Required. **Medi-Cal** and **TRICARE:** Not required.

Block 10. Lifetime Reserve Days. Under Medicare, each beneficiary has a lifetime reserve of 60

additional days of inpatient hospital services after using 90 days of inpatient hospital services during an occurrence of illness. **Medicare:** Required. **Medicare/Medicaid** and **Medicare/supplemental insurance:** Must be completed for patients. **Medicaid, Medi-Cal,** and **TRICARE:** Not required.

Block 11. Reserved for State Assignment. Leave blank.

Block 12. Patient's Name. Enter the patient's last name, first name, and middle initial. Avoid nicknames or aliases.

Block 13. Patient's Address. Enter the patient's street address, city, state, and zip code. **Private payers, some Medicaid programs, Medicare,** and **TRICARE:** Required. **Medi-Cal:** Not required.

Block 14. Patient's Birth Date. Enter the patient's date of birth in an eight-digit format (e.g., June 1, 20XX, becomes 060120XX). **Private payers** and **Medicare:** Required.

Block 15. Patient's Sex. Enter a capital "M" for male, or "F" for female. **Private payers** and **Medicare:** Required.

Block 16. Patient's Marital Status. S indicates single; M, married; P, life partner (also called domestic partner and significant other); D, divorced; W, widowed; X, legally separated; and U, unknown. Some **Private payers** and **TRICARE:** Enter marital status of the patient on date of registration as an inpatient or outpatient or at the start of care. **Medicaid, Medi-Cal,** and **Medicare:** Not required.

Block 17. Admission/Start of Care Date. Enter admission or start of care date. The electronic version requires an eight-character date in this format: 20XX 0710. **Medi-Cal:** Not required. **Medicaid, Medicare, third party payers,** and **TRICARE:** Required.

Block 18. Admission Hour. Enter the hour during which the patient was admitted for inpatient or outpatient care in two numeric characters using the 24-hour clock (e.g., midnight is 00 and noon is 12, 1 to 1:59 A.M. is 01, 1 to 1:59 P.M. is 13, 11:59 is shown as 23; Fig. 16−6). **Private payers** and **TRICARE:** Required. **Medicare** and **Medicare/Medi-Cal:** Not required.

Block 19. Admission Type. Enter the code indicating the priority of the inpatient admission. Coding structure: 1 = indicates emergency; 2 = urgent; 3 = elective; 4 = newborn; and 9 = information

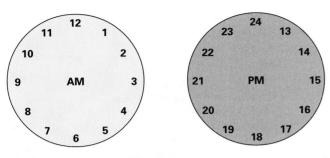

Figure 16-6. Clock face depicting standard A.M. time and clock face depicting P.M. military time.

not available. **Private payers, some Medicaid programs, Medicare,** and **TRICARE:** Required when inpatient claim submitted. **Medi-Cal:** Not required.

Block 20. Source of Admission. Enter the code indicating the source of the admission or outpatient service. **Medicare, private payers,** and **TRICARE:** Required. **Medicaid** and **Medi-Cal:** Not required. Codes are as follows:

Source of Admission Codes

1	Physician referral
2	Clinic referral
3	Health maintenance organization (HMO) referral
4	Transfer from a hospital
5	Transfer from a skilled nursing facility (SNF)
6	Transfer from another health care facility
7	Emergency department
8	Court/law enforcement
9	Information not available

	0	Transfer from psycho, substance abuse, or rehab hospital
	A	Transfer from a critical access hospital
	B	Transfer from another home health agency
	C	Readmission to some home health agency
	D–Z	Reserved for national assignment

Newborn Codes

1	Normal delivery
2	Premature delivery
3	Sick baby
4	Extramural birth
5–8	Reserved for national assignment
9	Information not available

Block 21. Discharge Hour. Enter hour when patient was discharged from inpatient care. Hours are indicated by two numeric characters using the 24-hour clock (e.g., midnight is 00 and noon is 12, 1 to 1:59 A.M. is 01, 1 to 1:59 P.M. is 13, 11:59 is shown as 23. See Figure 16-6). **Medicaid:** May be required. **Private payers** and **TRICARE:** Required. **Medi-Cal** and **Medicare:** Not required.

Block 22. Patient Status. Enter a code indicating the patient's disposition as of the ending date of service for the period of care reported. **Private payers, Medicaid, Medicare,** and **TRICARE:** Required for inpatient claims. **Medi-Cal:** Not required.

Patient Status Codes

01	Discharged to home or self-care (routine discharge)
02	Discharged/transferred to another short-term general hospital for inpatient care
03	Discharged/transferred to SNF
04	Discharged/transferred to an intermediate care facility
05	Discharged/transferred to another type of institution for inpatient care or referred for outpatient services to another institution
06	Discharged/transferred to home under care of organized home health service organization
07	Left against medical advice or discontinued care
08	Discharged/transferred to home under care of home intravenous therapy provider
09	Admitted as an inpatient to this hospital
10–19	Discharge to be defined at state level, if necessary
20	Expired
21–29	Expired, to be defined at state level, if necessary
30	Still a patient
31–39	Still a patient to be defined at state level, if necessary
40	Expired at home (for hospice care)
41	Expired in a medical facility such as a hospital, SNF, intermediate care facility, or freestanding hospice (for hospice care)
42	Expired, place unknown (for hospice care)
43–49	Reserved for national assignment
50	Discharged to hospice—home
51	Discharged to hospice—medical facility
52–60	Reserved for national assignment

Block 23. Medical Record Number. Enter the number assigned by the provider to the patient's medical record. **Private payers, Medicare,** and **TRICARE:** Required. **Some Medicaid programs:** May be required.

Blocks 24–30. Condition Codes. The codes help determine patient eligibility and benefits from primary or secondary insurance coverage and affect payer processing.

Condition Codes

01	Military service related
02	Condition is employment related
03	Patient covered by insurance not reflected here
04	Patient is HMO enrollee
05	Lien has been filed
06	End-stage renal disease (ESRD) patient in first 18 months of entitlement covered by employer group health insurance
07	Treatment of nonterminal condition for hospice patient
08	Beneficiary would not provide information concerning other insurance coverage
09	Neither patient nor spouse is employed
10	Patient and/or spouse is employed but no employer group health plan (EGHP) coverage exists
11	Disabled beneficiary, but no large group health plan (LGHP) coverage exists
12-14	Reserved for payer use only
15	Clean claim delayed in HCFA's processing system
16	Skilled Nursing Facility (SNF) transition exemption
17	Patient is homeless
18	Maiden name retained
19	Child retains mother's name
20	Beneficiary requested billing
21	Billing for denial notice
22	Patient on multiple drug regimen
23	Home caregiver available
24	Home intravenous therapy patient also receiving home health agency (HHA) services
25	Patient is a non-U.S. resident
26	Veterans Affairs–eligible patient chooses to receive services in Medicare-certified facility
27	Patient referred to a sole community hospital for a diagnostic laboratory test
28	Patient and/or spouse's EGHP is secondary to Medicare
29	Disabled beneficiary and/or family member's LGHP is secondary to Medicare
30	Reserved for national assignment
31	Patient is student (full-time day)
32	Patient is student (cooperative/work study program)
33	Patient is student (full-time night)
34	Patient is student (part-time)
35	Reserved for national assignment
36	General care patient in a special unit
37	Ward accommodation at patient's request
38	Semiprivate room not available
39	Private room medically necessary
40	Same-day transfer
41	Partial hospitalization
42	Continuing care not related to inpatient admission

Condition Codes *Continued*

43	Continuing care not provided within prescribed postdischarge window
44-45	Reserved for national assignment
46	TRICARE Nonavailability Statement on file
47	Reserved for TRICARE
48	Claims submitted by a TRICARE-authorized psychiatric residential treatment center (RTC) for children and adolescents
49-54	Reserved for national assignment.
55	SNF bed not available
56	Medical appropriateness. SNF admission was delayed more than 30 days after hospital discharge
57	SNF readmission
58-59	Reserved for national assignment
60	Reporting the stay was a day outlier
61	Requesting additional payment for the stay as a cost outlier
62	Payer code indicating bill was paid under a DRG
63-65	Payer only codes
66	Provider does not wish cost outlier payment
67	Beneficiary elects not to use lifetime reserve (LTR) days
68	Beneficiary elects to use lifetime reserve (LTR) days
69	Operating indirect medical education (IME) payment only
70	Self-administered epoetin (EPO) for home dialysis patient
71	Full care in dialysis unit
72	Self-care in dialysis unit
73	Self-care in dialysis training
74	Patient receiving dialysis services at home
75	Home dialysis— 100% payment
76	Backup in-facility dialysis
77	Provider accepts or is obligated/required due to a contractual arrangement or law to accept payment by a primary payer as payment in full
78	New coverage not implemented by HMO
79	Comprehensive outpatient rehabilitation facility (CORF) services provided offsite
80-99	Reserved for state assignment
A0	TRICARE External Partnership Program
A1	Early Periodic Screening Diagnosis Treatment/Child Health Assurance Program (EPSDT/CHAP)
A2	Physically handicapped children's program
A3	Special federal funding
A4	Family planning
A5	Disability
A6	Medicare pneumococcal pneumonia vaccine (PPV) services; influenza virus vaccine
A7	Induced abortion—danger to life
A8	Induced abortion—victim rape/incest
A9	Second opinion surgery
B0-B9	Reserved for national assignment
C0	Reserved for national assignment
C1	Approved as billed

Condition Codes *Continued*

C2	Automatic approval as billed based on focused review
C3	Partial approval
C4	Admission/services denied
C5	Postpayment review applicable
C6	Admission preauthorization
C7	Extended authorization
C8–C9	Reserved for national assignment
D0	Change to services dates
D1	Change to charges
D2	Changes in revenue codes/HCPCS
D3	Second or subsequent interim prospective payment system bill
D4	Change in grouper input
D5	Cancel to correct health insurance claim number (HICN) or provider identification number
D6	Cancel only to repay a duplicate or Office of the Inspector General (OIG) overpayment
D7	Change to make Medicare the secondary payer
D8	Change to make Medicare the primary payer
D9	Any other change
E0	Change in patient status
E1–L9	Reserved for national assignment
M0	All-inclusive rate for outpatient services (payer only code)
M1	Roster billed influenza virus vaccine (payer only code)
M2	HHA payment significantly exceeds total charges (payer only code)
M3–M9	Reserved for payer assignment
N0–W9	Reserved for national assignment
X0–Z9	Reserved for state assignment

Block 31. **Reserved for national assignment.**

Blocks 32–35. **Occurrence Codes and Dates.** Occurrence codes and dates are used to identify significant events relating to a bill that may affect payer processing (i.e., determination of liability, coordination of benefits, administration of subrogation clauses in benefit programs). The electronic version requires an eight-character date listing year, month, and day: 20XX0328. A total of seven occurrence codes and dates may be reported on a UB-92. **Private payers** or **Medicare:** Required.

Occurrence Codes and Dates

01	Auto accident
02	No-fault insurance involved including auto accident/other
03	Accident—tort liability
04	Accident—employment related
05	Other accident

Occurrence Codes and Dates *Continued*

06	Crime victim
07–08	Reserved for national assignment
09	Start of infertility treatment cycle
10	Last menstrual period
11	Onset of symptoms/illness
12	Date of onset for a chronically dependent individual (CDI) (HHA claims only)
13–16	Reserved for national assignment
17	Date outpatient occupational therapy plan established or last reviewed
18	Date of retirement of patient/beneficiary
19	Date of retirement of spouse
20	Guarantee of payment began
21	Utilization Review (UR) notice received
22	Date active care ended
23	Date of cancellation of hospice election period
24	Date insurance denied
25	Date benefits terminated by primary payer
26	Date SNF bed became available
27	Date of hospice certification or recertification
28	Date comprehensive outpatient rehabilitation plan established or last reviewed
29	Date outpatient physical therapy plan established or last reviewed
30	Date outpatient speech pathology plan established or last reviewed
31	Date beneficiary notified of intent to bill (accommodations)
32	Date beneficiary notified of intent to bill (diagnostic procedures or treatments)
33	First day of the Medicare coordination period for end-stage renal disease beneficiaries covered by an EGHP
34	Date of election of extended care services
35	Date treatment started for physical therapy
36	Date of inpatient hospital discharge for covered transplant patient
37	Date of inpatient hospital discharge for noncovered transplant patient
38	Date treatment started for home intravenous therapy
39	Date discharged on a continuous course of intravenous therapy
40	Scheduled date of admission
41	Date of first test for preadmission testing
42	Date of discharge (hospice only)
43	Scheduled date of canceled surgery
44	Date treatment started for occupational therapy
45	Date treatment started for speech therapy
46	Date treatment started for cardiac rehabilitation
47	Date cost outlier status begins
48–49	Payer codes
50–69	Reserved for state assignment
70–99	Reserved for occurrence span codes
A0	Reserved for national assignment

Occurrence Codes and Dates *Continued*

A1	Birthdate—insured A
A2	Effective date—insured A policy
A3	Benefits exhausted
A4–A9	Reserved for national assignment
B0	Reserved for national assignment
B1	Birthdate—insured B
B2	Effective date—insured B policy
B3	Benefits exhausted
B4–B9	Reserved for national assignment
C0	Reserved for national assignment
C1	Birthdate—insured C
C2	Effective date—insured C policy
C3	Benefits exhausted
C4–C9	Reserved for national assignment
D0–D9	Reserved for national assignment
E0	Reserved for national assignment
E1	Birthdate—insured D
E2	Effective date—insured D policy
E3	Benefits exhausted
E4–E9	Reserved for national assignment
F0	Reserved for national assignment
F1	Birthdate—insured E
F2	Effective date—insured E policy
F3	Benefits exhausted
F4–F9	Reserved for national assignment
G0	Reserved for national assignment
G1	Birthdate—insured F
G2	Effective date—insured F policy
G3	Benefits exhausted
G4–G9	Reserved for national assignment
H0–I9	Reserved for national assignment
J0–L9	Reserved for national assignment
M0–Z9	See Block 36 occurrence span codes

Block 36. **Occurrence Span Codes and Dates.** Enter code identifying occurrence that happened over a span of time. The electronic version requires an eight-character date listing year, month, and day (20XX0812). **Medicaid:** Complete when required. **Private payer, Medicare,** and **TRICARE:** Required.

Occurrence Span Codes and Dates

70	Qualifying stay dates (for SNF use only)
71	Prior stay dates
72	First/last visits
73	Benefit eligibility period
74	Noncovered level of care/leave of absence (LOA)
75	SNF level of care
76	Patient liability period
77	Provider liability period
78	SNF prior stay dates
79	Payer code
80–99	Reserved for state assignment

Occurrence Span Codes and Dates

Continued

M0	Peer review organization/utilization review (PRO/UR) approved stay dates (partial approval)
M1	Provider liability—no utilization
M2	Inpatient respite days
M3–W9	Reserved for national assignment
X0–Z9	Reserved for state assignment

Block 37. Internal Control Number (ICN)/Document Control Number (DCN). Enter the internal control number (ICN) or document control number (DCN) assigned to the original bill by the payer or the payer's intermediary. **Medicaid:** Depending on contract requirements, may be required. **Medi-Cal** and **private payers:** Not required. **Medicare:** Required. **TRICARE:** For reporting claim changes.

Block 38. Responsible Party Name and Address. Enter the name and address of the party responsible for the bill. **Private payers:** Required. **Medi-caid, Medi-Cal, Medicare,** or **TRICARE:** Not required.

Blocks 39–41. Value Codes and Amounts. Enter codes that have related dollar amounts that identify monetary data required for processing claims. **Medicaid:** May be required depending on state policy. **Private payer, Medicare,** and **TRICARE:** Complete when applicable. Enter the value codes as described below:

Value Codes

01	Most common semiprivate room rate
02	Hospital has no semiprivate rooms
03	Reserved for national assignment
04	Inpatient professional component charges that are combined billed
05	Professional component included in charges and also billed separately to carrier
06	Medicare blood deductible amount
07	Reserved for national assignment
08	Medicare lifetime reserve amount in the first calendar year
09	Medicare coinsurance amount in the first calendar year
10	Medicare lifetime reserve amount in the second calendar year
11	Medicare coinsurance amount for second calendar year
12	Working aged beneficiary/spouse with EGHP
13	End-stage renal disease beneficiary in a Medicare coordination period for an EGHP
14	No-fault insurance, including auto or other

Value Codes *Continued*

15	Workers' compensation
16	Public health service (PHS) or other federal agency
17	Outlier amount
18	Disproportionate share amount
19	Indirect medical education amount
20	Total prospective payment system capital payment amount
21	Catastrophic
22	Supplies
23	Recurring monthly income
24	Medicaid rate code
25–29	Reserved for national assignment—Medicaid
30	Preadmission testing
31	Patient liability amount
32–36	Reserved for national assignment
37	Pints of blood furnished
38	Blood deductible pints
39	Pints of blood replaced
40	New coverage not implemented by HMO (for inpatient claims only)
41	Black lung
42	Veterans affairs
43	Disabled beneficiary under age 65 with LGHP
44	Amount provider agreed to accept from primary insurer when this amount is less than total charges but greater than the primary insurer's payment
45	Accident hour
46	Number of grace days
47	Any liability insurance
48	Hemoglobin reading
49	Hematocrit reading
50	Physical therapy visits
51	Occupational therapy visits
52	Speech therapy visits
53	Cardiac rehabilitation visits
54–55	Reserved for national assignment
56	Skilled nurse—home visit hours (HHA only)
57	Home health aide—home visit hours (HHA only)
58	Arterial blood gas (PO_2/PA_2)
59	Oxygen saturation (O_2 SAT/oximetry)
60	HHA branch metropolitan statistical area (MSA)
61	Location where service is furnished (HHA and hospice)
62–65	Payer codes
66	Reserved for national assignment
67	Peritoneal dialysis
68	EPO—drug
70	Interest amount
71	Funding of ESRD networks
72	Flat rate surgery charge
73	Drug deductible
74	Drug coinsurance
75	Gramm-Rudman-Hollings reduction—for payers use only
76	Provider's interim rate

Value Codes *Continued*

77–79	Payer codes
80–99	Reserved for state assignment
A1	Deductible payer A
A2	Coinsurance payer A
A3	Estimated responsibility payer A
A4	Covered self-administrable drugs—emergency
A5	Covered self-administrable drugs—not self administered in form and situation furnished to patient
A6	Covered self-administrable drugs—diagnostic study and other
A7–AZ	Reserved for national assignment
B0	Reserved for national assignment
B1	Deductible payer B
B2	Coinsurance payer B
B3	Estimated responsibility payer B
B4–BZ	Reserved for national assignment
C0	Reserved for national assignment
C1	Deductible payer C
C2	Coinsurance payer C
C3	Estimated responsibility payer C
C4–CZ	Reserved for national assignment
C0–D2	Reserved for national assignment
D3	Estimated responsibility patient
D4–DZ	Reserved for national assignment
E0	Reserved for national assignment
E1	Deductible payer D
E2	Coinsurance payer D
E3	Estimated responsibility payer D
E4–EZ	Reserved for national assignment
F0	Reserved for national assignment
F1	Deductible payer E
F2	Coinsurance payer E
F3	Estimated responsibility payer E
F4–FZ	Reserved for national assignment
G0	Reserved for national assignment
G1	Deductible payer F
G2	Coinsurance payer F
G3	Estimated responsibility payer F
G4–GZ	Reserved for national assignment
H0–YZ	Reserved for national assignment
X0–ZZ	Reserved for national assignment

Block 42. Revenue Code. Enter a three- or four-digit code corresponding to each narrative description or standard abbreviation that identifies a specific accommodation, ancillary service, or billing calculation related to services billed. Revenue code 001 indicating a total must be the final entry on all bills. Revenue codes are an *important factor* when payment is considered by managed care contractors or private payers. Billing guidelines for revenue codes are extensive, so refer to the UB-92 *Manual* for detailed information. **Managed care:** Required since payment may be based on diagnosis, procedure, and revenue codes. For

example, codes 274, 275, 276, and 278 relate to implant of a pacemaker, lens, pin, or bolt. If the correct code is not used, payment will not be made for implant item if the cost is buried in supplies. Other items to be sure to code are special drugs for chemotherapy, cardiac balloons, cardiac catheters, and so on. **Medicare:** Required. All revenue codes from 001–999 must be preceded with an "0." The leading "0" is added automatically for electronic claims. Basic revenue codes end in "0." Detailed revenue codes end in 1–9. List revenue codes in ascending order. Do not repeat revenue codes on the same claim except when required by field or for coding more than one HCPCS code for the same revenue code item. **Medi-Cal:** Not required for outpatient services except when code 0001 is used to indicate Total Charge line.

Block 43. Revenue Description. This optional block helps separate and identify descriptions of each service. The description must identify the particular service code indicated in Block 44, the HCPCS/Rates block. **Third party payers** and **TRICARE:** Required **Medicare:** Not required. **Medicaid:** May be required depending on contract.

Block 44. HCPCS/Rates/Health Insurance Prospective Payment System (HIPPS) Rate Codes. Enter the applicable CPT or HCPCS code number and modifier (applicable to ancillary services for outpatient claims), HIPPS rate code, and two-digit modifier, or the accommodation rate for inpatient claims. Dollar values must include whole dollars, the decimal, and cents (e.g., $999.99). **Medicare:** Required. **Medicaid** or **private payers:** May be required depending on contract.

Block 45. Service Date. Enter the date the service was rendered for outpatient services in eight digits (e.g., 062320XX). See the patient's itemized bill for dates. The electronic version requires an eight-character date listing year, month, and day (e.g., 20XX0128). Inpatient dates are not required in this block. **Medicare:** Required. **Medicaid** and **private payers:** May be required depending on contract.

Block 46. Service Units. Enter the number of accommodation days, ancillary units, or visits when appropriate for each revenue code. This is itemized on the patient's detail bill. **Medicare and private payers:** Required.

Block 47. Total Charges. Enter the total charge pertaining to the related revenue codes (see Example 16–13). **Medicare** or **private payers:** Required.

Block 48. Noncovered Charges. Enter total noncovered charges for the primary payer pertaining to a particular revenue code. Personal items are not covered. **Medicaid, Medicare,** and **private payers:** Required. **Medi-Cal** and **TRICARE:** Not required.

Block 49. Unlabeled block. Reserved for national assignment.

Block 50. Payer Identification. Enter name and number identifying each payer organization from which the provider may expect some payment for the bill. Line 50A is used to report the primary payer. Line 50B is used for the secondary payer. Line 50C is used for the tertiary payer. **Medicaid, Medicare, private payers,** and **TRICARE:** Required. **Medi-Cal:** Enter "O/P MEDI-CAL" to indicate the type of claim and payer.

Block 51. Provider Number. Enter the number assigned to the provider by the payer. **Medicaid, Medicare,** and **private payers:** Required. **TRICARE:** Requires the zip code of the physical location of the provider plus the four-digit subidentification number.

Block 52. Release Information Certification Indicator. Enter code indicating if provider has patient's signature on file permitting release of data. Y = Yes; R = Restricted or modified release; and N = No release. **Medicaid:** May be required depending on contract. **Medicare, private payers,** and **TRICARE:** Required. **Medi-Cal:** Not required.

Block 53. Assignment of Benefits. Enter Y (yes, benefits assigned) or N (no, benefits not assigned). **Private payers** and **TRICARE:** Required. **Medicaid, Medi-Cal,** and **Medicare:** Not required.

Block 54. Prior Payments—Payers and Patient. Enter the amount of payment received on this bill prior to billing date. If payment has been received from other coverage, enter the amount on the same line as the other coverage "payer" listed in Block 50 (e.g., $100 should be entered as 100 00). *Do not* enter Medicare payments in this block; leave blank if not applicable. **Medicaid, Medi-Cal** and **Medicare:** Required.

Block 55. Estimated Amount Due. Enter the estimated amount due from the indicated payer according to the contract. **Medicaid, Medi-Cal, Medicare, private payers,** and **TRICARE:** Not required.

EXAMPLE 16–13

42 REV. CD.		43 DESCRIPTION	44 HCPCS/RATES	45 SERV.DATE	46.SERV.UNITS	47 TOTAL CHARGES	48 NON-COVERED CHARGES	49	
175		Neonatal ICU	1844.00		14	25816.00			1
250		Pharmacy				4083.20			2
258		IV Solutions–Pharmacy				3387.90			3
270		Med-Sur Supplies				15606.71			4
300		Laboratory				12958.40			5
310		Pathology Lab				47.10			6
320		OX X-Ray				950.00			7
360		OR Services				1800.00			8
370		Anesthesia				1392.37			9
390		Blood/Stor-Proc				630.30			10
402		Radiology Ultrasound				808.00			11
410		Respiratory SVC			22	8682.70			12
481		Cardiac Cath Lab				1139.60			13
920		Other DX SVS				36.00			14
									15
									16
									17
									18
									19
									20
									21
									22
001		Total				77338.28			23

517

Block 56. **Untitled block.** Reserved for state assignment.

Block 57. **Untitled block.** Reserved for national assignment.

Block 58. **Insured's Name.** Enter name of the patient or insured individual in whose name the insurance is issued. If billing for an infant, use the mother's name. If billing for an organ donor, enter the recipient's name and the patient's relationship to the recipient in Block 59. Otherwise leave blank. **Medicaid, Medicare, private payers,** and **TRICARE:** Required.

Block 59. **Patient's Relationship to Insured.** Enter code number indicating relationship of the patient to the insured individual identified in Block 58. **Medicaid, Medicare, private payers,** and **TRICARE:** Required.

Patient Relationship Codes

01	Patient is the insured
02	Spouse
03	Natural child/insured has financial responsibility
04	Natural child/insured does not have financial responsibility
05	Stepchild
06	Foster child
07	Ward of the court
08	Employee
09	Unknown
10	Handicapped dependent
11	Organ donor
12	Cadaver donor
13	Grandchild
14	Niece/nephew
15	Injured plaintiff
16	Sponsored dependent
17	Minor dependent of a minor dependent
18	Parent
19	Grandparent
20	Life partner
21–99	Reserved for national assignment

Block 60. **Certificate—Social Security Number—Health Insurance Claim—Identification Number.** Enter the insured's identification number assigned by the payer organization. Required by all programs.

Block 61. **Group Name.** Enter the group name or plan through which the health insurance coverage is provided to the insured. **Medicare** and **private payers**: Required. **Medi-Cal:** Not required.

TRICARE: Enter the sponsor's branch of service (e.g., USA, USAF).

Block 62. **Insurance Group Number.** Enter the insurance group number. **Private payers:** Required. **Medi-Cal** and **Medicare:** Not required. **TRICARE:** Enter the sponsor's military status and pay grade codes. **CHAMPVA:** Enter the veteran's military status code (e.g., "ACT" for active or "RET" for retired).

Block 63. **Treatment Authorization Codes.** Enter the treatment authorization request (TAR) number provided by the payer. **Medicare, private payers,** and **TRICARE:** Required. **Medi-Cal:** For services requiring a TAR, enter the 11-digit TAR Control Number. It is not necessary to attach a copy of the TAR to the claim.

Block 64. **Employment Status Code.** Enter the employment status code of the insured individual identified in Block 58. **Some Medicaid programs:** May be required. **Medi-Cal:** Not required. **Medicare** and **private payers**: Required. **TRICARE:** Enter the code that describes the employment status of the individual identified in Block 58.

Employment Status Codes

1	Employed full-time
2	Employed part-time
3	Not employed
4	Self-employed
5	Retired
6	On active military duty
7–8	Reserved for national assignment
9	Unknown

Block 65. **Employer Name.** Enter the employer's name for the individual listed in Block 58. **Medicaid**: May be required. **Medi-Cal:** Not required. **Medicare, private payers,** and **TRICARE:** Required.

Block 66. **Employer Location.** Enter the employer's location of the insured individual identified in Block 58. **Some Medicaid programs**: May be required. **Medi-Cal:** Not required. **Medicare, private payers,** and **TRICARE:** Required.

Block 67. **Principal Diagnosis Code.** Enter all numbers and letters of the ICD-9-CM code for the principal diagnosis, including fourth and fifth digits. Do not insert a decimal point. Required for all programs.

Blocks 68–75. Other Diagnosis Codes. Enter all numbers and letters of the ICD-9-CM codes that correspond to the patient's additional conditions that coexist at the time of admission or develop subsequently and have an effect on the treatment received or length of stay. Required for all programs. **Medi-Cal:** Not required.

Block 75. Enter DRG group number for inpatient claims.

Block 76. Admitting Diagnosis Code/Patient's Reason for Visit. Enter admitting diagnosis code, including fourth and fifth digits as stated by the physician at the time of admission for inpatient claims. For outpatient claims, enter the patient's stated reason for seeking care. Required for all programs.

Block 77. External Cause of Injury Code. If there is an external cause of injury, poisoning, or adverse effect, enter the diagnostic E code, including the third and fourth digits. **Medicare** and **private payers:** Not required.

Block 78. Unlabeled block. Reserved for state assignment.

Block 79. Procedure Coding Method Used. Enter appropriate code to identify the coding system used. **Medicaid, private payers,** and **TRICARE:** Required. **Medicare:** Not required.

Coding System Codes

1–3	Reserved for state assignment
4	CPT procedure codes
5	HCPCS codes
6–8	Reserved for national assignment
9	ICD-9-CM procedure codes

Block 80. Principal Procedure Codes and Date. Enter the procedure code for the principal procedure and date performed. The electronic version requires an eight-character date listing year, month, and day (20XX0425). **Medicaid, Medicare, private payers, TRICARE:** Required.

Block 81. Other Procedure Codes and Dates. Enter one or two additional major procedure codes and dates performed to identify significant procedures other than the principal procedure and cor-responding dates when procedures were performed. The electronic version requires an eight-character date listing year, month, and day (20XX0215). **Medicare, private payers,** and **TRICARE:** Required. **Medicaid:** May be required depending on contract.

Block 82. Attending Physician ID. Enter the name and/or provider number for the physician who has primary responsibility for the patient's care and treatment. This block is mandatory for radiologists. If the physician is a Medicaid or Medi-Cal provider, enter the state license number. Do not use a group provider number. Required by all programs.

Block 83. Other Physician ID. Enter the name and/or identification number of the licensed physician other than the attending physician. Required for all programs. **Medi-Cal:** On the upper line of Block 83, enter the individual nine-digit Medi-Cal provider number for the physician actually providing services. Do not use a group provider number or state license number.

Block 84. Remarks. Use this area to fulfill any reporting requirements, such as procedures that require additional information, justification for services, an emergency certification statement, or as an optional block for DRG group number for inpatient claims if not entered in Block 75. If it will not fit in this area, attach the statement to the claim. Required for all programs.

Block 85. Provider Representative Signature. Provider or authorized signer must sign and date claim. **Medicare, Medicaid, private payers,** and **TRICARE:** Required. For Medicare, a stamped signature is acceptable. For other programs, a facsimile signature may be acceptable after approval.

Block 86. Date Bill Submitted. Insert the date the claim is submitted to the insurance company or fiscal intermediary. **Medicaid, private payers,** and **TRICARE:** Required. **Medicare:** Not required.

Taking the hospital billing process a step further, Figure 16–5 illustrates which block of the UB-92 claim form is affected by the hospital department and employee. To become familiar with the UB-92 claim form, an assignment is presented in the *Workbook* asking you to divide the 86 blocks of information into six categories according to departmental input.

Diagnosis-Related Groups

History

The concept of diagnosis-related groups (DRGs) was developed by Professors John D. Thompson and Robert B. Fetter at Yale University and tested in New Jersey from 1977 to 1979. The goal was to develop a scheme of patient classification to be used in utilization review (UR).* Soon other applications were found in such areas as budgeting, planning, and reimbursement.

Because of inconsistencies and inadequacies in the original concept, a second set of DRGs was developed and has been used in New Jersey since 1982. Under the Medicare Prospective Payment System (PPS), the DRGs were implemented nationwide for all hospitalizations after the Tax Equity and Fiscal Responsibility Act of 1982 (TEFRA) was passed. The purpose of a DRG-based system used for Medicare reimbursement is to hold down rising health care costs. Therefore, Medicare reimbursement as a whole is expected to decrease significantly under the DRG payment system.

The Diagnosis-Related Groups System

The DRG system is a patient classification method that categorizes patients who are medically related with respect to diagnosis and treatment and who are statistically similar in length of stay. It is used to both classify past cases to measure the relative resources hospitals have expanded to treat patients with similar illnesses and to classify current cases to determine payment. This system changed hospital reimbursement from a fee-for-service system to a lump-sum, fixed-fee payment based on the diagnoses rather than on time or services rendered. The fees were fixed by a research team, which determined a national "average" fee for each of the principal discharge diagnoses. The classifications were formed from more than 10,000 ICD-9-CM codes that were divided into 25 basic **major diagnostic categories (MDCs).** These diagnoses were assigned a specific DRG number from 001 to 511 (as of the printing of this edition) and specific values commensurate with geographic areas, types of hospitals, depreciation values, teaching status, and other specific criteria. TRICARE and other private insurance that utilize DRGs use DRG numbers 600 to 900. Most MDCs are based on a particular organ system of the body. Within MDCs, DRGs are either

medical or surgical. Seven variables are responsible for DRG classifications:

▶ Principal diagnosis
▶ Secondary diagnosis (up to eight)
▶ Surgical procedures (up to six)
▶ Comorbidity and complications
▶ Age and sex
▶ Discharge status
▶ Trim points (number of hospital days for a specific diagnosis)

At the time of the initial admission review, the physician establishes a tentative diagnosis so that a tentative DRG can be assigned. The tentative DRG is assigned based on (1) admission diagnosis, (2) scheduled procedures, (3) age, and (4) known secondary diagnoses. An individual in the Health Information Management Department obtains the pertinent patient case history information listed above and codes the principal and secondary diagnoses and operative procedure(s). Using a computer software program called a **grouper,** this information is keyed in and the program calculates and assigns the DRG payment group. The grouper is not able to consider any differences between chronic and acute conditions. **Looping** is the grouper process of searching all listed diagnoses for the presence of any comorbid condition or complication or searching all procedures for operating room procedures or more specific procedures. If any factors that affect the DRG assignment change or are added, the new information is entered and the case is assigned to the new DRG.

Let's take an example of the case of a patient with chronic bronchitis who is admitted to the hospital with pneumonia; his medical record shows that he has had emphysema for many years. Refer to Figure 16–7, which lists the chronic obstructive lung disease diagnostic code as the principal diagnosis, with pneumonia as a secondary diagnosis (inaccurate DRG assignment). This would entitle the hospital to receive $2,723.66. However, if the pneumonia diagnostic code was listed as the principal diagnosis with two secondary diagnostic codes, emphysema and chronic bronchitis, then the hospital would be entitled to $3,294.17—$570 additional reimbursement with the use of the correct DRG assignment.

A case that cannot be assigned to an appropriate DRG because of an atypical situation is called a **cost outlier.** These atypical situations are as follows:

1. **Clinical outliers:**
   a. Unique combinations of diagnoses and surgeries causing high costs. These are more common than day outliers.
   b. Very rare conditions

---

*Review of hospital admissions to determine whether they are justified; this is discussed at the beginning of the chapter.

	42 REV. CD.	43 DESCRIPTION	44 HCPCS/RATES	45 SERV. DATE	46. SERV./UNITS	47 TOTAL CHARGES	48 NON-COVERED CHARGES	49	
1	175	Neonatal ICU	1844.00		14	25816.00			1
2	250	Pharmacy				4083.20			2
3	258	IV Solutions–Pharmacy				3387.90			3
4	270	Med-Sur Supplies				15606.71			4
5	300	Laboratory				12958.40			5
6	310	Pathology Lab				47.10			6
7	320	OX X-Ray				950.00			7
8	360	OR Services				1800.00			8
9	370	Anesthesia				1392.37			9
10	390	Blood/Stor-Proc				630.30			10
11	402	Radiology Ultrasound				808.00			11
12	410	Respiratory SVC			22	8682.70			12
13	481	Cardiac Cath Lab				1139.60			13
14	920	Other DX SVS				36.00			14
15									15
16									16
17									17
18									18
19									19
20									20
21									21
22									22
23	001	Total				77338.28			23

SAMPLE CASE HISTORY			
CORRECT DRG ASSIGNMENT		**INACCURATE DRG ASSIGNMENT**	
MDC 4: Respiratory System		MDC 4: Respiratory System	
Principal Diagnosis	Pneumonia (ICD9CM-486)	Principal Diagnosis	COPID (ICD9CM-496)
Secondary Diagnosis	Emphysema (ICD9CM-492.8)	Secondary Diagnosis	Pneumonia (ICD9CM-486)
Secondary Diagnosis	Chronic Bronchitis (ICD9CM-491.2)	Principal Operative Procedure	None
Principal Operative Procedure	None	Principal Operative Procedure	None
Secondary Operative Procedure	None	Secondary Operative Procedure	None
Age	69 Years	Age	69 Years
Discharge Status	Routine	Discharge Status	Routine
Sex	Male	Sex	Male
Length of Stay	15 Days	Length of Stay	15 Days
DRG	89	DRG	88
Trim Points	4–22 Days	Trim Points	3–19 Days
Rate	$3,294.17	Rate	$2,723.66

Figure 16–7. Sample case history showing correct and incorrect DRG assignment and the difference in payment between the two.

2. Long length of stay, referred to as *day outliers**
3. Low-volume DRGs

Inliers (hospital case falls below the mean average or expected length of stay):

1. Death
2. Leaving against medical advice (AMA)
3. Admitted and discharged on the same day

The current federal plan for outliers is the full DRG rate plus an additional payment for the services provided. An unethical practice, **DRG creep,** is to code a patient's DRG category for a more severe diagnosis than indicated by the patient's condition. This is also called upcoding.

In hospital billing, downcoding can also erroneously occur when sequencing several diagnoses (e.g., listing a normal pregnancy as the primary diagnosis for payment and complications in the secondary position when the patient remained in the hospital for an extended number of days). Additional examples are discussed in Chapter 5.

The amount of payment may be increased by documenting in the patient's medical record any comorbid conditions or complications. When referring to DRGs, the abbreviation CC is used to indicate such complications and/or comorbidities (not the more common interpretation found in patient charting, Chief Complaint). **Comorbidity** is defined

as a preexisting condition that will, because of its effect on the specific principal diagnosis, require more intensive therapy or cause an increase in length of stay by at least 1 day in approximately 75% of cases.

If a patient is admitted because of two or more conditions and the physician fails to indicate the "most resource-intensive" or "most specific" diagnosis as the principal diagnosis, the DRG assessment will be incorrect, resulting in decreased reimbursement to the health care facility (see Examples 16–14 and 16–15). It is the responsibility of the attending physician to decide on a principal diagnosis based on his or her best judgment.

EXAMPLE 16–14

A patient has had congestive heart failure for several years and is admitted with an admitting diagnosis of chest pain and principal diagnosis of anterior wall myocardial infarction (MI). While hospitalized, the patient experiences atrial fibrillation.

Principal diagnosis:	410.1	anterior wall myocardial infarction
Comorbid condition(CC):	428.0	congestive heart failure
Complication:	427.31	atrial fibrillation

---

*Day outliers are to be eliminated.

EXAMPLE 16–15

A patient has had chronic obstructive pulmonary disease (COPD) for the last 6 months and is admitted with an admitting diagnosis of chest pain and a principal diagnosis of anterior wall myocardial infarction (MI). While hospitalized, the patient experiences respiratory failure.

Principal diagnosis:	410.1	anterior wall myocardial infarction
Comorbid condition:	496	chronic obstructive pulmonary disease
Complication:	799.1	respiratory failure

Both examples would warrant additional payment because of comorbid conditions and complications.

DRG/ICD-9-CM Code Book is a good reference and code book presented in an easy-to-use binder and containing Volumes 1, 2, and 3 of ICD-9-CM. Sections are color-highlighted for maximum payment. Refer to Appendix B to locate publishers of ICD-9-CM code books.

Diagnosis-Related Groups and the Medical Assistant/Insurance Billing Specialist

Even though DRGs affect Medicare hospital payments, it is important to stress the role of the medical assistant in a physician's office when communicating the admitting diagnosis to the hospital. This can greatly affect the DRG assignment. The medical assistant should remember the following points:

1. Give all of the diagnoses, if there are more than one, when calling the hospital to admit a patient so the hospital personnel can use their expertise in listing the primary and secondary diagnoses.
2. Ask the physician to review the treatment or procedure in question when a hospital representative calls regarding a test, length of stay, or treatments ordered by the attending physician. The hospital needs this information to justify a higher-than-average bill to Medicare.
3. Get to know the hospital personnel on a first-name basis so that when the physician or patients have DRG-related questions, you can call on this hospital expert.

When the DRG system is implemented by other third party payers and/or segments of the population other than Medicare patients, you should contact them locally to assist you. It is important that records and hospital insurance claims contain the correct *principal diagnosis, detailed facts to support the principal diagnosis and complications, medical data to justify all procedures performed, the patient's age, and discharge diagnosis.*

Outpatient Classification

In late 2000 under the requirements of the Balanced Budget Act of 1997, the HCFA implemented a prospective payment system (PPS) for Medicare beneficiaries. This was a move from a cost-based reimbursement system to a line-item billing system for ambulatory surgery centers and hospital outpatient services. The HCFA has categorized outpatient services into an ambulatory payment classification system. Some Medicaid programs and private payers have embraced this system because of the escalation of outpatient costs.

Ambulatory Payment Classification System

Originally, ambulatory visit groups (AVGs) and then ambulatory patient groups (APGs) were developed as outpatient classification systems by Health Systems International (HSI). These groups were based on patient classifications (ICD-9-CM diagnoses, CPT and HCPCS procedures, age, and gender) rather than disease classifications. After that, ambulatory surgery categories (ASCs) were adopted replacing APGs for outpatient or one-day surgery cases that were derived from the surgery section of the CPT. ASCs used disease and procedural coding classification systems to supply the input to the computer program to assign ASCs.

Currently, the General Accounting Office (GAO) ordered Congress to begin conversion of surgical, radiology, and other diagnostic services to an APC system effective August 1, 2000, which replaces ASCs. There are approximately 451 APCs as of the printing of this edition that are subject to change in number in subsequent years.

APCs are applied to:

▶ Ambulatory surgical procedures
▶ Chemotherapy
▶ Clinic visits
▶ Diagnostic services and diagnostic tests
▶ Emergency department visits
▶ Implants
▶ Outpatient services furnished to nursing facility patients not packaged into nursing facility consolidated billing (services commonly furnished by hospital outpatient departments that nursing facilities are not able to provide [computed tomography, magnetic resonance imaging, ambulatory surgery])
▶ Partial hospitalization services for community mental health centers (CMHCs)
▶ Preventive services (colorectal cancer screening)
▶ Radiology, including radiation therapy
▶ Services for patients who have exhausted Part A benefits

▶ Services to hospice patient for treatment of a nonterminal illness

▶ Surgical pathology

Hospital Prospective Payment System

The development process for APCs is similar to that used for DRGs; however, the procedure code is the primary axis of classification, not the diagnosis code. The reimbursement methodology is based on median costs of services and facility cost to determine charge ratios in addition to copayment amounts. There is also an adjustment for area wage differences, and this is based on the hospital wage index currently used for inpatient services. This Hospital Prospective Payment System (HOPPS) may be updated annually, not periodically. An APC group may have a number of services or items packaged within it so that separate payment cannot be obtained.

APC Status

Categories of services have payment status indicators consisting of alpha code letters or symbols and these are:

Category	Payment Status Indicator
Medical visits to clinic or emergency department	V
Surgical services	T
Significant procedures	S
Ancillary services	X
Acquisition of corneal tissue	F
Current drug/biological pass-through payment	G
Device pass-through payment	H
New drug/biological pass-through payment	J
Payment under another fee schedule or rate	A
Inpatient only	C
Code not used by Medicare, service not covered	E
Service is packaged into APC rate	N
New technology APCs (range is 0970–0984)	#
Code unique to partial hospitalization	P

Partial hospitalization refers to a distinct and organized intensive psychiatric outpatient day treatment program designed to provide patients with profound and disabling mental health conditions an individual, coordinated, comprehensive, and multidisciplinary treatment program.

Types of APCs

The four types of APCs are:

1. *Surgical procedure APCs.* These are surgical procedures for which payment is allowed under the Prospective Payment System (PPS) (e.g., cataract removal, endoscopies, and biopsies). Surgical APCs are assigned based on CPT codes.
2. *Significant procedure APCs.* These consist of nonsurgical procedures that are the main reason for the visit and account for the majority of the time and services used during the visit (e.g., psychotherapy, computed tomography and magnetic resonance imaging, radiation therapy, chemotherapy administration, and partial hospitalization). Significant procedure APCs are selected based on CPT codes.
3. *Medical APCs.* These include encounters with a health care professional for evaluation and management services. The medical APC is determined by site of service (clinic or ED), level of the E/M service (CPT code), and diagnosis from one of 20 diagnostic categories (ICD-9-CM code).
4. *Ancillary APCs.* These involve diagnostic tests or treatments not considered to be significant procedure APCs (e.g., plain x-ray film, electrocardiograms, and cardiac rehabilitation). Ancillary APCs are assigned based on CPT codes.

It is possible that multiple APCs can be used when billing for a visit. Use of CPT modifiers for hospital outpatient visits affect APC payments so it is very important to accurately apply correct modifiers when applicable.

Most hospitals use a type of computer encoder program in which the CPT code is input and an APC group code number is assigned. For example, if CPT code number 99282 is input for a low level emergency department visit, the encoder assigns APC Group 610. Use of an unbundling reference book may be of help in assigning a CPT code, and it would be preferable to use the code that would generate the highest APC payment.

The data that hospitals submit during the first years of implementation of the APC system are vitally important to the revision of weights and other adjustments that affect payment in future years. The APC data that appear on the UB-92 claim form are shown in Figure 16–8.

RESOURCES ON THE INTERNET

 Refer to the *Federal Register* web site for up-to-date guidelines and policies at:

www.hcfa.gov

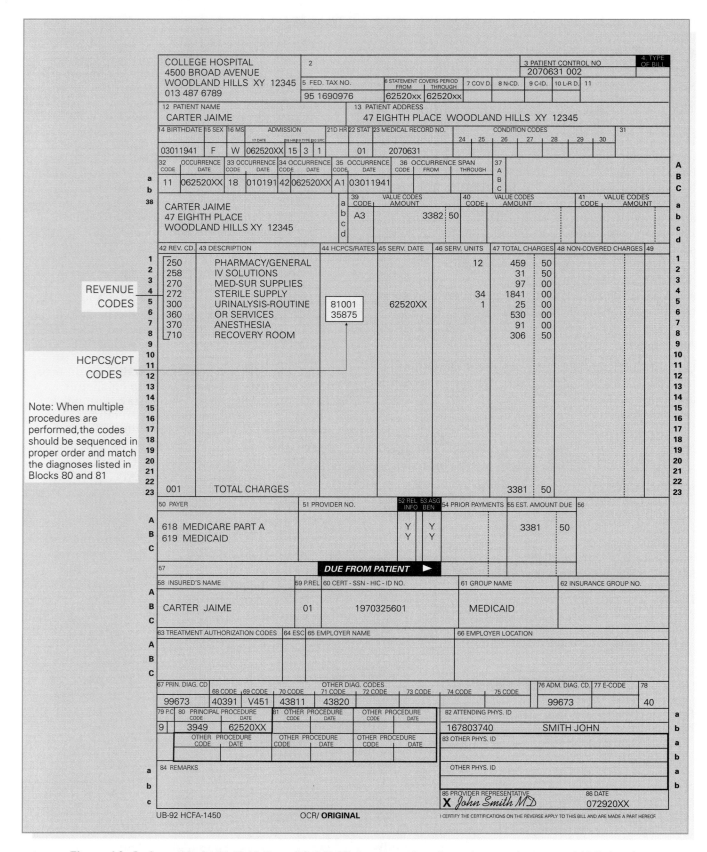

Figure 16–8. Scannable (red ink) Uniform Bill (UB-92) insurance claim form showing placement of APC data for an outpatient for submission to insurance company.

STUDENT ASSIGNMENT LIST

✔ Study Chapter 16.
✔ Answer the review questions in the *Workbook* to reinforce the theory learned in this chapter and to help prepare you for a future test.
✔ Complete the assignments in the *Workbook* to gain hands-on experience in analyzing and editing information from computer-generated UB-92 claim forms for inpatient and outpatient hospital billing. One of the assignments will assist you in further enhancing your diagnostic coding skills in relation to DRGs. These problems point out the value of coding properly in terms of proper diagnostic sequence, indicating the variance in payment.
✔ Turn to the Glossary at the end of this textbook for a further understanding of the Key Terms used in this chapter.

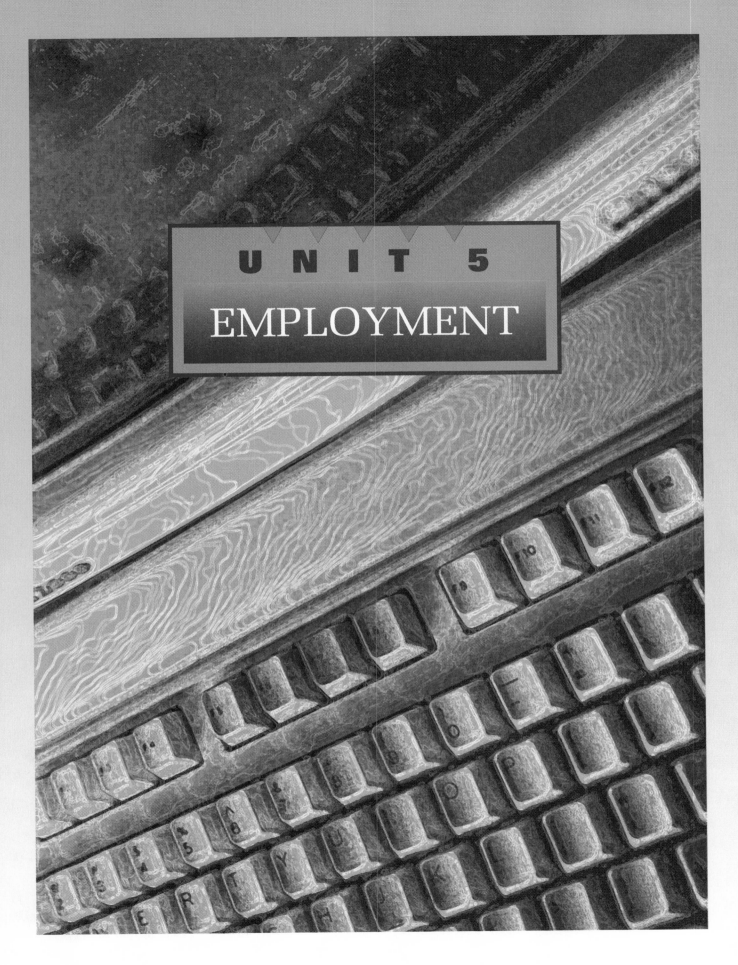

U N I T 5

EMPLOYMENT

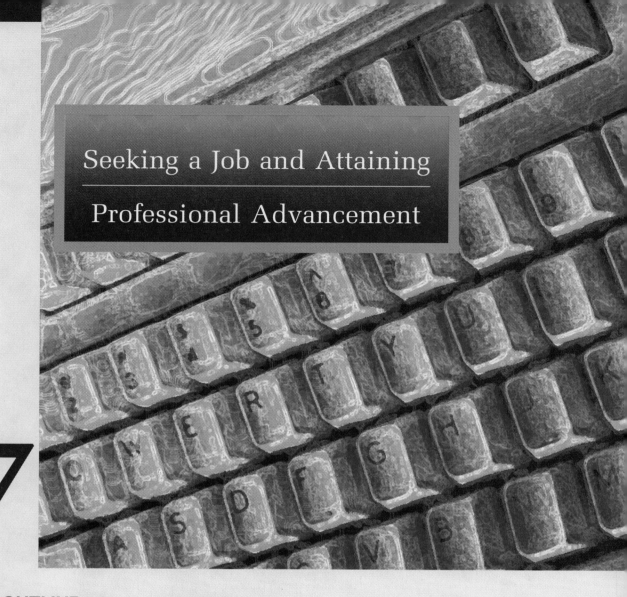

Seeking a Job and Attaining
Professional Advancement

17

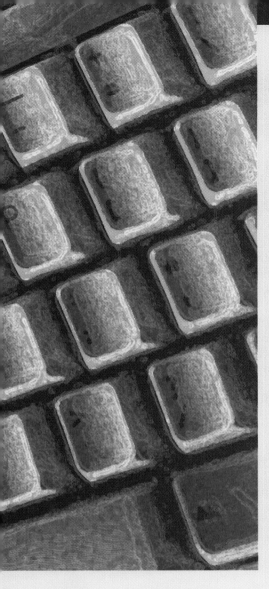

Professional Association of
Health Care Office Managers

Medical Group Management
Association

Keeping Current

Mentor

Networking

OBJECTIVES*

After reading this chapter you should be able to:

- Prepare to find a position as an insurance billing specialist, claims assistance professional, or electronic claims processor.
- Conduct a job search by listing prospective employers.
- Compose a letter of introduction to accompany the resume.
- Analyze education and experience to prepare a resume.
- Identify illegal interview questions.
- Prepare responses to interview questions.
- Assess responsibilities assigned to insurance billing and coding specialists, electronic claims processors, and claims assistance professionals.
- Contact computerized job search databases for on-line services.
- Explore the business aspects of self-employment.
- Search on line for employment opportunities.
- State types of certification and registration available to insurance billers, coders, and administrative medical assistants.

KEY TERMS

alien

application form

blind mailing

certification

Certified Claims Assistance Professional (CCAP)

Certified Coding Specialist (CCS)

Certified Coding Specialist—Physician (CCS-P)

Certified Electronic Claims Professional (CECP)

Certified Medical Assistant (CMA)

Certified Professional Coder (CPC)

chronologic resume

claims assistance professional (CAP)

coding specialist

combination resume

continuing education

cover letter

electronic claims processor (ECP)

employment agency

freelance

functional resume

interview

mentor

Nationally Certified Insurance Coding Specialist (NCICS)

networking

portfolio

continued

*Performance objectives and exercises for hands-on practical experience for this chapter appear in the *Workbook*.

Employment Opportunities

Insurance Billing Specialist

Employment opportunities are available throughout the United States for insurance billing specialists who attain coding skills, knowledge of insurance programs, and expertise in completing insurance claims accurately. In addition to the skills necessary for performance on the job, ask yourself the following questions to determine if you need to sharpen your job-seeking techniques:

▶ Are you motivated and interested in finding a job?
▶ Can you communicate effectively in an interview?
▶ Do you enjoy good health?
▶ Are you mature?
▶ Do you have good grooming and manners?

The increase in the required knowledge and volume of paperwork associated with insurance claims, medical record keeping, and state and government agencies means a corresponding increase in the need for an insurance billing specialist. Because an individual can choose a number of different types of positions, this chapter provides information on each.

Examples of generic job descriptions are shown in Figures 17–1 through 17–4 to illustrate what job duties, skills, and requirements might be encountered for various insurance billing and coding positions. Job descriptions include assisting managers, supervisors, and employers in recruiting, supervising, and evaluating individuals in these positions for salary upgrades. Companies have had to modify their job descriptions to address individuals with physical impairments who may fall under the Americans with Disabilities Act.

There are two ways to work—either employed by someone or self-employed (Fig. 17–5). In this career field, some of the choices are

▶ Insurance billing specialist
▶ Electronic claims processor
▶ Medicare or Medicaid billing specialist
▶ Claims assistance professional
▶ **Coding specialist (freelance or employed)**

Some hospital facilities and physicians prefer credentialed coders and/or insurance billers and advertise for

▶ **Certified Professional Coder (CPC)**
▶ **Certified Coding Specialist (CCS)**
▶ **Certified Coding Specialist—Physician (CCS-P)**
▶ **Certified Electronic Claims Processor (CECP)**
▶ **Certified Claims Assistance Professional (CCAPs)**
▶ Healthcare Reimbursement Specialist (HRS)
▶ **Nationally Certified Insurance Coding Specialist (NCICS)**
▶ **Registered Medical Coder (RMC)**

Becoming certified is certainly an essential goal if one seeks career advancement, and the steps to accomplish this as well as certification in other careers allied to this one are detailed at the end of this chapter.

GENERIC JOB DESCRIPTION FOR ENTRY LEVEL
INSURANCE BILLING SPECIALIST

Knowledge, skills, and abilities:
1. Minimum education level consists of certificate from one-year insurance billing course, associate degree, or equivalent in work experience and continuing education.
2. Knowledge of basic medical terminology, anatomy and physiology, diseases, surgeries, medical specialties, and insurance terminology.
3. Ability to operate word processing, computer, photocopy, and calculator equipment.
4. Written and oral communication skills including grammar, punctuation, and style.
5. Ability and knowledge to use procedure code books.
6. Ability and knowledge to use diagnostic code books.
7. Ability to type or key 45 to 60 wpm.
8. Abllity to work independently.
9. Certified Procedural Coder (CPC) or Certified Coding Specialist (CCS) status preferred.

Working conditions:
Medical office setting. Sufficient lighting.

Physical demands:
Prolonged sitting, standing and walking. Use of typewriter, wordprocessor, or computer equipment. Some stooping, reaching, climbing, and bending. Occasional lifting of _____lbs. to a height of 5 feet. Hearing and speech capabilities necessary to communicate with patients and staff in person and on telephone. Vision capable of viewing computer monitors, calculators, charts, forms, text, and numbers for prolonged periods.

Salary:
Employer would list range of remuneration for the position.

Job responsibilities:	**Performance standards:**
1. Abstracts medical information from patient records.	1.1 Uses knowledge of medical terminology, anatomy and physiology, diseases, surgeries, and medical specialties.
	1.2 Consults reference materials to clarify meanings of words.
	1.3 Meets accuracy and production requirements adopted by employer.
	1.4 Verifies with physician any vague information for accuracy.
2. Exhibits an understanding of ethical and medicolegal responsibilities related to insurance billing programs.	2.1 Observes policies and procedures related to confidentiality, medical records, release of information, retention of records, statute of limitations for claim submission.
	2.2 Meets standards of professional etiquette and ethical conduct.
	2.3 Recognizes and reports problems involving fraud, abuse, embezzlement, and forgery to appropriate individuals.

Figure 17–1. Generic job description for an insurance billing specialist.

(Illustration continued on following page)

3. Operates word processing, computers, or typewriter equipment to complete insurance claims.	3.1 Operates equipment skillfully and efficiently. 3.2 Evaluates condition of equipment and reports need for repair or replacement.
4. Follows employer's policies and procedures.	4.1 Punctual work attendance and is dependable. 4.2 Answers routine inquiries related to account balances and dates insurance forms submitted.
5. Completes and submits insurance claims accurately.	5.1 Updates insurance registration and account information. 5.2 Processes payments and posts to accounts accurately. 5.3 Handles correspondence related to insurance claims. 5.4 Reviews encounter forms for accuracy before submission to data entry. 5.5 Inserts data on insurance claims accurately. 5.6 Codes procedures and diagnoses accurately. 5.7 Telephones insurance companies with regard to delinquent claims. 5.8 Traces insurance claims. 5.9 Files appeals for denied claims. 5.10 Documents data from patients accurately. 5.11 Maintains separate insurance files.
6. Enhances knowledge and skills to keep up to date.	6.1 Attends continuing education activities. 6.2 Obtains current knowledge applicable to state and federal programs as they relate to insurance claim submission. 6.3 Keeps abreast of current changes in coding requirements from Medicare, Medicaid, and other third-party payers. 6.4 Assists with updating fee schedules and encounter forms with current codes. 6.5 Assists in the research of proper coding techniques to maximize reimbursement.
7. Employs interpersonal expertise to provide good working relationships with patients, employer, employees, and insurance companies.	7.1 Works with employer and employees cooperatively as a team. 7.2 Communicates effectively with patients and insurance companies regarding payment policies and financial obligations. 7.3 Executes job assignments with diligence and skill. 7.4 Assists staff with coding and reimbursement problems. 7.5 Assists other employees when needed. 7.6 Assists with giving fee estimates to patients when necessary.

Figure 17–1. *Continued*

GENERIC JOB DESCRIPTION FOR
A CLAIMS ASSISTANCE PROFESSIONAL

Knowledge, skills, and abilities:

1. Minimum education level consists of certificate from one-year insurance billing course, associate degree, or equivalent in work experience and continuing education.
2. Knowledge of basic medical terminology, anatomy and physiology, diseases, surgeries, medical specialties, and insurance terminology.
3. Ability to operate typewriter, word processing, or computer equipment as well as photocopy and calculator equipment.
4. Written and oral communication skills including grammar, punctuation, and style.
5. Ability and knowledge to use procedure code books.
6. Ability and knowledge to use diagnostic code books.
7. Ability to type or keyboard 45 to 60 wpm.
8. Ability to work independently.
9. Certified Claims Assistance Professional (CCAP) status preferred.

Working conditions:

Home office setting. Sufficient lighting and space to allow for at least 3 or more people.

Physical demands:

Prolonged sitting, standing, and walking. Use of typewriter, wordprocessor, or computer equipment. Some stooping, reaching, climbing, and bending. Occasional lifting of ____lbs. to a height of 5 feet. Hearing and speech capabilities necessary to communicate with clients in person and on telephone. Vision capable of viewing computer monitors, calculators, charts, forms, text, and numbers for prolonged periods.

Salary:

Client would pay a percentage of reimbursement or annual salary, hourly wage, or per claim fee.

Job responsibilities:	**Performance standards:**
1. Files secondary insurance claims and maintains insurance files.	1.1 Completes accurately and submits secondary insurance claims.
2. Tracks insurance claim payments received by clients.	2.1 Maintains files and traces insurance claims for clients.
3. Exhibits an understanding of ethical and medicolegal responsibilities related to insurance billing programs.	3.1 Observes policies and procedures confidentiality of medical records, release of information, retention of records, and statute of limitations for claim submission.

Figure 17–2. Generic job description for a claims assistance professional (CAP).

(Illustration continued on following page)

	3.2 Meets standards of professional etiquette and ethical conduct.
	3.3 Recognizes and reports problems involving fraud, abuse, embezzlement, and forgery to appropriate individuals.
4. Knowledge of medical terminology.	4.1 Explains data on insurance claim forms.
5. Knowledge of procedure and diagnostic code requirements as well as health insurance terminology.	5.1 Understands procedural and diagnostic codes and checks to see if correct codes were used.
6. Operates word processing, computers, or typewriter equipment to complete and submit secondary insurance claims.	6.1 Operates equipment skillfully and efficiently. 6.2 Evaluates condition of equipment and negotiates repair or replacement.
7. Employs interpersonal expertise to provide good working relationships with clients, medical office personnel, and insurance companies.	7.1 Works with clients, medical office personnel, and insurance companies with efficiency, diligence, and skill. 7.2 Communicates effectively with clients and insurance companies regarding payment policies. 7.3 Answers routine inquiries related to status of clients' accounts and dates insurance forms submitted.
8. Assists clients in challenging insurer's denials of payment of claims.	8.1 Handles correspondence related to denial of insurance payment. 8.2 Telephones insurance companies and medical offices with regard to delinquent claims.
9. Interacts with health personnel to render additional information to appeal a denied claim and obtains payment for clients depending on terms of the health insurance policy or program.	9.1 Files appeals for denied claims.
10. Enhances knowledge and skills to keep up to date.	10.1 Attends continuing education activities. 10.2 Obtains current knowledge applicable to private insurance and the Medicare program related to insurance claim submission and payments. 10.3 Keeps abreast of current changes in coding requirements from Medicare, Medicaid, and other third-party payers.

Figure 17–2. *Continued*

GENERIC JOB DESCRIPTION FOR
AN ELECTRONIC CLAIMS PROCESSOR

Knowledge, skills, and abilities:
1. Minimum education level consists of certificate from one-year insurance billing course, associate degree, or equivalent in work experience and continuing education.
2. Knowledge of basic medical terminology, anatomy and physiology, diseases, surgeries, medical specialties, and insurance terminology.
3. Ability to operate computer, modem, and printer as well as photocopy and calculator equipment.
4. Written and oral communication skills including grammar, punctuation, and style.
5. Ability and knowledge to use procedure code books.
6. Ability and knowledge to use diagnostic code books.
7. Ability to key 45 to 60 wpm.
8. Ability to work independently.
9. Certified Electronic Claims Processor (CECP) status preferred.

Working conditions:
Medical office setting. Sufficient lighting.

Physical demands:
Prolonged sitting, standing and walking. Use of computer equipment. Some stooping, reaching, climbing, and bending. Occasional lifting of _____lbs. to a height of 5 feet. Hearing and speech capabilities necessary to communicate with patients and staff in person and on telephone. Vision capabilities necessary to view computer monitors, calculators, charts, forms, text, and numbers for prolonged periods.

Salary:
Employer would list range of remuneration for the position.

Job responsibilities:	**Performance standards:**
1. Acts as a link between the medical provider or facility and insurance companies.	1.1 Uses knowledge of medical terminology, anatomy and physiology, diseases, surgeries, and medical specialties.
	1.2 Understands computer applications and equipment required to convert and transmit patient billing data electronically.
	1.3 Consults reference materials to clarify meanings of words.
	1.4 Meets accuracy and production requirements adopted by employer.
	1.5 Verifies with physician any vague information for accuracy.
	1.6 Reduces volume of paperwork and variety of claim forms providers need to submit claims for payment.
2. Converts patient billing data into electronically readable formats.	2.1 Inputs data and transmits insurance claims accurately, either directly or through a clearinghouse.
	2.2 Answers routine inquiries related to account balances and dates insurance data transmitted to insurance carriers.

Figure 17–3. Generic job description for an electronic claims processor (ECP).

(Illustration continued on following page)

2.3 Updates and maintains software applications with requirements of clearinghouses and insurance carriers.

3. Uses software that eliminates common claim filing errors, provides clean claims to insurance carriers, expedites payments to providers or facilities, and follows up on delinquent or denied claims.

3.1 Codes procedures and diagnoses accurately.
3.2 Telephones insurance companies about delinquent claims.
3.3 Traces insurance claims.
3.4 Files appeals for denied claims.

4. Exhibits an understanding of ethical and medicolegal responsibilities related to insurance billing programs and plans.

4.1 Observes policies and procedures related to confidentiality, medical records, release of information, retention of records, and statute of limitations for claim submission.
4.2 Meets standards of professional etiquette and ethical conduct.
4.3 Recognizes and reports problems involving fraud, abuse, embezzlement, and forgery to appropriate individuals.

5. Operates computer equipment to complete insurance claims.

5.1 Operates equipment skillfully and efficiently.
5.2 Evaluates condition of equipment and reports need for repair or replacement.

6. Follows employer's policies and procedures.

6.1 Must have punctual work attendance and be dependable.

7. Enhances knowledge and skills to keep up to date.

7.1 Attends continuing education skills activities.
7.2 Obtains current knowledge applicable to state and federal programs as they relate to transmission of insurance claims.
7.3 Keeps abreast of current changes in coding requirements from Medicare, Medicaid, and other third-party payers. Assists in the research of proper coding techniques to maximum reimbursement.

8. Employs interpersonal expertise to provide good working relationships with patients, employer, employees, and insurance companies.

8.1 Works with employer and employees cooperatively as a team.
8.2 Communicates effectively with patients and insurance companies regarding payment policies and financial obligations.
8.3 Executes job assignments with diligence and skill.
8.4 Assists staff with coding and reimbursement problems.
8.5 Assists other employees when needed.
8.6 Assists with giving fee estimates to patients when necessary.

Figure 17–3. *Continued*

GENERIC JOB DESCRIPTION FOR CODERS

POSITION TITLE

Health Information/Medical Record Technician; Coder and Specialist for an acute and/or ambulatory care setting.

DEPARTMENT

Health Information/Medical Record.

JOB SUMMARY

Codes information from the medical records of patients to generate a clinical patient care database for the facility. Assures the maintenance and accuracy of diagnostic and procedural statistics for the facility as well as optimum appropriate reimbursement from third party payers, by the timely coding of diagnoses and procedures using the required classification systems.

SPECIFIC RESPONSIBILITIES

Reviews and screens the entire medical record to abstract medical, surgical, laboratory, pharmaceutical, demographic, social and administrative data from the medical record in a timely manner.

Ensures providers that all diagnoses and procedures that may impact the facility's reimbursement are identified and attested to by the physician, if appropriate, sequenced correctly, and coded in an accurate and ethical manner for optimum reimbursement. Determines correct codes for routine, and/or new or unusual diagnoses and procedures not clearly listed in ICD-9-CM and CPT.

Consults with physicians for clarifications of clinical data when encountering conflicting or ambiguous information. Keeps abreast of regulatory changes affecting coded information required by the Health Care Financing Administration, the office of Statewide Health Planning Department, and others, as appropriate; and applies current Uniform Hospital Discharge Data Set (UHDDS) definitions for code selection.

Maintains knowledge of current information related to third party reimbursement regulations and seeks continuing education in all phases of coding acumen.

Participates in the Coding Team's regular meetings with the objective of solving problems, brain-storming, educating physicians and others as to the coding policies and procedures of the facility, as well as promoting consistency of data collected.

Achieves a balance in quality and quantity, with a goal of maintaining both elements at a prescribed level of efficiency.

Abides by AHIMA's established code of ethical principles to safeguard the public and contribute within the scope of the profession to quality and efficiency in health care, thus promoting ethical conduct.

OTHER SPECIFIC OR POTENTIAL DUTIES/RESPONSIBILITIES FOR THIS POSITION:

Identifies any loss of revenue by failure to charge for any procedures, supplies, injections or other services, and then submits the missed charges.

Verifies all fee sheets to assure that all charges, appropriate modifiers, dates of injury, E code(s) as well as referring physicians' license numbers (when required) have been documented.

Assigns Diagnosis-Related Groups (DRGs) after identifying not only the principal diagnosis (reason for admission) but also significant complications and/or comorbidities as well as operating room procedures following comparison of relative weights in the DRG GROUPER software, and selection of the highest reimbursement allowable among alternative principal diagnoses documented in the record.

Identifies and abstracts information from medical records for special studies and audits, internal and external.

Assists physicians, ancillary, and administrative personnel with retrieving patient care information for research, planning and marketing projects. Answers questions regarding DRGs as well as disease and procedure classification systems.

Figure 17–4. Generic job description for a coder. (From Stewart SP: Generic job description for coders. J CHIA, 1992. Reprinted with permission from California Health Information Association, Fresno, CA.)

(Illustration continued on following page)

Generates reports using a computer report-writer to retrieve coded and abstracted information from the provider's data processing system.

Orients and instructs new personnel and/or students from health information/medical record technology/administration programs, on unit operations, coding and abstracting activities.

DESCRIPTION OF SKILLS:

I. TECHNICAL SKILLS REQUIRED:

   A. Experience with and knowledge of instructional notations and conventions of ICD-9-CM and CPT HCPCS classification systems; and ability to follow the detailed guidelines related to their use in assigning single, and sequencing multiple, diagnosis and procedure codes for appropriate reimbursement and data collection.

   B. Ability to read handwritten and transcribed documents in the medical record, interpret information, and enter complete and accurate data into an on-line computer system.

   C. Comprehensive knowledge of medical diagnostic and procedural terminology required.

   D. College level understanding of disease processes, anatomy and physiology necessary for assigning accurate numeric and alpha-numeric codes.

   E. Knowledge of federal, state and local government regulations and requirements which pertain to patient care information.

   F. Knowledge of legalities and confidentiality issues involved with release of clinical or billing information.

   G. Knowledge of third party payer reimbursement requirements and an understanding of relative values for multimedical specialties, encounters, and procedures in acute care and ambulatory care settings.

II. DECISION-MAKING/
    RESEARCH SKILLS REQUIRED:

   A. Ability to query, analyze and determine the type of data needed to meet the request for information.

   B. Ability to communicate technical and clinical information concerning patient care and classification systems at different levels; i.e., physicians, ancillary, and administrative personnel.

   C. Ability to apply policies and procedures regarding data security and confidentiality to protect the inappropriate release of information.

   D. Ability to exercise judgement with minimal supervision.

III. ORGANIZATIONAL SKILLS REQUIRED:

   A. Ability to assume responsibility for compilation of clinical data related to inpatient and outpatient encounters including diagnoses, procedures, physicians and services.

   B. Remains current with periodic updates of all coding manuals and guidelines in accordance with federal, state and local regulations.

   C. Ability to manage time schedules, deadlines, multiple requests and priorities, and to maintain productivity.

IV. INTERPERSONAL SKILLS REQUIRED:

   A. Communicates effectively, orally and in writing, with physicians, nurses and peers (both inter- and intra-departmentally) and with external organizations.

   B. Communicates medical information with consideration of ethical and professional standards.

   C. Upholds standards of confidentiality regarding patients, personnel and physicians.

V. EDUCATION AND
   EXPERIENCE REQUIRED:

   A. High school diploma.

   B. Completion of an accredited program for coding certification or an accredited health information medical record technology program. A Certified Coding Specialist (CCS), a Certified Coding Specialist —Physician-based(CCS-P), a Registered Health Information Technician (RHIT), or a Registered Health Information Administrator (RHIA) preferred, with current affiliation with the American Health Information Management Association.

   C. Continuing education in health information management is required. ■

Figure 17–4. *Continued*

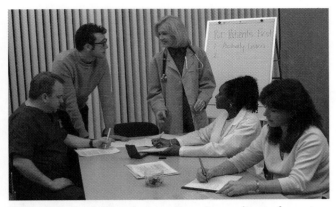

Figure 17–5. Staff conference discussing applicants for potential interviews.

Claims Assistance Professional

If you wish to establish self-employment as a **claims assistance professional (CAP)** in addition to some of the aforementioned positions, contact local hospitals to see whether they have patients who require insurance help. Also call on small employers to see whether they need assistance in explanation of their health insurance policies and/or need to enhance insurance benefits.

Job Search

There are several ways to seek employment. The applicant may wish to be employed by a physician, hospital, medical facility, insurance company, or managed care organization. He or she may choose to be self-employed or may even choose some type of combination situation. Here are suggested ways to search for a job.

1. Join a professional organization, as mentioned later in this chapter, to network with others in the same career field and to hear about job openings (Fig. 17–6). Put a notice about your availability in the chapter newsletter.
2. Attend meetings and workshops in this career field to keep up to date and network with others.
3. Contact the school placement personnel, complete the necessary paperwork, and leave a resume on file if you have just completed a course at a community college or trade school.
4. Spread the word to those who work in medical settings and those who might hear of openings in medical facilities, such as classmates, instructors, school counselors, relatives, and friends.
5. Contact pharmaceutical representatives who visit physicians' offices and hospitals for employment information or leads.

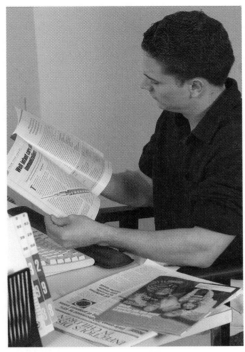

Figure 17–6. Student scanning a professional journal for job leads.

6. Visit public and private **employment agencies** including temporary and temp to permanent agencies. Before signing up with an agency, ask whether the employer or the applicant pays the agency fee.
7. Inquire at state and federal government offices and their employment agencies.
8. Look for part-time employment that might lead to a permanent full-time position.
9. Check bulletin boards frequently in personnel offices of hospitals and clinics for posted job offerings.
10. Go to your local medical society to see if it has a provision for supplying job leads.
11. Consult the *Yellow Pages* of the telephone directory or medical society roster for names of professional offices and hospitals to contact with an introductory telephone call or letter.
12. Send a **blind mailing** of the resume, including a cover letter, to possible prospects. A blind mailing means to send information to employers that you do not know personally and who have not advertised for a job opening. This may result in a positive response with either a request to complete an application form or an invitation for an interview.
13. Go to the local library and look through Dunn and Bradstreet's *Million Dollar Directory* and the *Middle Market Directory* for information on potential employers in many cities.

14. Visit the chamber of commerce and ask for some of their publications that contain membership directories, names of major professional employers in specific areas, and brochures describing regional facts.
15. Subscribe to the principal newspaper of the city where employment is desired. Read help wanted ads in the classified section. Positions of interest might be listed as insurance billing specialist, reimbursement manager, insurance claims manager, insurance coordinator, insurance biller, coding/reimbursement specialist, reimbursement coordinator, coder/abstracter, electronic claims processor, and so on.
16. Telephone job hot lines of large medical clinics in your area.
17. Visit unannounced ("cold calls") at job locations.
18. Explore the Internet's World Wide Web.

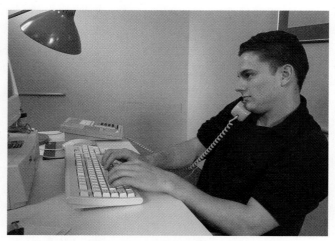

Figure 17–7. Student doing an on-line job search.

On-Line Job Search

Because of vast communication available via the Internet's World Wide Web, newspaper and magazine classified advertisements may become resources of the past. An individual with a computer and modem can access on-line services. Many web sites on the Internet incorporate text, sound, graphics, animation, and video. It is possible to locate potential employers at their web sites who are offering jobs to health care workers by using various search engines. At some sites, you can find detailed descriptions of posted positions and locate opportunity postings by location or employer. You may be able to find and respond to a specific job of interest by delivering an on-line resume, attaching a cover letter, and updating your posting as often as needed. Some web sites allow you to receive e-mailed job alerts.

There are several ways to gain access to the Internet. Your school may allow you to access the Internet on campus. Many libraries have computers with free Internet service. If you have a computer at home, you may wish to subscribe to either a commercial on-line service (e.g., America Online) with Internet access or an Internet service in your locale (Fig. 17–7).

Internet

Once on line, go to a web index to locate a search engine that lists different options to explore, such as Yahoo (www.yahoo.com), Infoseek (www.infoseek.go.com), or Alta Vista (www.altavista.com). One of the resources will be Career Magazine (www.careermag.com/careermag/), which lets you browse through hundreds of national job openings in a variety of fields. Check out America's Job Bank (www.ajb.dni.us) and E-Span Employment Database Search (www.espan.com/), which have job postings that you can browse according to field, location, and career type. Go to PracticeNet (www.practice-net.com), which provides descriptions of medical practice opportunities. This 24-hour service names the recruiter, location, and an 800 number to contact. MedSearch America is another health employment service that posts jobs for hospitals, managed care organizations (MCOs), and pharmaceutical companies. Job seekers can send their resumes via e-mail for free on-line posting. MedSearch has two on-line addresses (www.medsearch.com and gopher://gopher.medsearch.com).

If you subscribe monthly to a commercial on-line service, you can network by posting a notice on a bulletin board with your resume or a note that you are looking for a particular type of position in a given locale.

Register with a computerized job search company. A firm in Irvine, California, American Computerized Employment Service,* has entered the job placement field with a trademarked system called TeleRecruiting. Job candidates may register without charge and complete an extensive profile questionnaire listing experience, skills, job-related factors, maximum commuting distance, and flextime requirements. The firm acts as a liaison between employers and applicants. Employers use a touch-tone telephone to access the computer and

---

*American Computerized Employment Service, 17801 Main Street, Suite A, Irvine, CA 92714. Telephone 714-250-0221.

search for candidates. They pay either an annual subscription, pay-per-search, or package search fee.

If you wish to read about career options on the Internet, obtain a book by Joyce Lain Kennedy entitled *Hook Up, Get Hired! The Internet Job Search Revolution* published by John Wiley & Sons, New York. Another source of information is a book entitled *Buying and Starting Your Medical Billing Service* (http://www.sellingdoctors.com/book/book. html).

Job Fairs

Annual community events feature job fairs at community colleges and technical trade schools or sponsored by professional associations. Job recruiters set up booths with information about their companies and available positions; however, they do not have much time to spend with each job seeker. Thus, it is wise to come prepared and practice a 30-second introduction before attending. This introduction should consist of a quick overview of your career goals, experience, skills, training, education, and personal strengths. Be sure and explain what you can offer the employer. These events are usually day long and you may wish to investigate a number of participating employer's booths.

Go prepared by carrying a binder or folder with plenty of copies of your resume to give to the company representatives you meet. They should be neat, clean, and not folded, wrinkled, or coffee-stained. Take a pen, pencil, and notepad to obtain information. Research the employers attending so you know which ones you will visit and can appear confident, enthusiastic, interested, and knowledgeable to the job recruiter.

Take home the business card and brochure of anyone you talk to who genuinely interests you. After the fair, send that person a follow-up letter to reaffirm your interest.

Application

When visiting a potential employer, ask for an **application** form to complete and inquire if the facility keeps potential job applicants on file and for how long (Fig. 17–8). Study each question carefully before answering, because the employer may evaluate the application itself to determine whether the applicant can follow instructions. Furnish as much information as possible, and if a question does not apply or cannot be answered, insert "no," "none," "NA" (not applicable), or "DNA" (does not apply). When visiting a potential employer for an application form, be sure you

have prepared in advance for an interview in case an opportunity arises on that first visit.

In completing an application form, follow these guidelines:

1. Read the whole application form, since some instructions may appear on the last page or last line.
2. Read the fine print and instructions: "Please print," "Put last name first," or "Complete in your own handwriting." This indicates ability to follow directions or instructions.
3. Print if your handwriting is poor, and abbreviate only when there is lack of space.
4. Complete the application in ink unless pencil is specified.
5. Refer to data from a portfolio, sample application form, or resume that has been checked for accuracy; use this information to copy onto each new application form. Be neat.
6. List correct dates of previous employment so that if the employer should seek to verify this, it will be accurate. If a question is presented asking the reason for leaving a position, leave it blank and discuss this during the interview.
7. Name specific skills, such as procedural coding, diagnostic coding, knowledge of insurance programs, completing the HCFA-1500 claim form, typing or keyboarding (number of words per minute), and speaking a second language.
8. When a question is asked about salary amount, write in "negotiable" or "flexible" and then discuss this during the interview.
9. Sign the application after completion.
10. Reread the entire form, word for word, to find any errors of omission or commission. This avoids having to apologize during an interview for a mistake.

Letter of Introduction

Individuals spend days in perfecting a resume but throw together a *letter of introduction* or **cover letter** in minutes. This is a mistake. The main goal of the cover letter is to get the employer to take notice of the potential employee and resume so an interview appointment can be made. Letters should be typed, addressed to a specific person, and customized to each potential employer. If the advertisement gives a telephone number, call and ask for the name of the person doing the interviewing so the letter can include that person's name. When the name is unknown, use "Dear Sir or Madam" or "To Whom It May Concern," or a less formal "Hello" or "Good Morning."

APPLICATION FOR POSITION / Medical or dental office
AN EQUAL OPPORTUNITY EMPLOYER

(in answering questions, use extra blank sheet if necessary)

No employee, applicant, or candidate for promotion, training or other advantage shall be dicriminated against (or given preference) because of race, color, religion, sex, age, physical handicap, veteran status, or national origin.

PLEASE READ CAREFULLY AND WRITE OR PRINT ANSWERS TO ALL QUESTIONS. DO NOT TYPE.

Date of application: *7-2-XX*

A. PERSONAL INFORMATION

Name - Last *Velasquez,*	First *Jennifer*	Middle *M.*	Social Security No. *361 20 4915*	Area code/phone no. *(013) 439-9800*

Present address: Street *1234 Martin Street, Woodland Hills* (Apt.#) — State *XY* — Zip *12345* — How long at this address?: *10 years*

Previous address: Street — City — State — Zip — Person to notify in case of emergency or accident - name: *John Velasquez*
From: — To: — Address: — Telephone: *013-439-9800*

B. EMPLOYMENT INFORMATION

For what position are you applying?: *insurance biller* — ☒Full-time ☐Part-time ☐Either — Date available for employment?: *7-6-XX* — Wage/salary expectations: *negotiable*

List hrs./days you prefer to work *M-F 8-5 PM* — List any hrs./days you are not available: (Except for times required for religious practices or observances) — Can you work overtime, if necessary? ☒Yes ☐No

Are you employed now? ☐Yes ☒No — If so, may we inquire of your present employer?: ☐No ☐Yes, if yes: Name of employer: — Phone number: ( )

Have you ever been bonded? ☐Yes ☒No — If required for position, are you bondable? ☒Yes ☐No ☐Uncertain — Have you applied for a position with this office before? ☒No ☐Yes If Yes, when?:

Referred by / or where did you learn of this job?:

Can you, upon employment, submit verification of your legal right to work in the United States? ☒Yes ☐No
Submit proof that you meet legal age requirement for employment? ☒Yes ☐No

Language(s) applicant speaks or writes (if use of a language other than english is relevant to the job for which the applicant is applying: *Spanish*

C. EDUCATION HISTORY

	Name and address of schools attended (include current)	Dates From — Thru	Highest grade/ level completed	Diploma/degree(s) obtained/areas of study
High school	*ABC High School, Woodland Hills, XY*	*1990–1994*	*12*	*Diploma*
College	*Vocational-Tech School*	*1995*		Degree/major *Certificate*
Post graduate	*Montana State University*	*1995–97*		Degree/major *24 credits*
Other				Course/diploma/license/ certificate

Specific training, education, or experiences which will assist you in the job for which you have applied. *See résumé*

Future educational plans *Continuing education-preparing for certification*

D. SPECIAL SKILLS

CHECK BELOW THE KINDS OF WORK YOU HAVE DONE:			
☐ BLOOD COUNTS	☐ DENTAL ASSISTANT	☒ MEDICAL INSURANCE FORMS	☐ RECEPTIONIST
☐ BOOKKEEPING	☐ DENTAL HYGIENIST	☒ MEDICAL TERMINOLOGY	☒ TELEPHONES
☒ COLLECTIONS	☐ FILING	☐ MEDICAL TRANSCRIPTION	☒ TYPING
☒ COMPOSING LETTERS	☐ INJECTIONS	☐ NURSING	☐ STENOGRAPHY
☐ COMPUTER INPUT	☐ INSTRUMENT STERILIZATION	☐ PHLEBOTOMY(draw blood)	☐ URINALYSIS
OFFICE EQUIPMENT USED: ☒ COMPUTER	☐ DICTATING EQUIPMENT	☒ POSTING	☐ X-RAY
		☒ WORD PROCESSOR	☒ OTHER *calculator*

Other kinds of tasks performed or skills that may be applicable to position: — Typing speed *60 wpm* — Shorthand speed

ORDER # 72-110 • © 1976 BIBBERO SYSTEMS, INC. • PETALUMA, CA. • (Rev. 1/95)
TO REORDER CALL TOLL FREE: (800) BIBBERO (800-242-2376) OR FAX (800) 242-9330

MFG IN U.S.A.

(PLEASE COMPLETE OTHER SIDE)

Figure 17–8. Application for Position/Medical or Dental Office form. (Reprinted with permission from Bibbero Systems, Inc., Petaluma, CA. Phone: 800-242-2376. Fax: 800-242-9330.)

E. EMPLOYMENT RECORD

| LIST MOST RECENT EMPLOYMENT FIRST | May we contact your previous employer(s) for a reference? ☒ Yes ☐ No |

| 1) Employer St. John's Outpatient Clinic | Worked performed. Be specific: ins biller—see résumé |

| Address: Street 24 Center St. City Woodland Hills, State XY Zip code 12345 | |

| Phone number (013) 782-0155 | |

| Type of business outpt hospital/clinic | Dates Mo. Yr. Mo. Yr. From 2 97 To 8 2000 | |

| Your position ins billing specialist | Hourly rate/salary Starting $9/hr Final $11.50/hr | |

| Supervisor's name Candice Johnson | |

| Reason for leaving Professional advancement | |

| 1) Employer Eastern Airlines | Worked performed. Be specific: |

| Address: Street City Orlando, State Florida Zip code | |

| Phone number (013) 350-7000 | Dates Mo. Yr. Mo. Yr. From 1 88 To 12 89 | |

| Type of business airline transportation | Hourly rate/salary Starting Final | |

| Your position receptionist | |

| Supervisor's name Gary Stevens | |

| Reason for leaving career change | |

| 1) Employer | Worked performed. Be specific: |

| Address: Street City State Zip code | |

| Phone number ( ) | Dates Mo. Yr. Mo. Yr. From To | |

| Type of business | Hourly rate/salary Starting Final | |

| Your position | |

| Supervisor's name | |

| Reason for leaving | |

F. REFERENCES — FRIENDS / ACQUAINTANCES NON-RELATED

| (1) _furnished upon request_ Name | Address | Telephone number | (☐ Work ☐ Home) | Occupation | Years acquainted |

| (1) Name | Address | Telephone number | (☐ Work ☐ Home) | Occupation | Years acquainted |

Please feel free to add any information which you feel will help us consider you for employment

READ THE FOLLOWING CAREFULLY, THEN SIGN AND DATE THE APPLICATION

"I certify that all answers given by me on this application are true, correct and complete to the best of my knowledge. I acknowledge notice that the information contained in this application is subject to check. I agree that, if hired, my continued employment may be contingent upon the accuracy of that information. If employed, I further agree to comply with Company/Office rules and regulations."

Signature: _Jennifer M. Velasquez_ Date: 7-2-XX

Figure 17–8. *Continued*

Do not repeat everything in the resume. Begin with an attention-grabber, and get right to the point so the employer knows what is wanted and why. The letter should explain how the applicant's qualifications and skills would benefit the employer. Use key words that appear in the "position wanted" ad. End the letter by requesting an interview and be sure to enclose a resume. Always include a telephone number and the time of day when you are available.

Reread the letter for typos and errors in grammar, punctuation, and spelling. Avoid the use of "I" in the sentence structure (Fig. 17−9).

Resume

A **resume** is a data sheet designed to sell job qualifications to prospective employers. There are several formats from which to choose:

▶ **Chronologic resume** gives recent experiences first with dates and descriptive data for each job.
▶ **Functional resume** states the qualifications or skills an individual is able to perform.
▶ **Combination resume** summarizes the applicant's job skills as well as educational and employment history. Combination style is the best choice for an insurance billing specialist (Fig. 17−10).

The ideal length for a resume is one page. It can be typed on a 10 × 14-inch page and reduced to letter size. The resume should be keyed or typed, not handwritten, on high-quality, wrinkle-free bond off-white or white paper; single spaced internally with double spacing between main headings; and balanced spacing for all four margins. Laser-printed resumes give a professional appearance.

Under the Civil Rights Act of 1964, enforced by the Equal Employment Opportunity Commission, information about height, weight, birth date, marital status, Social Security number, and physical condition may be omitted. Additional items to omit are salary requirements, reason for leaving jobs, date of resume preparation, date available to begin work, references, and vague references to time gaps. Hobbies and outside interests that would relate to the profession might be included. Membership and/or leadership positions held in professional organizations related to the medical field might be mentioned. A photograph is not necessary but might be included if it will be of

Figure 17−9. Suggested content for a letter of introduction to accompany a resume.

Street Address
City, State, ZIP code
Date of letter

John Doe, MD or
Personnel Director
Street Address
City, State, ZIP code

Dear Dr. Doe:

Paragraph 1: Explain where you heard about the position and say you are writing for a position mentioned in the advertisement.

Paragraph 2: Name two or more qualifications of great interest to the prospective employer. State reasons you are interested in this specialty, location, or type of work. Mention if experienced or trained for this career field.

Paragraph 3: Refer the reader to the resume or application form enclosed.

Paragraph 4: Close the letter by asking for an interview and suggesting a date and time or that you will call for an appointment. If requesting further information about the job opening, enclose a self-addressed, stamped envelope as a courtesy. Do not end the letter with a vague statement but give the reader a specific action to take.

Sincerely yours,

(handwritten signature)

Type name

Enclosure

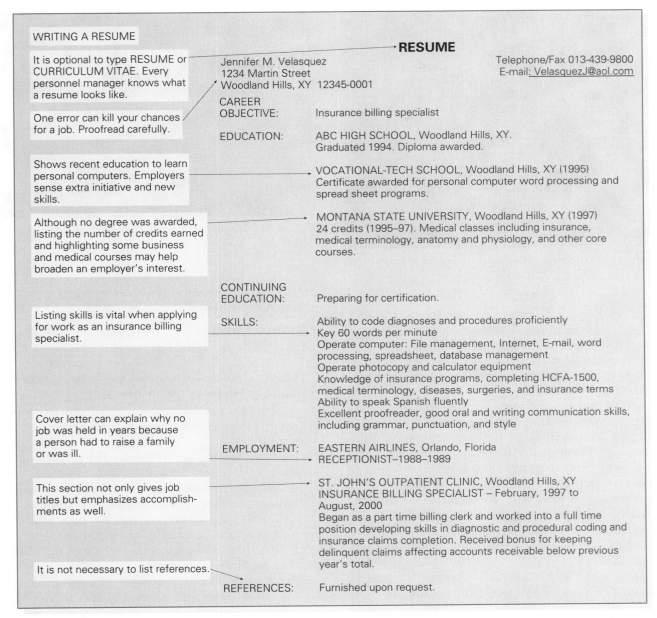

WRITING A RESUME

It is optional to type RESUME or CURRICULUM VITAE. Every personnel manager knows what a resume looks like.

One error can kill your chances for a job. Proofread carefully.

Shows recent education to learn personal computers. Employers sense extra initiative and new skills.

Although no degree was awarded, listing the number of credits earned and highlighting some business and medical courses may help broaden an employer's interest.

Listing skills is vital when applying for work as an insurance billing specialist.

Cover letter can explain why no job was held in years because a person had to raise a family or was ill.

This section not only gives job titles but emphasizes accomplishments as well.

It is not necessary to list references.

RESUME

Jennifer M. Velasquez
1234 Martin Street
Woodland Hills, XY 12345-0001

Telephone/Fax 013-439-9800
E-mail: VelasquezJ@aol.com

CAREER OBJECTIVE: Insurance billing specialist

EDUCATION: ABC HIGH SCHOOL, Woodland Hills, XY.
Graduated 1994. Diploma awarded.

VOCATIONAL-TECH SCHOOL, Woodland Hills, XY (1995)
Certificate awarded for personal computer word processing and spread sheet programs.

MONTANA STATE UNIVERSITY, Woodland Hills, XY (1997)
24 credits (1995–97). Medical classes including insurance, medical terminology, anatomy and physiology, and other core courses.

CONTINUING EDUCATION: Preparing for certification.

SKILLS: Ability to code diagnoses and procedures proficiently
Key 60 words per minute
Operate computer: File management, Internet, E-mail, word processing, spreadsheet, database management
Operate photocopy and calculator equipment
Knowledge of insurance programs, completing HCFA-1500, medical terminology, diseases, surgeries, and insurance terms
Ability to speak Spanish fluently
Excellent proofreader, good oral and writing communication skills, including grammar, punctuation, and style

EMPLOYMENT: EASTERN AIRLINES, Orlando, Florida
RECEPTIONIST–1988–1989

ST. JOHN'S OUTPATIENT CLINIC, Woodland Hills, XY
INSURANCE BILLING SPECIALIST – February, 1997 to August, 2000
Began as a part time billing clerk and worked into a full time position developing skills in diagnostic and procedural coding and insurance claims completion. Received bonus for keeping delinquent claims affecting accounts receivable below previous year's total.

REFERENCES: Furnished upon request.

Figure 17–10. Example of the combination-format resume stressing education and skills. Personal data may be excluded as a result of the Civil Rights Act of 1964, enforced by the EEOC.

value to the interviewer for recall purposes (Fig. 17–11).

The format may include the following:

▶ *Title*. Resume, Personal Datasheet, Biographic Sketch, or Curriculum Vitae.

▶ *Heading*. At the beginning of the resume, the applicant's name, address, and telephone number are entered.

▶ *Summary*. This may be a statement as to why the employer would be interested in this applicant. Use action words as shown in Figure 17–10 and avoid the personal pronoun.

▶ *Education*. Name high school, college, and any business school attended, city and state, degree, and date received. List in reverse chronologic order. Grade average and awards or scholastic honors may be included.

▶ *Professional Experience*. Name all employers in reverse chronologic order with addresses, telephone numbers, and dates of employment. Include summer, full-time, part-time, and temporary jobs as well as externship and volunteer work.

▶ *Skills*. List typing or keyboarding words per minute, computer equipment operated,

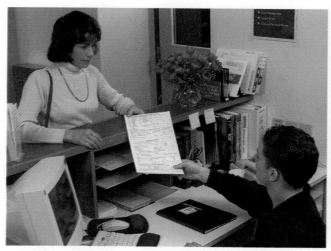

Figure 17–11. Student delivering a resume to a potential job site.

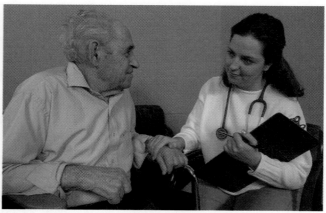

Figure 17–12. Insurance billing student at an externship site.

experience in medical software programs, accurate procedure and diagnostic coding, expertise in insurance claims completion and submission, knowledge of medical terminology, bookkeeping (posting charges, payments, and adjustments to accounts receivable journal), experience in preparing appeals for denied claims, resubmittal of delinquent claims, ability to explain insurance programs and plans (i.e., benefits, requirements, and submission of claims), ability to abstract information from patients medical and financial records, and ability to review insurance payments. If you are fluent in another language, insert this information. Telephone skills might also be mentioned.

▶ *References.* Type in the phrase "Furnished upon request." Prepare approximately five references on a separate sheet and be sure to contact the persons referenced *before* an interview.

▶ *Final Details.* It is acceptable to fax a resume to an employer who advertises a job opening but gives no guidelines on how to submit the resume. In a competitive employment market where time is of the essence, it is wise to use every advantage possible (Fig. 17–12).

Proofread the resume carefully for spelling, punctuation, grammar, and typographic errors. Ask a friend or professional individual with excellent English skills to read and critique it. Remember that the resume is only a foot in the door and not what is going to land that job for you—you are!

PROCEDURE: Creating an Electronic Resume

Once a medical position has been discovered some basic steps to go on line with a resume are:

1. Compose a resume using a word processor with accurate spelling features and then save in a job search file.
2. Discard traditional resume-writing techniques, such as focusing on action verbs. Instead, think descriptive nouns, such as medical biller, education, experience, skills, knowledge, and abilities.
3. Avoid the use of decorative graphics and complex typefaces, underlining, or italics.
4. Forget the one-page rule; electronic resumes may be three to four pages.
5. Refer to the word processor manual to convert the cover letter and resume to ASCII (American Standard Code for Information Interchange; pronounced AS-kee), to plain text, which can be read by most personal computers.
6. Study on-line guides presenting special procedures for sending e-mail and files. Some e-mail programs allow binary files to be sent, whereas others only allow ASCII text files.
7. Use the word processing software's "copy and paste" feature and enter the information into e-mail or "attach a file" to the e-mail message.
8. Do not post a letter of introduction when posting a resume to a bulletin board.
9. Upload the resume to post on line using the file transfer feature of the software following the computer manual directions. When sending the resume over an on-line service or from a

computer to a dial direct bulletin board, the ASCII file is all that is required.

If the file is sent across the Internet, it should be doctored up in a technical form—encoded by the sender and decoded by the receiver. Take the following steps to prepare a plain ASCII text file.

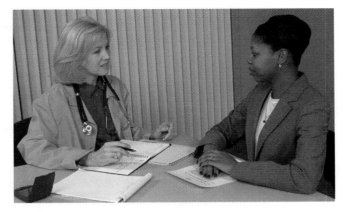

Figure 17–13. Student being interviewed for an insurance billing position.

PROCEDURE: Preparing a Resume in ASCII

1. Create the message using WordPerfect or Word software. Make certain all lines are no more than 65 characters in length. Put a space at the beginning of each blank line between paragraphs.
2. Proofread the resume and save it as plain ASCII text, referring to the word processing software manual for directions.
3. Log onto the bulletin board to upload the ASCII text. Go to the message menu and follow the bulletin board's directions.
4. Select or type "All" or "Resume posting" from the bulletin board's message menu for the recipient and subject.
5. Upload the resume following the software manual's directions for the communications program being used.
6. Customize the resume by typing in additional information related to the specific job. Depending on the bulletin board, a "Message Edit" menu or the next available line will appear issuing message-editing commands.

Interview

After looking for a potential employer, preparing a resume, and completing an application, the final step in landing a job is the face-to-face interview. An **interview** is a formal consultation with questions by an employer to evaluate the qualifications of a prospective job applicant (Fig. 17–13). It is important to make the best impression possible to the prospective employer as soon as you walk through the door. Hiring depends on positive qualities. Concentrate on good grooming and a fresh, relaxed appearance. Display a warm, positive attitude. Use proper grammar, avoid using slang, and maintain eye contact.

A female applicant should wear a clean skirt, dress, or tailored suit and nylon stockings with low-heeled pumps. A man should wear a clean dark suit or sport coat, conservative necktie, white shirt, plain slacks, plain socks, and well-shined shoes. Men should avoid a lot of facial hair, long hair, earrings, and heavy aftershave lotion. Women should have a conservative hair style, wear jewelry sparingly, and avoid heavy makeup, low-cut necklines, sleeveless dresses, strong perfume, and dark or bright nail polish. Do not smoke or chew gum. Use a proper deodorant. Eliminate nervous habits. It has been found that when applicants have similar skills and education, the decision to hire has been based on physical appearance at the interview.

Figure 17–14 is an example of an interview evaluation and reference investigation form. This form points out the areas an interviewer observes and how impressions are rated.

Research beforehand to know whether the salary (when offered) is acceptable. If you wish to ask questions about fringe benefits, do not appear to be too interested in them.

Choose the right time for the interview and arrive promptly. It has been found that late Monday and Friday afternoons between 4:00 P.M. and 5:00 P.M. are not good times for interviews because Mondays are usually catch-up, heavily scheduled days and Fridays are getaway days. Research has proved that the likelihood of hiring the last person interviewed for a position is greater than that of hiring those interviewed first.

Role playing is a good method to use to prepare for an interview. Give a friend a list of questions to ask you, then try to answer the questions, spontaneously without stumbling. Videotape or audiotape the session, if possible, to see and/or hear what the employer will experience.

Questions an interviewer might ask about personal life (marital status), family planning,

INTERVIEW EVALUATION AND REFERENCE INVESTIGATION FORM, MEDICAL or DENTAL OFFICE	SUMMARY OF EVALUATION	
	POINTS FROM APPLICATION AND INTERVIEW	
	POINTS FROM REFERENCES	
	TOTAL POINTS	
NAME OF APPLICANT DATE	OVERALL IMPRESSION	

RATING: GOOD – 2 POINTS
FAIR – 1 POINT
POOR – 0 POINTS

POSITION APPLIED FOR:

			GOOD	FAIR	POOR
FROM APPLICATION FOR POSITION, GAUGE APPLICANT IN FOLLOWING AREAS					
A P P L I C A T I O N S E C T I O N R E F E R E N C E	1.	STABILITY (REMAINED IN ONE PLACE OF RESIDENCE AND ONE JOB FOR A REASONABLE LENGTH OF TIME)?			
	2.	HEALTH?			
	3.	THE PROPER EDUCATIONAL BACKGROUND TO FILL THE POSITION?			
	4.	LEGIBLE HANDWRITING?			
	5.	AN EMPLOYMENT HISTORY THAT POINTS TOWARD DEPENDABILITY?			
	6.	LIMITATION ON WORKING HOURS?			
	7.	THE PROPER EXPERIENCE AND / OR SKILLS TO FILL THE POSITION?			
	8.	SALARY REQUIREMENT COMMENSURATE WITH POSITION?			
FROM THE PERSONAL INTERVIEW – (SHOULD BE SPECIFIC QUALITIES – OBJECTIVE)					
9. SUFFICIENT CAPABILITY TO HANDLE ANY SITUATION THAT MAY ARISE WHEN ALONE IN OFFICE?					
10. AN APPROPRIATE ATTITUDE TOWARD WORK?					
11. AN APPROPRIATE VOICE, DICTION, GRAMMAR?					
12. POISE?					
13. SELF CONFIDENCE (NOT OVER-CONFIDENCE)?					
14. TACT?					
15. SUFFICIENT MATURITY FOR JOB?					
16. AN ABILITY TO EXPRESS ONESELF WELL?					
17. AN INITIATIVE OR INTEREST IN LEARNING?					
18. APPROPRIATE APPEARANCE (NEAT, CLEAN; SUITABLE TO BUSINESS)					
19. ENERGY, VITALITY AND PERCEIVED ABILITY TO HANDLE PRESSURE OF POSITION?					
20. EAGERNESS TO OBTAIN THE POSITION IN QUESTION?					
		COLUMNAR TOTALS			
			GRAND TOTAL		

DIRECTIONS FOR USE OF FORM:

1. Look over your ratings. A zero score on any one VITAL question should automatically eliminate applicant. Add up the total rating points and enter in the SUMMARY OF EVALUATION BLOCK in the upper right-hand corner of this page.
2. After finishing all interviews, choose the "best bets" and check their references using the reverse side of this form.
3. Enter, as above, the results of your reference check and then your overall impression. (E – Excellent, G – Good, F – Fair, P – Poor)

FORM # 72-120 © 1987 BIBBERO SYSTEMS, INC. • PETALUMA, CA. • TO REORDER CALL TOLL FREE: (800) BIBBERO (800-242-2376) OR FAX (800) 242-9330 (REV. 7/87)

Figure 17–14. Example of an Interview Evaluation and Reference Investigation form. (Reprinted with permission from Bibbero Systems, Inc., Petaluma, CA. Phone: 800-242-2376. Fax: 800-242-9330.)

NOTES:

	REFERENCE INVESTIGATION		
1.	OFFICE CONTACTED	PHONE: ( )	DATE
	PERSON CONTACTED		
	HOW LONG HAVE YOU KNOWN THIS PERSON?		
	BETWEEN WHAT DATES WAS THIS PERSON EMPLOYED BY YOU?	FROM TO	
	WHAT TYPE OF WORK DID THIS PERSON DO FOR YOU?	TITLE OF POSITION:	SATISFACTORILY?
	WAS THIS PERSON CONSISTENTLY COOPERATIVE?	WHAT WERE SHORTCOMINGS?	
	DID THIS PERSON GET ALONG WELL WITH OTHERS?		
	WAS THIS PERSON TRUSTWORTHY / DEPENDABLE?		ATTENDANCE RECORD:
	WHY DID THIS PERSON LEAVE YOUR EMPLOY?		SALARY LEVEL:
	WOULD YOU REHIRE THIS PERSON?		
	NOTES:		
			RATING:
2.	OFFICE CONTACTED	PHONE: ( )	DATE
	PERSON CONTACTED		
	HOW LONG HAVE YOU KNOWN THIS PERSON?		
	BETWEEN WHAT DATES WAS THIS PERSON EMPLOYED BY YOU?	FROM TO	
	WHAT TYPE OF WORK DID THIS PERSON DO FOR YOU?	TITLE OF POSITION:	SATISFACTORILY?
	WAS THIS PERSON CONSISTENTLY COOPERATIVE?	WHAT WERE SHORTCOMINGS?	
	DID THIS PERSON GET ALONG WELL WITH OTHERS?		
	WAS THIS PERSON TRUSTWORTHY / DEPENDABLE?		ATTENDANCE RECORD:
	WHY DID THIS PERSON LEAVE YOUR EMPLOY?		SALARY LEVEL:
	WOULD YOU REHIRE THIS PERSON?		
	NOTES:		
			RATING:
3.	OFFICE CONTACTED	PHONE: ( )	DATE
	PERSON CONTACTED		
	HOW LONG HAVE YOU KNOWN THIS PERSON?		
	BETWEEN WHAT DATES WAS THIS PERSON EMPLOYED BY YOU?	FROM TO	
	WHAT TYPE OF WORK DID THIS PERSON DO FOR YOU?	TITLE OF POSITION:	SATISFACTORILY?
	WAS THIS PERSON CONSISTENTLY COOPERATIVE?	WHAT WERE SHORTCOMINGS?	
	DID THIS PERSON GET ALONG WELL WITH OTHERS?		
	WAS THIS PERSON TRUSTWORTHY / DEPENDABLE?		ATTENDANCE RECORD:
	WHY DID THIS PERSON LEAVE YOUR EMPLOY?		SALARY LEVEL:
	WOULD YOU REHIRE THIS PERSON?		
	NOTES:		
			RATING:

INTERVIEWER _____   DATE: _____

Figure 17–14. *Continued*

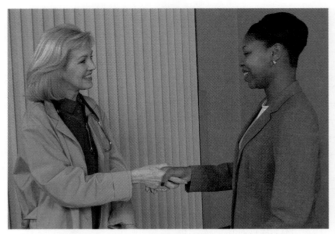

Figure 17–15. Job applicant concluding an interview with an office manager.

pregnancy, provision for child care, religious preference, club memberships, height, weight, dependents, age (birth date), ethnic background, maiden name, native language, physical or psychiatric problems, a spouse being employed and the earnings, credit rating, and home and automobile ownership, family planning, and pregnancy are illegal and do not have to be answered. If an employer wishes to know whether an applicant smokes, this is not considered discriminatory. Three suggestions of handling an illegal question are

1. Answer the question and ignore the fact you know it is illegal.
2. Answer with "I think the question is not relevant to the requirements of this position."
3. Refuse to answer and contact the nearest Equal Employment Opportunity Commission (EEOC) office.

Shake the interviewer's hand at the conclusion of the meeting (Fig. 17–15). Ask how long it will be before a job offer or a denial is forthcoming and then leave with a "thank you." If the job is offered at the interview and the applicant is not sure about accepting, ask "How soon do you need to know?" This will allow time to think and compare job offers before making a commitment.

Portfolio

Prepare in advance for the interview by organizing a **portfolio.** Assemble letters of recommendation (from former employers, teachers, family physician, professional friends, community leaders), school diplomas or degrees, transcripts, certificates, names and addresses of references, extra copies of the resume, Social Security card, timed typing test certified by an instructor, some neatly

typed insurance claim forms with evidence of coding skills, and any other items related to prior education and work experience.

Alien

Any **alien** employee must have on file with his or her employer an Employment Eligibility Verification Form I-9. This form can be obtained by writing the Immigration and Naturalization Service (INS) at 425 I Street, NW, Washington, DC 20536. Within 3 days of hiring an alien, the employee must show one of the following: a naturalization certification (citizen papers), an alien registration receipt card, a temporary resident receipt card, or an employment authorization card. One of these items should be in the portfolio in the event it is requested by the prospective employer during the interview.

Follow-Up Letter

Write a follow-up letter indicating thanks for the interview and restating interest in the position (Fig. 17–16). This keeps the applicant's name before the potential employer. If no response is heard within the time frame given, telephone to express continued interest in the position.

Self-Employment

Setting Up an Office

When an individual wishes to be his or her own boss **(self-employment),** it is usually wise to get at least 2 years of experience in the chosen career before undertaking this task. Preferably an individual should begin as an insurance billing specialist and then proceed to becoming an **electronic claims processor (ECP).** For the individual who wants to work as a claims assistance professional, some experience in public relations as well as having a strong insurance background is desirable. For an outpatient coding specialist, it is vital to have outpatient hospital and physician billing experience in several specialties before becoming a coding expert. For a hospital coding specialist, hospital inpatient and outpatient coding experience is necessary.

One must have something to offer clients when marketing and selling one's services and skills. Only with years of experience can this knowledge and expertise be gained. Full-time commitment, hard work, dedication, and many long hours to obtain clients will be encountered when beginning a business.

In addition, money is needed for equipment, computer software, overhead, taxes, stationery,

Street Address
City, State, ZIP code
Date of letter

John Doe, MD or
Personnel Director
Street Address
City, State, ZIP code

Dear Dr. Doe:

Thank you for spending your valuable time yesterday to interview me for
the insurance billing specialist position in your clinic.

I hope that you will allow me the opportunity to prove my abilities as I feel
that I am able to perform the work with expertise. Meeting your staff was
most enjoyable and it would certainly be pleasurable working with them as
a team.

I am looking forward to hearing from you in the near future.

Sincerely yours,

(handwritten signature)

Type name

Figure 17–16. Example of a thank-you letter sent after an interview.

preprinted statements, HCFA-1500 claim forms, and myriad other expenses. It is vital to have sufficient funds to run the business for a period of 1 year or more. It is imperative that this be accrued before vacating a full-time job. This will help eliminate a lot of fear and anxiety over not having enough business clients. A common reason for business failure is running out of the money necessary to keep the business going. It may take a year or more to begin seeing a profit, so one must be patient.

If you work a while before striking out independently, contacts will be made on the job that will often help build clientele. Networking is extremely important when one tries to establish a successful business. Many times it is who the individual knows that may get a foot in the potential client's door. Networking may open up many opportunities.

An insurance billing specialist can work as an independent contractor to have flexible hours, work from home, and reduce a medical practice's overhead. Some communities prohibit residents from telecommuting or operating a home-based business, although most allow it with restrictions. Working at home requires self-discipline, and one must develop a schedule and stick to it. Good time management is essential. It takes additional hours to advertise, obtain clients, bill, and perform the bookkeeping tasks. Figure 17–17 is a checklist of tasks that must be done to establish a new business.

It is always wise to rent a post office box. Never use a home address because this encourages patients who might visit at inconvenient hours. In some regions, business licenses are not issued for residential areas if clients come to the door. To get around this issue, a post office box becomes essential.

Publications available about starting your own claims processing or medical billing service are listed in Appendix B.

Finances

If an individual has had no experience or is not strong in marketing skills and small business accounting, courses may be taken to gain knowledge and instill confidence in these areas. Attend workshops and lectures on starting a business that are offered by financial institutions, universities, community colleges, or private institutions.

It would be wise to seek the services of a lawyer, accountant, or both before legally establishing a business and making appropriate selection of the tax options involved. Establish detailed financial records from the very beginning, even if an accountant is to be hired. Obtain simplified bookkeeping software for use on the computer. Expert advice is essential and will help develop a successful business; without it, a business could fail.

Establishing a business in a home may result in some deductions, so obtain the Internal Revenue

---

NEW BUSINESS CHECKLIST

__1. Decide what address you will use, since you may wish to obtain a post office box number instead of using your home address.

__2. Obtain a business license from the business license section of your city hall. Regulations vary in each city licensing office. You might have to obtain a home occupation permit from the planning department and have it signed by your landlord if you are renting. The city may have guidelines on hours of business, pedestrian and vehicular activity, noise, and so forth in the residential area.

__3. File a fictitious business name (Doing Business As–DBA) at the county clerk's office by obtaining the proper form for completion. If you use your given name, you do not have to file a fictitious business name.

__4. Publish the fictitious name in a local newspaper.

__5. If you have employees, contact the Internal Revenue Service (IRS) for an employer identification number and/or tax information. Obtain the booklet *Tax Guide for Small Business* No. 334 to determine business expenses that are deductible. Depending on how you set up your business, some possible tax breaks are as follows: depreciation of office equipment; declaring a room of your home as an office; subscriptions to professional publications; dues to professional associations; expenses associated with your automobile; telephone, photocopying, office supplies (stationery, books, typewriter ribbons, and so on); promotion and advertising (postage, meals with business associates, and so on); and any expenses pertaining to meetings, conventions, workshops, or seminars (registration fees, lodging, meals, transportation, parking, and so forth).

__6. If you have no employees, contact the Franchise Tax Board for the form used for estimating state withholding taxes for yourself. This must be filed quarterly. If you build up your business and have employees, obtain the proper forms and information for employees (state income tax, and state disability and unemployment insurance).

__7. Obtain the insurance that you need: health insurance, disability insurance, life insurance, liability insurance, worker's compensation (if you have employees), and so forth. Insurance is available to protect you against loss of material called "Release of Information Insurance" or "Errors and Omissions Insurance" with a "Hold Harmless" clause. You might want to consider a retirement IRA or Keogh plan.

__8. Contact the telephone company for information regarding lines for phone, fax equipment and computer modem. Inquire about custom or special calling services such as call waiting and so forth. Do this early because there is often a delay in hook-up. You might consider using your existing telephone number and switching to a business listing. This allows you to be listed in the *Yellow Pages* of your telephone directory.

__9. Open a bank account. If you want your telephone number on your checks, put the checks on hold until the telephone is confirmed. Some banks require a business license and Doing Business As documents to open an account. Take these documents with you to the bank.

__10. Order business cards, stationery, billing forms, and reference books. Design a logo for the business.

__11. Begin to advertise your business by some of the following methods: newspaper, radio, flyers, announcements, signs, word of mouth, and letters to prospects (hospitals, clinics, and physician's offices).

Additional points to consider if expanding to a location outside of a home:

__12. Check the zoning of the location at your city hall's planning department or, if you are in the county, the county's planning department. Sign a lease contingent on proper zoning and on meeting all federal, state, county, and city building safety and health requirements. Inquire about parking and sign restrictions at the planning department. Find out if you need any permits (building permit, certificate of occupancy, health permit, and so forth). City and county offices may require a sign permit for new signs and changes on old ones.

__13. If you have opened an office at a location, make a deposit for water, gas, and electricity. Rent, renovation, and janitorial or trash services must be considered.

__14. Call the assessor's office and ask to be put on the mailing list for business property tax (inventory tax).

__15. Contact the various inspectors: health, building, and safety, and sign to have all completed work inspected and the necessary permits signed off.

Figure 17–17. New business checklist. (Modified from Diehl MO, Fordney MT: Medical Keyboarding, Typing, and Transcribing Techniques and Procedures. Philadelphia, WB Saunders, 1997.)

Service (IRS) publication No. 587 entitled "Business Use of Your Home." Self-employment tax on net income is due each year. Quarterly estimated tax payments are required once the net income amounts to $500 or more. Keep receipts and complete records of income and expenses, because these are extremely important for IRS purposes.

Paycheck stubs, copies of hours worked, and identifying data on clients must be retained for the period of time stipulated by the IRS. The following is a record retention schedule.

Bank statements: 3 years
Canceled checks: permanently
Expired contracts: 7 years
Financial statements: permanently
General correspondence: 2 years
Payroll records and summaries: 7 years
Tax returns, worksheets, and other tax documents: permanently

Keep a record of business travel expenses and document mileage. Travel log books are available at stationery stores.

Equipment

When setting up a business at home or in a small office, certain items must be purchased. Necessary equipment to consider are a computer, medical software, modem, printer, telephone answering machine, fax machine, photocopy machine, office furniture, filing cabinet, and calculator. It is imperative to install a separate telephone line for clients or patients calling in. For transmitting claims electronically, a telephone line will be needed to operate with the computer modem. An optional item might be a postage meter. Research equipment costs and maintenance options before purchase or lease and find out how much it costs for service contracts.

It is possible to obtain a low-interest government Small Business Administration (SBA) loan for starting a business. Loans are also available to physically challenged persons who qualify.

Insurance

Business owners find it necessary to protect income and property from unexpected loss. If the business grows and employees are hired, workers' compensation insurance must be obtained. Some types of insurance to investigate are

▶ Property insurance in case of fire, theft, or a disaster
▶ Disability insurance if one becomes unable to work because of illness or injury
▶ Health insurance
▶ Life insurance
▶ Business interruption insurance. (In case of fire, it would take time and money to re-create data. Backed-up data should be stored off site.)
▶ Professional liability insurance

Marketing, Advertising, Promotion, and Public Relations

Marketing refers to how a business is presented or advertised to promote sales. Depending on the section of the public that is targeted, marketing strategies vary. When promoting a medical billing service, develop a well-organized marketing plan and follow basic guidelines to reach a specific target audience.

Ways to market a business and the reasons for marketing strategies are presented in Exhibit 17–1.

Insurance billing and coding specialists market to those who will use their services in the community, such as physicians (family practitioners, surgeons, psychiatrists, psychologists, physical therapists), small hospitals, clinics, laboratories, podiatrists, and chiropractors. However, claims assistance professionals' target audience is the consumer and Medicare recipients.

Obtain figures to help convince clients that the service you are offering is better and can do more for their business than what they presently have—save them time and money! Stress being honest, reliable, committed, efficient, and professional, and offer them something they cannot do for themselves.

Contracts or Agreements

Develop a contract or agreement when dealing with some facilities, such as an acute care hospital, whose legal department may review it before signing. This can clarify job responsibilities and help eliminate misunderstandings. Put everything in writing. A contract needs to define the following:

▶ Who does the coding?
▶ Will claims be filed electronically?
▶ What is the per claim processing fee?
▶ Who is responsible for rebilling?
▶ Who will handle collection procedures (follow-up telephone calls or letters)?
▶ Who pays for rebilling, photocopying of records, mailing fees, and clearinghouse charges?
▶ Under whose name will bills be sent to patients?
▶ Will the billing service phone number appear on the statement or will a toll-free number or local number be used?
▶ How will the telephone be answered?
▶ What are the charges for coding consultation services?
▶ What are the coverage arrangements due to absence or illness?

If there is any change in the terms of the agreements, write a letter outlining the new terms. Some contracts may include a statement on confidentiality assuring the contracting facility that all patient data will be handled in a confidential manner. Long-term contracts are preferred over short-term contracts, so it is important to put in dates of validity. When the contract expires, renegotiation is in order.

Documentation

If you are hired as a coding specialist, keep written records of the numbers of hours worked, the quantity of work done each day, and the corrections applied to the work by officials in the contracting facility or hospital. Retain any written coding guideline from the contracting facility or hospital.

Statements and Pricing

A variety of methods are used to price services, such as a percentage of reimbursement or an

EXHIBIT 17–1

Strategy	Reason
Obtain professionally printed stationery and business cards.	Enhance professional image.
Pass out business cards at professional meetings.	Advertises availability and services.
Develop a business name and a logo for the company.	Enables potential clients to remember you.
Ensure accuracy of all printed materials.	When items are not professionally assembled or proofread to eliminate misspelling errors, a potential client receives a negative image of the company.
Develop a professional flyer and distribute it to medical facilities and physicians' offices.	Introduces company name, advertises services, and describes benefits.
Follow up with a personal visit or telephone call.	A friendly voice and professional image offers personal services and lets potential clients know you are available and interested.
Advertise in the journal or newsletter of the country medical society and state medical association.	Potential clients read such publications and advertisements of this nature lend to your credibility.
Place on advertisement in the newspaper or on cable television.	Circulates business within the county.
Put an ad in the *Yellow Pages*.	Solicits wider range of prospective clients.
Network with members of professional organizations.	Word of mouth advertising can be the best public relations tool, especially if done by professional peers.
Network via computer using the Internet's World Wide Web, Prodigy, CompuServe, America Online, and Genie bulletin boards for this career field.	Offers wide range of contacts.
Check with established businesses to determine whether they are overloaded with work, the owner needs a vacation, or help is needed in a temporary situation because of illness.	Present your services as a help, not a threat to current office staff.

annual, hourly, or per claim fee. Deciding on which method depends on the type of client being served and the work to be done. Claims assistance professionals bill in 15-minute increments. Telephone other billing and insurance services preferably outside the area to see how they are charging because in-area competitors may be reluctant to divulge that information.

Professional Associations: Certification and Registration

Because of specialization in the allied health careers, more exacting professional requirements have evolved. Certification and registration are two ways of exhibiting professional standards. **Certification** is a statement issued by a board or associa-

tion verifying that a person meets professional standards. **Registration** may be accomplished in two methods, as an entry in an official registry or record that lists names of persons in an occupation who have satisfied specific requirements or by attaining a certain level of education and paying a registration fee. In the latter, if there are certain requirements for registration, then an unregistered person may be prevented from working in a career for which he or she is otherwise qualified.

A number of certifications are available on a national level, depending on how you wish to specialize.

American Association of Medical Assistants

In some medical practices, job duties may overlap (e.g., a front office assistant might carry out receptionist responsibilities as well as billing and coding duties). Many of these assistants obtain certification or become registered by national associations. In some states, there may be certification by a state organization. To become a **Certified Medical Assistant (CMA),** one must have graduated from a medical assisting program accredited by the Commission on Accreditation of Allied Health Education Programs (CAAHEP) and then apply to take the national certifying examination in medical assisting. Applications, membership, and further information may be obtained from

American Association of Medical Assistants, Inc. (AAMA)
20 N. Wacker Drive
Chicago, IL 60606
Telephone: 1-800-228-2262
Web site: www.aama.ntl.org

American Medical Technologists

To become a **Registered Medical Assistant (RMA),** one must take the certification examination offered by the American Medical Technologists (AMT). For further information, contact

Registered Medical Assistant/AMT
710 Higgins Road
Park Ridge, IL 60068
Telephone: 847-823-5169
E-mail: amtmail@aol.com
Web site: www.amt1.com

National Electronic Biller's Alliance

There are organizations that offer certifications as an insurance billing specialist. A *Healthcare Reimbursement Specialist* (HRS) certification is obtained after successfully completing an open-book examination offered by

National Electronic Biller's Alliance (NEBA)
2226-A Westborough Boulevard, #504
South San Francisco, CA 94080
Telephone: (415) 577-1190
Fax (415) 577-1290
E-mail: mmedical@aol.com
Web site: www.nebazone.com

Nationally Certified Insurance Coding Specialist

A *Nationally Certified Insurance Coding Specialist* (NCICS) certification is one of many allied health career certifications offered by the National Center for Competency Testing (NCCT). The NCCT is an independent testing agency that develops and maintains a certification testing process to provide competent and unbiased evaluation of an individual's knowledge. The examination is given a psychometric evaluation every three years. There are two sections: Classical Test Theory and Item Response Theory. The test is administered and proctored monthly across the United States at many school sites. It meets industrial standards. To maintain current status of certification, one **continuing education** unit (CEU) per year is required. Information may be obtained from the following:

National Center for Competency Testing
7007 College Boulevard, Suite 250
Overland Park, KS 66211
Telephone: 800-875-4404
Fax: 913-498-1243
E-mail: Visit web site
Web site: www.ncctinc.com

American Association of Medical Billers

A national organization for individuals who bill for physicians and clinics is the American Association of Medical Billers (AAMB). It has established two national certification programs for medical billers. The Certified Medical Biller (CMB) examination is a 2-hour examination written for physician's office billers and other outpatient facilities. The Certified Medical Billing Specialist (CMBS) examination is a 3-hour examination. Both examinations include multiple-choice questions and case studies. Information on membership may be obtained by writing, telephoning, or e-mailing.

American Association of Medical Billers (AAMB)
P.O. Box 44614
Los Angeles, CA 90044-0614
Telephone: 323-778-4352
Fax: 323-778-2814
E-mail: AAMB@aol.com
Web site: billers.com/aamb/page2.html

International Billing Association

An organization established in 1992 for professional billing businesses or services that support the billing services industry is the International Billing Association, Inc. (IBA). This trade association was formed to promote the general welfare of the billing industry. IBA is working to give the billing industry a unified voice and to structure effective communication with the Health Care Financing Administration and the health care industry. Members agree to abide by a strict code of ethics. A pilot certification program was offered by the California chapter in the latter part of 1996 and was a model for a national certification program. After completing a comprehensive program and taking the proficiency test, a passing candidate receives the title *Certified Medical Billing Association* (CMBA). For complete information about eligibility requirements for membership and its benefits, contact

International Billing Association, Inc.
7315 Wisconsin Avenue, Suite 424 East
Bethesda, MD 20814
Telephone: 301-961-8680
E-mail: micheles@biller.com
Web site: www.biller.com

American Academy of Professional Coders

If you decide to specialize as a coder, certification by examination from two national associations is available. Visit the CCS Prep! Column web site www.ADVANCEforHIM.com to help you prepare for the examination offered by the American Academy of Professional Coders (AAPC). It features a quiz consisting of questions and answers that may be taken for review. For information regarding membership, independent study programs, and becoming a Certified Professional Coder (CPC), or a Certified Professional Coder-Hospital (CPC-H), contact the following organization:

American Academy of Professional Coders (AAPC)
145 West Crystal Avenue
Salt Lake City, UT 84115
Telephone: 1-800-626-CODE
E-mail: aapc@worldnet.att.net
Web site: www.aapcnatl.org

American Health Information Management Association

If you would like information about becoming a Certified Coding Specialist (CCS), or a Certified Coding Specialist—Physician (CCS-P), contact the following organization:

American Health Information Management Association (AHIMA)
P.O. Box 97349
Chicago, IL 60690-7349
Telephone: 1-800-335-5535
E-mail: info@ahima.mhs.compuserve.com
Web site: www.ahima.org

To become a member of the AHIMA Society for Clinical Coding (SCC), write or telephone (1-800-574-1027) for an application and datasheet.

Individuals who become certified by either of these associations must participate in an ongoing program of continuing education in health information management to increase their knowledge of coding and the changes taking place in various insurance programs (e.g., Medicare, Medicaid,

TRICARE). Depending on the policies of the certifying association, the individual goes through a process of **recertification** either annually or every 3 to 5 years by meeting established requirements. For example, AAPC's annual renewal requires 18 continuing education credits and payment of a fee.

Medical Management Institute

The Medical Management Institute (MMI) provides a yearly Registered Medical Coder (RMC) program governed by the National Coding Standards Committee. A student is assigned a class advisor and mailed all course work, test booklets, and educational material including audiocassette tapes of the class. On completion of the course work, an individual must make a passing grade on an examination to receive the RMC registered title. Then students are required to attain recertification within 3 months of the expiration date.

Information may be obtained from the following:

Medical Management Institute
1125 Cambridge Square
Alpharetta, GA 30004-1863
Telephone: 800-334-5724
E-mail: bobby.carvell@ipractice.md
Web site: www.theinstitute.com

Alliance of Claims Assistance Professionals

For information on membership and how to obtain titles such as a Certified Claims Assistance Professional (CCAP) or Certified Electronic Claims Professional (CECP), contact

Alliance of Claims Assistance Professionals (ACAP)
c/o Susan A. Dressler, CCAP
873 Brentwood Drive
West Chicago, IL 60185
Telephone: 877-275-8765
Fax: (630) 690-0377
E-mail: askus@claims.org
Web site: www.claims.org

American Guild of Patient Account Management

Another national, state, and regional organization is the American Guild of Patient Account Management (AGPAM). This organization promotes the recognition of patient account managers who are responsible for the management of patient accounts in hospitals and in physicians' practices. A certification program is offered for hospital and medical business office personnel in either managerial or technical (nonmanagerial) careers. The AGPAM self-study course leads to designation as any one of the following: Certified Patient Account Technician (CPAT), Certified Clinic Account Technician (CCAT), Certified Patient Account Manager (CPAM), or Certified Clinic Account Manager (CCAM). Standard examinations are administered twice a year. For information on eligibility requirements, application forms, and information, write to

American Guild of Patient Account Management (AGPAM)
National Certification Examination Program
1101 Connecticut Avenue, NW, Suite 700
Washington, DC 20036
Telephone: 202-857-1179
E-mail: Scott_Hall@dc.sba.com
Web site: www.agpam.org

Professional Association of Health Care Office Managers

If working in a managerial or supervisory capacity, you may wish to become a member of a national association for medical office managers of small-group and solo practices called **Professional Association of Health Care Office Managers (PAHCOM).** For further information about the examination to obtain credentials as a Certified Medical Office Manager (CMOM), write to

Professional Association of Health Care Office Managers (PAHCOM)
461 E. Ten Mile Road
Pensacola, FL 32534-9712
Telephone: 1-800-451-9311
E-mail: pahcom@pahcom.com
Web site: www.pahcom.com

Medical Group Management Association

A national organization that supports the development of medical practice administration is Medical Group Management Association (MGMA). Membership is available to persons working in the group management field. It has groups that are focused by specialty and profession; for example, an individual may belong to the Cardiovascular and Thoracic Surgery group as well as the Financial Management group. An affiliated organization is American College of Medical Practice Executives (ACMPE). It is a professional organization for group practice administrators with three levels of membership. The primary or entry level is called a nominee. After successfully completing a 6- to 7-hour examination, a nominee moves to certified member and is eligible to use the initials CMPE (Certified Medical Practice Executive) after his or her name. The final level is fellow and requires the completion of either a mentoring project or

thesis. It offers a professional certification process that aims at personal development and provides the employer with a baseline when searching for candidates for a new position. Information may be obtained from the following:

Medical Group Management Association (MGMA)
(Affiliate Organization American College of Medical Practice Executives [ACMPE])
104 Inverness Terrace East
Englewood, CO 80112
Telephone: 303-397-7869
Fax: 303-643-4427
E-mail: acmpe@mgma.com
Web site: www.mgma.com/acmpe

Keeping Current

Membership in any of the aforementioned organizations helps in keeping up to date. Most of these associations have student as well as active and associate membership categories. You can inquire whether there is a local chapter or state organization affiliated with the national association. Benefits of belonging to a professional organization in addition to certification and recertification include problem solving, continuing education, and employment opportunities. Local meetings can keep you knowledgeable by providing guest speakers on topics of current interest. The newsletters and journals published by these organizations keep you abreast of current trends either as a subscriber or as a benefit when becoming a member.

Mentor

A valuable vehicle for career development is to find a **mentor** in the business. A mentor is a guide or teacher who offers advice, criticism, wisdom, guidance, and perspective to an inexperienced but promising protégé to help reach a life goal. Decide what kind of help you want, such as technical, general feedback, managerial, and so on. Then look for a mentor whose background, values, and style are similar to yours. Be willing to face criticism with a positive attitude and express gratitude when excellence is praised.

Networking

Another avenue to pursue for career development is to *network*. **Networking** is the exchange of information or services among individuals, groups, or institutions and making use of professional contacts. To do this, join as many organizations as possible, because when you are self-employed, it can be difficult to keep abreast of ongoing changes in the insurance industry. Many of the professional organizations publish monthly newsletters and/or quarterly journals, offer certification, and plan national conventions, state conferences, and regional meetings. In addition to the organizations mentioned in this chapter, some additional ones to contact are

Health Care Management Association of Southern California
P.O. Box 27771
Santa Ana, CA 92799

Healthcare Financial Management Association (HFMA)
Two Westbrook Corporate Center, Suite 700
Westchester, IL 60154-5700

For Claims Assistance Professionals, attend local meetings for Medicare recipients. Join local volunteer service organizations and the chamber of commerce to network with others. Contact the LEADS Club at (800) 783-3761 or The National Association of Female Executives at (800) 669-1002 for potential client leads and networking.

RESOURCES ON THE INTERNET

JOB SEARCH RESOURCES:
Yahoo
   www.yahoo.com/
Infoseek
www.infoseek.go.com
Alta Vista
   www.altavista.com
Career Magazine
   www.careermag.com/careermag/
America's Job Bank
   www.ajbb.dni.us
E-Span Employment Database Search
   www.espan.com/
PracticeNet
   www.practice-net.com
MedSearch
   www.medsearch.com
   gopher://gopher.medsearch.com
PROFESSIONAL ORGANIZATION WEBSITES:
American Association of Medical Assistants
   www.aama.ntl.org
American Medical Technologists
   www.amtl.com
   e-mail: amtmail@aol.com

National Electronic Biller's Alliance
   www.nebazone.com
   e-mail: mmedical@aol.com
National Center for Competency Testing
   www.ncctinc.com
American Association of Medical Billers
   www.billers.com/aamb/page2.html
   e-mail: aamb@aol.com
International Billing Association
   www.biller.com
   e-mail: micheles@biller.com
American Academy of Professional Coders
   www.aapcnatl.org
   e-mail: aapc@worldnet.att.net
American Health Information Management Association
   www.ahima.org
   e-mail: info@ahimma.mhs.compuserve.com
Medical Management Institute
   www.theinstitute.com
   e-mail: bobby.carvell@ipractice.md
Alliance of Claims Assistance Professionals
   www.claims.org
   e-mail: askus@claims.org
American Guild of Patient Account Management
   www.agpam.org
   e-mail: Scott_Hall@dc.sba.com
Professional Association of Health Care Office Managers
   www.pahcom.com
   e-mail: pahcom@pahcom.com
Medical Group Management Association
   www.mgma.com/acmpe
   e-mail: acmpe@mgma.com

STUDENT ASSIGNMENT LIST

✔ Study Chapter 17.
✔ Answer the review questions in the *Workbook* to reinforce the theory learned in this chapter and to help prepare you for a future test.
✔ Complete the assignments in the *Workbook* to give you hands-on experience in completing an application for a position as an insurance billing specialist, preparing and typing a resume, composing a cover letter to go with the resume, having someone evaluate you during an interview, and typing a follow-up thank-you letter after being interviewed.
✔ Turn to the Glossary at the end of this textbook for a further understanding of the Key Terms used in this chapter.

The list of names and addresses presented here for each state has been compiled for your use in submitting insurance claim forms to state or federal programs. In addition, insurance commissioners' state offices are included if a question, problem, or complaint arises that needs to be resolved. Addresses for state boards of medical examiners are included in case medicolegal information is sought at a state level. State addresses for workers' compensation are given in case there is need to obtain forms and guidelines or for cases that are being settled or appealed. Insurance companies across the nation handle workers' compensation insurance; they are too numerous to include in this textbook. Federal workers' compensation district office addresses for each state may be used when submitting insurance claims for a federal worker injured while working.

The information contained in this Appendix has been reorganized so the reader can locate information quickly and easily. Look for the name of your state and then check the subheadings, which are arranged alphabetically, for the program or plan name and address.

The list of names and addresses in this Appendix has been compiled from state and federal references published in 2000. Because fiscal intermediaries (insurance carriers) for state and federal programs (i.e., CHAMPVA, Medicaid, Medicare, TRICARE) change as contracts expire, it is always wise to use the telephone directory and call to verify addresses when in doubt as to their accuracy.

This textbook will be revised every 2 years, and these lists will continue to be updated as necessary.

ALABAMA

CHAMPVA Claim Office
CHAMPVA Center
4500 Cherry Creek Drive, South
P. O. Box 65024
Denver, CO 80206-9024

Insurance Commissioner State Office
Insurance Commissioner
201 Monroe Street, #1700 (36104)
P. O. Box 303351
Montgomery, AL 36130-3351

Maternal and Child Health Program
Bureau of Family Health Services
RSA Tower, Suite 1368
201 Monroe Street
P. O. Box 303017
Montgomery, AL 36130-3017

Children's Rehabilitation Services
2129 East South Boulevard
P. O. Box 11586
Montgomery, AL 36111-0586

Medicaid Fiscal Agent
Electronic Data Systems Corporation
P. O. Box 7604
Montgomery, AL 36107

Medicare Durable Medical Equipment
Palmetto Government Benefits Administrators
Medicare DMERC Operations
P. O. Box 100141
Columbia, SC 29202-3141

Medicare Fiscal Agent or Carrier
Blue Cross-Blue Shield of Alabama
Medicare Claims Administration
P. O. Box 995
Birmingham, AL 35298

State Board of Medical Examiners
Alabama State Board of Medical Examiners
848 Washington Avenue (36104)

P. O. Box 946
Montgomery, AL 36101-0946

TRICARE Claim Office
Palmetto Government Benefits Administrators
P. O. Box 7031
Florence, SC 29020-7031

Veterans Affairs Installation
Alabama Medical Centers:

Birmingham 35233 (700 S. 19th Street)
Montgomery 36109 (215 Perry Hill Road)
Tuscaloosa 35404 (3701 Loop Road East)
Tuskegee 36083 (2400 Hospital Road)

Workers' Compensation Federal District Office
Office of Workers' Compensation Programs
214 North Hogan Street, Suite 1006
Jacksonville, FL 32202

Workers' Compensation State Plan Office
Workmen's Compensation Division
Department of Industrial Relations
Industrial Relations Building
649 Monroe Street
Montgomery, AL 36131

ALASKA

CHAMPVA Claim Office
CHAMPVA Center
4500 Cherry Creek Drive, South
Box 65024
Denver, CO 80206-9024

Insurance Commissioner State Office
Division of Insurance
Department of Commerce and Economic Development
P. O. Box 110805
Juneau, AK 99811-0805

Maternal and Child Health Program
Alaska Department of Health & Social Services
Maternal Child and Family Health
1231 Gambell Street
Anchorage, AK 99501-4627

Special Needs Programs Administration
Alaska Department of Health & Social Services
Division of Public Health
1231 Gambell Street
Anchorage, AK 99501-4627

Medicaid Fiscal Agent
First Health (EC)
P. O. Box 240808
Anchorage, AK 99524-0808

Medicare Durable Medical Equipment
CIGNA Medicare Region D DMERC
P. O. Box 690
Nashville, TN 37202

Medicare Fiscal Agent or Carrier
Noridian Mutual Insurance Company
4305 13th Avenue, SW
Fargo, ND 58103

State Board of Medical Examiners
Alaska State Medical Board
3601 C Street, Suite 722
Anchorage, AK 99503-5986

TRICARE Claim Office
Palmetto Government Benefits Administrators
P. O. Box 870001
Surfside Beach, SC 29587-8701

Veterans Affairs Installation
Alaska Outpatient Clinic and Regional Office
2925 De Barr Road
Anchorage, AK 99508-2989

Workers' Compensation Federal District Office
Office of Workers' Compensation Programs
1111 Third Avenue, Suite 615
Seattle, WA 98101

Workers' Compensation State Plan Office
Division of Workers' Compensation
Department of Labor
P. O. Box 25512
Juneau, AK 99802-5512

AMERICAN SAMOA

Insurance Commissioner State Office
Insurance Commissioner
Office of the Governor
Pago Pago, AS 96799

Maternal and Child Health Program
Division of Preventive and Environmental Health
Government of American Samoa
Pago Pago, AS 96799

Medicare Durable Medical Equipment
Connecticut General Life Insurance
DMERC-CIGNA Medicare
P. O. Box 690
Nashville, TN 37320

Medicare Fiscal Agent or Carrier
Noridian Mutual Insurance Company
4305 13th Street
Fargo, ND 58103

Workers' Compensation State Plan Office
Workmen's Compensation Commission
Office of the Governor
American Samoa Government
Pago Pago, AS 96799

ARIZONA

CHAMPVA Claim Office
CHAMPVA Center
4500 Cherry Creek Drive, South
P. O. Box 65024
Denver, CO 80206-9024

Insurance Commissioner State Office
Director of Insurance
2910 North 44th Street, Suite 210
Phoenix, AZ 85018-7256

Maternal and Child Health Program
Community/Family Health Services
2927 North 35th Avenue
Phoenix, AZ 85017

Office of Women's and Children's Health
Arizona Department of Health
2927 North 35th Avenue
Phoenix, AZ 85017

Medicaid Fiscal Agent
Arizona Health Care Cost Containment System
P. O. Box 25520
Phoenix, AZ 85002-9949

Medicare Durable Medical Equipment
CIGNA Medicare Region D DMERC
P. O. Box 690
Nashville, TN 37202

Medicare Fiscal Agent or Carrier
Noridian Mutual Insurance Company
4305 13th Avenue
Fargo, ND 58103

State Board of Medical Examiners
Arizona Board of Medical Examiners
9545 East Doubletree Ranch Road
Phoenix, AZ 85258

Arizona Board of Osteopathic Examiners in Medicine and Surgery
9535 East Doubletree Ranch Road
Scottsdale, AZ 85258-5539

TRICARE Claim Office
Except for the Yuma area:
TRICARE Central Regions 7/8
Palmetto Government Benefits Administrators
P. O. Box 8700026
Surfside Beach, SC 29587-8726

Yuma area:
P. O. Box 870001
Surfside Beach, SC 29587-8701

Veterans Affairs Installation
Arizona Medical Centers:
  Phoenix 85012 (650 E. Indian School Road)
  Prescott 86313 (500 Highway 89, North)
  Tucson 85723 (3601 S. 6th Avenue)

Workers' Compensation Federal District Office
Office of Workers' Compensation Programs
71 Stevenson Street, 2nd Floor
San Francisco, CA 94105

Workers' Compensation State Plan Office
Industrial Commission of Arizona
800 W. Washington Street (85007-2922)
P. O. Box 19070
Phoenix, AZ 85005-9070

ARKANSAS

CHAMPVA Claim Office
CHAMPVA Center
4500 Cherry Creek Drive, South

P. O. Box 65024
Denver, CO 80206-9024

Insurance Commissioner State Office
Department of Insurance
1200 West 3rd Street
Little Rock, AR 72201-1904

Maternal and Child Health Program
Section of Maternal and Child Health
Arkansas State Department of Health
4815 W. Markham, Slot 41
Little Rock, AR 72205-3867

Children's Medical Services
Arkansas Department of Human Services
P. O. Box 1437, Slot 526
Little Rock, AR 72203

Medicaid Fiscal Agent
Electronic Data Systems (EC)
P. O. Box 8036
Little Rock, AR 72203-2501

Medicare Durable Medical Equipment
Palmetto Government Benefits Administrators
Medicare DMERC Operations
P. O. Box 100141
Columbia, SC 29202-3141

Medicare Fiscal Agent or Carrier
Medicare/Arkansas Blue Cross and Blue Shield
601 Gaines Street (72201)
P. O. Box 1418
Little Rock, AR 72203-1418

State Board of Medical Examiners
Arkansas State Medical Board
2100 Riverfront Drive, Suite 200
Little Rock, AR 72202-1793

TRICARE Claim Office
Except a small part of Arkansas in the Naval Hospital, Millington, TN, service area:
Wisconsin Physicians Service
P. O. Box 8999
Madison, WI 53708-8999

The Millington area address is:
Palmetto Government Benefits Administrators
P. O. Box 202000
Florence, SC 29502-2000

Veterans Affairs Installation
Arkansas Medical Centers:
  Fayetteville 72703 (1100 N. College Avenue)
  Little Rock 72205 (4300 W. 7th Street)

Workers' Compensation Federal District Office
Office of Workers' Compensation Programs
525 Griffin Street, Room 100
Dallas, TX 75202

Workers' Compensation State Plan Office
Workers' Compensation Commission
Fourth & Spring Streets
P. O. Box 950
Little Rock, AR 72203-0950

CALIFORNIA

California Medical Services
(Known in other states as Maternal and Child Health Program)
Childrens Medical Services
California State Department of Health
714 P Street, Room 323
Sacramento, CA 95814

Maternal & Child Health
California State Department of Health Services
714 P Street, Room 476
Sacramento, CA 95814

CHAMPVA Claim Office
CHAMPVA Center
4500 Cherry Creek Drive, South
P. O. Box 65024
Denver, CO 80206-9024

Insurance Commissioner State Office
Commissioner
Department of Insurance
300 Capitol Mall, Suite 1500
Sacramento, CA 95814

Medi-Cal Fiscal Agent
Medi-Cal Fiscal Intermediary
P. O. Box 15700
Sacramento, CA 95852-1700

Medicare Durable Medical Equipment
CIGNA Medicare Region D DMERC
P. O. Box 690
Nashville, TN 37202

Medicare Fiscal Agent or Carrier
National Heritage Insurance Company
Medicare Claims Department
450 West East Avenue (95926)
P. O. Box 2804
Chico, CA 95927-2804

State Board of Medical Examiners
Medical Board of California
1426 Howe Avenue, Suite 54
Sacramento, CA 95825-3236

Osteopathic Medical Board of California
2720 Gateway Oaks Drive, Suite 350
Sacramento, CA 95833-3500

TRICARE Claim Office
Palmetto Government Benefits Administrators
TRICARE Claims
P. O. Box 870001
Surfside Beach, SC 29587-8701

Unemployment Compensation Disability & State Disability Offices

Chico
645 Salem, 95928-5576
P. O. Box 8190, 95297-8190

City of Industry
17171 East Gale Avenue,
Suite 110, 91745-1810
P. O. Box 60006, 91716-0006

Eureka
490 K Street, Suite 201, 95501-1529
P. O. Box 4986, 95502-4986

Fresno
2550 Mariposa, Room 1080A, 93707-0032
P. O. Box 32, 93721-2270

Long Beach
4300 Long Beach, Suite 600, 90807-2011
P. O. Box 469, 90801-0469

Los Angeles
221 North Figueroa Street, Suite 200, 90012-2652
P. O. Box 513096, 90051-1096

Oakland
7700 Edgewater Road, Suite 210, 94621-3018
P. O. Box 1857, 94604-1857

Redding
615 Locust, 96099-2711
P. O. Box 991898, 96099-1898

Riverside
1190 Palmyrita, Suite 100, 92507-1908
P. O. Box 59903, 92517-1903

Sacramento
5009 Broadway, 95820-1613
P. O. Box 13140, 95813-3140

San Bernardino
371 W. 3rd Street, Room 101, 92401-1818
P. O. Box 781, 92402-0781

San Diego
8977 Activity Road, Building B, Suite 200, 92126-4427
P. O. Box 120831, 92112-0831

San Francisco
1625 Van Ness Avenue, Suite 400
P. O. Box 193534, 94119-3534

San Jose
297 W. Hedding Street, 95110-1628
P. O. Box 637, 95106-0637

Santa Ana
28 Civic Center Plaza, Room 735, 92701-4024
P. O. Box 1466, 92702-1466

Santa Barbara
128 E. Ortega, 93101-1631
P. O. Box 1529, 93102-1529

Santa Rosa
50 D Street, Room 325, 95404-4757
P. O. Box 700, 95402-0700

Stockton
528 N. Madison Street, 95202-1917
P. O. Box 201006, 95201-9006

Van Nuys
15400 Sherman Way, Room 500, 91406
P. O. Box 10402, Van Nuys, CA 91410-0402

Woodland Hills
21210 Erwin, 91367-3714
P. O. Box 4256, 91365-4256

Veterans Affairs Installation
California Medical Centers:
   Bakersfield 93301 (1801 Westwind Drive)
   Fresno 93703 (2615 E. Clinton Avenue)
   Livermore 94450 (4951 Arroyo Road)
   Loma Linda 92357 (11201 Benton Street)
   Long Beach 90822 (5901 E. 7th Street)
   Los Angeles 90012 (351 E. Temple Street)
   Martinez 94553 (150 Muir Road)
   Palo Alto 94304 (3801 Miranda Avenue)
   San Diego 92161 (3350 La Jolla Village Drive)
   San Francisco 94121 (4150 Clement Street)
   Santa Barbara 93110 (4440 Calle Real)
   Sepulveda 91343 (16111 Plummer Street)
   West Los Angeles 90073 (11301 Wilshire Blvd.)

Workers' Compensation Federal District Office
Office of Workers' Compensation Programs
71 Stevenson Street, 2nd Floor (94105)
P. O. Box 3769
San Francisco, CA 94119-3769

Workers' Compensation State Plan Offices
Department of Industrial Relations
Division of Workers' Compensation
455 Golden Gate Avenue, 9th Floor
San Francisco, CA 94102

Workers' Compensation Appeals Board
45 Fremont Street, Suite 410
San Francisco, CA 94105

CANADA

CHAMPVA Claim Office
CHAMPVA Center
4500 Cherry Creek Drive, South
P. O. Box 65024
Denver, CO 80206-9024

TRICARE Claim Office
Wisconsin Physician Service
P. O. Box 7985
Madison, WI 53707-7985

COLORADO

CHAMPVA Claim Office
CHAMPVA Center
4500 Cherry Creek Drive, South
P. O. Box 65024
Denver, CO 80206-9024

Insurance Commissioner State Office
Commissioner of Insurance
1560 Broadway, Suite 850
Denver, CO 80202

Maternal and Child Health Program
Family and Community Health Services

Colorado Department of Public Health and Environment
4300 Cherry Creek Drive, South
Denver, CO 80246-1530

Adolescent and School Health Section
Colorado Department of Public Health and Environment
4300 Cherry Creek Drive, South
Denver, CO 80246-1530

Medicaid Fiscal Agent
Blue Cross and Blue Shield
P. O. Box 173300
Denver, CO 80217

Medicare Durable Medical Equipment
Palmetto Government Benefits Administrators
Medicare DMERC Operations
P. O. Box 10041
Columbia, SC 29202-3141

Medicare Fiscal Agent or Carrier
Noridian Mutual Insurance Company
4305 13th Avenue, SW
Fargo, ND 58103

State Board of Medical Examiners
1560 Broadway, Suite 1300
Denver, CO 80220-5140

TRICARE Claim Office
Palmetto Government Benefits Administrators
P. O. Box 870027
Surfside Beach, SC 29587-8727

Veterans Affairs Installation
Colorado Medical Centers:
   Denver 80220 (1055 Clermont Street)
   Fort Lyon 81038 (C Street)
   Grand Junction 81501 (2121 North Avenue)

Workers' Compensation Federal District Office
Office of Workers' Compensation Programs
1801 California Street, Suite 915
Denver, CO 80202

Workers' Compensation State Plan Office
Division of Workers' Compensation
1515 Arapahoe Street, Suite 500
Denver, CO 80202-2117

Industrial Claims Appeal Office
1515 Arapahoe Street
Denver, CO 80202

CONNECTICUT

CHAMPVA Claim Office
CHAMPVA Center
4500 Cherry Creek Drive, South
P. O. Box 65024
Denver, CO 80206-9024

Insurance Commissioner State Office
Commissioner
Department of Insurance
P. O. Box 816
Hartford, CT 06412-0816

Maternal and Child Health Program
Department of Public Health
Family Health Services Division
410 Capitol Avenue, MS 11FHS
P. O. Box 340308
Hartford, CT 06134-0308

MCH and CSCHN
Department of Public Health
410 Capitol Avenue, MS 11MAT
P. O. Box 340308
Hartford, CT 06134-0308

Medicaid Fiscal Agent
Electronic Data Systems Corporation
P. O. Box 2941
Hartford, CT 06104-2941

Medicare Durable Medical Equipment
United Health Care Insurance Company
(formerly MetraHealth, Inc.)
P. O. Box 6800
Wilkes-Barre, PA 18773-6800

Medicare Fiscal Agent or Carrier
Blue Cross and Blue Shield of Florida, Inc.
(aka First Coast Service Options, Inc.)
Medicare Part B
Jacksonville, FL 32231

State Board of Medical Examiners
Connecticut Medical Examining Board
P. O. Box 340308
Hartford, CT 06134-0308

TRICARE Claim Office
Palmetto Government Benefits Administrators (PGBA)
P. O. Box 7011
Camden, SC 29020-7011

Veterans Affairs Installation
Connecticut Health System
  Newington 06111 (555 Willard Avenue)
  West Haven 06516 (950 Campbell Avenue)

Workers' Compensation Federal District Office
Office of Workers' Compensation Programs
JFK Federal Office Building, Room E-260
Boston, MA 02203

Workers' Compensation State Plan Office
Workers' Compensation Commission
21 Oak Street
Hartford, CT 06106

DELAWARE

CHAMPVA Claim Office
CHAMPVA Center
4500 Cherry Creek Drive, South
P. O. Box 65024
Denver, CO 80206-9024

Insurance Commissioner State Office
Commissioner
Department of Insurance
841 Silver Lake Boulevard

P. O. Box 7007
Dover, DE 19904

Maternal and Child Health Program
Family Health Services
Delaware Division of Public Health
P. O. Box 637
Dover, DE 19903

Medicaid Fiscal Agent
Electronic Data Systems Corporation
P. O. Box 907
New Castle, DE 19720

Medicare Durable Medical Equipment
United Health Care Insurance Company
(formerly MetraHealth, Inc.)
P. O. Box 6800
Wilkes-Barre, PA 18773-6800

Medicare Fiscal Agent or Carrier
Blue Cross and Blue Shield of Texas
Dba. Trail Blazer Health Enterprises, Inc.
P. O. Box 660031
Dallas, TX 75266-0031

State Board of Medical Examiners
Delaware Board of Medical Practice
861 Silver Lake Blvd., Cannon Building, Suite 203
P. O. Box 1401
Dover, DE 19903-1401

TRICARE Claim Office
Palmetto Government Benefits Administrators (PGBA)
P. O. Box 7011
Camden, SC 29020-7011

Veterans Affairs Installation
Medical Center
1601 Kirkwood Highway
Wilmington, DE 19805

Workers' Compensation Federal District Office
Office of Workers' Compensation Programs
Gateway Building, Room 15200
3535 Market Street
Philadelphia, PA 19104

Workers' Compensation State Plan Office
Industrial Accident Board
4425 N. Market Street, 3rd Floor
Wilmington, DE 19802

DISTRICT OF COLUMBIA

CHAMPVA Claim Office
CHAMPVA Center
4500 Cherry Creek Drive, South
P. O. Box 65024
Denver, CO 80206-9024

Insurance Commissioner State Office
Insurance Administration
810 First Street, NE, Suite 701
Washington, DC 20002

Maternal and Child Health Program
Office of Maternal and Child Health

825 N. Capitol Street, NW, 3rd Floor
Washington, DC 20002

Medicaid Fiscal Agent
First Health
122 Y. Street, NW, #600
Washington, DC 20001

Medicare Durable Medical Equipment
Assigned:
AdminaStar Federal, Inc.
Attn: DMERC Operations
P. O. Box 7027
Indianapolis, IN 46207-7027

Nonassigned:
P. O. Box 7031
Indianapolis, IN 46207-7931

Medicare Fiscal Agent or Carrier
Trail Blazer Health Enterprises, Inc.
P. O. Box 660031
Dallas, TX 75266-0031

State Board of Medical Examiners
District of Columbia Board of Medicine
825 North Capitol Street, NE, 2nd Floor, Room 2224
Washington, DC 20002

TRICARE Claim Office
Palmetto Government Benefits Administrators (PGBA)
P. O. Box 7011
Camden, SC 29020-7011

Veterans Affairs Installation
District of Columbia Medical Center
50 Irving Street, NW
Washington, DC 20422

Workers' Compensation Federal District Office
Office of Workers' Compensation Programs
800 N. Capitol Street, NW, Room 800
Washington, DC 20211

Workers' Compensation State Plan Office
Department of Employment Services
Office of Workers' Compensation
1200 Upshur Street, NW, 3rd Floor
Washington, DC 20011

FLORIDA

CHAMPVA Claim Center
CHAMPVA Center
4500 Cherry Creek Drive, South
Box 65024
Denver, CO 80206-9024

Insurance Commissioner State Office
Commissioner
The Capitol, Plaza Level II
Tallahassee, FL 32399-0300

Maternal and Child Health Program
Division of Children's Medical Services
Department of Health
2020 Capitol Circle, SE, Mail Bin A
Tallahassee, FL 32399-0700

Division of Family Health Services
Department of Health
Family Health Services
Capitol Circle Office Complex
4025 Esplanade Way
Tallahassee, FL 32399-1723

Medicaid Fiscal Agent
UNISYS (EC)
P. O. Box 7072
Tallahassee, FL 32314-7072

Medicare Durable Medical Equipment
Palmetto Government Benefits Administrators
Medicare DMERC Operations
P. O. Box 100141
Columbia, SC 29202-3141

Medicare Fiscal Agent or Carrier
Blue Cross and Blue Shield of Florida
Medicare Part B
P. O. Box 2078
Jacksonville, FL 32231-0048

State Board of Medical Examiners
Florida Board of Medicine, Department of Health
Medical Quality Assurance
4052 Bald Cypress Way, BIN #C03
Tallahassee, FL 32399-1753

Florida Board of Osteopathic Medicine
Department of Health
4052 Bald Cypress Way, SE, BIN #C06
Tallahassee, FL 32399-1753

TRICARE Claim Office
Palmetto Government Benefits Administrators
P. O. Box 7032
Camden, SC 29020-7032

Veterans Administration Installation
Florida Medical Centers:
  Bay Pines 33708 (10000 Bay Pines Blvd., North)
  Gainesville 32608 (1601 Southwest Archer Road)
  Lake City 32025 (801 5. Marion Street)
  Miami 33125 (1201 N.W. 16th Street)
  Tampa 33612 (13000 Bruce B. Downs Blvd.)
  West Palm Beach 33410 (7305 N. Military Trail)

Workers' Compensation Federal District Office
Office of Workers' Compensation Programs
214 North Hogan Street, Suite 1006
Jacksonville, FL 32202

Workers' Compensation State Plan Office
Division of Workers' Compensation
Department of Labor and Employment Security
301 Forrest Building
2728 Centerview Drive
Tallahassee, FL 32399-0680

GEORGIA

CHAMPVA Claim Office
CHAMPVA Center
4500 Cherry Creek Drive, South

P. O. Box 65024
Denver, CO 80206-9024

Insurance Commissioner State Office
Commissioner
Department of Insurance
704 West Tower
2 Martin L. King, Jr. Drive
Atlanta, GA 30334

Maternal and Child Health Program
Georgia Department of Human Resources
2 Peachtree Street, NW, Suite 11-206
Atlanta, GA 30303-3142

Family Health Branch
2 Peachtree Street, NW, Suite 11-414
Atlanta, GA 30303-3142

Medicaid Fiscal Agent
Electronic Data Systems Corporation
P. O. Box 105013
Tucker, GA 30085

Medicare Durable Medical Equipment
Palmetto Government Benefits Administrators
Medicare DMERC Operations
P. O. Box 100141
Columbia, SC 29202-3141

Medicare Fiscal Agent or Carrier
Blue Cross Blue Shield of Alabama
Medicare Claims Administration
P. O. Box 830139
Birmingham, AL 35283-0139

State Board of Medical Examiners
Georgia Composite State Board of Medical Examiners
2 Peachtree Street, NW, 6th Floor
Atlanta, GA 30303

TRICARE Claim Office
Palmetto Government Benefits Administrators
P. O. Box 7032
Camden, SC 29020-7032

Veterans Administration Installation
Georgia Medical Centers:
  Augusta 30904 (1 Freedom Way)
  Decatur 30033 (1670 Clairmont Road)
  Dublin 31021 (1826 Veterans Blvd.)

Workers' Compensation Federal District Office
Office of Workers' Compensation Programs
214 North Hogan Street, Suite 1006
Jacksonville, FL 32202

Workers' Compensation State Plan Office
State Board of Workers' Compensation
270 Peachtree Street, NW, 6th Floor
Atlanta, GA 30303-1205

GUAM

Insurance Commissioner State Office
Commissioner
Department of Revenue and Taxation
Government of Guam

Building 13-3m 1st Floor
Mariner Avenue
Tiyan, Barrigada, GU 96913

Maternal and Child Health Program
Department of Public Health & Social Services
Bureau of Family Health and Nursing Services
P. O. Box 2816
Hagatna, GU 96932

Medicare Durable Medical Equipment
CIGNA Medicare Region D DMERC
P. O. Box 690
Nashville, TN 37202

Medicare Fiscal Agent or Carrier
Noridian Mutual Insurance Company
4305 13th Avenue, SW
Fargo, ND 58103

Medicare Railroad Retiree Carrier
Medicare Part B claims are handled by claim service centers. For the address and toll-free number of the office nearest you, call the Railroad Retirement Board listed in your telephone directory under U.S. Government.

State Board of Medical Examiners
Guam Board of Medical Examiners
Health Professional Licensing Office
P. O. Box 2816
Hagatna, GU 96932

Veterans Affairs Installation
Veterans Affairs Clinic
U.S. Naval Hospital
313 Farenholt Road
Agana Heights, GU 96919

Workers' Compensation State Plan Office
Worker's Compensation Commission
Department of Labor
Government of Guam
108 E Street (96913)
P. O. Box 9970
Tamuning, GU 96930-2970

HAWAII

CHAMPVA Claim Office
CHAMPVA Center
4500 Cherry Creek Drive, South
P. O. Box 65024
Denver, CO 80206-9024

Insurance Commissioner State Office
Commissioner
Department of Insurance
250 S. King Street, 5th Floor
Honolulu, HI 96813-3614

Maternal and Child Health Program
Family Health Services Division
Hawaii State Department of Health
1250 Punchbowl Street, Room 216
Honolulu, HI 96813

CSHCN Branch
Hawaii State Department of Health
741 Sunset Avenue
Honolulu, HI 96816

Medicaid Fiscal Agent
Hawaii Medical Service Association (EC)
P. O. Box 860
Honolulu, HI 96808

Medicare Durable Medical Equipment
CIGNA Medicare Region D DMERC
P. O. Box 690
Nashville, TN 37202

Medicare Fiscal Agent or Carrier
Noridian Mutual Insurance Company
4305 13th Avenue, SW
Fargo, ND 58103

State Board of Medical Examiners
Hawaii Board of Medical and Osteopathic Examiners
Department of Commerce and Consumer Affairs
1010 Richards Street (98613)
P. O. Box 3469
Honolulu, HI 96801

TEMPORARY DISABILITY INSURANCE
Department of Labor & Industrial Relations
Disability Compensation Division

Hawaii
State Office Building
75 Aupuni Street
Hilo, HI 96720

Kauai
State Office Building
3060 Eiwa Street
Lihue, HI 96766

Maui
State Office Building, #2
2264 Aupuni Street
Wailuku, HI 96793

Oahu
830 Punchbowl Street, Suite 210
P. O. Box 3769
Honolulu, HI 96812-3769

West Hawaii
Ashikawa Building
P. O. Box 49
Kealakekua, HI 96750

TRICARE Claim Office
Palmetto Government Business Administration
P. O. Box 870001
Surfside Beach, SC 29587-8701

Veterans Affairs Installation
Hawaii Medical Center and Regional Office
300 Ala Moana Blvd., Room 1352
P. O. Box 50188

Honolulu 96850-0001
Medical Office: (808) 566-1000
Regional Office: From Oahu: (808) 566-1000
From Hawaiian neighbor islands, 1-800-827-1000

From Guam, 475-8387
From American Samoa, 1-1-800-844-7928

Workers' Compensation Federal District Office
Office of Workers' Compensation Programs
71 Stevenson Street (94105)
P. O. Box 3769
San Francisco, CA 94119-3769

Workers' Compensation State Plan Office
Disability Compensation Division
Department of Labor and Industrial Relations
830 Punchbowl Street, Room 211
P. O. Box 3769
Honolulu, HI 96812

Labor and Industrial Relations Appeals Board
888 Mililani Street, Room 400
Honolulu, HI 96813

IDAHO

CHAMPVA Claim Office
CHAMPVA Center
4500 Cherry Creek Drive, South
P. O. Box 65024
Denver, CO 80206-9024

Insurance Commissioner State Office
Director
Department of Insurance
700 W. State Street, 3rd Floor
P. O. Box 83720
Boise, ID 83720-0043

Maternal and Child Health Program
Children's Special Health Program
Idaho Department of Health and Welfare
450 W. State Street
P. O. Box 83720
Boise, ID 83720-0036

Public Health Services
Idaho Department of Health and Welfare
450 W. State Street
P. O. Box 83720
Boise, ID 83720-0036

Medicaid Fiscal Agent
Electronic Data Systems (EC)
P. O. Box 23
Boise, ID 83707

Medicare Durable Medical Equipment
CIGNA Medicare Region D DMERC
P. O. Box 690
Nashville, TN 37202

Medicare Fiscal Agent or Carrier
CIGNA Medicare Claims Office
2 Vantage Way, Metro Exchange Bldg.
Nashville, TN 37228

Medicare Railroad Retiree Carrier
United Health Care Insurance Company
P. O. Box 10066
Augusta, GA 30999-0001

State Board of Medical Examiners
Idaho State Board of Medicine
Statehouse Mall
1755 Westgate Drive, Suite 140 (83704)
P. O. Box 83720
Boise, ID 83720-0058

TRICARE Claim Office
Northern Idaho (Benewah, Bonner, Boundary, Kootenai, Shoshone, and Latah Counties)
Foundation Health Federal Services, Inc.
Wisconsin Physician Services
TRICARE Northwest
P. O. Box 8929
Madison, WI 53708-8929

Except for 6 counties in Northern Idaho
Palmetto Government Benefits Administrators
P. O. Box 870028
Surfside Beach, SC 29587-8728

Veterans Affairs Installation
Idaho Medical Center
500 West Fort Street
Boise, ID 83702

Workers' Compensation Federal District Office
Office of Workers' Compensation Programs
4010 Federal Office Building
1111 Third Avenue, Suite 615
Seattle, WA 98101

Workers' Compensation State Plan Office
Industrial Commission
317 Main Street
P. O. Box 83720
Boise, ID 83720-0041

ILLINOIS

CHAMPVA Claim Office
CHAMPVA Center
4500 Cherry Creek Drive, South
P. O. Box 65024
Denver, CO 80206-9024

Insurance Commissioner State Office
Director
Department of Insurance
320 W. Washington Street, 4th Floor
Springfield, IL 62767-0001

Maternal and Child Health Program
Office of Family Health
Illinois Department of Public Health
535 W. Jefferson Street
Springfield, IL 62702-5058

Division of Specialized Care for Children, UIC
University of Illinois at Chicago
2815 W. Washington, Suite 300
P. O. Box 19481
Springfield, IL 62794-9481

Medicaid Fiscal Agent
Department of Public Aid (Hospital)
P. O. Box 19105
Springfield, IL 62793-9105

Medicare Durable Medical Equipment
Assigned:
AdminaStar Federal, Inc.
Attn: DMERC Operations
P. O. Box 7027
Indianapolis, IN 46207-7027

Nonassigned:
P. O. Box 7031
Indianapolis, IN 46207-7931

Medicare Fiscal Agent or Carrier
Wisconsin Physicians Services
Insurance Corporation
P. O. Box 1787
Madison, WI 53701

State Board of Medical Examiners
Illinois Department of Professional Regulation
100 W. Randolph Street, Suite 9-300
Chicago, IL 60601

TRICARE Regions 2/5 Claims
Palmetto Government Benefits Administrators (PGBA)
P. O. Box 7021
Camden, SC 29020-7021

Veterans Affairs Installation
Illinois Medical Centers:
  Chicago 60611 (Lakeside, 333 E. Huron St.)
  Chicago 60612 (Westside, 820 S. Damen Avenue, P. O. Box 8195)
  Danville 61832 (1900 E. Main Street)
  Hines 60141 (Roosevelt Road & 5th Avenue)
  Marion 62959 (2401 W. Main Street)
  North Chicago 60064 (3001 Green Bay Road)

Workers' Compensation Federal District Office
Office of Workers' Compensation Programs
230 S. Dearborn Street, 8th Floor
Chicago, IL 60604

Workers' Compensation State Plan Office
Industrial Commission
100 W. Randolph Street, Suite 8-200
Chicago, IL 60601

INDIANA

CHAMPVA Claim Office
CHAMPVA Center
4500 Cherry Creek Drive, South
P. O. Box 65024
Denver, CO 80206-9024

Insurance Commissioner State Office
Commissioner
Department of Insurance
311 W. Washington Street, Suite 300
Indianapolis, IN 46204-2787

Maternal and Child Health Program
Children's Special Health Care Services
Indiana State Department of Health
2 N. Meridian Street, Section 7-B
Indianapolis, IN 46204

State Department of Health
2 N. Meridian Street, Section 7-C
Indianapolis, IN 46204

Medicaid Fiscal Agent
Department of Family Independence
402 W. Washington Street, #W363
Indianapolis, IN 46204

Medicare Durable Medical Equipment
Assigned:
AdminaStar Federal Incorporated
Attn: DMERC Operations
P. O. Box 7027
Indianapolis, IN 46207-7027

Nonassigned:
P. O. Box 7031
Indianapolis, IN 46207-7931

Medicare Fiscal Agent or Carrier
Part B Participating:
Medicare Part B/AdminaStar Federal
P. O. Box 6160
Indianapolis, IN 46250-6160

Part B Nonparticipating:
Assigned:
AdmininaStar Federal
P. O. Box 6026
Indianapolis, IN 46206-6026

Nonassigned:
AdminaStar Federal
P. O. Box 7073
Indianapolis, IN 46206-7073

State Board of Medical Examiners
Indiana Health Professions Bureau
402 W. Washington Street, Room 041
Indianapolis, IN 46204

TRICARE Regions 2/5 Claims
Palmetto Government Benefits Administrators (PGBA)
P. O. Box 7021
Camden, SC 29020-7021

Veterans Affairs Installation
Indiana Medical Centers:

  Fort Wayne 46805 (2121 Lake Avenue)
  Indianapolis 46202 (1481 W. 10th Street)
  Marion 46953 (1700 E. 38th Street)

Workers' Compensation Federal District Office
Office of Workers' Compensation Programs
1240 E. Ninth Street, Room 851
Cleveland, OH 44199

Workers' Compensation State Plan Office
Worker's Compensation Board
402 W. Washington Street, Room W196
Indianapolis, IN 46204

IOWA

CHAMPVA Claim Office
CHAMPVA Center
4500 Cherry Creek Drive, South

P. O. Box 65024
Denver, CO 80206-9024

Insurance Commissioner State Office
Commissioner
Division of Insurance
330 East Maple Street
Des Moines, IA 50319-0065

Maternal and Child Health Program
Family Services Bureau
Iowa Department of Public Health
321 East 12th Street, Lucas Building
Des Moines, IA 50319-0075

Child Health Specialty Clinics
University of Iowa Hospital School
100 Hawkins Drive, Room 247
Iowa City, IA 52242-1011

Medicaid Fiscal Agent
UNISYS (EC)
P. O. Box 14421
Des Moines, IA 50306

Medicare Durable Medical Equipment
CIGNA Medicare Region D DMERC
P. O. Box 690
Nashville, TN 37202

Medicare Fiscal Agent or Carrier
Noridian Mutual Insurance Company
4305 13th Avenue
Fargo, ND 58103

State Board of Medical Examiners
Iowa State Board of Medical Examiners
400 SW 8th Street, Suite C
Des Moines, IA 50309-4686

TRICARE Claim Office
Palmetto Government Benefits Administrators
P. O. Box 870030
Surfside Beach, SC 29587-8730

Veterans Administration Installation
Iowa Medical Centers:

  Des Moines 50310 (3600 30th & Euclid Avenue)
  Iowa City 52246 (601 Highway 6 West)
  Knoxville 50138 (1515 W. Pleasant Street)

Workers' Compensation Federal District Office
Office of Workers' Compensation Programs
City Center Square
1100 Main Street, Suite 750
Kansas City, MO 64105

Workers' Compensation State Plan Office
Division of Workers' Compensation
Workforce Development Department
1000 E. Grand Avenue
Des Moines, IA 50319

KANSAS

CHAMPVA Claim Office
CHAMPVA Center
4500 Cherry Creek Drive, South

Box 65024
Denver, CO 80206-9024

Insurance Commissioner State Office
Commissioner
Department of Insurance
420 S.W. 9th Street
Topeka, KS 66612-1678

Maternal and Child Health Program
Services for CSHCN
Kansas Department of Health & Environment
900 S.W. Jackson, 10th Floor, 1005 N, LSOB
Topeka, KS 66612-1290

Medicaid Fiscal Agent
Electronic Data Systems Federal Corp. (EC)
P. O. Box 3571
Topeka, KS 66601

Medicare Durable Medical Equipment
CIGNA Medicare Region D DMERC
P. O. Box 690
Nashville, TN 37202

Medicare Fiscal Agent or Carrier
Blue Cross and Blue Shield of Kansas, Inc.
1133 Topeka Avenue (66629)
P. O. Box 239
Topeka, KS 66601

State Board of Medical Examiners
Kansas State Board of Healing Arts
235 S.W. Topeka Blvd.
Topeka, KS 66603-3068

TRICARE Claim Office
Palmetto Government Benefits Administrators
P. O. Box 870030
Surfside Beach, SC 29587-8730

Veterans Affairs Installation
Kansas Medical Centers:

  Leavenworth 66048 (4101 S. 4th Street, Trafficway)
  Topeka 66622 (2200 SW Gage Blvd.)
  Wichita 67218 (5500 E. Kellogg)

Workers' Compensation Federal District Office
Office of Workers' Compensation Programs
City Center Square
1100 Main Street, Suite 750
Kansas City, MO 64106

Workers' Compensation State Plan Office
Division of Workers' Compensation
Department of Human Resources
800 S.W. Jackson Street, Suite 600
Topeka, KS 66612-1227

KENTUCKY

CHAMPVA Claim Office
CHAMPVA Center
4500 Cherry Creek Drive, South
Box 65024
Denver, CO 80206-9024

Insurance Commissioner State Office
Commissioner
Department of Insurance
215 West Main Street
P. O. Box 517
Frankfort, KY 40602-0517

Maternal and Child Health Program
Division of Adult and Child Health
Department for Health Services
275 E. Main Street, HSB 2R
Frankfort, KY 40621-0001

Kentucky Commission for CSHCN
982 Eastern Parkway
Louisville, KY 40217

Medicaid Fiscal Agent
Department for Medicaid Services
275 East Main Street, 6WA
Frankfort, KY 40621-0001

Medicare Durable Medical Equipment
Palmetto Government Benefits Administrators
Medicare DMERC Operations
P. O. Box 100141
Columbia, SC 29202-3141

Medicare Fiscal Agent or Carrier
AdminaStar Federal, Inc.
9901 Linn Station Road
Louisville, KY 40223-3824

State Board of Medical Examiners
Kentucky Board of Medical Licensure
Hurstbourne Office Park
310 Whittington Parkway, Suite 1B
Louisville, KY 40222-4916

TRICARE Claim Office
Palmetto Government Benefits Administrators (PGBA)
P. O. Box 7021
Camden, SC 29020-7021

Veterans Affairs Installation
Kentucky Medical Centers:

  Lexington 40511 (2250 Leestown Road)
  Louisville 40206 (800 Zorn Avenue)

Workers' Compensation Federal District Office
Office of Workers' Compensation Programs
214 North Hogan Street, Suite 1006
Jacksonville, FL 32202

Workers' Compensation State Plan Office
Department of Workers' Claims
Perimeter Park West, Building C
1270 Louisville Road
Frankfort, KY 40601

LOUISIANA

CHAMPVA Claim Office
CHAMPVA Center
4500 Cherry Creek Drive, South
P. O. Box 65024
Denver, CO 80206-9024

Insurance Commissioner State Office
Commissioner
Department of Insurance
P. O. Box 94214
Baton Rouge, LA 70804-9214

Maternal and Child Health Program
Children's Special Health Services
Office of Public Health
P. O. Box 60630
New Orleans, LA 70160

Maternal and Child Health Section
Office of Public Health
P. O. Box 60630
New Orleans, LA 70160

Medicaid Fiscal Agent
UNISYS Corp. (EC)
P. O. Box 91020
Baton Rouge, LA 70821

Medicare Durable Medical Equipment
Palmetto Government Benefits Administrators
Medicare DMERC Operations
P. O. Box 100141
Columbia, SC 29202-3141

Medicare Fiscal Agent or Carrier
Arkansas Blue Cross and Blue Shield
601 Gaines Street
Little Rock, AR 72201

State Board of Medical Examiners
Louisiana State Board of Medical Examiners
630 Camp Street
P. O. Box 30250
New Orleans, LA 70190-0250

TRICARE Claim Office
Western two-thirds, mainly west of Baton Rouge:
Wisconsin Physicians Service
P. O. Box 8999
Madison, WI 53708-8999

Eastern third of the state, including Baton Rouge and New Orleans:
Palmetto Government Benefits Administrators
P. O. Box 7032
Camden, SC 29520-7032

Veterans Affairs Installation
Louisiana Medical Centers:
   Alexandria 71306 (P. O. Box 69004)
   New Orleans 70112 (1601 Perdido Street)
   Shreveport 71101 (510 E. Stoner Avenue)

Workers' Compensation Federal District Office
Office of Workers' Compensation Programs
525 Griffin Street, Room 100
Dallas, TX 75202

Workers' Compensation State Plan Office
Department of Labor
Office of Workers' Compensation
P. O. Box 94040
Baton Rouge, LA 70802-9040

MAINE

CHAMPVA Claim Office
CHAMPVA Center
4500 Cherry Creek Drive, South
P. O. Box 65024
Denver, CO 80206-9024

Insurance Commissioner State Office
Department of Professional and Financial Regulation
Bureau of Insurance
State House, Station #34
Augusta, ME 04333-0034

Maternal and Child Health Program
Division of Community and Family Health
Department of Human Services
State House Station #11
151 Capitol Street
Augusta, ME 04333-0011

Medicaid Fiscal Agent
Medical Assistance Claims Processing M500
Bureau of Med SVCS-249
Western Avenue
Augusta, ME 04333-0001

Medicare Durable Medical Equipment
United Health Care Insurance Company
(formerly MetraHealth)
P. O. Box 6800
Wilkes-Barre, PA 18773-6800

Medicare Fiscal Agent or Carrier
National Heritage Insurance Company
450 West East Avenue
Chico, CA 95973

State Board of Medical Examiners
Maine Board of Osteopathic Licensure
2 Bangor Street, 2nd Floor
137 State House Station
Augusta, ME 04333-0137

Maine Board of Osteopathic Licensure
Two Bangor Street
142 State House Station
Augusta, ME 04333-0142

TRICARE Claim Office
Palmetto Government Benefits Administrators (PGBA)
P. O. Box 7011
Camden, SC 29020-7011

Veterans Affairs Installation
Maine Medical Center
1 VA Center
Togus, ME 04330

Workers' Compensation Federal District Office
Office of Workers' Compensation Programs
JFK Federal Office Building, Room E-260
Boston, MA 02203

Workers' Compensation State Plan Office
Workers' Compensation Board
Deering Building
State House Station #27
Augusta, ME 04333-0027

MARYLAND

CHAMPVA Claim Office
CHAMPVA Center
4500 Cherry Creek Drive, South
P. O. Box 65024
Denver, CO 80206-9024

Insurance Commissioner State Office
Commissioner
Insurance Administration
525 St. Paul Place, 7th Floor
Baltimore, MD 21202-2272

Maternal and Child Health Program
Specialty Care, Office of Children's Health
Department of Health and Mental Hygiene
201 W. Preston Street, Room 319
Baltimore, MD 21201

Maternal Health and Family Planning
Department of Health and Mental Hygiene
201 W. Preston Street, Room 318
Baltimore, MD 21201

Medicaid Fiscal Agent
Medical Care Operations Administration
Claims Department
201 West Preston Street
P. O. Box 1935
Baltimore, MD 21203

Medicare Durable Medical Equipment
Assigned:
AdminaStar Federal, Inc.
Attn: DMERC Operations
P. O. Box 7027
Indianapolis, IN 46207-7027

Nonassigned:
P. O. Box 7031
Indianapolis, IN 46207-7931

Medicare Fiscal Agent or Carrier
Montgomery and Prince George's counties:
Xact Medicare Services (EC)
P. O. Box 890101
Camp Hill, PA 17089-0101

Rest of State:
Trail Blazer Health Enterprisers, Inc.
P. O. Box 660031
Dallas, TX 75266-0031

State Board of Medical Examiners
Maryland Board of Physician Quality Assurance
4201 Patterson Avenue, 3rd Floor
P. O. Box 2571
Baltimore, MD 21215-0095

TRICARE Claim Office
Palmetto Government Benefits Administrators (PGBA)
P. O. Box 7011
Camden, SC 29020-7011

Veterans Affairs Installation
Maryland Medical Centers:

  Baltimore 21201 (Prosthetic Assesment Information Center, 103 E. Gay Street)

  Baltimore 21201 (10 N. Greene Street)
  Fort Howard 21052 (9600 N. Point Road)
  Perry Point 21902

Workers' Compensation Federal District Office
Office of Workers' Compensation Programs
800 N. Capitol Street, NW, Room 800
Washington, DC 20211

Workers' Compensation State Plan Office
Workers' Compensation Commission
6 N. Liberty Street
Baltimore, MD 21201-3785

MASSACHUSETTS

CHAMPVA Claim Center
CHAMPVA Center
4500 Cherry Creek Drive, South
P. O. Box 65024
Denver, CO 80206-9024

Insurance Commissioner State Office
Commissioner
Division of Insurance
470 Atlantic Avenue, 6th Floor
Boston, MA 02210-2223

Maternal and Child Health Program
Bureau of Family & Community Health
Massachusetts Department of Public Health
250 Washington Street, 5th Floor
Boston, MA 02108-4619

Medicaid Fiscal Agent
UNISYS Corp.
P. O. Box 9102
Somerville, MA 02145-9101

Medicare Durable Medical Equipment
United Health Care Insurance Company
(formerly MetraHealth)
P. O. Box 6800
Wilkes-Barre, PA 18773-6800

Medicare Fiscal Agent or Carrier
National Heritage Insurance Company
450 West East Avenue
Chico, CA 95973

State Board of Medical Examiners
Massachusetts Board of Registration in Medicine
Ten West Street, 3rd Floor
Boston, MA 02111

TRICARE Claim Office
Palmetto Government Benefits Administrators
P. O. Box 7011
Camden, SC 29020-7011

Veterans Affairs Installation
Massachusetts Medical Centers:

  Bedford 01730 (200 Springs Road)
  Boston 02130 (150 S. Huntington Avenue)
  Brockton 02301 (940 Belmont Street)
  Northampton 01053 (421 N. Main Street)
  West Roxbury 02132 (1400 VFW Parkway)

Workers' Compensation Federal District Office
Office of Workers' Compensation Programs
JFK Federal Building, Room E-260
Boston, MA 02203

Workers' Compensation State Plan Office
Department of Industrial Accidents
600 Washington Street, 7th Floor
Boston, MA 02111

MICHIGAN

CHAMPVA Claim Office
CHAMPVA Center
4500 Cherry Creek Drive, South
P. O. Box 65024
Denver, CO 80206-9024

Insurance Commissioner State Office
Commissioner
Department of Commerce
P. O. Box 30220
Lansing, MI 48909-7720

Maternal and Child Health Program
CSHCS Planning Division
Medical Services Administration
P. O. Box 30479
Lansing, MI 48909-7979

Michigan Department of Public Health
3423 N. Martin L. King, Jr., Blvd., Room 218
P. O. Box 30195
Lansing, MI 48909-0195

Medicaid Fiscal Agent
Medical Services Administration
P. O. Box 30042
Lansing, MI 48909

Medicare Durable Medical Equipment
Assigned:
AdminaStar Federal, Inc.
Attn: DMERC Operations
P. O. Box 7027
Indianapolis, IN 46207-7027

Nonassigned:
P. O. Box 7031
Indianapolis, IN 46207-7931

Medicare Fiscal Agent or Carrier
Wisconsin Physicians Service
Insurance Corp.
P. O. Box 1787
Madison, WI 53701

State Board of Medical Examiners
Michigan Board of Medicine
611 W. Ottawa Street, 4th Floor (48933)
P. O. Box 30670
Lansing, MI 48909-8170

Michigan Board of Osteopathic Medicine and Surgery
611 West Ottawa Street, 4th Floor (48933)
P. O. Box 30670
Lansing, MI 48909-8170

TRICARE Claim Office
Palmetto Government Benefits Administrators
P. O. Box 7021
Camden, SC 29020-7021

Veterans Affairs Installation
Michigan Medical Centers:
  Ann Arbor 48105 (2215 Fuller Road)
  Battle Creek 49016 (5500 Armstrong Road)
  Detroit 48201 (4646 John R. Street)
  Iron Mountain 49801 (325 East H. Street)
  Saginaw 48602 (1500 Weiss Street)

Workers' Compensation Federal District Office
Office of Workers' Compensation Programs
1240 East Ninth Street, Room 851
Cleveland, OH 44199

Workers' Compensation State Plan Office
Bureau of Workers' Disability Compensation
P. O. Box 30016
Lansing, MI 48909

MINNESOTA

CHAMPVA Claim Office
CHAMPVA Center
4500 Cherry Creek Drive, South
P. O. Box 65024
Denver, CO 80206-9024

Insurance Commissioner State Office
Commissioner
Department of Commerce
133 E. 7th Street
St. Paul, MN 55101-2362

Maternal and Child Health Program
Division of Family Health
Minnesota Department of Health
P. O. Box 64882
Minneapolis, MN 55164-0882

Medicaid Fiscal Agent
Department of Human Services (EC)
P. O. Box 64166
St. Paul, MN 55164

Medicare Durable Medical Equipment
Assigned:
AdminaStar Federal, Inc.
Attn: DMERC Operations
P. O. Box 7027
Indianapolis, IN 46207-7027

Nonassigned:
P. O. Box 7031
Indianapolis, IN 46207-7931

Medicare Fiscal Agent or Carrier
Wisconsin Physicians Services
Insurance Corp.
P. O. Box 1787
Madison, WI 53701

State Board of Medical Examiners
Minnesota Board of Medical Practice
2829 University Avenue SE, Suite 400
Minneapolis, MN 55414-3246

TRICARE Claim Office
Palmetto Government Benefits Administrators
P. O. Box 870029
Surfside Beach, SC 29587-8729

Veterans Affairs Installation
Minnesota Medical Centers:
  Minneapolis 55417 (One Veterans Drive)
  St. Cloud 56303 (4801 8th Street, North)

Workers' Compensation Federal District Office
Office of Workers' Compensation Programs
230 S. Dearborn Street, 8th Floor
Chicago, IL 60604

Workers' Compensation State Plan Offices
Workers' Compensation Division
Department of Labor and Industry
443 Lafayette Road
St. Paul, MN 55155-4319

Workers' Compensation Court of Appeals
25 Constitution Avenue, Suite 405
St. Paul, MN 55155

MISSISSIPPI

CHAMPVA Claim Office
CHAMPVA Center
4500 Cherry Creek Drive, South
P. O. Box 65024
Denver, CO 80206-9024

Insurance Commissioner State Office
Commissioner
Department of Insurance
1804 Walter Sillers Building
P. O. Box 79
Jackson, MS 39205

Maternal and Child Health Program
Children and Adolescent Health
Mississippi State Health Department
2423 N. State Street
P. O. Box 1700
Jackson, MS 39215-1700

CSHCN Program
Mississippi State Health Department
2423 N. State Street
P. O. Box 1700
Jackson, MS 39215-1700

Medicaid Fiscal Agent
111 East Capitol Street, Suite 400 (39201)
P. O. Box 23077
Jackson, MS 38225-3077

Medicare Durable Medical Equipment
Palmetto Government Benefits Administrators
Medicare DMERC Operations
P. O. Box 100141
Columbia, SC 29202-3141

Medicare Fiscal Agent or Carrier
Blue Cross and Blue Shield of Alabama
Medicare Claims Administration

P. O. Box 830139
Birmingham, AL 35283-0139

State Board of Medical Examiners
Mississippi State Board of Medical Licensure
1867 Crane Ridge Drive, Suite 200 B
Jackson, MS 39216

TRICARE Claim Office
Palmetto Government Benefits Administrators
P. O. Box 7032
Camden SC 29020-7032

Veterans Affairs Installation
Mississippi Medical Centers:
  Biloxi 39531 (400 Veterans Ave.)
  Jackson 39216 (1500 E. Woodrow Wilson Drive)

Workers' Compensation Federal District Office
Office of Workers' Compensation Programs
214 North Hogan Street, Suite 1006
Jacksonville, FL 32202

Workers' Compensation State Plan Office
Workers' Compensation Commission
1428 Lakeland Drive
P. O. Box 5300
Jackson, MS 39296-5300

MISSOURI

CHAMPVA Claim Office
CHAMPVA Center
4500 Cherry Creek Drive, South
P. O. Box 65024
Denver, CO 80206-9024

Insurance Commissioner State Office
Director of Insurance
301 W. High Street, 6 North
P. O. Box 690
Jefferson City, MO 65102-0690

Maternal and Child Health Program
Bureau of Special Health Care Needs
Missouri Department of Health
930 Wildwood Drive
P. O. Box 570
Jefferson City, MO 65102-0570

Division of Maternal, Child & Family Health
Missouri Department of Health
930 Wildwood Drive
P. O. Box 570
Jefferson City, MO 65102-0570

Medicaid Fiscal Agent
Missouri Medicaid
P. O. Box 5600
Jefferson City, MO 65102

Medicare Durable Medical Equipment
CIGNA Medicare Region D DMERC
P. O. Box 690
Nashville, TN 37202

Medicare Fiscal Agent or Carrier
Eastern Missouri:

Arkansas Blue Cross and Blue Shield
601 Gaines Street
Little Rock, AR 72201

Western Missouri:
Blue Cross and Blue Shield of Kansas, Inc.
1133 Topeka Avenue (66629)
P. O. Box 239
Topeka KS 66601

State Board of Medical Examiners
Missouri State Board of Registration for the Healing Arts
3605 Missouri Boulevard (65109)
P. O. Box 4
Jefferson City, MO 65102

TRICARE Claim Offices
St. Louis area:
Palmetto Government Benefits Administrators
P. O. Box 7021
Camden, SC 29020-7021

Except for St. Louis area:
Palmetto Government Benefits Administrators
P. O. Box 870030
Surfside Beach, SC 29587-8730

Veterans Affairs Installation
Missouri Medical Centers:
  Columbia 65201 (800 Hospital Drive)
  Kansas City 64128 (4801 Linwood Blvd.)
  Poplar Bluff 63901 (1500 N. Westwood Blvd.)
  St. Louis 63106 (John Cochran Division, 915 N. Grand Blvd.)
  St. Louis 63125 (#1 Jefferson Barracks Division)

Workers' Compensation Federal District Office
Office of Workers' Compensation Programs
City Center Square
1100 Main Street, Suite 750
Kansas City, MO 64105

Workers' Compensation State Plan Office
Division of Workers' Compensation
Department of Labor and Industrial Relations
3315 W. Truman Blvd.
P. O. Box 58
Jefferson City, MO 65102-0058

MONTANA

CHAMPVA Claim Office
CHAMPVA Center
4500 Cherry Creek Drive, South
P. O. Box 65024
Denver, CO 80206-9024

Insurance Commissioner State Office
Commissioner
Department of Insurance
126 N. Sanders (59601)
Mitchell Building, Room 270
P. O. Box 4009
Helena, MT 59604-4009

Maternal and Child Health Program
Children's Special Health Services

Department of Public Health & Human Sciences
1400 Broadway, Cogswell Bldg.
P. O. Box 202951
Helena, MT 59620

Family and Community Health Bureau
Department of Public Health and Human Sciences
1400 Broadway, Cogswell Bldg.
P. O. Box 202951
Helena, MT 59620

Medicaid Fiscal Agent
Consultec, Inc. (EC)
34 N. Last Chance Gulch (59601)
P. O. Box 8000
Helena, MT 59604

Medicare Durable Medical Equipment
CIGNA Medicare Region D DMERC
P. O. Box 690
Nashville, TN 37202

Medicare Fiscal Agent or Carrier
Blue Cross and Blue Shield of Montana, Inc.
P. O. Box 4310
Helena, MT 59604

State Board of Medical Examiners
Montana Board of Medical Examiners
Arcade Building, Lower Level
111 N. Jackson
P. O. Box 200513
Helena, MT 59620-0513

TRICARE Claim Office
Palmetto Government Benefits Administrators
P. O. Box 870031
Surfside Beach, SC 29587-8731

Veterans Affairs Installation
Montana Centers and Regional Office:
  Fort Harrison 59636 (William Street off Highway 12 W)
  Miles City 59301 (210 S. Winchester)

Workers' Compensation Federal District Office
Office of Workers' Compensation Programs
1801 California Street, Suite 915
Drawer 3558
Denver, CO 80202

Workers' Compensation State Plan Office
Employment Relations Division
Department of Labor and Industry
P. O. Box 8011
Helena, MT 59604-8011

NEBRASKA

CHAMPVA Claim Office
CHAMPVA Center
4500 Cherry Creek Drive, South
P. O. Box 65024
Denver, CO 80206-9024

Insurance Commissioner State Office
Director

Department of Insurance
941 O Street, Suite 400
Lincoln, NE 68508-3690

Maternal and Child Health Program
Division of Family Health
Nebraska Department of Health and Human Services
301 Centennial Mall South
P. O. Box 95044
Lincoln, NE 68509-5044

Special Services for Children and Adults
Nebraska Department of Health and Human Services
301 Centennial Mall South
P. O. Box 95044
Lincoln, NE 68509-5044

Medicaid Fiscal Agent
Department of Social Services (EC)
301 Centennial Mall South, 5th Floor (68508)
P. O. Box 95026
Lincoln, NE 68509-5026

Medicare Durable Medical Equipment
CIGNA Medicare Region D DMERC
P. O. Box 690
Nashville, TN 37202

Medicare Fiscal Agent or Carrier
Blue Cross and Blue Shield of Kansas, Inc.
1133 SW Topeka Blvd. (66629)
P. O. Box 239
Topeka, KS 66601

State Board of Medical Examiners
Board of Examiners in Medicine & Surgery
301 Centennial Mall South
P. O. Box 94986
Lincoln, NE 68509-4986

TRICARE Claim Office
Palmetto Government Benefits Administrators
P. O. Box 870027
Surfside Beach, SC 29587-8727

Veterans Affairs Installation
Nebraska Medical Centers:
  Grand Island 68803 (2201 N. Broadwell Avenue)
  Lincoln 68510 (600 S. 70th Street)
  Omaha 68105 (4101 Woolworth Avenue)

Workers' Compensation Federal District Office
Office of Workers' Compensation Programs
City Center Square
1100 Main Street, Suite 750
Kansas City, MO 64105

Workers' Compensation State Plan Office
Workers' Compensation Court
State House, 12th Floor
P. O. Box 98908
Lincoln, NE 68509-8908

NEVADA

CHAMPVA Claim Office
CHAMPVA Center

4500 Cherry Creek Drive, South
P. O. Box 65024
Denver, CO 80206-9024

Insurance Commissioner State Office
Commissioner
Division of Insurance
1665 Hot Springs Road, Suite 152
Carson City, NV 89706-0646

Maternal and Child Health Program
Family Health Services
Nevada State Health Division
505 E. King Street, Room 200
Carson City, NV 89710-4792

Medicaid Fiscal Agent or Carrier
Blue Cross & Blue Shield of Nevada
P. O. Box 12127
Reno, NV 89510-2127

Medicare Durable Medical Equipment
CIGNA Medicare Region D DMERC
P. O. Box 690
Nashville, TN 37202

Medicare Fiscal Agent or Carrier
Noridian Mutual Insurance Company
4305 13th Avenue, SW
Fargo, ND 58103

State Board of Medical Examiners
Nevada State Board of Medical Examiners
1105 Terminal Way, Suite 301 (89502)
P. O. Box 7238
Reno, NV 89510

Nevada State Board of Osteopathic Medicine
2950 E. Flamingo Road, Suite E-1
Las Vegas, NV 89121-5208

TRICARE Claim Office
Palmetto Government Benefits Administrators
P. O. Box 870033
Surfside Beach, SC 29587-8733

Veterans Affairs Installation
Nevada Medical Center:
  Las Vegas 89106 (1700 Vegas Drive)
  Reno 89520 (1000 Locust Street)

Workers' Compensation Federal District Office
Office of Workers' Compensation Programs
71 Stevenson Street, 2nd Floor (94105)
P. O. Box 3769
San Francisco, CA 94119-3769

Workers' Compensation State Plan Office
Division of Industrial Insurance Relations
400 W. King Street, Suite 400
Carson City, NE 89703

NEW HAMPSHIRE

CHAMPVA Claim Office
CHAMPVA Center
4500 Cherry Creek Drive, South

P. O. Box 65024
Denver, CO 80206-9024

Insurance Commissioner State Office
Commissioner
Department of Insurance
56 Old Suncook Road
Concord, NH 03301-5151

Maternal and Child Health Program
Maternal and Child Health
Department of Health and Human Services
6 Hazen Drive
Concord, NH 03301

Bureau of Special Medical Services
New Hampshire Department of Health and Human
Services
6 Hazen Drive
Concord, NH 03301

Medicaid Fiscal Agent
Electronic Data Systems Federal Corporation (EC)
P. O. Box 2001
Concord, NH 03302-2001

Medicare Durable Medical Equipment
United Health Care Insurance Co.
(formerly MetraHealth)
P. O. Box 6800
Wilkes-Barre, PA 18773-6800

Medicare Fiscal Agent or Carrier
National Heritage Insurance Company
450 West East Avenue
Chico, CA 95973

State Board of Medical Examiners
New Hampshire Board of Medicine
2 Industrial Park Drive, Suite 8
Concord, NH 03301-8520

New Hampshire Board of Registration in Medicine
Health & Welfare Building
6 Hazen Drive
Concord, NH 03301

TRICARE Claim Office
Palmetto Government Benefits Administrators
P. O. Box 7011
Camden, SC 29020-7011

Veterans Affairs Installation
New Hampshire Medical Center
718 Smyth Road
Manchester, NH 03104

Workers' Compensation Federal District Office
Office of Workers' Compensation Programs
JFK Federal Building, Room E-260
Boston, MA 02203

Workers' Compensation State Plan Office
Department of Labor
Division of Workers' Compensation
State Office Park South
95 Pleasant Court
Concord, NH 03301

NEW JERSEY

CHAMPVA Claim Office
CHAMPVA Center
4500 Cherry Creek Drive, South
P. O. Box 65024
Denver, CO 80206-9024

Insurance Commissioner State Office
Commissioner
Department of Insurance
20 West State Street
P. O. Box 325
Trenton, NJ 08625-0325

Maternal and Child Health Program
Adm MCHS-Family Health Services
State Department of Health and Senior Services
50 E. State Street
P. O. Box 364
Trenton, NJ 08625-0364

Special Child and Adult Health Services
State Department of Health and Senior Services
50 E. State Street
P. O. Box 364
Trenton, NJ 08625-0364

Medicaid Fiscal Agent
UNISYS, CN
P. O. Box 4808
Trenton, NJ 08650-4808

Medicare Durable Medical Equipment
United Health Care Insurance Co.
(formerly MetraHealth)
P. O. Box 6800
Wilkes-Barre, PA 18773-6800

Medicare Fiscal Agent or Carrier
Veritus Medicare Services
120 Fifth Avenue, Suite P5101
Pittsburgh, PA 15222-30999

State Board of Medical Examiners
New Jersey State Board of Medical Examiners
140 E. Front Street, 2nd Floor (08608)
P. O. Box 183
Trenton, NJ 08625-0183

Temporary Disability Insurance
New Jersey Department of Labor
Division of Temporary Disability Insurance
CN 387
Trenton, NJ 08625-0387

TRICARE Claim Office
Palmetto Government Benefits Administrators
P. O. Box 7011
Camden, SC 29020-7011

Veterans Affairs Installation
New Jersey Medical Centers:
  East Orange 07018 (385 Tremont Avenue)
  Lyons 07939 (151 Knollkroft Road)

Workers' Compensation Federal District Office
Office of Workers' Compensation Programs

201 Varick Street, Room 750
P. O. Box 566
New York, NY 10014-0566

Workers' Compensation State Plan Office
Department of Labor
Division of Workers' Compensation
P. O. Box 381
Trenton, NJ 08625-0381

NEW MEXICO

CHAMPVA Claim Office
CHAMPVA Center
4500 Cherry Creek Drive, South
P. O. Box 65024
Denver, CO 80206-9024

Insurance Commissioner State Office
Superintendent
Department of Insurance
P. O. Drawer 1269
Santa Fe, NM 87504-1269

Maternal and Child Health Program
Children's Medical Services
Department of Health, PHD
Family Health Bureau
1190 St. Francis Drive
P. O. Box 26110
Santa Fe, NM 87502

Department of Health, PHD
Family Health Bureau
525 Camino de los Marquez, Suite 6
Santa Fe, NM 87501

Medicaid Fiscal Agent
Consultec, Inc. (EC)
P. O. Box 25700
Albuquerque, NM 87125-0700

Medicare Durable Medical Equipment
Palmetto Government Benefits Administrators
Medicare DMERC Operations
P. O. Box 10041
Columbia, SC 29202-3141

Medicare Fiscal Agent or Carrier
Arkansas Blue Cross and Blue Shield
601 Gaines Street
Little Rock, AR 72201

State Board of Medical Examiners
New Mexico State Board of Medical Examiners
Lamy Building, 2nd Floor
491 Old Santa Fe Trail
Santa Fe, NM 87501

New Mexico Board of Osteopathic Medical Examiners
2055 South Pacheco, Suite 400
P. O. Box 25101
Santa Fe, NM 87504

TRICARE Claim Office
Palmetto Government Benefits Administrators
P. O. Box 870032

Surfside Beach, SC 29587-8732

Veterans Affairs Installation
New Mexico Medical Center:
    Albuquerque 87108 (1501 San Pedro Street, SE)

Workers' Compensation Federal District Office
Office of Workers' Compensation Program
525 Griffin Street, Room 100
Dallas, TX 75202

Workers' Compensation State Plan Office
Workers' Compensation Administration
2410 Centre Street, S.E.
P. O. Box 27198
Albuquerque, NM 87125-7198

NEW YORK

CHAMPVA Claim Office
CHAMPVA Center
4500 Cherry Creek Drive, South
P. O. Box 65024
Denver, CO 80206-9024

Disability Benefits Bureau
See Temporary Disability Insurance

Insurance Commissioner State Office
Consumer Services Bureau
NYS Insurance Department
Agency Bldg. 1-ESP
Empire State Plaza
Albany, NY 12257

Consumer Services Bureau
NYS Insurance Department
65 Court Street #7
Buffalo, NY 14202

Consumer Services Bureau
NYS Insurance Department
25 Beaver Street
New York, NY 10014-2319

Maternal and Child Health Program
Division of Family and Local Health
New York State Department of Health
Corning Tower Building, Room 890
Albany, NY 12237-0621

Bureau of Child and Adolescent Health
New York State Department of Health
Corning Tower Building, Room 821
Albany, NY 12237

Medicaid Fiscal Agent
Computer Sciences Corporation (EC)
P. O. Box 4444
Albany, NY 12204-0444

Medicare Durable Medical Equipment
United Health Care Insurance Company
(formerly MetraHealth)
P. O. Box 6800
Wilkes-Barre, PA 18773-6800

Medicare Fiscal Agent or Carrier
Counties of Bronx, Columbia, Delaware, Dutchess, Greene, Kings, Nassau, New York, Orange, Putnam, Richmond, Rockland, Suffolk, Sullivan, Ulster, and Westchester

Empire Blue Cross and Blue Shield (EC)
622 Third Avenue
New York, NY 10017

County of Queens
Group Health, Inc. (EC)
88 West End Avenue
New York, NY 10023

Rest of the state:
Blue Cross and Blue Shield of Western New York, Inc.
P. O. Box 5236
Binghamton, NY 13905-5236

State Board of Medical Examiners
New York State Board for Medicine
Cultural Education Center, Room 3023
Empire State Plaza
Albany, NY 12230

New York Board for Professional Medical Conduct
New York State Department of Health
433 River Street, Suite 303
Troy, NY 12180-2299

Temporary Disability Insurance
Workers' Compensation Board
Disability Benefits Bureau
100 Broadway (Menands)
Albany, NY 12241

TRICARE Claim Office
Palmetto Government Benefits Administrators
P. O. Box 7011
Camden, SC 29020-7011

Veterans Affairs Installation
New York Medical Centers:

  Albany 12208 (113 Holland Avenue)
  Batavia 14020 (222 Richmond Avenue)
  Bath 14810 (76 Veterans Avenue)
  Bronx 10468 (130 W. Kingsbridge Road)
  Brooklyn 11209 (800 Poly Place)
  Buffalo 14215 (3495 Bailey Avenue)
  Canandaigua 14424 (400 Fort Hill Avenue)
  Castle Point 12511 (Route 9D)
  Montrose 10548 (138 Albany Post Road)
  New York City 10010 (423 E. 23rd Street)
  Northport 11768 (79 Middleville Road)
  St. Albans 11425 (179 Street & Linden Blvd.)
  Syracuse 13210 (800 Irvine Avenue)

Workers' Compensation Federal District Office
Office of Workers' Compensation Programs
201 Varick Street, Room 750
P. O. Box 566
New York, NY 10014-0556

Workers' Compensation State Plan Office
Workers' Compensation Board

100 Broadway-Menands
Albany, NY Y2241

NORTH CAROLINA

CHAMPVA Claim Office
CHAMPVA Center
4500 Cherry Creek Drive, South
P. O. Box 65024
Denver, CO 80206-9024

Insurance Commissioner State Office
Commissioner
Department of Insurance
Dobbs Building
430 N. Salisbury Street
P. O. Box 26387
Raleigh, NC 27611

Maternal and Child Health Program
Division of Women's and Children's Health
Department of Health and Human Services
1916 Mail Service Center
Raleigh, NC 27699-1916

Children & Youth Section
Department of Health and Human Services
1916 Mail Service Center
Raleigh, NC 27699-1916

Medicaid Fiscal Agent
Electronic Data Systems Federal Corporation (EC)
4905 Wateredge Drive (27606)
P. O. Box 30968
Raleigh, NC 27622

Medicare Durable Medical Equipment
Palmetto Government Benefits Administrators
Medicare DMERC Operations
P. O. Box 100141
Columbia, SC 29202-3141

Medicare Fiscal Agent or Carrier
CIGNA Medicare
P. O. Box 671
Nashville, TN 37202

State Board of Medical Examiners
North Carolina Medical Board
1201 Front Street (27609)
P. O. Box 20007
Raleigh, NC 27619-0007

TRICARE Claim Office
Palmetto Government Benefits Administrators
P. O. Box 7021
Camden, SC 29020-7021

Veterans Affairs Installation
North Carolina Medical Centers:

  Asheville 28805 (1100 Tunnel Road)
  Durham 27705 (508 Fulton Street)
  Fayetteville 28301 (2300 Ramsey Street)
  Salisbury 28144 (1601 Brenner Avenue)

Workers' Compensation Federal District Office
Office of Workers' Compensation Programs

214 North Hogan Street, Suite 1006
Jacksonville, FL 32202

Workers' Compensation State Plan Office
Industrial Commission
Dobbs Building
430 N. Salisbury Street
Raleigh, NC 27611

NORTH DAKOTA

CHAMPVA Claim Office
CHAMPVA Center
4500 Cherry Creek Drive, South
P. O. Box 65024
Denver, CO 80206-9024

Insurance Commissioner State Office
Commissioner
Department of Insurance
600 E. Boulevard Avenue, Dept. 401
Bismarck, ND 58505-0320

Maternal and Child Health Program
Children's Special Health Services
North Dakota Department of Human Services
600 E. Boulevard Avenue, Dept. 325
Bismarck, ND 58505-0269

Division of Maternal and Child Health
North Dakota Department of Health
600 E. Boulevard Avenue, Dept. 301
Bismarck, ND 58505-0200

Medicaid Fiscal Agent
Department of Human Services (EC)
Medical Services
600 East Avenue
Bismarck, ND 58505-0261

Medicare Durable Medical Equipment
CIGNA Medicare Region D DMERC
P. O. Box 690
Nashville, TN 37202

Medicare Fiscal Agent or Carrier
Blue Cross and Blue Shield of North Dakota
4305 13th Avenue, SW (58103)
P. O. Box 6706
Fargo, ND 58108

State Board of Medical Examiners
North Dakota State Board of Medical Examiners
City Center Plaza
418 E. Broadway, Suite 12
Bismarck, ND 58501

TRICARE Claim Office
Palmetto Government Benefits Administrators
P. O. Box 870031
Surfside Beach, SC 29587-8731

Veterans Affairs Installation
North Dakota Medical Center
2101 North Elm Street
Fargo, ND 58102

Workers' Compensation Federal District Office
Office of Workers' Compensation Programs
1801 California Street, Suite 915
Denver, CO 80202

Workers' Compensation State Plan Office
Workers' Compensation Bureau
500 E. Front Avenue
Bismarck, ND 58504-5685

OHIO

CHAMPVA Claim Office
CHAMPVA Center
4500 Cherry Creek Drive, South
P. O. Box 65024
Denver, CO 80206-9024

Insurance Commissioner State Office
Director
Department of Insurance
2100 Stella Court
Columbus, OH 43215-1067

Maternal and Child Health Program
Division of Family and Community Health Services
Ohio Department of Public Health
246 N. High Street
P. O. Box 118
Columbus, OH 43216-0118

Ohio Department of Public Health
Bureau for Children with Medical Handicaps
P. O. Box 1603
Columbus, OH 43216-1603

Medicaid Fiscal Agent
Ohio Department of Human Services
P. O. Box 1461
Columbus, OH 43216-1461

Medicare Durable Medical Equipment
Assigned:
AdminaStar Federal, Inc.
Attn: DMERC Operations
P. O. Box 7027
Indianapolis, IN 46207-7027

Nonassigned:
P. O. Box 7031
Indianapolis, IN 46207-7931

Medicare Fiscal Agent or Carrier
Nationwide/Medicare
P. O. Box 16788
Columbus, OH 43216-6788

State Board of Medical Examiners
State Medical Board of Ohio
77 S. High Street, 17th Floor
Columbus, OH 43266-0315

TRICARE Claim Office
Palmetto Government Benefits Administrators
P. O. Box 7021
Camden, SC 29020-7021

Veterans Affairs Installation
Ohio Medical Centers:
  Brecksville 44141 (10000 Brecksville Road)
  Chillicothe 45601 (17273 State Route 104)
  Cincinnati 45220 (3200 Vine Street)
  Cleveland 44106 (10701 East Blvd.)
  Dayton 45428 (4100 W. 3rd Street)

Workers' Compensation Federal District Office
Office of Workers' Compensation Programs
1240 E. Ninth Street, Room 851
Cleveland, OH 44199

Workers' Compensation State Plan Office
Industrial Commission
30 W. Spring Street
Columbus, OH 43215-0581

Bureau of Workers' Compensation
30 W. Spring Street
Columbus, OH 43266-0581

OKLAHOMA

CHAMPVA Claim Office
CHAMPVA Center
4500 Cherry Creek Drive, South
P. O. Box 65024
Denver, CO 80206-9024

Insurance Commissioner State Office
Commissioner
Department of Insurance
3814 North Santa Fe
P. O. Box 53408
Oklahoma City, OK 73152-3408

Maternal and Child Health Program
Maternal and Child Health Service
Oklahoma State Department of Health
1000 NE Tenth Street
Oklahoma City, OK 73117-1299

Family Support Services
Department of Human Services
P. O. Box 25352
Oklahoma City, OK 73125

Medicaid Fiscal Agent
UNISYS Corp.
201 NW 63rd, Suite 100 (73116)
P. O. Box 54740
Oklahoma City, OK 73154

Medicare Durable Medical Equipment
Palmetto Government Benefits Administrators
Medicare DMERC Operations
P. O. Box 100141
Columbia, SC 29202-3141

Medicare Fiscal Agent or Carrier
Arkansas Blue Cross and Blue Shield
601 Gaines Street
Little Rock, AR 72201

State Board of Medical Examiners
Oklahoma State Board of Medical Licensure &

Supervision
5104 N. Francis, Suite C 73118
P. O. Box 18256
Oklahoma City, OK 73154-0256

Oklahoma State Board of Osteopathic Examiners
4848 N. Lincoln Blvd., Suite 100
Oklahoma City, OK 73105-3321

TRICARE Claim Office
Wisconsin Physicians Service
P. O. Box 8999
Madison WI 53708-8999

Veterans Affairs Installation
Oklahoma Medical Centers:
  Muskogee 74401 (1011 Honor Heights Drive)
  Oklahoma City 73104 (921 NE 13th Street)

Workers' Compensation Federal District Office
Office of Workers' Compensation Programs
525 Griffin Street, Room 100
Dallas, TX 75202

Workers' Compensation State Plan Office
Oklahoma Workers' Compensation Court
1915 N. Stiles Avenue
Oklahoma City, OK 73105-4904

OREGON

CHAMPVA Claim Office
CHAMPVA Center
4500 Cherry Creek Drive, South
P. O. Box 65024
Denver, CO 80206-9024

Insurance Commissioner State Office
Director
Department of Consumer and Business Services
350 Winter Street, NE, Room 440-2
Salem, OR 97310-0765

Maternal and Child Health Program
Oregon State Health Division
800 NE Oregon Street, Suite 850
Portland, OR 97232

Child Development and Rehabilitation Center
P. O. Box 574
Portland, OR 97207-0574

Medicaid Fiscal Agent
Office of Medical Assistance Program
P. O. Box 14955
Salem, OR 97309

Medicare Durable Medical Equipment
CIGNA Medicare Region D DMERC
P. O. Box 690
Nashville, TN 37202

Medicare Fiscal Agent or Carrier
Noridian Mutual Insurance Company
4305 13th Avenue SW
Fargo, ND 58108-6702

State Board of Medical Examiners
Oregon Board of Medical Examiners
620 Crown Plaza
1500 SW First Avenue
Portland, OR 97201-5826

TRICARE Claim Office
Wisconsin Physician Service
TRICARE Northwest
P. O. Box 8929
Madison, WI 53708-8929

Veterans Affairs Installation
Oregon Medical Centers:
   Portland 97201 (3710 SW U.S. Veterans Hospital Road)
   Roseburg 97470 (913 NW Garden Valley Blvd.)

Workers' Compensation Federal District Office
Office of Workers' Compensation Programs
1111 Third Avenue, Suite 615
Seattle, WA 98101

Workers' Compensation State Plan Office
Department of Consumer and Business Services
Workers' Compensation Division
350 Winter Street NE, Room 21
Salem, OR 97310-0220

Workers' Compensation Board
2250 McGilcrist SE
Salem, OR 97310

PENNSYLVANIA

CHAMPVA Claim Office
CHAMPVA Center
4500 Cherry Creek Drive, South
P. O. Box 65024
Denver, CO 80206-9024

Insurance Commissioner State Office
Commissioner
Insurance Department
1326 Strawberry Square, 13th Floor
Harrisburg, PA 17120

Maternal and Child Health Program
Division of Maternal and Child Health
Pennsylvania Department of Health
Room 733, Health and Welfare Building
P. O. Box 90
Harrisburg, PA 17108

Pennsylvania Department of Health
Division of CSHCN
Room 724, Health and Welfare Building
P. O. Box 90
Harrisburg, PA 17108

Medicaid Fiscal Agent
Department of Public Welfare
515 Health and Welfare Bldg.
7th and Forster Streets (17120)
P. O. Box 2675
Harrisburg, PA 17105-2675

Medicare Durable Medical Equipment
United Health Care Insurance Company

(formerly MetraHealth)
P. O. Box 6800
Wilkes-Barre, PA 18773-6800

Medicare Fiscal Agent or Carrier
HGS Administrators
(formerly Xact Medicare Services)
P. O. Box 890065
Camp Hill, PA 17089-0065

Part B/Eastern PA:
P. O. Box 890418
Camp Hill, PA 17089

Part B/Western PA:
P. O. Box 890318
Camp Hill, PA 17089

State Board of Medical Examiners
Pennsylvania State Board of Medicine
124 Pine Street (17101)
P. O. Box 2649
Harrisburg, PA 17105-2649

Pennsylvania State Board of Osteopathic Medicine
124 Pine Street (17101)
P. O. Box 2649
Harrisburg, PA 17105-2649

TRICARE Claim Office
Palmetto Government Benefits Administrators
P. O. Box 7011
Camden, SC 29020-7011

Veterans Affairs Installation
Pennsylvania Medical Centers:
   Altoona 16602 (2907 Pleasant Valley Road)
   Butler 16001 (325 New Castle Road)
   Coatesville 19320 (1400 Black Horse Hill Road)
   Erie 16504-1596 (135 E. 38th Street)
   Lebanon 17042 (1700 South Lincoln Avenue)
   Philadelphia 19104 (University & Woodland Avenues)
   Pittsburgh 15215 (Delafield Road.)
   Pittsburgh 15206 (7180 Highland Drive)
   Pittsburgh 15240 (University Drive C)
   Wilkes-Barre 18711 (1111 East End Blvd.)

Workers' Compensation Federal District Office
Office of Workers' Compensation Programs
Gateway Building, Room 15200
3535 Market Street
Philadelphia, PA 19104

Workers' Compensation State Plan Office
Bureau of Workers' Compensation
Department of Labor and Industry
1171 S. Cameron Street, Room 324
Harrisburg, PA 17104-2501

Workers' Compensation Appeal Board
901 North 7th Street, 3rd Floor South
Harrisburg, PA 17102-0034

PUERTO RICO

CHAMPVA Claim Office
CHAMPVA Center
4500 Cherry Creek Drive, South

P. O. Box 65024
Denver, CO 80206-9024

Insurance Commissioner State Office
Commissioner
Office of the Commission of Insurance
Fernandez Juncos Station
1607 Ponce de Leon Avenue
P. O. Box 8330
San Juan, PR 00910-8330

Maternal and Child Health Program
CSHCN Director
Puerto Rico Department of Health
Call Box 70184
San Juan, PR 00936-8184

Maternal Child Health Director
Puerto Rico Department of Health
Call Box 70184
San Juan, PR 00936-8184

Medicare Durable Medical Equipment
Palmetto Government Benefits Administrators
Medicare DMERC Operations
P. O. Box 100141
Columbia, SC 29202-3141

Medicare Fiscal Agent or Carrier
Triple-S, Inc.
Call Box 71391
San Juan, PR 00936-1391

State Board of Medical Examiners
Board of Medical Examiners of Puerto Rico
Kennedy Avenue, ILA Building, Hogar del Obrero
Portuario, Piso 8, Puerto Nuevo (00920)
P. O. Box 13969
San Juan, PR 00908

Temporary Disability Insurance
Department of Labor and Human Resources
Bureau of Employment Security
Disability Insurance Program
Prudencio Rivera Martinez Building
505 Munoz Rivera Avenue
Hato Rey, PR 00918

TRICARE Claim Office
Wisconsin Physicians Service
P. O. Box 7985
Madison, WI 53707-7985

Veterans Affairs Installation
Puerto Rico Medical Center
10 Casia Street
San Juan, PR 00927

Workers' Compensation Federal District
Office of Workers' Compensation Programs
201 Varick Street, Room 750
P. O. Box 566
New York, NY 10014-0566

Workers' Compensation State Plan Office
Corporation of the State Insurance Fund
G. P. O. Box 365028
San Juan, PR 00936-5028

Industrial Commission
G. P. O. Box 364466
San Juan, PR 00936-4466

RHODE ISLAND

CHAMPVA Claim Office
CHAMPVA Center
4500 Cherry Creek Drive, South
P. O. Box 65024
Denver, CO 80206-9024

Insurance Commissioner State Office
Commissioner
Insurance Division
233 Richmond Street, Suite 233
Providence, RI 02903-4233

Maternal and Child Health Program
Division of Family Health
Rhode Island Department of Health
Three Capitol Hill, Room 302
Providence, RI 02908-5097

Medicaid Fiscal Agent
Electronic Data Systems Federal Corporation
P. O. Box 2009
Warwick, RI 02887

Medicaid Rhode Island
Medical Services Department
600 New London Avenue
Cranston, RI 02920-3037

Medicare Durable Medical Equipment
United Health Care Insurance Company
(formerly MetraHealth)
P. O. Box 6800
Wilkes-Barre, PA 18773-6800

Medicare Fiscal Agent or Carrier
Blue Cross and Blue Shield of Rhode Island (EC)
444 Westminster Street
Providence, RI 02903-3279

State Board of Medical Examiners
Rhode Island Board of Licensure & Discipline
Department of Health
Cannon Building, Room 205
Three Capitol Hill
Providence, RI 02908-5097

Temporary Disability Insurance
Department of Employment and Training
Temporary Disability Insurance Division
P. O. Box 1028
Providence, RI 02901-1028

TRICARE Claim Office
Palmetto Government Benefits Administrators
P. O. Box 7011
Camden, SC 29020-7011

Veterans Affairs Installation
Rhode Island Medical Center
830 Chalkstone Avenue
Providence, RI 02908

Workers' Compensation Federal District Office
Office of Workers' Compensation Programs
JFK Federal Office Building, Room E-260
Boston, MA 02203

Workers' Compensation State Plan Office
Department of Labor and Training
Division of Workers' Compensation
610 Manton Avenue
P. O. Box 20190
Providence, RI 02920-0942

Workers' Compensation Court
1 Dorrance Plaza
Providence, RI 02903

SOUTH CAROLINA

CHAMPVA Claim Office
CHAMPVA Center
4500 Cherry Creek Drive, South
P. O. Box 65024
Denver, CO 80206-9024

Insurance Commissioner State Office
Director
Department of Insurance
1612 Marion Street (24201)
P. O. Box 100105
Columbia, SC 29202-3105

Maternal and Child Health Program
Bureau of Maternal and Child Health
Department of Health & Environmental Control
Mills/Jarrett Complex
1751 Calhoun Street
P. O. Box 101106
Columbia, SC 29211

Division of Children's Rehabilitative Services
Department of Health & Environmental Control
Mills/Jarrett Complex
1751 Calhoun Street
P. O. Box 101106
Columbia, SC 29211

Medicaid Fiscal Agent
Department of Human Services (EC)
P. O. Box 8206
Columbia, SC 29202-8206

Medicare Durable Medical Equipment
Palmetto Government Benefits Administrators
Medicare DMERC Operations
P. O. Box 100141
Columbia, SC 29202-3141

Medicare Fiscal Agent or Carrier
Medicare Part B
Blue Cross and Blue Shield of South Carolina (EC)
Dba. Palmetto Government Benefits Administrators
P. O. Box 100190
Columbia, SC 29202-3190

State Board of Medical Examiners
South Carolina State Board of Medical Examiners
Department of Labor, Licensing, and Regulation

110 Centerview Drive, Suite 202 (29210)
P. O. Box 11289
Columbia, SC 29211-1289

TRICARE Claim Office
Palmetto Government Benefits Administrators
P. O. Box 7032
Camden, SC 29020-7032

Veterans Affairs Installation
South Carolina Medical Centers:
  Charleston 29401 (109 Bee Street)
  Columbia 29209 (6439 Garners Ferry Road)

Workers' Compensation Federal District Office
Office of Workers' Compensation Programs
214 North Hogan Street, Suite 1006
Jacksonville, FL 32202

Workers' Compensation State Plan Office
Workers' Compensation Commission
1612 Marion Street
P. O. Box 1715
Columbia, SC 29202-1715

SOUTH DAKOTA

CHAMPVA Claim Office
CHAMPVA Center
4500 Cherry Creek Drive, South
P. O. Box 65024
Denver, CO 80206-9024

Insurance Commissioner State Office
Director
Division of Insurance
Department of Commerce and Regulation
118 W. Capitol Avenue
Pierre, SD 57501-2000

Maternal and Child Health Program
Children's Special Health Services
South Dakota Department of Health
615 East 4th Street
Pierre, SD 57501-3185

Office of Family Health
South Dakota Department of Health
615 East 4th Street
Pierre, SD 57501-3185

Medicaid Fiscal Agent
Department of Social Services (EC)
Office of Medicaid/Richard F. Kneip Building
700 Governors Drive
Pierre, SD 57501-2291

Medicare Durable Medical Equipment
CIGNA Medicare Region D DMERC
P. O. Box 690
Nashville, TN 37202

Medicare Fiscal Agent or Carrier
Noridian Mutual Insurance Company
4305 13th Avenue SW
Fargo, ND 58103

State Board of Medical Examiners
South Dakota State Board of Medical & Osteopathic
Examiners
1323 S. Minnesota Avenue
Sioux Falls, SD 57105

TRICARE Claim Office
P. O. Box 870031
Surfside Beach, SC 29587-8731

Veterans' Affairs Installation
South Dakota Medical Centers:

  Fort Meade 57741 (113 Comanche Road)
  Hot Springs 57747 (500 N. 5th Street)
  Sioux Falls 57117 (2501 W. 22nd Street)

Workers' Compensation Federal District Office
Office of Workers' Compensation Programs
1801 California Street, Suite 915
Denver, CO 80202

Workers' Compensation State Plan Office
Division of Labor and Management
Department of Labor
Kneip Building, Third Floor
700 Governors Drive
Pierre, SD 57501-2291

TENNESSEE

CHAMPVA Claim Office
CHAMPVA Center
4500 Cherry Creek Drive, South
P. O. Box 65024
Denver, CO 80206-9024

Insurance Commissioner State Office
Commissioner
Department of Commerce and Insurance
500 James Robertson Parkway, 5th Floor
Nashville, TN 37243-0565

Maternal and Child Health Program
Maternal and Child Health
Tennessee Department of Health
5th Floor, Cordell Hull Building
425 5th Avenue, North
Nashville, TN 37247-4701

Medicaid Fiscal Agent
Electronic Data Systems Federal Corp.
729 Church Street, 3rd Floor
Nashville, TN 37243

Medicare Durable Medical Equipment
Palmetto Government Benefits Administrators
Medicare DMERC Operations
P. O. Box 100141
Columbia, SC 29202-3141

Medicare Fiscal Agent or Carrier
CIGNA Medicare
P. O. Box 1465
Nashville, TN 37202-1465

State Board of Medical Examiners
Tennessee Board of Medical Examiners
1st Floor, Cordell Hull Building

425 5th Avenue North
Nashville, TN 37247-1010

Tennessee State Board of Osteopathic Examiners
1st Floor, Cordell Hull Building
425 5th Avenue North
Nashville, TN 37247-1010

TRICARE Claim Office
Palmetto Government Benefits Administrators
P. O. Box 7032
Camden, SC 29020-7032

Veterans Affairs Installation
Tennessee Medical Centers:

  Memphis 38104 (1030 Jefferson Avenue)
  Mountain Home 37684 (Sidney & Lamont Streets)
  Murfreesboro 37129 (3400 Lebanon Road)
  Nashville 37212 (1310 24th Avenue, South)

Workers' Compensation Federal District Office
Office of Workers' Compensation Program
214 North Hogan Street, Suite 1006
Jacksonville, FL 32202

Workers' Compensation State Plan Office
Workers' Compensation Division
Department of Labor
710 James Robertson Parkway
Andrew Johnson Tower, Second Floor
Nashville, TN 37243-0661

TEXAS

CHAMPVA Claim Office
CHAMPVA Center
4500 Cherry Creek Drive, South
P. O. Box 65024
Denver, CO 80206-9024

Insurance Commissioner State Office
Commissioner
Department of Insurance
333 Guadalupe Street
P. O. Box 149104
Austin, TX 78714-9104

Maternal and Child Health Program
Bureau of Children's Health
Texas Department of Health
1100 W. 49th Street
Austin, TX 78756-3199

Medicaid Fiscal Agent
National Heritage Insurance Company
P. O. Box 200555
Austin, TX 78720-0555

Medicare Durable Medical Equipment
Palmetto Government Benefits Administrators
Medicare DMERC Operations
P. O. Box 100141
Columbia, SC 29202-3141

Medicare Fiscal Agent or Carrier
Part B Participating:
Medicare/Blue Cross and Blue Shield of Texas, Inc.

Dba. Trail Blazer Health Enterprises, Inc.
P. O. Box 660031
Dallas, TX 75266-0031

Part B Nonparticipating:
Blue Cross and Blue Shield of Texas
P. O. Box 660094
Dallas, TX 75266-0094

State Board of Medical Examiners
Texas State Board of Medical Examiners
333 Guadalupe, Tower 3, Suite 610 (78701)
P. O. Box 2018
Austin, TX 78768-2018

TRICARE Claim Office
*For William Beaumont Catchment area and Cannon
AFB, New Mexico catchment area ZIP codes that fall in
Texas:*
Palmetto Government Benefits Administrators
P. O. Box 870032
Surfside Beach, SC 29587-8732

*Except William Beaumont catchment area and Cannon
AFB, New Mexico, catchment area ZIP codes that fall in
Texas:*
Wisconsin Physicians Services
P. O. Box 8999
Madison, WI 53708-8999

Veterans Affairs Installation
Texas Medical Centers:

   Amarillo 79106 (6010 Amarillo Blvd., West)
   Big Spring 79720 (300 Veterans Blvd.)
   Bonham 75418 (1201 E. Ninth Street)
   Dallas 75216 (4500 S. Lancaster Road)
   Houston 77030 (2002 Holcombe Blvd.)
   Kerrville 78028 (3600 Memorial Blvd.)
   Marlin 76661 (1016 Ward Street)
   San Antonio 78284 (7400 Merton Minter Blvd.)
   Temple 76504 (1901 Veterans Memorial Drive)
   Waco 76711 (4800 Memorial Drive)

Workers' Compensation Federal District Office
Office of Workers' Compensation Program
525 Griffin Street, Room 100
Dallas, TX 75202

Workers' Compensation State Plan Office
Workers' Compensation Commission
Southfield Building, MS-4C
4000 South IH 35
Austin, TX 78704-7491

UTAH

CHAMPVA Claim Office
CHAMPVA Center
4500 Cherry Creek Drive, South
P. O. Box 65024
Denver, CO 80206-9024

Insurance Commissioner State Office
Commissioner
Department of Insurance
State Office Building, Suite 3110
Salt Lake City, UT 84114-6901

Maternal and Child Health Program
Community and Family Health Services
Utah Department of Health
P. O. Box 144610
Salt Lake City, UT 84114-4610

Community & Family Health Services Division
Utah Department of Health
P. O. Box 142001
Salt Lake City, UT 84114-2001

Medicaid Fiscal Agent
Bureau of Medicaid Operations
P. O. Box 143106
Salt Lake City, UT 84114-3106

Medicare Durable Medical Equipment
CIGNA Medicare Region D DMERC
P. O. Box 690
Nashville, TN 37202

Medicare Fiscal Agent or Carrier
Medicare/Blue Cross and Blue Shield of Utah
P. O. Box 30269, Dept. 14
Salt Lake City, UT 84130-0269

State Board of Medical Examiners
Utah Department of Commerce
Division of Occupational & Professional Licensure
Heber M. Wells Building, 4th Floor
160 East 300 South (84102)
P. O. Box 146741
Salt Lake City, UT 84114-6741

TRICARE Claim Office
Palmetto Government Benefits Administrators
P. O. Box 870032
Surfside Beach, SC 29587-8732

Veterans Administration Installation
Utah Medical Center
500 Foothill Drive
Salt Lake City, UT 84148

Workers' Compensation Federal District Office
Office of Workers' Compensation Program
1801 California Street, Suite 915
Denver, CO 80202

Workers' Compensation State Plan Office
Industrial Accident Division
Labor Commission
P. O. Box 146610
Salt Lake City, UT 84114-6610

VERMONT

CHAMPVA Claim Office
CHAMPVA Center
4500 Cherry Creek Drive, South
P. O. Box 65024
Denver, CO 80206-9024

Insurance Commissioner State Office
Commissioner
Department of Banking, Insurance, and Securities
and Health Care Administration
89 Main Street, Drawer 20
Montpelier, VT 05620-3101

Maternal and Child Health Program
Children with Special Health Care Needs
Vermont Department of Health
108 Cherry Street
P. O. Box 70
Burlington, VT 05402

Maternal and Child Health
Vermont Department of Health
108 Cherry Street
P. O. Box 70
Burlington, VT 05402-0070

Medicaid Fiscal Agent
Electronic Data Systems Federal Corporation (EC)
P. O. Box 888
Williston, VT 05495-0888

Medicare Durable Medical Equipment
United Health Care Insurance Co.
(formerly MetraHealth)
P. O. Box 6800
Wilkes-Barre, PA 18773-6800

Medicare Fiscal Agent or Carrier
National Heritage Insurance Company
450 West East Avenue
Chico, CA 95973

State Board of Medical Examiners
Vermont Board of Medical Practice
One Prospect Street
Montpelier, VT 05609-1106

Vermont Board of Osteopathic Physicians and Surgeons
26 Terrace Street
Drawer 09
Montpelier, VT 05609-1106

TRICARE Claim Office
Palmetto Government Benefits Administrators
P. O. Box 7011
Camden, SC 29020-7011

Veterans Affairs Installation
Vermont Medical Center
215 North Main Street
White River Junction, VT 05009

Workers' Compensation Federal District Office
Office of Workers' Compensation Programs
JFK Federal Office Building, Room E-260
Boston, MA 02203

Workers' Compensation State Plan Office
Department of Labor and Industry
National Life Building
Drawer 20
Montpelier, VT 05620-3401

VIRGIN ISLANDS

CHAMPVA Claim Office
CHAMPVA Center
4500 Cherry Creek Drive, South
P. O. Box 65024
Denver, CO 80206-9024

Insurance Commissioner State Office
Director
Division of Banking and Insurance
1131 King Street, Suite 101
Christiansted
St. Croix, VI 00820

Maternal and Child Health Program
Department of Health MCH and CSHCN
ElaineCo Building Complex, 2ND Floor
St. Thomas, VI 00802

Maternal and Child Health and Children with Special
Health Care Needs
3012 Vitraco Mall
Estate Golden Rock
Christiansted
St. Croix, VI 00820-4320

Medicare Durable Medical Equipment
Palmetto Government Benefits Administrators
Medicare DMERC Operations
P. O. Box 100141
Columbia, SC 29202-3141

Medicare Fiscal Agent or Carrier
Medicare/Triple-S, Inc.
Call Box 71391
San Juan, Puerto Rico 00936-1391

Medicare Railroad Retiree Carrier
Medicare Part B Claims are handled by claim service
centers. For the address and toll-free number of the office nearest you, call the Railroad Retirement Board
listed in your telephone directory under U.S. Government.

State Board of Medical Examiners
Virgin Islands Board of Medical Examiners
Virgin Islands Department of Health
48 Sugar Estate
St. Thomas, VI 00802

Veterans Affairs Installation
For information on VA benefits call 1-800-827-1000

Workers' Compensation Federal District Office
Office of Workers' Compensation Programs
201 Varick Street, Room 750
P. O. Box 566
New York, NY 10014-0566

Workers' Compensation State Plan Office
Department of Labor
Workers' Compensation Division
3012 Vitraco Mall, Golden Rock
Christiansted
St. Croix, VI 00820-4466

VIRGINIA

CHAMPVA Claim Office
CHAMPVA Center
4500 Cherry Creek Drive, South
Box 65024
Denver, CO 80206-9024

Insurance Commissioner State Office
Commissioner
State Corporation Commission
Bureau of Insurance
1300 E. Main Street
P. O. Box 1157
Richmond, VA 23218

Maternal and Child Health Program
Office of Family Health Services
1500 E. Main Street, Suite 104
Richmond, VA 23219

CSHCN Program
Division of Child and Adolescent Health
1500 E. Main Street, Suite 138
P. O. Box 2448
Richmond, VA 23219

Medicaid Fiscal Agent
HCFA
P. O. Box 27444
Richmond, VA 23261

Medicare Durable Medical Equipment
Assigned:
AdminaStar Federal, Inc.
Attn: DMERC Operations
P. O. Box 70727
Indianapolis, IN 46207-7027

Nonassigned:
P. O. Box 7031
Indianapolis, IN 46207-7931

Medicare Fiscal Agent or Carrier
Blue Cross and Blue Shield of Texas
Dba. Trail Blazer Health Enterprises, Inc.
P. O. Box 660031
Dallas, TX 75266-0031

State Board of Medical Examiners
Virginia Board of Medicine
6606 W. Broad Street, 4th Floor
Richmond, VA 23230-1717

TRICARE Claim Offices
Certain Northern Virginia ZIP codes located near the Washington, DC, area and a few ZIP codes in the northeast part of West Virginia:
Palmetto Government Benefits Administrators
P. O. Box 7011
Camden, SC 29020-7011

Most of Virginia:
Palmetto Government Benefits Administrators
P. O. Box 7021
Camden, SC 29020-7021

Veterans Affairs Installation
Virginia Medical Centers:

Hampton 23667 (100 Emancipation Drive)
Richmond 23249 (1201 Broad Rock Road)
Salem 24153 (1970 Roanoke Blvd.)

Workers' Compensation Federal District Office
Office of Workers' Compensation Programs

800 N. Capitol Street, NW, Room 800
Washington, DC 20211

Workers' Compensation State Plan Office
Workers' Compensation Commission
1000 DMV Drive (23220)
P. O. Box 1794
Richmond, VA 23214

WASHINGTON

CHAMPVA Claim Office
CHAMPVA Center
4500 Cherry Creek Drive, South
Box 65024
Denver, CO 80206-9024

Insurance Commissioner State Office
Commissioner
Insurance Building-Capitol Campus
P. O. Box 40255
Olympia, WA 98504-0255

Maternal and Child Health Program
Maternal and Child Health
Washington State Department of Health
P. O. Box 47880
Olympia, WA 98504-7880

Washington State Department of Health
Community and Family Health
P. O. Box 47880, Industrial Center, Building 8
Olympia, WA 98504-7880

Medicaid Fiscal Agent
Department of Social & Health Services
Office of Provider Services
P. O. Box 9248
Olympia, WA 98507-9248

Medicare Durable Medical Equipment
CIGNA Medicare Region D DMERC
P. O. Box 690
Nashville, TN 37202

Medicare Fiscal Agent or Carrier
Noridian Mutual Insurance Company
4305 13th Avenue SW
Fargo, ND 58103

State Board of Medical Examiners
Washington Medical Quality Assurance Commission
1300 S.E. Quince Street (98501)
P. O. Box 47866
Olympia, WA 98504-7866

Washington State Board of Osteopathic Medicine and Surgery
Washington State Department of Health
1300 S.E. Quince Street (98501)
P. O. Box 47870
Olympia, WA 98504-7870

TRICARE Claim Office
Wisconsin Physicians Service
TRICARE Northwest

P. O. Box 8929
Madison, WI 53708-8929

Veterans Affairs Installation
Washington Medical Centers:

Seattle 98108 (1660 S. Columbian Way)
Spokane 99205 (N. 4815 Assembly Street)
Tacoma 98493 (9600 Veterans Drive, SW, American Lake)
Walla Walla 99362 (77 Wainwright Drive)

Workers' Compensation Federal District Office
Office of Workers' Compensation Programs
1111 Third Avenue, Suite 615
Seattle, WA 98101

Workers' Compensation State Plan Office
Board of Industrial Insurance Appeals
2430 Chandler Court, SW
P. O. Box 42401
Mail Stop FN 21
Olympia, WA 98504

Department of Labor and Industry
Headquarters Building
P. O. Box 44001
Olympia, WA 98504-4100

WEST INDIES

CHAMPVA Claim Office
CHAMPVA Center
4500 Cherry Creek Drive, South
P. O. Box 65024
Denver, CO 80206-9024

TRICARE Claim Office
Wisconsin Physicians Service
P. O. Box 7985
Madison, WI 53707-7985

WEST VIRGINIA

CHAMPVA Claim Office
CHAMPVA Center
4500 Cherry Creek Drive, South
P. O. Box 65024
Denver, CO 80206-9024

Insurance Commissioner State Office
Commissioner
Department of Insurance
1124 Smith Street
P. O. Box 50540
Charleston, WV 25305-0540

Maternal and Child Health Program
Office of Maternal and Child Health
West Virginia Department of Health
350 Capitol Street, Room 427
Charleston, WV 25301-3714

Division of Children's Specialty Care
Office of Maternal and Child Health

350 Capitol Street
Charleston, WV 25301-1757

Medicaid Fiscal Agent
Department of Health and Human Resources
Capitol Complex Bldg 6-350
Capitol Street, Suite 251
Charleston, WV 25301

Medicare Durable Medical Equipment
Assigned:
AdminaStar Federal, Inc.
Attn: DMERC Operations
P. O. Box 7027
Indianapolis, IN 46207-7027

Nonassigned:
P. O. Box 7031
Indianapolis, IN 46207-7931

Medicare Fiscal Agent or Carrier
Nationwide Mutual Insurance Company
Medicare General Correspondence
P. O. Box 16788
Columbus, OH 43216-6788

State Board of Medical Examiners
West Virginia Board of Medicine
101 Dee Drive
Charleston, WV 25311

West Virginia Board of Osteopathy
334 Penco Road
Weirton, WV 26062

TRICARE Claim Offices
Northern tip of West Virginia:
Palmetto Government Benefits Administrators
P. O. Box 7011
Camden, SC 29020-7011

Most of West Virginia:
Palmetto Government Benefits Administrators
P. O. Box 7021
Camden, SC 29020-7021

Veterans Affairs Installation
West Virginia Medical Centers:

Beckley 25801 (200 Veterans Avenue)
Clarksburg 26301 (1 Medical Center Drive)
Huntington 25704 (1540 Spring Valley Drive)
Martinsburg 25401 (Route 9)

Workers' Compensation Federal District Office
Office of Workers' Compensation Programs
Gateway Building, Room 15200
3535 Market Street
Philadelphia, PA 19104

Workers' Compensation State Plan Office
Bureau of Employment Programs
Workers' Compensation Division
4700 MacCorkle Avenue, SE (25304)
Executive Offices
P. O. Box 3151
Charleston, WV 25332-1416

Workers' Compensation Appeal Board
104 Dee Drive
P. O. Box 2628
Charleston, WV 25329

WISCONSIN

CHAMPVA Claim Office
CHAMPVA Center
4500 Cherry Creek Drive, South
P. O. Box 65024
Denver, CO 80206-9024

Insurance Commissioner State Office
Commissioner
Office of the Commissioner of Insurance
121 E. Wilson Street (53702)
P. O. Box 7873
Madison, WI 53707-7873

Maternal and Child Health Program
Children with Special Health Care Needs
Wisconsin Division of Health
One West Wilson Street
P. O. Box 2659
Madison, WI 53701-2659

Medicaid Fiscal Agent
Electronic Data Systems Federal Corporation (EC)
6406 Bridge Road
Madison, WI 53784-1846

Medicare Durable Medical Equipment
Assigned:
AdminaStar Federal, Inc.
Attn: DMERC Operations
P. O. Box 7027
Indianapolis, IN 46207-7027

Nonassigned:
P. O. Box 7031
Indianapolis, IN 46207-7931

Medicare Fiscal Agent or Carrier
Wisconsin Physicians Service
P. O. Box 1787
Madison, WI 53701

State Board of Medical Examiners
Wisconsin Medical Examining Board
Department of Regulation & Licensing
1400 E. Washington Avenue (53703)
P. O. Box 8935
Madison, WI 53708-8935

TRICARE Claim Office
Palmetto Government Benefits Administrators
P. O. Box 7021
Camden, SC 29020-7021

Veterans Affairs Installation
Wisconsin Medical Centers:

Madison 53705 (2500 Overlook Terrace)
Milwaukee 53295 (5000 W. National Avenue)
Tomah 54660 (500 E. Veterans Street)

Workers' Compensation Federal District Office
Office of Workers' Compensation Programs
230 S. Dearborn Street, 8th Floor
Chicago, IL 60604

Workers' Compensation State Plan Office
Labor and Industry Review Commission
P. O. Box 8126
Madison, WI 53708

Workers' Compensation Division
Department of Workforce Development
201 E. Washington Avenue, Room 161
P. O. Box 7901
Madison, WI 53707-7901

WYOMING

CHAMPVA Claim Office
CHAMPVA Center
4500 Cherry Creek Drive, South
P. O. Box 65024
Denver, CO 80206-9024

Insurance Commissioner State Office
Commissioner
Department of Insurance
Herschler Building
122 W. 25th Street, 3rd Floor East
Cheyenne, WY 82002-0440

Maternal and Child Health Program
Maternal and Child Health
Division of Public Health
Hathaway Building, Room 465
Cheyenne, WY 82002-0480

CSHCN
Division of Public Health
Hathaway Building, Room 467
Cheyenne, WY 82002-0480

Medicaid Fiscal Agent
Division of Health & Medical Service
6101 Yellowstone Road, #259B
Cheyenne, WY 82002

Medicare Durable Medical Equipment
CIGNA Medicare Region D DMERC
P. O. Box 690
Nashville, TN 37202

Medicare Fiscal Agent or Carrier
Noridian Mutual Insurance Company
4305 13th Avenue SW
Fargo, ND 58103

State Board of Medical Examiners
Wyoming Board of Medicine
Colony Building
211 West 19th Street, 2nd Floor
Cheyenne, WY 82002

TRICARE Claim Office
Palmetto Government Benefits Administrators
P. O. Box 870030
Surfside Beach, SC 29587-8730

Veterans Affairs Installation

Wyoming Medical Centers:

  Cheyenne 82001 (2360 E. Pershing Blvd.)

  Sheridan 82801 (1898 Fort Road)

Workers' Compensation Federal District Office

Office of Workers' Compensation Programs

1801 California Street, Suite 915

Denver, CO 80202

Workers' Compensation State Plan Office

Workers' Compensation Division

East Wing, Herschler Building, 2nd Floor

122 W. 25th Street

Cheyenne, WY 82002-0700

Entries are listed as follows: Title, edition if any, comments if any (in parentheses), author (in parentheses), date of publication or production where appropriate, and publisher. Look through the subject matter headings on this page, then review entries within the sections you select, note the name of the publisher or manufacturer, and then find this under "Name and Addresses of Resources" at the end of this Appendix.

INDEX

Automation
Billing
Certification
Charges
Claims Assistance Professionals
Coding
Collections
Compliance
Delinquent and Denied Claims
Diagnosis Related Groups
Diagnostic and Procedure Handbooks for Terminology (DPT)
Dictionaries and Glossaries
Disability Benefit Programs
Disability Income Insurance
Documentation, Medical
Education and Training
Electronic Data Interchange
Ethics
Fees, Reimbursement, Charges
Fraud and Abuse
HCFA-1500 Claim Form
HCFA Common Procedure Coding System (HCPCS)
Health Insurance
Health Maintenance Organizations/Preferred Provider Organizations
Hospital Insurance Claims
Insurance Directories
Law and Ethics

Managed Care
Medicaid
Medical Management
Medicare
Preferred Provider Organizations
Reimbursement
Relative Value Studies
Self-Employment
TRICARE
Videotapes
Workers' Compensation
Workshops and Seminars

RESOURCE LIST

AUTOMATION
See *Electronic Data Interchange*

BILLING
See *also Fees, Reimbursement, Charges*

Newsletters
The Health Care Biller (monthly publication), Aspen Publishers, Inc.

Reference Guides
Health Care Billing: A Guide to Billing Office Policies & Practices (Health Care Billing Manual), (monthly publication), Aspen Publishers, Inc.

Reports
"Countdown to UB-92" (monthly publication), Aspen Publishers, Inc.
"40 Tips Health Care Billers Can't Live Without" (monthly publication), Aspen Publishers, Inc.

CERTIFICATION
Certification Study Guide for CPAM/CCAM Exams. American Guild of Patient Account Management
Certified Coding Specialist Certification Guide. American Health Information Management Association
Certified Professional Coder/CPC-Hospital Outpatient. Independent Study Programs. American Academy of Professional Coders

annually), (Context Software Systems), McGraw-Hill Healthcare Management Group

ICD-9-CM International Classification of Diseases, 9th Revision, Clinical Modification, Volumes 1 and 2, Volumes 1, 2 and 3, or Binder Version or Hard Bound Version, Practice Management Information Corporation

ICD-9-CM to CPT Radiology Cross Code, R. B. Holt

ICD-9-CM Coding Handbook (Faye Brown), 2000, American Hospital Association

ICD-9-CM Coding in a SNAP (alphabetical listing of over 1700 commonly used diagnosis codes updated annually), (Ann G. Uniack), Skilled Nursing Assessment Programs (SNAP)

ICD-9 Coding—Introduction (Catalog #211), Medical Business Resource Center

ICD-9 Coding—Late Effects, V Codes (Catalog #212), Medical Business Resource Center

ICD-9 Coding—Special Tables, E Codes (Catalog #213), Medical Business Resource Center

ICD-10, The International Statistical Classification of Diseases and Related Health Problems, Tenth Revision, Volume 1 (World Health Organization), 1992, distributed by Medicode/Ingenix Publishing Group

ICD-10 Made Easy, 1999, Medicode/Ingenic Publishing Group

Interventional Radiology Coder (This company publishes code books for ambulatory surgery procedures, emergency services, and laboratory tests), Medical Learning Incorporated

The Interventional Radiology Coding User's Guide (updated annually), The Society of Cardiovascular and Interventional Radiology

Introduction to Coding (Catalog #200), Medical Business Resource Center

Key Questions in Cardiopulmonary Coding, American Health Consultants, Inc.

Key Questions in Medicare Coding, American Health Consultants, Inc.

Key Questions in Oncology Coding, American Health Consultants, Inc.

Key Questions in Orthopaedic Coding, American Health Consultants, Inc.

Key Questions in Surgical Coding, American Health Consultants, Inc.

Medical Terminology—Basic (Catalog #229/230), Medical Business Resource Center

Medical Terminology—Body Systems (Catalog #231), Medical Business Resource Center

Medical Terminology—Body Systems II (Catalog #232), Medical Business Resource Center

Modifiers Made Easy (annually published), Medicode/Ingenix Publishing Group

National Correct Coding Guide (updated annually), St. Anthony/Ingenix Publishing Group

National Correct Coding Primer (Part B News), United Communications Group

Orthopaedic ICD-9-CM Expanded, American Academy of Orthopaedic Surgeons

Post Binder Hospital Version, The Educational Annotation of ICD-9-CM, Volumes 1, 2, 3 (updated annually), Channel Publishing, Ltd.

Principles of CPT Coding, 1999, American Medical Association

Principles of ICD-9-CM Coding, 1999, American Medical Association

Procedure Coding, American College of Emergency Physicians

Soft Cover Hospital Version, The Educational Annotation of ICD-9-CM, Volumes 1, 2, 3, (updated annually), Channel Publishing, Ltd.

Soft Cover Physician Version, The Educational Annotation of ICD-9-CM, Volumes 1 and 2 (soft cover), Channel Publishing, Ltd.

Specialty Coding Manuals, Medical Management Institute

St. Anthony's Coding and Payment Guide (books are available for the following specialties: podiatry services, radiology services, and behavioral health science), St. Anthony/Ingenix Publishing Group

St. Anthony's Coding Companion (books are available for the following specialties: cardiology, general surgery, obstetrics/gynecology, ophthalmology, orthopedics, otorhinolaryngology), St. Anthony/Ingenix Publishing Group

St. Anthony's Color-Coded Annotated ICD-9-CM Code Book, St. Anthony/Ingenix Publishing Group

St. Anthony's Guide to APC and ASC Groups, St. Anthony/Ingenix Publishing Group

St. Anthony's ICD-9-CM Code Book for Home Health Services, Nursing Homes & Hospices, St. Anthony/Ingenix Publishing Group

St. Anthony's ICD-9-CM Code Book for Physician Compliance, Combined Volumes 1 and 2, in 3-hole binder with indexes and color coded for maximum reimbursement, St. Anthony/Ingenix Publishing Group

St. Anthony's Medicare Reimbursement Guide for Radiology Services: The Coding, Billing and Coverage Guide, St. Anthony/Ingenix Publishing Group

St. Anthony's Updatable ICD-9-CM Code Book, St. Anthony/Ingenix Publishing Group

St. Anthony's Updatable ICD-9-CM Code Book for Outpatient Services, St. Anthony/Ingenix Publishing Group

St. Anthony's Updatable ICD-9-CM Code Book for Physician Compliance, St. Anthony/Ingenix Publishing Group

Using CPT for Cardiothoracic Reimbursement: A Manual for Surgeons and Insurance Billing Specialists, Society of Thoracic Surgeons

Code Cards

"Code-Its" (compiled list of most common ICD-9-CM codes in each specialty. Request specialty—family practice, cardiology, ears/nose/throat, obstetrics/gynecology, urology, pediatrics, podiatry, cardiovascular surgery, ophthalmology, laminated cards), Karen Zupko & Associates

Code Journals

CPT Assistant (four issues), American Medical Association

Code Hotlines

Hotlines for Coding and Billing, St. Anthony's Hotline, (703) 836–9471, St. Anthony/Ingenix Publishing Group

Code Newsletters

AAPC News, American Academy of Professional Coders

Clinical Coding and Reimbursement (published annually), St. Anthony/Ingenix Publishing Group

The Coding Connection, Group Health Management Corporation

Coding News, Unicor Medical, Inc.

How to Get Paid (features Medicare, coding, and third party payer information, monthly), Opus Communications

Physicians Payment Update (includes center section specific to coding strategies), American Health Consultants, Inc.

Reimbursement Updated, Medicode/Ingenix Publishing Group

St. Anthony's Coding and Reimbursement (newsletters for the following: behavior health services, cardiovascular, ear/nose/throat and allergy, general surgery, nonphysician practitioner, obstetrics/gynecology, ophthalmology, orthopaedics, pediatrics, physicians, radiology), St. Anthony/Ingenix Publishing Group

St. Anthony's Hospital Fast Payment Report Newsletter, St. Anthony/Ingenix Publishing Group

St. Anthony's ICD-9-CM Coding for Reimbursement, St. Anthony/Ingenix Publishing Group

Code Research and Review Services

St. Anthony's Operative Report and Coding, Research and Review Service, St. Anthony/Ingenix Publishing Group

Code Software

Alpha II ICD-9 Coder, Unicor Medical, Inc.

Claims Editor, Context Software Systems, Inc.

Code Master Plus, Code Master Corporation

CODELINK, Context Software Systems, Inc.

Codelink for Ophthalmology (Context Software Systems), McGraw-Hill Healthcare Management Group

Codelink for Oral & Maxillofacial Surgery (Context Software Systems), McGraw-Hill Healthcare Management Group

Codelink for Orthopaedics (Context Software Systems), McGraw-Hill Healthcare Management Group

Codelink Software (CPT, HCPCS, and ICD-9-CM codes), (Context Software Systems), McGraw-Hill Healthcare Management Group

Code-Search, Diagnostic Data, Inc

Diagnostic ICD-9-Code Software (Context Software Systems), McGraw-Hill Healthcare Management Group

ICD-9-CM (floppy disk), American Medical Association

ICD-9-CM Volume I Software and HCPCS Level II Software, Opus Communications

InfoCoder (ICD-9-CM encoder), Channel Publishing, Ltd.

MCSS CPT and HCPCS Software (ADP Business Assessments), MedSmart

MCSS CPT and ICD-9 and HCPCS Software (ADP Business Assessments), MedSmart

MCSS CPT and ICD-9 Software (ADP Business Assessment), MedSmart

MCSS ICD-9 Software (ADP Business Assessment), MedSmart

Medcoder Idea Planners, Inc.

Medical Code Software System MCSS Automated Code Finder (searches CPT, ICD-9, and HCPCS), MCSS CPT Software (ADP Business Assessments), MedSmart

Omnicode and lCD Coder, SRC Systems

QuickCODE, Dr. P's Software, Inc.

RBRVS FEECALC (calculates physicians' payments under the Medicare RBRVS fee schedule, upgraded periodically), United Communications Group

Surgical Cross Coder (CPT and ICD-9 Codes), Medicode/Ingenix Publishing Group

COLLECTIONS

Successful Billing and Collection Handbooks, Conomikes Reports, Inc.

Newsletters

Health Care Collector (monthly), Aspen Publishers, Inc.

How to Get Paid, Opus Communications

Software

Appeal Solutions (450 appeal letters), 1998, Appeal Solutions

COMPLIANCE

See also *Fraud and Abuse*

Compliance Guide to Electronic Health Records, A Practical Reference to Legislation, Codes, Regulations, and Industry Standards, 2001, Faulkner & Gray, Inc.

Health Care Fraud and Abuse, 2000, American Medical Association

Medicare Billing Compliance Guide (updated annually), St. Anthony/Ingenix Publishing Group

Medicare Billing Compliance Reference Manual (updated annually), St. Anthony/Ingenix Publishing Group

Medicare Rules and Compliance Regulations, 1999, Medical Management Institute

National Correct Coding Guide (updated annually), St. Anthony/Ingenix Publishing Group

The National Correct Coding Manual (updated annually), Medical Management Institute

St. Anthony's Complete Guide to Part B Billing and Compliance, St. Anthony/Ingenix Publishing Group

DELINQUENT AND DENIED CLAIMS

Collections from Insurance Carriers

Collections Made Easy! A Comprehensive Guide for Medical and Dental Professionals (Michael J. Berry), Practice Management Information Corporation

DIAGNOSIS RELATED GROUPS

St. Anthony's Clinical Coder, St. Anthony/Ingenix Publishing Group

St. Anthony's DRG Optimizer, St. Anthony/Ingenix Publishing Group

St. Anthony's DRG Working Guidebook, St. Anthony/Ingenix Publishing Group

DIAGNOSTIC AND PROCEDURE HANDBOOKS FOR TERMINOLOGY

These medical books may be of some assistance as references for researching medical terminology when doing diagnostic and procedural coding.

Diagnostic Procedures Handbook Including Keyword Index (Franklin A. Michota, Jr., MD), 2001, Lexi-Comp

The Merck Manual of Diagnosis and Therapy, Merck Sharp and Dohme Research Laboratories, 1999, distributed by MedSmart

DICTIONARIES AND GLOSSARIES

Dorland's Illustrated Medical Dictionary (W. B. Saunders), 2000, Harcourt Health Sciences/W. B. Saunders

Health Insurance Terminology: A Glossary of Health Insurance Terms, Health Insurance Association of America

Stedman's Medical Dictionary, 2000, Lippincott/Williams & Wilkins

Taber's Cyclopedic Medical Dictionary (Clayton L. Thomas, editor), 2001, F. A. Davis Company

DISABILITY BENEFIT PROGRAMS

Booklets and Pamphlets

Obtain from the state disability programs for the following states: California, Hawaii, New Jersey, New York, Puerto Rico, Rhode Island. See Appendix A for state addresses.

Newsletters

Unemployment Insurance Reports With Social Security (weekly), Commerce Clearing House, Inc.

Disability Income Insurance

Disability Income Insurance: An Overview of Income Protection Insurance, Health Insurance Association of America

DOCUMENTATION, MEDICAL

Documentation and Reimbursement for Physician Offices (Lynn Kuehn and LaVonne Wieland), 1999, American Health Information Management Association

Medical Documentation, Streamlining an Essential Clinical Process, Medicode/Ingenix Publishing Group

Physician Documentation for Reimbursement (Gabrielle M. Kotoski and Melinda S. Stegman), 1994, Aspen Publishers, Inc.

EDUCATION AND TRAINING

Audiocassette Tapes

Individual Health Insurance, Parts A and B, Group Life & Health Insurance, Parts A, B, and C, Long-Term Care, Health Insurance Association of America

Books

Basic CPT/HCPCS Coding (Sherri A. Mallett), 2000, American Health Information Management Association

Basic ICD-9-CM Coding (Lou Ann Schraffenberger), 2000, American Health Information Management Association

Basic ICD-9-CM for Physician Office Coding (Anita Hazelwood and Carol Venable), 2001, American Health Information Management Association

Basic Keyboarding for the Medical Office Assistant (Edna Moss), 1995, Delmar Publishers, Inc.

Case Study Workbook (for advanced coder), (Patricia Morin-Spatz), 2001, MedBooks

Coding Curriculum Guide, American Health Information Management Association

Coding Skills for the Medical Assistant (Joy Renfro), 1993, American Association of Medical Assistants

Coding Workbook for the Physician's Office (published annually), (Alice G. Covell), Delmar Publishers, Inc.

Complete Coding Tutor 2001, St. Anthony/Ingenix Publishing Group

CP "Teach," Instructors Manual (published annually), (Patricia Morin-Spatz), MedBooks

CP "Teach," Workbook (published annually), (Patricia Morin-Spatz), MedBooks

CP "Teach" Expert Coding Made Easy! Textbook (published annually), (Patricia Morin-Spatz), MedBooks

CPT: Beyond the Basics (self-study, four lessons), (Gail I. Smith), 2000, American Health Information Management Association

CPT Coding Workbook for the Student, Medical Learning Incorporated

CPT/HCPCS for Physician Office Coding (Therese M. Jorwic), 2000, American Health Information Management Association

Glencoe Medical Insurance Coding Workbook (Nenna L. Bayes, Joanne Valerius, Cindy Keller), 2001, Glencoe/McGraw-Hill

ICD-9-CM: Beyond the Basics (self-study, four lessons), (Ellen Anderson and Toula Nichols), American Health Information Management Association

Intermediate CPT/HCPCS for Physician Office Coding (Donna M. Didier), 2000, American Health Information Management

Med-Index Self-Tests (Coding Instructions), Medicode/Ingenix Publishing Group

Module II, The Advanced Coder, California Health Information Association

Multispecialty Medical Coding Workbook (updated annually), (Sandra Soerries), Soerries Enterprises

Step-by-Step Medical Coding (Carol J. Buck), 1998, Harcourt Health Sciences/W. B. Saunders

Steps to Coding with ICD-9-CM for Long Term Care, 2000, California Health Information Association

Steps to Coding with ICD-9-CM Module I, The Beginning Coder, California Health Information Association

Courses

See also *Videotapes; Workshops and Seminars; Courses*

CPT-4 Clinic: Basic Procedural Coding, St. Anthony/Ingenix Publishing Group

Electronic Medical Claims, Strategic Decisions Plus

Evaluation and Management Training (2-hour training session), (Sandra Soerries), Soerries Enterprises

ICD-9-CM Clinic: Basic Diagnostic Coding, St. Anthony/Ingenix Publishing Group

Multispecialty Medical Coding Workbook (updated annually), (Sandra Soerries), Soerries Enterprises

Physician Reimbursement Clinic: Managing Payment, Billing & Coding in the RBRVS Era, St. Anthony/Ingenix Publishing Group

S. O. S. for the Medical Office (12-hour training session), (Sandra Soerries), Soerries Enterprises

St. Anthony's Basic ICD-9-CM Coding: Self-Directed Training for the Physician Office Professional, four audiocassette tapes and workbook, St. Anthony/Ingenix Publishing Group

The 3-in-1 Coding Workshop: ICD-9-CM, CPT and HCPCS Level II, St. Anthony/Ingenix Publishing Group

ELECTRONIC DATA INTERCHANGE
Books

Automated Medical Payments Directory (updated annually), Faulkner & Gray, Inc.

Compliance Guide to Electronic Health Records, A Practical Reference to Legislation, Codes, Regulations, and Industry Standards, 2001, Faulkner & Gray, Inc.

Claims Processing Bulletin Board Service

Claims Wizard Software, Info Alliance

Computer Bulletin Board for Claims Professionals, Info Alliance

Electronic Medical Claims Presentation Manual, Strategic Decisions Plus

Health Care Software Sourcebook, Aspen Publishers, Inc.

ETHICS

See also *Law and Ethics*

Code of Medical Ethics, Current Opinions with Annotations, 2001, American Medical Assocation

FEES, REIMBURSEMENT, CHARGES

"Fees on Disk" Software (specialties: cardiology, dermatology, family/general practice, internal medicine, ob/gyn/surgery), HealthCare Consultants of America, Inc.

Health Care Billing and Collections Forms, Checklists and Guidelines (Health and Administration Development Group), 1997, Aspen Publishers, Inc.

Health Care Financial Transactions Manual (Thomas C. Fox, Carol Colborn, Carl Krasik, and Joseph W. Metro), revised periodically, West Group

"Medirisk Physician Fee Schedules," (reports are available for 30 specialties and all geographic regions), St. Anthony/Ingenix Publishing Group

Physician Fee Analyzer Plus, Medicode/Ingenix Publishing Group

Physicians Fee & Coding Guide, A Comprehensive Fee and Coding Reference (updated annually), (James R. Lyle and Hoyt W. Torras), HealthCare Consultants of America

Physicians' Fee Reference (available in book and on disk, updated annually), Wasserman Medical Publishers Limited

Physician Fees, A Comprehensive Guide for Fee Schedule Review and Management (updated annually), Practice Management Information Corporation

Reimbursement Manual for the Medical Office (a comprehensive guide to coding, billing and fee management), (James R. Davis), 2001, Practice Management Information Corporation

Reimbursement Strategies, Master the Payment Cycle Today, Medicode/Ingenix Publishing Group

RVP Fees: Primary Care (software program), McGraw-Hill Healthcare Management Group

RVP Fees, Version 3.1 (software program), McGraw-Hill Healthcare Management Group

What Are My Fees? A Physician's Guide to the Complete Local Medicare Fee Schedule, McGraw-Hill Healthcare Management Group

What Are My Fees? A Physician's Guide to the Complete National Medicare Fee Schedule (Cambridge Health Economics Group), McGraw-Hill Healthcare Management Group

FRAUD AND ABUSE

See also *Videotapes*

"Consumer Fraud—Medicare and Home Medical Equipment" (pamphlet 1992:332.525), United States Government Printing Office

Health Care Fraud and Abuse, A Physician's Guide to Compliance, 2000, American Medical Association

Health Care Fraud and Abuse (revised annually), (Paul P. Cacioppo), West Group

HCFA COMMON PROCEDURE CODING SYSTEM (HCPCS)

HCPCS Common Proceduring Coding System (non-CPT-4 portion). Order document number 01706000307-3 from U. S. Government Printing Office

HCPCS, HCFA Common Procedure Coding System, spiral bound version or binder version, (annual publication), Practice Management Information Corporation

HCPCS Level II Code Book (updated annually), Wasserman Medical Publishers, Limited

HCPCS Level II Codes (published annually), St. Anthony/Ingenix Publishing Group

HCPCS Level II, National Codes (published annually), (Context Software Systems), McGraw-Hill Healthcare Management Group

HCPCS, Medicare's National Level II Codes, Medicode/Ingenix Publishing Group

St. Anthony's HCPCS Report Newsletter, St. Anthony/Ingenix Publishing Group

HEALTH INSURANCE
Books

The Business of Insurance, 1993, Health Insurance Association of America

From Patient to Payment: Insurance Procedures for the Medical Office (Rhoda Collins), 1998, Glencoe/McGraw-Hill

Glencoe Medical Insurance (Cindy Keller, Nenna L. Bayes, Joanne Valerius), 2001, Glencoe/McGraw-Hill

Mastering the Reimbursement Process (L. Lamar Blount and Joanne M. Waters), 2001, American Medical Association

Understanding Medical Insurance: A Step by Step Guide (JoAnn C. Rowell), 1998, Delmar Publishers, Inc.

HEALTH MAINTENANCE ORGANIZATIONS/ PREFERRED PROVIDER ORGANIZATIONS

See *Managed Care*

HOSPITAL INSURANCE CLAIMS

APC Claims Auditor (updated annually), St. Anthony/Ingenix Publishing Group

APC Payment Manual (updated annually), St. Anthony/ Ingenix Publishing Group

APC Reference Manual (updated annually), St. Anthony/ Ingenix Publishing Group

APC Pocket Guide (updated annually), St. Anthony/ Ingenix Publishing Group

Complete Guide to APCs (updated annually), St. Anthony/Ingenix Publishing Group

DRG Compliance Auditor (updated annually), St. Anthony/Ingenix Publishing Group

DRG Companion (updated annually), St. Anthony/Ingenix Publishing Group

DRG Guidebook (updated annually), St. Anthony/Ingenix Publishing Group

Hospital Chargemaster Guide (updated annually), St. Anthony/Ingenix Publishing Group

Outpatient Procedures Resource Book (updated annually), St. Anthony/Ingenix Publishing Group

UB-92 Editior (updated annually), St. Anthony/Ingenix Publishing Group

Newsletter

Health Care Biller (monthly), Aspen Publishers, Inc.

INSURANCE DIRECTORIES

Health Insurance Carrier Directory, A Comprehensive Guide to Insurance Carriers & Claims Processing, binder or spiral-bound versions (annual publication), Practice Management Information Corporation

Insurance Directory (updated annually), Medicode/Ingenix Publishing Group

Physicians' Insurance Reference (updated annually), Wasserman Medical Publishers, Limited

LAW AND ETHICS

See also *Ethics*

Books

Glencoe Law & Ethics for Medical Careers (Karen Judson and Sharon Blesie Hicks), 1999, Glencoe/McGraw-Hill

Health Care Fraud and Abuse (revised annually), (Paul P. Cacioppo), West Group

Law, Liability & Ethics for Medical Office Personnel (Myrtle R. Flight), Delmar Publishers, Inc.

Medicolegal Forms with Legal Analysis, American Medical Association

Newsletters

In Confidence (6 issues/year), American Health Information Management Association

Patient Confidentiality, Alphabetical Guide to the Release of Medical Information (updated annually), Medicode/Ingenix Publishing Group

Software

Black's Law Dictionary (electronic edition, 3.5″ or 5.25″ disks), (Henry Campbell Black), West Group

MANAGED CARE

Conomikes Managed Care Handbook, Conomikes Associates, Inc.

CPT Guidebook for Managed Care, 1997, St. Anthony/Ingenix Publishing Group

Criteria for Participating in Managed Care Systems, How to Evaluate a Managed Care System Contract, American Medical Association

Doctors Resource Service (DRS) (publication, videocassette, audiocasette, mailed every 6 weeks), American Medical Association

HMO/PPO Directory (published annually), Medical Economics Publishing

The Managed Care Handbook, A Comprehensive Guide to Preparing Your Practice for the Managed Care Revolution, Practice Management Information Corporation

Managed Care Organizer (system for referencing plan contracts and requirements, monitoring plan utilization, providing in-plan referrals, tracking referrals, and calculating and comparing plan profitability), St. Anthony/Ingenix Publishing Group

Managed Care Resource Guide (quarterly), Managed Care Information Center

The Managed Health Care Handbook (Peter R. Kongsvedt), 2001, Aspen Publishers, Inc.

Managing Managed Care for the Physician's Office (Carol K. Richards), 1991, American Association of Medical Assistants

Negotiating Managed Care Contracts (Medical Management Institute), 1994, McGraw-Hill Health Care Management Group

The Physician's Guide to Managed Care (David B. Nash), 1994, Aspen Publishers, Inc.

Physician's Guide to Managed Care, A Comprehensive Guide to Managed Competition, Managed Care, and Global Budgeting (James R. Lyle and Hoyt W. Torras), 1993, HealthCare Consultants of America, Inc.

Newsletters

CCH Monitor, The Newsletter of Managed Care (biweekly), Commerce Clearing House, Inc.

CCH Pulse, The Health Care Reform Newsletter (bimonthly), Commerce Clearing House, Inc.

Physician's Managed Care Report (monthly), American Health Consultants, Inc.

MEDICAID

Bulletins

Obtain from State Intermediary. See Appendix A for the address in your state.

CD-ROM

The Medicare and Medicaid Guide, Volumes 1–5 updated weekly and CD-ROM updated monthly, Commerce Clearing House, Inc.

The Medicare/Medicaid Library (CD-ROM monthly subscription with modem access to bulletin board service, which contains updates to *Federal Register*), Information Handling Services (IHS) Regulatory Products

Newsletters

California Medi-Cal Guide (monthly), Commerce Clearing House, Inc.

MEDICAL MANAGEMENT

Managing Medical Office Personnel, a Comprehensive Guide to Personnel Management in the Medical Practice, 2001, Practice Management Information Corporation

Newsletters

Conomikes Reports On Medical Practice Management (monthly), Conomikes Associates, Inc.

The Doctor's Office (monthly), Opus Communications

Journal of CHIA (includes articles on coding, reimbursement, and legal issues; directed to hospitals and ambulatory surgery centers, monthly), California Health Information Association

Medical Office Manager, Medical Office Manager

The Physician's Advisory (monthly), Advisory Publications

Physician's Marketing & Management (monthly), American Health Consultants, Inc.

Uncommon Sense (monthly), Practice Performance Publishing, Inc.

MEDICARE

Books

Commerce Clearing House and the American Medical Association Physicians' Medicare Guide (every other month), Commerce Clearing House, Inc.

Complete Guide to Medicare Coverage Issues (updated annually), St. Anthony/Ingenix Publishing Group

Guide to RBRVS for Primary Care Physicians (also other RVS fee guides and insurance publications), HealthCare Consultants of America, Inc.

Key Questions in Medicare Coding, American Health Consultants

Make Medicare Work For You (updated to include RBRVS) (James R. Lyle and Hoyt W. Torras), 1992, HealthCare Consultants of America, Inc.

Medicare at a Glance: How Carriers Scrutinize Your Procedural Coding, Medicode/Ingenix Publishing Group

Medicare Billing Guide (published annually), Medicode/Ingenix Publishing Group

The Medicare Coverage Issues Manual (Denise L. Knaus), McGraw-Hill HealthCare Management Group

Medicare RBRVS: The Physicians' Guide Book, 1994, American Medical Association

Medicare Rules & Regulations, Volumes 1 through 8 (updated as necessary), (Context Software Systems, Inc.), McGraw-Hill HealthCare Management Group

Medicare Rules & Regulations, A Survival Guide to Policies, Procedures and Payment Reform, 2001, Practice Management Information Corporation

The Medicare Survival Guide (Denise L. Knaus), McGraw-Hill HealthCare Management Group

Part B Answer Book, Medicare Billing Rules from A to Z (updated quarterly), United Communications Group

Part B Pocket Billing Guide (updated quarterly), United Communications Group

The ProSTAT Guide to Medicare (Philip L. Bear), Medicode/Ingenix Publishing Group

St. Anthony's Color-Coded Medicare Coverage Manual (with color-coded prompts), St. Anthony/Ingenix Publishing Group

St. Anthony's Complete Guide to Medicare Coverage Issues, St. Anthony/Ingenix Publishing Group

St. Anthony's Complete Guide to Part B Billing and Compliance, St. Anthony/Ingenix Publishing Group

St. Anthony's Guide to Ambulatory Surgery Center Payment Groups, St. Anthony/Ingenix Publishing Group

St. Anthony's Medicare Billing Compliance Guide and Monitor, St. Anthony/Ingenix Publishing Group

St. Anthony's Medicare Billing and Compliance Source Book, St. Anthony/Ingenix Publishing Group

St. Anthony's Medicare Correct Coding and Payment Manual, St. Anthony/Ingenix Publishing Group

St. Anthony's Medicare Outpatient Reference Manual, St. Anthony/Ingenix Publishing Group

St. Anthony's Medicare Reimbursement Guide for Radiology Services. The Coding, Billing and Coverage Reference, St. Anthony/Ingenix Publishing Group

St. Anthony's Medicare Unbundling Guidebook, Understanding Medicare's National Correct Coding Policy, St. Anthony/Ingenix Publishing Group

Bulletins

Obtain from State intermediary. See Appendix A to obtain the address for your state.

CD-ROM

The Medicare and Medicaid Guide, Volumes 1 through 5 updated weekly and CD-ROM updated monthly, Commerce Clearing House, Inc.

The Medicare/Medicaid Library, IHS Regulatory Products

Newsletters

Conomike's Medicare Hotline (monthly), Conomike's Reports, Inc.

Medicare Review (monthly), Shannon Publications, Inc.

Part B News (bimonthly), United Communications Group

Physicians' Medicare Guide Newsletter (every other month), Commerce Clearing House, Inc.

PREFERRED PROVIDER ORGANIZATIONS

See *Managed Care*

REIMBURSEMENT

See *Fees, Reimbursement, Charges*

RELATIVE VALUE STUDIES

Relative Value Studies with Regard to Radiology (write for information), American College of Radiology

Resource Based Relative Value Scale (RBRVS), Physicians Fee Schedule, Addendum E, page 63852, *Federal Register,* Stock No. 069-001-00063-7, December 2, 1993, United States Government Printing office

St. Anthony's Complete RBRVS, (updated annually), St. Anthony/Ingenix Publishing Group

St. Anthony's Relative Values for Physicians, St. Anthony/Ingenix Publishing Group

SELF-EMPLOYMENT

Audiotapes

Electronic Medical Claims Marketing Strategies, Strategic Decisions Plus

Books

Health Service Businesses on your Home-Based P/C (Rick Benzel), (may be purchased from Oxford Medical Systems), Windcrest/McGraw-Hill

Independent Medical Coding (Donna Avila-Weil and Rhonda Regan), 1999, Rayve Productions, Inc.

Magazines

Home Office Computing (monthly), Home Office Computing

Marketing

Brochure Collection (24 sample pieces), Strategic Decisions Plus

Newsletter

PRO Claimer Analyst (monthly), Strategic Decisions Plus

Software

Eazy Quote, Strategic Decisions Plus
PowerLeads for Medical Claims Businesses, InfoAlliance

TRICARE

Bulletins

Obtain from State Intermediary. See Appendix A for the address in your state.

Newsletters

Understanding CHAMPUS, Volume 1, (updated as needed), Commerce Clearing House, Inc.

VIDEOTAPES

"Beginning ICD-9-CM," 2-hour videotape, binder, and workbook, Channel Publishing, Ltd.

"The Case for Case Management," Health Insurance Association of America

"Coding for Quality," ICD-9-CM Level 1 (26 videotapes); Introduction to CPT (3 videotapes), Healthcare Management Advisors, Inc.

"E & M Coding & Documentation," ChartCare Solutions

"Fighting Fraud," Health Insurance Association of America

"ICD-10" (HealthMarket International), Medical Learning Incorporated

"Medicare Part B: Putting an End to Fraud & Abuse," 8 minutes, Blue Shield of California

"Protecting Tomorrow: Long-Term Care," Health Insurance Association of America

"Understanding Limiting Charges, Benefits of Medicare Part B Beneficaries," 8 minutes, Blue Shield of California

WORKERS' COMPENSATION

Guides to the Evaluation of Permanent Impairment, 1994, American Medical Association

Healthcare Management Guidelines Return-to-Work Planning (Milliman and Robertson, Inc.), distributed by St. Anthony/Ingenix Publishing Group

Official California Workers' Compensation Medical Fee Schedule, (California Medical Fee Schedule), State of California

WORKSHOPS AND SEMINARS

American Health Information Management Association
Conomikes Reports, Inc.
Medical Management Institute
Medical Management Information Services, Inc.
The Reimbursement Manager Training Program (RMTP), Medicode/Ingenix Publishing Group
St. Anthony's Seminars
   Advanced Cardiovascular Coding
   Ambulatory Surgery Coding Clinic
   Ambulatory Training Series
   Cardiovascular Coding Workshop
   CPT-4 Hospital Clinic
   Emergency Medicine Workshop
   Ob/Gyn Coding Workshop
   Ophthalmology Coding Workshop
   Orthopaedic Coding Workshop
   Physician Billing & Reimbursement
   Radiology Coding & Reimbursement
   Three-In-One Coding Clinic
United Communications Group
See also *Education and Training, Courses,* which offer prior approval and continuing education units.

NAMES AND ADDRESSES OF RESOURCES

Advisory Publications, P.O. Box 551, Norristown, PA 19404
Phone: (610) 941-4488
Web: www.smartpracticemanagement.com

American Academy of Orthopaedic Surgeons,
6300 N. River Road, Rosemont, IL 60018-4226
Phone: (800) 346-AAOS, (800) 626-6726, or (708) 823-7186
Fax: (708) 823-8125
Web: www.aaos.org

American Academy of Pediatrics, 141 N.W. Point Boulevard, P.O. Box 927, Elk Grove Village, IL 60009-0927
Phone: (800) 433-9016 or (708) 228-5005
Web: www.aap.org

American Academy of Professional Coders,
309 West 700 South, Salt Lake City, UT 84101
Phone: (800) 626-CODE
Web: www.aapcnatl.org

American Association of Medical Assistants,
20 N. Wacker Drive, Suite 1575, Chicago, IL 60606
Phone: (800) 228-2262
Web: www.aama-natl.org

American College of Emergency Physicians,
P.O. Box 619911, Dallas, TX 75261
Phone: (800) 798-1822
Web: www.acep.org

American College of Radiology RVS, 1891 Preston White Drive, Reston, VA 22090

American College of Rheumatology, 60 Executive Park South, Suite 150 Atlanta, GA 30329
Phone: (404) 633-3777

American Guild of Patient Account Management,
National Certification Examination Program,
1101 Connecticut Avenue, NW, Suite 700, Washington, DC 20036

American Health Consultants, Inc., 3525 Piedmont Road, NE, Bldg. 6, Suite 400, (30305), P.O. Box 740060, Department 1203, Atlanta, GA 30374-9822
Web: www.ahcpub.com/online.html

American Health Information Management Association,
Books and publications:
233 North Michigan Avenue, Suite 2150
Chicago, IL 60601-5519
Phone: (312) 233-1100 or (800) 335-5535

Certification information:
Attention: AHIMA Coordinator, Professional Examination Service, 475 Riverside Drive, New York, NY 10115
Phone: (212) 870-3136
Web: www.ahima.org

American Medical Association, 515 N. State Street, P.O. Box 930876, Atlanta, GA 31193-0876
Phone: (800) 621-8335
Web: www.ama-assn.org

American Psychiatric Press, Inc., 1400 K Street, NW, Washington, DC 20005
Phone: (800) 368-5777
Web: www.appi.org

American Society for Parenteral and Enteral Nutrition, 8630 Fenton Street, Suite 412, Silver Spring, MD 20910-3805
Phone: (301) 587-6315

Appeal Solutions, 703 Blue Oak, Lewisville, TX 75067
Phone: (888) 399-4925

Aspen Publishers, Inc., 7201 McKinney Circle (21704) P.O. Box 990, Frederick, MD 21705-9727
Phone: (800) 638-8437
Web: www.aspenpub.com

Blue Shield of California, Fraud & Abuse Unit, P.O. Box 2807, Chico, CA 95927
Phone: (916) 896-7055

California Health Information Association, 5108 E. Clinton Way, Suite 113, Fresno, CA 93727-0538
Phone: (800) 247-8907
Web: www.california.hia.org

California Medical Fee Schedule, Department 05445, P.O. Box 39000, San Francisco, CA 94139

Channel Publishing, Ltd., 4750 Longley Lane, Suite 110, Reno, NV 89502
Phone: (800) 248-2882
Web: www.channelpublishing.com

ChartCare Solutions, 7803 N. 12th Avenue, Phoenix, AZ 85021
Phone: (800) 449-1272
Web: www.chirocode.com

Code Master Corporation, 10 South Riverside Plaza, Chicago, IL 60611

Commerce Clearing House, Inc., 4025 West Peterson Avenue (60646), P.O. Box 5490, Chicago, IL 60680-9882
Phone: (800) 835-5224
Web: www.cch.com

Commission on Professional Hospital Activities (CPHA) P.O. Box 1809, Ann Arbor, MI 48106
Phone: (313) 769-6511

Conomikes Associates, Inc., 151 Kalmus Drive, Suite B150, Costa Mesa, CA 92626-9627
Phone: (800) 421-6512
Web: www.conomikes.com

Context Software Systems, Inc., 241 S. Frontage Road, Suite 38, Burr Ridge, IL 60521
Phone: (800) 783-3378 or (708) 654-8800

F. A. Davis Company/Publishers, 1915 Arch Street, Philadelphia, PA 19103
Phone: (800) 323-3555
Web: www.fadavis.com

Delmar Publishers, Inc., 3 Columbia Circle Drive, P.O. Box 15015, Albany, NY 12212-5015
Phone: (800) 347-7707
Web: www.DelmarAlliedHealth.com

DiagnostIC Data, Inc., 20 Balfour Drive, West Hartford, CT 06117
Phone: (800) 999-6405
Web: www.diagdata.com

Dr. P's Software, Inc., 3525 S. National, Suite 110, Springfield, MI 65807

Entrepreneur, 6001 D Landerhaven, Cleveland, OH 44124

Faulkner & Gray, Inc., 11 Penn Plaza, 17th floor, New York, NY 10117-0373
Phone: (800) 535-8403
Web: www.faulkner&gray.com

Glencoe, Macmillan/McGraw-Hill, P.O. Box 508, Columbus, OH 43216
Phone: (800) 334-7344
Web: www.glencoe.com

Group Health Management Corporation, P.O. Box 12929, Tucson, AZ 85732

Harcourt Health Sciences/Mosby, 11830 Westline Industrial Drive, St. Louis, MO 63146
Phone: (800) 633-6699
Fax: (314) 432-1380
Web: www.harcourthealth.com

Harcourt Health Sciences/W. B. Saunders, 6277 Sea Harbor Drive, Orlando, FL 32821-9989
Phone: (800) 545-2522
Fax: (800) 874-6418
Web: www.harcourthealth.com

HCIA Inc., 300 East Lombard Street, Baltimore, MD 21202
Phone: (800) 568-3282
Web: www.solution.com

HealthCare Consultants of America, Inc., 1054 Claussen Road, Augusta, GA 30907
Phone: (888) 738-7494 or (706) 738-2078
Fax: (706) 722-9869
Web: www.hcca.com

Healthcare Management Advisors, Inc., 1091-C Cambridge Square, Atlanta, GA 30201-1844
Phone: (800) 875-8HMA
Web: www.hma.com

Health Insurance Association of America, 1021 F Street, NW, Suite 500, Washington DC 20004-1204
Phone: 202-824-1600
Web: www.hiaa.org

Health Market International, 4885 Lone Oak Court, Ann Arbor, MI 48108
Phone: (313) 665-1360

Dr. R. B. Holt, 2182 E. Sublette Place, Sandy, UT 84093-1056

Home Office Computing, P.O. Box 51344, Boulder, CO 80321-1344

William J. Hunt, MD, 3540 Forest Hill Boulevard, West Palm Beach, FL 33406

Idea Planners, Inc., 2075 San Marino Way, North, Clearwater, FL 34623

InfoAlliance, 6701 Seybold, Suite 219, Madison, WI 53719

Information Handling Services (IHS) Regulatory Products, 6160 S. Syracuse Way, Englewood, CO 80110
Phone: (800) 525-5539 or (303) 267-0543
Web: www.ihshealth.com

KFC Medical Systems, Inc., 713 St. Louis Avenue, Long Beach, CA 90804

Lexi-Comp, Hudson, OH
Phone: (800) 837-LEXI
Web: www.lexi.com

Lippincott/Williams & Wilkins, 530 Walnut Street, Philadelphia, PA 19106-3621
Phone: (800) 777-2295
Web: www.LWW.com

Managed Care Information Center, 3100 Highway 138, Wall Township, NJ 07719-1442

McGraw-Hill Healthcare Management Group, 1221 Avenue of the Americas, New York, NY 10020

MedBooks, 101 West Buckingham Road, Richardson, TX 75081
Phone: (800) 443-7397
Web: www.medbooks.com

Medical Business Resource Center, 1221 E. Osborn Road, Suite 101, Phoenix, AZ 85014

Medical Economics Publishing, 5 Paragon Drive, Montvale, New Jersey 07645
Phone: (800)-432-4570
Web: www.memag.com

Medical Learning Incorporated, 245 East Sixth Street, Suite 502, St. Paul, MN 55101
Phone: (800) 252-1578
Fax: (612) 224-4694
Web: www.medlearn.com

Medical Management Information Services, Inc., 6475 E. Pacific Coast Highway, Suite 409 (90802), P.O. Box 33-409, Long Beach, CA 90801

Medical Management Institute, 11405 Old Roswell Road, Alpharetta, Georgia 30004
Phone: (800) 334-5724
Web: www.institute.md and www.codingbooks.com

Medical Office Manager, P.O. Box 500845, Atlanta, GA 31150

Medicode/Ingenix Publishing Group, 5225 Wiley Post Way, Suite 500 (84116-2889), P.O. Box 27116, Salt Lake City, UT 84152-6l80
Phone: (800) 999-4600
Web: www.medicode.com

MedSmart, 1590 S. Milwaukee Avenue, Suite 212, Libertyville, IL 60048

Opus Communications, 100 Hoods Lane, P.O. Box 1168, Marblehead, MA 01945
Phone: (800) 650-6787
Web: www.hcmarketplace.com

Oxford Medical Systems, 230 Nortland Boulevard, Suite 223, Cincinnati, OH 45246

Practice Management Information Corporation, 4727 Wilshire Boulevard, Los Angeles, CA 90010
Phone: (800) MED-SHOP
Web: http://medicalbookstore.com

Practice Performance Publishing, Inc., 2508 E. Willow, Suite 302, Long Beach, CA 90806

Professional Practice Builders, 2000 Ticonderoga Drive, San Mateo, CA 94402
Phone: (415) 573-0109

Rayve Productions, Inc., (800) 852-4890

Shannon Publications, Inc., Northcreek Place 1, 9441 LBJ Freeway, Suite 510, Box 2, Dallas, TX 75243-9940
Phone: (800) 578-4888

Skilled Nursing Assessment Programs (SNAP), P.O. Box 574, San Anselmo, CA 94979
Phone: (415) 454-5752
Fax: (415) 453-6029

The Society of Cardiovascular and Interventional Radiology, 10201 Lee Highway, Suite 500, Fairfax, VA 22030
Phone: (703) 691-1805
Web: www.scvir.org

Society of Thoracic Surgeons, 401 N. Michigan Avenue, Chicago, IL 60611-4267
Phone: (312) 644-6610
Web: www.sba.com

Soerries Enterprises, 8318 S. Outer Belt Road, Oak Grove, MO 64075
Phone: (816) 690-8996

SRC Systems, 14785 Omicron Drive, Texas Research Park, San Antonio, TX 78245-3201

St. Anthony/Ingenix Publishing Group, 11410 Isaac Newton Square, Reston, VA 22090 and P.O. Box 96561, Washington, DC 20044-4212
Phone: (800) 632-0123 or (703) 904-3900
Fax: (703) 706-5830
Web: www.st-anthony.com

St. Anthony's Seminars, 5224 Juliette Street, Springfield, VA 22151
Phone: (800) 632-0123
Web: www.st-anthony.com

State of California, Department of Industrial Relations, Division of Workers' Compensation, 455 Golden Gate Avenue, Room 5182, San Francisco, CA 94102

Strategic Decisions Plus, P.O. Box 2108, Silverthorne, CO 80498

Unicor Medical, Inc., 4160 Carmichael Road, Suite 101, Montgomery, AL 36106
Phone: (800) 825-7421 or (205) 260-8150
Web: http://www.unicormed.com

United Communications Group, 11300 Rockville Pike, Suite 1100 (20852), P.O. Box 90608, Washington, DC 20077-7637
Phone: (800) 929-4824

United States Government Printing Office, Superintendent of Documents, Washington, DC 20402
Web: www.pueblo.gsa.gov

Wasserman Medical Publishers, Limited, 3036 S. 92nd Street, P.O. Box 27365, West Allis, WI 53227
Phone: (800) 669-3337
Web: www.medfees.com

West Group, 620 Opperman Drive, P.O. Box 64526, Eagan, MN 55123-1396
Phone: (800) 328-9352
Web: www.westgroup.com

Windcrest /McGraw-Hill, Blue Ridge Summit, PA
  17294-0850
Karen Zupko & Associates, 980 N. Michigan Avenue,
  #1325, Chicago, IL 60611

Phone: (312) 642-5616
Web: www.karenzupko.com

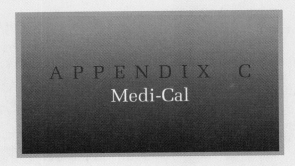

APPENDIX C
Medi-Cal

CHAPTER OUTLINE

OBJECTIVES*

After reading this appendix, you should
be able to:

- Define key terms and abbreviations inherent to Medi-Cal.
- Identify the patient's Medi-Cal benefits identification card and list important information to obtain from the card.
- Describe the point of service device and state how it relates to the recipient's eligibility and share of cost.
- List important information to obtain from the patient's Medi-Cal identification card.
- State how to verify a patient's Medi-Cal eligibility.
- Explain how to identify patients covered by Medi-Cal prepaid health plans.

---

*Performance objectives and exercises for hands-on practical experience for this chapter
appear in the *Workbook*.

- Understand the benefits and nonbenefits of Medi-Cal.
- Explain when it is necessary to use and how to complete a Treatment Authorization Request Form.
- List basic Medi-Cal claim procedure guidelines.
- State how to collect information and process claim forms for Medi-Cal patients who have additional coverage.
- Explain how to minimize the number of insurance forms rejected because of improper completion.
- Identify the Medi-Cal time limit for submitting claims.
- Identify when an over-1-year Medi-Cal claim will be accepted by the fiscal intermediary.
- Edit the Uniform Bill (UB-92) Outpatient Claim Form.
- Explain entries shown on a Remittance Advice Details document.
- Identify information on a Resubmission Turnaround Document.
- State when to use and how to complete a Claims Inquiry Form.

KEY TERMS

Medi-Cal terms are used when reading updates to the program policy manuals, which are available via the Internet or in hard copy by annual subscription. However, during lectures and in some publications about the Medi-Cal program, abbreviations are used rather than complete terms or phrases. Therefore, it is important to study both thoroughly. In addition to the key terms given in Chapter 12 used for Medicaid and Other State Programs, the following key terms and abbreviations are emphasized for study from Appendix C that are specific to the Medi-Cal program.

accounts receivable (A/R) transaction

Aid to the Blind (AB)

Aid to Families with Dependent Children (AFDC)

Aid to the (permanently) Disabled (ATD)

automated eligibility verification system (AEVS)

benefits identification card (BIC)

California Children's Services (CCS)

Child Health and Disability Prevention Program (CHDP)

claim control number (CCN)

Claims and eligibility real-time software (CERTS)

Claims Inquiry Form (CIF)

Comprehensive Perinatal Services Program (CPSP)

computer media claims (CMC)

County Medical Services Program (CMSP)

Department of Health Services (DHS)

durable medical equipment (DME)

Electronic Data Systems (EDS) Corporation

electronic funds transfer (EFT)

eligibility verification confirmation (EVC)

Genetically Handicapped Persons Program (GHPP)

medically indigent (MI)

medically needy (MN)

nursing facility (NF)

Old Age Survivors, Health and Disability Insurance (OASHDI) Program

point of service (POS) device or network

presumptive eligibility (PE)

Provider Telecommunications Network (PTN)

Remittance Advice Details (RAD)

Resubmission Turnaround Document (RTD)

share of cost (SOC)

Treatment Authorization Request (TAR) form

Voice Drug TAR System (VDTS)

For the history of Medicaid and basic knowledge about how the welfare system works, read Chapter 12, Medicaid and Other State Programs, before reading Appendix C. As mentioned in Chapter 12, in California the Medicaid program is known as Medi-Cal and became effective on March 1, 1966. Medi-Cal is administered by the California State **Department of Health Services (DHS)**, a department of the California State Human Relations Agency. The information in this appendix is a brief overview of the Medi-Cal program with basic guidelines for most regions in California. For additional current detailed information on policies and procedures supplied by the current fiscal intermediary, refer to either an updated *Medi-Cal Provider Manual for Medical Services* or go online to obtain the information at www.medi-cal.ca.gov.

Types of Medi-Cal Plans

Managed Care Plans

The Medi-Cal program has evolved into health care plans (HCPs) that fall into one of several managed care plan (MCP) models:

▶ MCP: County Organized Health System (COHS)
▶ MCP: Fee-for-Service/Managed Care (FFS/MC)
▶ MCP: Geographic Managed Care (GMC)
▶ MCP: Prepaid Health Plans (PHP)
▶ MCP: Primary Care Case Management (PCCM)
▶ MCP: Special Projects
▶ MCP: Two-Plan Model

Individuals covered under these plans must seek treatment from facilities contracted under the MCP, except in emergencies. Otherwise, services will not be reimbursed by Medi-Cal. If service is not available through contracted facilities and the patient seeks care outside of the plan, a denial letter from the health plan must accompany the Medi-Cal claim.

Descriptions of Managed Care Plans

The *MCP: County Organized Health System (COHS)* is a local agency created by a county board of supervisors to contract with the Medi-Cal program. Enrolled recipients choose their health care provider from among all COHS providers.

The *MCP: Fee-for-Service/Managed Care (FFS/MC)* program requires specific Medi-Cal recipients to enroll in state-contracted FFS/MC Networks (FFS/MCN) administered by selected rural counties. Enrollees may select a primary care provider (PCP) who will manage their health care. The PCP provides primary care services and referrals for all necessary specialty services through an ongoing patient–physician relationship. The county is paid a case management fee for creating the provider network, establishing enrollee outreach services, and monitoring use.

The *MCP: Geographic Managed Care (GMC)* program model was established to provide medical and dental care for Medi-Cal recipients in speci-

fied aid code categories for a capitated fee. Each county may have different guidelines as to the delivery of the dental care; that is, either a recipient may choose between various dental MCPs or may receive dental care on a fee-for-service basis.

The *MCP: Prepaid Health Plan (PHP)* was established to allow Medi-Cal recipients to enroll in health maintenance organizations (HMOs) as an alternative to the Medi-Cal fee-for-service program. PHPs are required to render, on a capitated at-risk basis, all basic Medi-Cal covered benefits. PHPs provide case management, prevention, and health maintenance services. These plans have membership services and member grievance procedures. PHPs render care to privately insured individuals as well as Medi-Cal recipients.

The *MCP: Primary Care Case Management (PCCM)* program contractors case manage medical care for a voluntarily enrolled population of Medi-Cal recipients. PCCM plans are capitated for most outpatient services. Prior approval requests must be obtained for noncapitated services requiring authorization under the fee-for-service program, except acute inpatient facility psychiatric services and Adult Day Health Care (ADHC) services. PCCM contractors also assume an additional responsibility to arrange and authorize inpatient services, which are reimbursed fee-for-service by Medi-Cal. Contracts participate in program savings through a savings sharing agreement with the Department of Health Services (DHS).

The *MCP: Special Projects* are new managed care county programs or pilot projects to extend coordinated, competent care to identified populations. These special projects are designed to improve recipients health status and to avoid unnecessary costs.

The *MCP: Two-Plan Model* is when the DHS contracts with two managed care plans in each of 12 California counties to provide medical services to most Medi-Cal recipients in each county. Each county offers a local initiative plan and a commercial plan. Local initiative plans are operated by a locally developed comprehensive managed care organization. Commercial plans are operated by nongovernmental managed health care organizations. Medi-Cal recipients may enroll in either plan.

Medi-Cal Eligibility

Individuals in the following groups are entitled to benefits under the Medi-Cal program:

▶ Californians who qualify for **Old Age Survivors, Health and Disability Insurance (OASHDI) program**

▶ **Aid to Families with Dependent Children (AFDC)**
▶ **Aid to the Blind (AB)**
▶ **Aid to the (permanently) Disabled (ATD)**
▶ **Medically needy (MN)** people whose incomes are above the assistance level but who are unable to provide mainstream medical care and are eligible as **medically indigent (MI).**

Share of Cost

Some medically needy patients have a dollar amount (liability) to meet each month called **share of cost (SOC).** This is the amount of money that must be paid by the patient each month before any Medi-Cal benefits will begin.

Identification Card

The State of California Department of Health Services issues a plastic **benefits identification card (BIC)** to each Medi-Cal recipient when the individual is declared eligible for benefits (Fig. C–1). County welfare departments may issue paper Medi-Cal cards in exceptional cases for temporary use (i.e., retroactive eligibility). A person may have a Medi-Cal card, but this does not indicate proof of eligibility.

Eligibility Verification

It is the provider's responsibility to verify that the person to receive care is eligible for the month service is rendered and is the individual to whom the card was issued. Eligibility, which is verified at the first of the month, is valid for the entire month of service. Inspect the card and look for the following key points.

▶ Recipient's identification number may be numeric or alphanumeric.
▶ Issue date on the card must match the issue date on the recipient's master file accessed through the Medi-Cal point of service network.
▶ Recipient's date of birth on the card must match the recipient's date of birth on the recipient's master file, accessed through the point of service network.

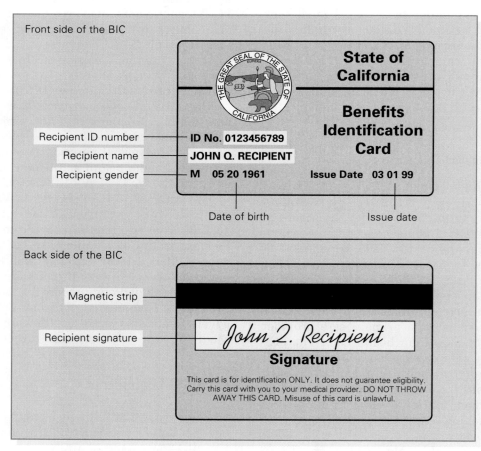

Figure C–1. Medi-Cal sample plastic Benefits Identification Card (BIC). This is a white card with blue letters on front and black letters on back.

▶ Recipient's signature located on the back of the BIC is used to verify the recipient's identification. This should be compared to the signature on a valid California driver's license, a California identification card issued by the Department of Motor Vehicles, another acceptable picture identification card, or another credible document of identification.

Verification Methods

Methods by which to verify eligibility and perform SOC and Medi-Service transactions are listed below:

▶ **Point of service (POS)** device. This is a piece of equipment interfaced with an analog telephone line. It has swipe card capabilities, or data may be manually input. It is used to identify recipient eligibility, obtain SOC liability status, key in SOC payment toward balance, reserve Medi-Services, perform Family PACT (planning, access, care, and treatment) client eligibility transactions, and submit pharmacy or HCFA-1500 insurance claims.

An **eligibility verification confirmation (EVC)** number on a printout from the POS device verifies that an inquiry was received and eligibility information was transmitted. The insurance billing specialist should keep the eligibility verification confirmation number in the recipient's file and use it as proof of eligibility for the entire month. When a Medi-Cal recipient is limited to receive certain medical services, a restriction message is returned from the Medi-Cal host computer after verification of eligibility. Document that the services relate to the applicable restriction (i.e., date of service and name of provider who prescribed limited services). Never bill Medi-Cal for the SOC that a patient pays. Instead enter the amount paid into the POS system and indicate the amount on the HCFA-1500 claim form. This will let the Medi-Cal fiscal intermediary know that the patient has paid and clear the SOC, allowing the recipient to become eligible for Medi-Cal benefits. Figure C−2 illustrates SOC and Medi-Service printouts from the POS device.

▶ **Claims and eligibility real-time software (CERTS).** This is computer software that allows providers to electronically verify recipient eligibility, clear SOC liability, reserve Medi-Services, perform Family PAC client eligibility transactions, and submit pharmacy or HCFA-1500 claims using a personal computer. A modem and telephone line are required. An EVC number on a printout from the software verifies that an inquiry was received and eligibility information was transmitted.

▶ **Computer software.** This may be existing software modified by a vendor or a vendor-supplied software package capable of performing the transactions. An EVC number verifies that an inquiry was received and eligibility information was transmitted.

▶ **Automated eligibility verification system (AEVS).** This is an interactive voice response system allowing providers to access recipient eligibility, clear SOC, and/or reserve a Medi-Service. A touch-tone telephone is required. An EVC number verifies that an inquiry was received and eligibility information was transmitted. However, this system is not able to perform SOC or Medi-Service transactions.

Receipt of an EVC number does not guarantee claim payment. Carefully review all information returned with the eligibility response to ensure that services are covered under the recipient eligibility.

Medi-Cal Benefits

The basic medical benefits provided under Medi-Cal include the following:

▶ Physician services
▶ Inpatient or outpatient hospital services in any approved hospital
▶ Laboratory and x-ray services
▶ Nursing home services
▶ Home health care
▶ Private duty nursing
▶ Outpatient clinic services
▶ Dental services (through Delta Dental, called Denti-Cal)
▶ Hearing aids
▶ Drugs and medical supplies
▶ Optometric services and eye appliances
▶ Physical therapy and other diagnostic, preventive, or rehabilitative services and equipment
▶ Medicare deductible and premium payment. Medi-Cal also pays the full deductible under Medicare Part A and buys into Medicare Part B by paying the monthly premiums for those who are older than 65, disabled, or blind. These persons are called Medicare/Medi-Cal recipients (see Chapter 11, Medicare).
▶ Obstetric services. The **Comprehensive Perinatal Services Program (CPSP)** offers a wide range of services to pregnant Medi-Cal recipients from conception through 60 days after the month of delivery.

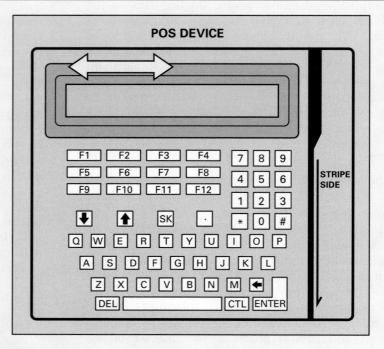

POS DEVICE: SHARE OF COST PRINTOUT

EDS TRAINING 3213 PROSPECT PARK TERMINAL

XX-02-15
01:44:35

PROVIDER NUMBER:
HSC30175G

TRANSACTION TYPE: SHARE OF COST

RECIPIENT ID:
607357101

YEAR AND MONTH OF BIRTH:
1964-10

DATE OF ISSUE:
XX-02-01

DATE OF SERVICE:
XX-02-15

CASE NUMBER:

PROCEDURE CODE:
90945

PATIENT APPLIED AMOUNT:
$50.00

TOTAL BILLED AMOUNT:
$100.00

LAST NAME: JOHNSO.
AMOUNT DEDUCTED: $50.00
SHARE OF COST HAS BEEN MET.

POS DEVICE: MEDI-SERVICE PRINTOUT

EDS 10050 OLSON DRIVE TERMINAL T309006

XX-02-15
17:16:36

PROVIDER NUMBER:
HSC30175G

TRANSACTION TYPE: MEDI-SERVICES

RECIPIENT ID:
607357101

YEAR AND MONTH OF BIRTH:
1966-12

DATE OF ISSUE:
XX-02-01

DATE OF SERVICE:
XX-02-15

PROCEDURE CODE:
A2000

LAST NAME: JOHNSO. MEDI SVC
RESERVATION APPLIED.

Figure C–2. Point of Service (POS) device and two examples of printouts: Share of Cost and Medi-Service.

In addition to maternity services, certified providers may be reimbursed for nutritional, psychosocial, and health education services, case coordination, client orientation, and vitamin and mineral supplements. A federal/state program designed to ease access to prenatal care is called **presumptive eligibility (PE)**. It allows the provider to offer immediate temporary coverage for prenatal care to low-income pregnant women pending a formal Medi-Cal application.

Medi-Services

Medi-Services are certain services supplied by chiropractors, psychologists, acupuncturists, podiatrists, occupational therapists, speech pathologists, and audiologists. Most recipients eligible for Medi-Cal are allowed two Medi-Services per calendar month.

Prior Approval

Telecommunications Networks

The **Provider Telecommunications Network (PTN)** is an automated voice-response system that allows the provider to use the telephone to obtain checkwrite, claim, and prior authorization (TAR) information for services rendered through the Medi-Cal program, **County Medical Services Program (CMSP), Child Health and Disability Prevention Program (CHDP), California Children's Services (CCS), and Genetically Handicapped Persons Program (GHPP)**. If a provider chooses to use the PTN, it must be the primary source of checkwrite (issuing of Medi-Cal payment check), claim, and TAR information. Providers are automatically enrolled in the PTN and assigned a seven-digit provider identification number (PIN) that must be used to access the PTN on a touch-tone telephone.

Treatment Authorization Request

Certain procedures and services require prior approval from the Medi-Cal field office consultant. The approval process is begun by either completing a **Treatment Authorization Request (TAR)** Form 50-1 (Fig. C–3) or accessing the Medi-Cal web site via the Internet to electronically transmit an e-TAR.

To find out whether a particular service requires a TAR, refer to the *Medi-Cal Provider Manual for Medical Services* or go to the Medi-Cal web site at www.medi-cal.ca.gov. Find the TAR benefit/nonbenefit list that indicates what services require a TAR or are not a benefit. Some, but not all, of the TAR-required services are as follows:

- Long-term care facility services
- Some vision services
- Inpatient hospital services
- Home health agency services
- Chronic hemodialysis services
- Some transportation services
- Some **durable medical equipment (DME)**, medical supplies, or prosthetic/orthotic appliances
- Hearing aids
- Some pharmacy services
- Some surgical procedures

Response to a form-generated TAR takes 10 to 15 days, but an e-TAR has a quicker response time. Once an e-TAR is submitted, it is electronically routed to the appropriate field office for a decision (adjudication). Providers can return to the web site to check TAR status (approved, denied, deferred). A TAR Transmittal Form MC3020 may be completed to help track submitted TARs or to appeal a TAR. Check with the field office to determine if and when faxed TARs will be accepted, because policies vary from one office to another.

If the request for hospitalization of a patient is approved, a copy of the approved TAR should be faxed or sent to the hospital before admission of the patient. In some cases, it is not possible to obtain a TAR in advance of hospital admission or initiation of a treatment program. In these cases, authorization may be obtained by telephone or fax. Call the local department of health services field office to receive approval, and then complete and submit a TAR Form 50-1 to the field office, indicating that it was already authorized by including

- Date authorized
- Name of person who gave authorization
- Approximate time of day at which authorization was given
- Verbal number stated by the field office

Do not bill the fiscal intermediary with the verbal TAR number.

A **Voice Drug TAR System (VDTS)** is also available and linked to the Medi-Cal Drug Units to permit the processing of TARs after completion of a recording. VDTS can *only* be used to request *urgent* and *initial* drug TARs, to inquire about the status of previously entered drug TARs, or to inquire whether a patient is receiving continual care with a drug.

STATE USE ONLY (1)

SERVICE CATEGORY

CONFIDENTIAL PATIENT INFORMATION

(1A) FOR F.I. USE ONLY

CCN

TYPEWRITER ALIGNMENT Elite Pica

TREATMENT AUTHORIZATION REQUEST

STATE OF CALIFORNIA DEPARTMENT OF HEALTH SERVICES

F.I. USE ONLY (40) (41) (42) (43)

TYPEWRITER ALIGNMENT Elite Pica

(PLEASE TYPE) FOR PROVIDER USE (2A) (PLEASE TYPE)

VERBAL CONTROL NO.	TYPE OF SERVICE REQUESTED		REQUEST IS RETROACTIVATE?		IS PATIENT MEDICARE ELIGIBLE?		PROVIDER PHONE NO.
(1B)	(2) DRUG	OTHER	YES	NO	YES	NO	AREA
		X		X		X	(013) 555-1111

(32A) PATIENT'S AUTHORIZED REPRESENTATIVE (IF ANY) ENTER NAME AND ADDRESS

(3) PROVIDER NO. HSC12345F

(2B) PROVIDER NAME AND ADDRESS

PLEASE TYPE YOUR NAME AND ADDRESS HERE

SMITH, SUSAN MD
727 ELM BLVD
ANYTOWN, CA 90101

30 83

FOR STATE USE

(33) PROVIDER; YOUR REQUEST IS:

1 APPROVED AS REQUESTED · DENIED · DEFERRED

2 APPROVED AS MODIFIED (ITEMS MARKED BELOW AS AUTHORIZED MAY BE CLAIMED) · JACKSON VS RANK PARAGRAPH CODE

BY *John Doe*

MEDI-CAL CONSULTANT

I.D. # (34) 0 1 DATE (35) 0 8 2 0 X X REVIEW COMMENTS INDICATOR 44

NAME AND ADDRESS OF PATIENT

PATIENT NAME (LAST, FIRST, M. I.) (4) APPLEGATE, NANCY

MEDI-CAL IDENTIFICATION NO. (5) 253971060 CHECK DIGIT (6)

STREET ADDRESS 1515 RIVER ROAD

SEX (7) F AGE 32 DATE OF BIRTH (8) 06 18 65

CITY, STATE, ZIP CODE SACRAMENTO, CA 95822

(8A) PATIENT STATUS: X HOME · BOARD AND CARE · SNF/ICF · ACUTE HOSPITAL

PHONE NUMBER AREA (013) 545-1123

COMMENTS/ EXPLANATION

DIAGNOSIS DESCRIPTION: ENDOMETRIOSIS

(8B) ICD-9-CM DIAGNOSIS CODE 617.9

MEDICAL JUSTIFICATION:

(8C) VISTA HOSPITAL - 1200 MAPLE ST., ANYTOWN, CA

UNCONTROLLABLE ENDOMETRIOSIS

RETROACTIVE AUTHORIZATION GRANTED IN ACCORDANCE WITH SECTION 51003 (B)

(36) 1 2 3 4 5 6

	AUTHORIZED YES	NO	APPROVED UNITS	SPECIFIC SERVICES REQUESTED	UNITS OF SERVICE	PROCEDURE OR DRUG CODE	QUANTITY	CHARGES
1	(9) X		(10) 3	(10A) DAYS: 3 HOSPITAL DAYS REQUESTED	(10B)	(11)	(12) 3	$ (12A)
2	13 X		14 1	HYSTERECTOMY	1	15 5815070	16 1	$ 1300.00
3	17		18			19	20	$
4	21		22			23	24	$
5	25		26			27	28	$
6	29		30			31	32	

TO THE BEST OF MY KNOWLEDGE, THE ABOVE INFORMATION IS TRUE, ACCURATE AND COMPLETE AND THE REQUESTED SERVICES ARE MEDICALLY INDICATED AND NECESSARY TO THE HEALTH OF THE PATIENT.

Susan Smith *MD* *8-10-XX*

(39A) SIGNATURE OF PHYSICIAN OR PROVIDER · TITLE · DATE

AUTHORIZATION IS VALID FOR SERVICES PROVIDED

(37) FROM DATE 0 9 0 1 X X (38) TO DATE 0 9 3 0 X X

TAR CONTROL NUMBER

(39B) OFFICE 12 · SEQUENCE NUMBER 61240229 · PI 0

NOTE: AUTHORIZATION DOES NOT GUARANTEE PAYMENT. PAYMENT IS SUBJECT TO PATIENT'S ELIGIBILITY. BE SURE THE IDENTIFICATION CARD IS CURRENT BEFORE RENDERING SERVICE. SEND TO FIELD SERVICES (F.I. COPY)

SEE YOUR PROVIDER MANUAL FOR ASSISTANCE REGARDING THE COMPLETION OF THIS FORM. 50-1 12/87

Figure C–3. Example of a Medi-Cal Treatment Authorization Request form completed by a primary care physician for preauthorization of a professional service.

PROCEDURE: Completing a Treatment Authorization Request Form 50-1

The following item numbers and descriptions correspond to Figure C–3.

1. Leave blank.
1A. The fiscal intermediary inserts a **claim control number (CCN)** in this box.
1B. Verbal Control Number is generally left blank unless this number is obtained by telephone.
2. Enter an "X" in the appropriate boxes to show Drug or Other, Retroactive Request, and/or Medicare eligibility status.
2A. Enter the provider's area code and telephone number.
2B. Enter the provider's name and complete address.
3. Enter the nine-digit Medi-Cal rendering provider number. When requesting authorization for an elective hospital admission, the hospital provider number must be entered in this box. The hospital name may be placed in the Medical Justification area.
4. Enter the patient's last name, first name, middle initial, address, and telephone number.
5. Enter the recipient's Medi-Cal identification number from the BIC. The county code and aid code must be entered above this box. Do not use any characters (dashes, hyphens, special characters) in the remaining blank positions of the Medi-Cal ID field or in the Check Digit box (Fig. C–4).
6. Insert the letter P to indicate pending if the patient's Medi-Cal eligibility is not yet

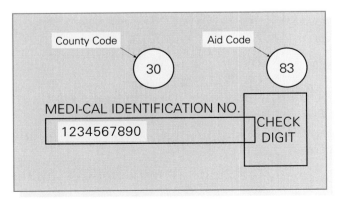

Figure C–4. Block 5 of the Treatment Authorization Request (50-1) form. Leave check digit block blank. This example shows placement of the county code and aid code on the form above Block 5.

established and the Medi-Cal number is unknown.

7. Use a capital M for male, or F for female, obtained from the BIC. Enter the patient's age in the AGE box.
8. Enter the recipient's date of birth in six-digit format. If not available, enter the year of the recipient's birth preceded by "0101."
8A. Patient's status: Enter an X if patient is an inpatient in a nursing facility Level A (NF-A) or **nursing facility (NF-B)** Level B. Enter the name of the facility in the Medical Justification area of the form.
8B. Diagnosis: Enter the description of the diagnosis and its code from the diagnostic code book.
8C. Medical justification: Provide sufficient supporting information for the consultant to determine whether the service is medically justified. If necessary, attach documentation. Enter name of the hospital or nursing facility Level A or B. Requests by nonmedical providers must include the name and telephone number of the prescriber (placed in the lower left corner of this box).
9. Leave blank. Consultant will indicate if the service line item is authorized.
10. Approved Units. Leave blank. Consultant will indicate the number of times the procedure, item, or days have been authorized.
10A. Specific Services Requested: Indicate the name of the procedure, item, or service requested.
10B. Units of Service: Leave blank.
11. Enter the procedure code (five-digit CPT with two-digit modifier or five-character HCPCS when necessary). When requesting hospital days, the stay must be requested on the first line of the TAR with the provider entering the word "DAY(S)."
12. Enter the number of times a procedure or service is requested or the number of hospital days requested.
12A. Indicate the dollar amount of the provider's usual and customary charge for the service(s) requested.
13–32. Additional TAR lines 2 through 6.
32A. Enter the name and address of the patient's authorized representative, representative payee, conservator over the person, legal representative, or other representative handling the recipient's medical and personal affairs, if applicable.
33–36. Leave blank. Consultant's determination and comments will be entered in this section. The TAR must show the consultant's

signature. Comments/Explanation lines: List the approved procedures or any further information the provider must submit with the HCFA-1500 claim.

37–38. Leave blank. Consultant will indicate valid dates of authorization.

39A. Signature of physician or provider: the provider or authorized representative must sign and date the form.

39B. Leave blank. Medi-Cal field office consultant will enter a two-digit prefix and a one-digit suffix to the preimprinted eight-digit number. This 11-digit number must be entered on the HCFA-1500 claim form when the service is billed, indicating prior authorization has been obtained. PI means pricing information and is to be left blank. *Do not attach a copy of the TAR to the HCFA-1500 claim form.*

40–43. Leave blank.

Claim Procedure

Fiscal Intermediaries

Two fiscal intermediaries are contracted by the state of California to receive and audit claims for payment of medical services and to make payments to providers of services. When the contract expires, these intermediaries may change, but at present they are (1) **Electronic Data Systems (EDS) Corporation** in Sacramento, California, for hospital billing and outpatient professional services and (2) Delta dental (formerly California Dental Services) for dental services under Denti-Cal. For the address of EDS, refer to Appendix A.

Copayment

Current law requires Medi-Cal recipients to make a nominal copayment for most outpatient services, some emergency department services, and some prescribed drugs. Copayment is never required for the following:

▶ Any person 18 years of age or younger
▶ Any woman receiving perinatal care
▶ Any child in AFDC foster care
▶ Any person who is an inpatient in a health facility (e.g., hospital, skilled nursing facility, intermediate care facility)
▶ Any service for which payment by Medi-Cal is $10 or less
▶ Emergency services or family planning services and supplies; the health care provider has the

MEDI-CAL COPAYMENT CRITERIA

Services Subject to Copayment	Copayment Fee	Exceptions to Fee
NONEMERGENCY SERVICES PROVIDED IN AN EMERGENCY ROOM A nonemergency service is defined as "any service not required for alleviation of severe pain or in the immediate diagnosis and treatment of severe medical conditions which, if not immediately diagnosed and treated, would lead to disability or death." Such services provided in an emergency room are subject to copayment.	$5.00	1. Persons age 18 or under. 2. Any woman during pregnancy and the postpartum period (through the end of the month in which the 60-day period following termination of pregnancy ends) 3. Persons who are inpatients in a health facility (hospital, skilled nursing facility or intermediate care facility)
OUTPATIENT SERVICES Physician, optometric, chiropractic, psychology, speech therapy, audiology, acupuncture, occupational therapy, podiatric, surgical center, hospital or outpatient clinic, physical therapy.	$1.00	4. Any child in AFDC-Foster care 5. Any service for which the program's payment is $10 or less 6. Any hospice patient
DRUG PRESCRIPTIONS Each drug prescription or refill.	$1.00	7. Family planning services and supplies

Figure C–5. Medi-Cal copayment criteria.

option to collect or not collect copayment at the time at which emergency service is rendered. Figure C–5 lists the services subject to copayment, copayment fees, and exclusions.

Time Limit

Medi-Cal claims must be submitted within 6 months from the end of the month of service to be reimbursed at 100% of the Medi-Cal maximum allowable. To be eligible for full reimbursement on late claims, one of the approved billing limit exception codes (1-8 or A) shown in the provider manual must be used in Field 22 of the HCFA-1500 claim form. Claims submitted more than 6 months after the month of service are reimbursed at the following reduced rates.

100% 1–6 months after the month of service
75%   7–9 months after the month of service
50%   10–12 months after the month of service
0%   Over 1 year from the month of service

An over-1-year (OOY) claim may be submitted with appropriate documentation or justification attached using exception code 8 for one of the following reasons:
▶ Retroactive eligibility
▶ Court order
▶ State of administrative hearing
▶ County error
▶ Department of Health Services approval
▶ Reversal of decision on appealed TAR
▶ Medicare/other health coverage

Helpful Billing Tips

When submitting an insurance claim for surgical procedures performed, the Medi-Cal global fee includes the preoperative visit seven days before surgery, the surgical procedure, and the postoperative care (0, 10, 30, or 90 days). This differs from standard surgical and Medicare global package policies.

Medi-Cal and Other Coverage

Medi-Cal and Private Insurance

Medi-Cal is considered the payer of last resort, and the physician must bill all other insurance carriers first and then Medi-Cal. Have the patient sign an assignment of benefits form for the other insurance. After payment is received from the other insurance carrier, include a copy of the other insurance EOB when submitting the Medi-Cal claim.

Medi-Cal and Medicare

Outpatient claims for recipients eligible for both Medicare and Medi-Cal coverage must always be billed to Medicare before Medi-Cal. These claims may be referred to as *crossover claims* because after being processed by Medicare, claims are automatically crossed over to the Medi-Cal fiscal intermediary for final processing, unless 100% of the claim was paid by Medicare. The claim *must be assigned*, or it will not be crossed over. Hardcopy billing instructions for Medicare Part B crossover claims are different from the instructions for submitting standard Medicare or Medi-Cal claims. When submitting a crossover claim, on the HCFA-1500 claim form, enter an "X" in both the Medicaid and Medicare boxes of Block 1 to identify the claim as a crossover. Enter the Medicare claim number from the identification card in Block 1a. Include the Medi-Cal recipient identification number in either Block 9a or Block 32, depending on the circumstances of the case (Fig. C–6). The Medi-Cal provider identification number appears in Block 31.

Medi-Cal and TRICARE

If a Medi-Cal patient is also covered by TRICARE, bill TRICARE first. Then bill Medi-Cal and attach the TRICARE Summary Payment Voucher to the claim form (see Chapter 13).

Computer Media Claims

The **computer media claims (CMC)** system permits submission of Medi-Cal claims via telecommunication through magnetic tape or diskette and modem. A variety of computer software formats are acceptable. The *Medi-Cal CMC Technical Manual* and the Medi-Cal web site at www.medi-cal.ca.gov contains the latest specifications to update existing systems.

Health Insurance Claim Form HCFA-1500

After verifying Medi-Cal eligibility using one of the aforementioned methods, complete an HCFA-1500 claim form and mail it to the fiscal intermediary in the blue and white envelope provided by EDS.

Instructions for Completing the HCFA-1500 Claim Form for the Medi-Cal Program

Basic instructions on how to complete the HCFA-1500 claim form for the Medicaid program and guidelines on how to prepare the document for optical scanning equipment are given in Chapter 6.

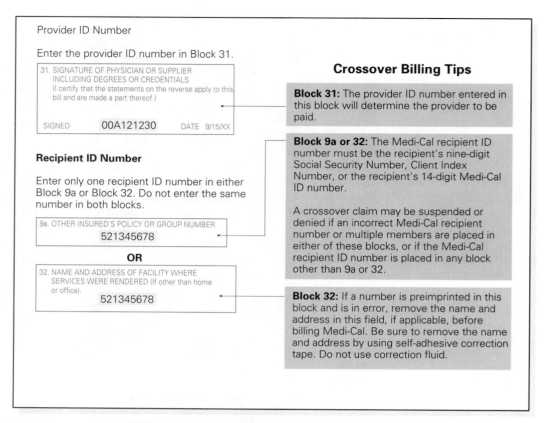

Figure C–6. Medicare/Medi-Cal crossover billing tips for completing the HCFA-1500 insurance claim form.

To learn the Medi-Cal block requirements for claim submission, use the HCFA-1500 template shown in Figure C–7. Refer to basic Medicaid instructions in Chapter 6 and the detailed instructions for the following blocks. Do not type to the right of the bar code because the fiscal intermediary inserts a claim number in that space.

Block 6. Generally, leave blank. For a claim submitted for a child younger than 2 months of age using the mother's identification card, check the box for child.

Block 10b. Not required by Medi-Cal.

Block 10c. Not required by Medi-Cal.

Block 10d. Enter the amount of the patient's SOC for the procedure, service, or supply. Do not enter a decimal point (.) or dollar sign ($); for example, $95.00 should be shown as 9500.

Block 11d. Check "Yes" if recipient has Other Health Coverage (OHC). OHC includes private insurance carriers, prepaid health plans (PHPs), and health maintenance organizations (HMOs). Eligibil-

ity under Medicare or Medi-Cal managed care plan (MCP) is NOT considered Other Health Coverage. If OHC has paid, enter the amount in the right side of this block (e.g., $50.00 should be shown as 5000).

Block 13. The EVC number may be entered here.

Block 17a. Enter the Medi-Cal nine-digit pro-vider number (not UPIN) or state license number of the referring provider or nonphysician practitioner working under the supervision of a physician.

Block 19. Enter remarks or a statement certifying the claim includes emergency services.

Block 20. Leave blank if not applicable. Check "Yes" box if the claim includes fees for outside laboratory tests and state in Block 19 that a specimen was sent to an unaffiliated laboratory.

Block 21. Only two diagnostic codes (primary and secondary) are accepted.

Block 22. Medicare status codes are required for Charpentier claims. In all other circumstances, these codes are optional. The Medicare status codes are:

APPROVED OMB 0936-006

HEALTH INSURANCE CLAIM FORM

6 Digits

PLEASE DO NOT STAPLE IN THIS AREA

CARRIER

1. MEDICARE	MEDICAID	CHAMPUS	CHAMPVA	GROUP HEALTH PLAN	FECA BLK LUNG	OTHER	1a. INSURED'S I.D. NUMBER (FOR PROGRAM IN ITEM 1)
(Medicare #)	[X] (Medicaid #)	(Sponsor's SSN)	(VA File #)	(SSN or ID)	(SSN)	(ID)	MEDI-CAL ID NUMBER

2. PATIENT'S NAME (Last Name, First Name, Middle Initial)
PATIENT'S COMPLETE NAME

3. PATIENT'S BIRTH DATE MM DD YYYY   SEX
DATE OF BIRTH M [ ] SEX F [ ]

4. INSURED'S NAME (Last Name, First Name, Middle Initial)
MOTHER'S NAME FOR NEWBORN

5. PATIENT'S ADDRESS (No., Street)
PATIENT'S COMPLETE ADDRESS

6. PATIENT RELATIONSHIP TO INSURED
Self [ ] Spouse [ ] Child [ ] Other [ ]

7. INSURED'S ADDRESS (No., Street)
N/A

CITY PATIENT'S CITY   STATE ST

8. PATIENT STATUS N/A
Single [ ] Married [ ] Other [ ]
Employed [ ] Full-Time Student [ ] Part-Time Student [ ]

CITY N/A   STATE N/A

ZIP CODE PATIENT'S ZIP   TELEPHONE (include Area Code) ( )PATIENT'S PHONE

ZIP CODE N/A   TELEPHONE (include Area Code) ( )N/A

9. OTHER INSURED'S NAME (Last Name, First Name, Middle Initial)
N/A

10. IS PATIENT'S CONDITION RELATED TO:

11. INSURED'S POLICY GROUP OR FECA NUMBER
N/A

a. OTHER INSURED'S POLICY OR GROUP NUMBER
N/A

a. EMPLOYMENT? (CURRENT OR PREVIOUS)
[ ] YES [ ] NO

a. INSURED'S DATE OF BIRTH MM DD YYYY   SEX
N/A   M [ ] F [ ]

b. OTHER INSURED'S DATE OF BIRTH MM DD YYYY   SEX
N/A   M [ ]N/A F [ ]

b. AUTO ACCIDENT? PLACE (State)
N/A [ ] YES [ ] NO N/A

b. EMPLOYER'S NAME OR SCHOOL NAME
N/A

c. EMPLOYER'S NAME OR SCHOOL NAME
N/A

c. OTHER ACCIDENT?
N/A [ ] YES [ ] NO

c. INSURANCE PLAN NAME OR PROGRAM NAME
N/A

d. INSURANCE PLAN NAME OR PROGRAM NAME
N/A

10d. RESERVED FOR LOCAL USE
PATIENT'S SHARE OF COST

d. IS THERE ANOTHER HEALTH BENEFIT PLAN?
OTHER COVERAGE/DOLLAR AMOUNT
[ ] YES [ ] NO If yes, return to and complete item 9 a-d.

READ BACK OF FORM BEFORE COMPLETING AND SIGNING THIS FORM.
12. PATIENT'S OR AUTHORIZED PERSON'S SIGNATURE I authorize the release of any medical or other information necessary to process this claim. I also request payment of government benefits either to myself or to the party who accepts assignment below.
SIGNED N/A   DATE N/A

13. INSURED'S OR AUTHORIZED PERSON'S SIGNATURE I authorize payment of medical benefits to the undersigned physician or supplier for services described below.
SIGNED EVC Number

14. DATE OF CURRENT: MM DD YYYY   ILLNESS (First symptom) OR INJURY (Accident) OR PREGNANCY (LMP)
DATE OF ONSET

15. IF PATIENT HAS HAD SAME OR SIMILAR ILLNESS GIVE FIRST DATE MM DD YYYY
N/A

16. DATES PATIENT UNABLE TO WORK IN CURRENT OCCUPATION MM DD YYYY   TO MM DD YYYY
FROM N/A

17. NAME OF REFERRING PHYSICIAN OR OTHER SOURCE
NAME OF REFERRING PROVIDER

17a. I.D. NUMBER OF REFERRING PHYSICIAN
REFERRING PROVIDER NUMBER

18. HOSPITALIZATION DATES RELATED TO CURRENT SERVICES MM DD YYYY   TO MM DD YYYY
FROM FROM DOS   THRU DOS

19. RESERVED FOR LOCAL USE
REMARKS/EMERGENCY CERTIFICATION STATEMENT

20. OUTSIDE LAB? $CHARGES
OUTSIDE LAB
[ ] YES [ ] NO   N/A | N/A

21. DIAGNOSIS OR NATURE OF ILLNESS OR INJURY (RELATE ITEMS 1,2,3 OR 4 TO ITEM 24E BY LINE)
1. PRIMARY ICD 9-CM   3. N/A
2. SECONDARY ICD 9-CM   4. N/A

22. MEDICAID RESUBMISSION CODE
MEDICARE STATUS ZONE   ORIGINAL REF. NO. N/A

23. PRIOR AUTHORIZATION NUMBER
TAR CONTROL NUMBER   11-digit

24. A DATE(S) OF SERVICE						B Place of Service	C Type of Service	D PROCEDURES, SERVICES, OR SUPPLIES (Explain Unusual Circumstances) CPT/HCPCS | MODIFIER	E DIAGNOSIS CODE	F $ CHARGES	G DAYS OR UNITS	H EPSDT Family Plan	I EMG	J COB	K RESERVED FOR LOCAL USE
From MM	DD	YYYY	To MM	DD	YYYY										
DATE OF SERVICE FROM 6 Digits			DATE OF SERVICE			POS N/A		PRO-CEDURE CODE MOD N/A	N/A	SERVICE CHARGES	QUANTITY	FP/CHDP	EMER CERT	BILLING LIMIT	RENDERING PROVIDER NUMBER

25. FEDERAL TAX I.D. NUMBER   SSN EIN
N/A   [ ] [ ]

26. PATIENT'S ACCOUNT NO.
PATIENT ACCOUNT NUMBER

27. ACCEPT ASSIGNMENT? (For govt. claims, see back)
[ ] YES [ ] NO N/A

28. TOTAL CHARGE
$ TOTAL CHARGES

29. AMOUNT PAID
$ TOTAL DEDUCTIONS

30. BALANCE DUE
$ NET AMT BILLED

31. SIGNATURE OF PHYSICIAN OR SUPPLIER INCLUDING DEGREES OR CREDENTIALS (I certify that the statements on the reverse apply to this bill and are made a part thereof.)
SIGNATURE OF PROVIDER OR PERSON AUTHORIZED
SIGNED   DATE

32. NAME AND ADDRESS OF FACILITY WHERE SERVICES WERE RENDERED (if other than home or office)
FACILITY PROVIDER NUMBER

33. PHYSICIAN'S, SUPPLIER'S BILLING NAME, ADDRESS, ZIP CODE AND PHONE #
PROVIDER NAME
ADDRESS
CITY, STATE, ZIP
PROVIDER PHONE NUMBER
MEDI-CAL PROVIDER #   GRP# N/A

(APPROVED BY AMA COUNCIL ON MEDICAL SERVICE 8/88)   PLEASE PRINT OR TYPE
FORM HCFA (12 90)
FORM OCWP 1500   FORM RRB 1500

REORDER FROM STANDARD REGISTER FORM NO HC0901B-2

PATIENT AND INSURED INFORMATION

PHYSICIAN OR SUPPLIER INFORMATION

Figure C-7. HCFA-1500 claim form illustrating Medi-Cal required fields.

Code Explanation

0	Younger than 65, does not have Medicare coverage		by Medicare intermediary
*1	Benefits exhausted	8	Noncovered services
*2	Utilization committee denial or physician non-certification	*9	PSRO denial
		*L	Medi/Medi Charpentier (rebill): Benefit limitations
*3	No prior hospital stay	*R	Medi/Medi Charpentier (rebill): Rates
*4	Facility denial		
*5	Noneligible provider	*T	Medi/Medi Charpentier (rebill): Both rates and benefit limitations
*6	Noneligible recipient		
*7	Medicare benefits denied or cut short		

Note: A permanent injunction (Charpentier v. Belshe [Coye/Kizer]) filed December 29, 1994, allows providers to rebill Medi-Cal for supplemental payment for Medicare/Medi-Cal Part B services, excluding physician services (e.g., G0001 venipuncture or laboratory tests). All Charpentier rebilled claims must have been first processed as Medi/Medi crossover claims.

Block 23. Enter the 11-digit TAR control number, if applicable.

Block 24A. Enter dates, using six digits.

Block 24B. Refer to page 201 in Chapter 6.

Block 24C. Not required by Medi-Cal.

Block 24E. Not required by Medi-Cal.

Block 24H. Enter code for family planning (FP) or CHDP services. Leave blank if not applicable.

Code Description

1	Family planning/sterilization (sterilization consent form must be attached)	2	Family planning/other
		3	CHDP screening related

Block 24I. Enter an "X" if the claim is billed for emergency services, and attach an emergency certification statement or enter a statement in Block 19.

Block 24J. Enter code that corresponds with billing limit exception and include the required documentation (see Medi-Cal provider manual).

Block 24K. Enter the nine-digit Medi-Cal provider number of the rendering provider if different from the billing provider number in Block 33.

Block 25. Not required by Medi-Cal.

Block 32. Enter only the facility's nine-digit provider number. Do not include the name and address of the facility.

Block 33. Enter the individual or group nine-character Medi-Cal provider number in the PIN# area as shown in Figure C–8.

To delete specific information from Blocks 24A through K on the HCFA-1500 claim form, draw a thin black line through the entire line but do not obliterate. Enter the correct information on another line. Use white paper tape or dry line tape to block out and correct a typed error in all other blocks. There is no need to write "See Attachments" because the equipment stamps the same assigned claim number on all accompanying sheets until the equipment recognizes another bar code. Keep the small printout from the POS device for the physician's records and, in general, do not use it as an attachment. If for some reason you need to send it to the fiscal intermediary, attach it to a standard-size sheet of paper noting the EVC number in Block 13.

Uniform Bill (UB-92) Outpatient Claim Form

The Uniform Bill (UB-92) claim form is used by institutional facilities (e.g., inpatient and outpatient departments, rural health clinics, chronic

33. PHYSICIAN'S, SUPPLIER'S BILLING NAME, ADDRESS, ZIP CODE AND PHONE #

COLLEGE CLINIC
4567 BROAD AVENUE
WOODLAND HILLS XY 12345 0001
013 486 9002

PIN#   ZZR12005F   GRP#

Figure C–8. Block 33 of the HCFA-1500 insurance claim form indicating the location for insertion of an individual or group nine-character Medi-Cal provider number.

---

*Documentation required.

dialysis services, and adult day health care) to submit claims for outpatient services.

Instructions for Completing the UB-92 Claim Form

When editing a computer-generated UB-92 claim form, refer to basic Medi-Cal block-by-block information about completion of the UB-92 claim form in Chapter 16. Figure 16–5 shows a completed UB-92 claim form; however, because Medi-Cal guidelines vary from the block-by-block illustration shown, you must refer to the block-by-block Medi-Cal instructions in that chapter. Outpatient claims are submitted in an orange envelope, and inpatient claims are submitted in a red envelope provided the by the EDS.

After Claim Submission

Remittance Advice Details

An RAD, formerly known as Explanation of Benefits and Remittance Advice (EOB/RA), accompanies all Medi-Cal payment vouchers (checks) sent to the physician. Five categories of adjudicated claims appear on an RAD:

1. Adjustments
2. Payments or approvals
3. Denials
4. Suspends
5. Accounts receivable (A/R) transactions.

Some categories of adjudicated claims are shown in Chapter 12, Figure 12–7 illustrating the Medi-Cal resolution process.

Electronic RADs are transmitted via computer to providers who have individual agreements with the fiscal intermediary. The State Controller's Office also sends a hard copy of the RAD.

Providers receiving RADs should reconcile each claim transaction to their records. Claim payments are posted as credits to the patient's ledger card. Negative adjustments are posted as debits to the patient's ledger card. It is important that each claim being reported, or not reported, be accounted for, that the necessary follow-up be performed, and that all the rules governing timelines be followed.

Adjustments

When overpayments or underpayments occur, an adjustment is initiated and two lines appear on the RAD. The first line indicates a "take back" of the original payment (original CCN); the second line reflects the correct payment of the claim (new CCN). The net amount between the two lines is the adjustment. CCNs are assigned to identify and track claims as they move through the claims processing system.

Approvals or Payments

If an original claim or a previously denied claim is approved for payment, it is listed on the RAD. If a reduction in the billed amount is warranted, the explanation will be given by means of a three-digit code.

Electronic Funds Transfer

Through **electronic funds transfer (EFT)**, providers may have their payments deposited directly into their bank accounts, and paper warrants will not be generated. However, the provider will receive an RAD document. This system will be phased in to enrollees, so it is important to keep abreast of the latest information through Medi-Cal bulletins.

Denials

Denial of claims is shown only on the RAD. Review denied claims to ensure they are correct. If a physician believes that the claim was incorrectly denied, he or she should submit a Claims Inquiry Form (CIF) for reconsideration of the claim. Until the claim is resubmitted for processing, it is no longer in the system. When the claim is resubmitted, it will be given a new CCN and be processed as a new claim in the system. For translations of the RAD codes and billing tips on how to correct denied claims, refer to the *Medi-Cal Provider Manual for Medical Services.*

Suspends

A claim requiring special handling or correction of errors is placed in temporary suspense and may be referred to as a *suspend*. Claims in suspense for 30 days or more are listed. Suspends should be referenced to determine whether an RTD was issued. There are several general explanation codes for suspended claims. Such a listing does not explain the reason but lets the physician know that the claim was received by the fiscal intermediary. *Do not* send CIFs for claims that have been temporarily suspended.

Accounts Receivable Transactions

An accounts receivable (A/R) transaction is a miscellaneous transaction as a result of a cost settlement, state audit, or refund check received by the fiscal intermediary. A three-digit code indicates the reason for the A/R transaction. A/R transactions show when it is necessary to recover funds from a provider or, in certain situations, to pay funds to a provider. The A/R system is used in financial transactions pertaining to:

▶ Recoupment of interim payments
▶ Withholds against payments to providers according to state instructions
▶ Payments to providers according to state instructions

Amounts may be either positive or negative amounts that correspond to the increase or decrease in the amount of the Medi-Cal voucher (check). An adjustment may be initiated by the provider, fiscal intermediary, or the state. Some adjustments refer to previously paid claims that may be adjusted if an error in payment occurred. A/R transactions are posted to the appropriate suspense account.

Resubmission Turnaround Document

The fiscal intermediary sends a **Resubmission Turnaround Document,** the RTD 65-1, to providers when the submitted claim form has questionable or missing information. This document eliminates the need for providers to resubmit the entire claim form to correct a limited number of errors. The RTD must be completed and returned to the fiscal intermediary by the date specified on the RTD.

PROCEDURE: Completing the Resubmission Turnaround Document

Part A of the RTD describes the information that requires correction, and part B corrects the suspended claim. To complete an RTD, either type or handwrite the correct data on the appropriate line in the Correct Information section of Part B. The data should be entered exactly as required on the claim form (i.e., no dashes, all dates in six-digit format). If a line is correct, it is not necessary to repeat the data; leave blank that line of the Correct Information section. Providers must return Part B of the RTD to the fiscal intermediary, but *do not* mail RTDs in the same envelope with claims. Refer to the *Medi-Cal Medical Services Provider Manual* for the address. Figure C−9 shows a correctly completed RTD, and the following item numbers and descriptions correspond to the figure. The top of the form contains instructions for completing the form.

1. Information block: The name of the claim form box in question.
2. Submitted information: Questionable or missing information on the claim as entered into the Medi-Cal system.
3. Service code: Procedure code, medical supply code, or drug code for the services under inquiry.
4. Error code: See Item 7. RTD error codes are *not* the same as the remittance advice denial codes. Note that 0012 indicates that "the number given on the claim as the TAR control number is not numeric or has an incorrect number of digits."
5. Beginning date of service: Date the service was rendered.
6. Corrected information: If the information in Item 2 needs to be corrected, the correct information may be noted here for the provider's records. The actual correction of the information that is sent to the fiscal intermediary is entered in Item 21.
7. Error description: This is the full explanation of the code that appears in Item 4. Compare this with your copy of the claim to assist you in identifying the error; the error description will be helpful.
8. Provider's name and address.
9. Provider's identification number.
10. Final notice: This is for the fiscal intermediary's use only.
11. Date of notice.
12. Number of pages in RTD.
13. Service date(s)/provider reference number.
14. Preprinted information that identifies the patient, Medi-Cal identification number, medical records number, total charges, and specific CCN.
15. Correspondence reference number: leave blank.
16. Provider's identification number.
17. Provider's name.
18. Patient's Medi-Cal identification number entered by the provider on the original claim.
19. Patient's name.
20. For fiscal intermediary's use only.
21. Enter correct information (Part B of the RTD) in the numbered box that corresponds with the error line in the Information Block (Item 1 in Part A). If the information in Part A is correct, leave the corresponding line blank. When entering correct information, enter all characters (numbers and letters) exactly as they would be entered on the claim. Corrected information on the RTD must be the same alphabetic or numeric format required on the claim form (i.e., date of birth: June 6, 1968, would be entered 060668). Claims cannot be processed if the corrected information is not accurate or is not shown in the required format.

RESUBMISSION TURNAROUND DOCUMENT

INSTRUCTIONS: Listed in Section "A" are error(s) found on the original claim. To expedite payment, type the correct information in the numbered Box of Section "B" that corresponds to numbered line in Section "A", sign and date the form, and return Section "B" (bottom portion) to F.I. Please respond promptly as the claim cannot be paid unless your corrections are received by October 30, 1999. See your provider manual for assistance regarding the completion of this form.

INFORMATION BLOCK	SUBMITTED INFORMATION	SERVICE CODE	ERROR CODE	BEG DOS - PATIENT NAME - COR INFO
TAR CONTROL NUMBER A1123456789			0012	XX/08/01 Smith, Mike
①	②	③	④	⑤ ⑥

⑦ ERROR DESCRIPTION

0012 - THE NUMBER GIVEN ON THE CLAIM AS THE TAR CONTROL NUMBER IS NOT NUMERIC OR HAS AN INCORRECT NUMBER OF DIGITS

PROVIDER NAME AND ADDRESS

⑨ PROVIDER NUMBER
XXXXXXXXX

FINAL NOTICE ⑩

ABC PROVIDER
123 ANY STREET
ANYTOWN, CA 95000
⑧

⑪ DATE
August 30, 20XX

PAGE OF
1 ⑫ 1

SERVICE DATE(S) / PROVIDER REFERENCE NO.
August 15, 20XX ⑬

RETAIN THIS PORTION

PATIENT NAME ⑭	MEDI-CAL ID NUMBER	MEDICAL RECORDS NO.	TOTAL CHARGES	CLAIM CONTROL NUMBER
SMITH, MIKE	1234567899	123455	$1575.00	0170626097022

DETACH AND RETURN TO APPROPRIATE F.I.

DO NOT STAPLE IN BAR AREA

CORRESPONDENCE REFERENCE NUMBER - F.I. USE ONLY
⑮

4

PROVIDER NUMBER
XXXXXXXXX ⑯

FINAL NOTICE
AUGUST 30, 1999

CORRECT INFORMATION MUST BE ENTERED ON THE SAME LINE AS THE ERROR SHOWN IN SECTION "A"

F.I. USE ONLY

PROVIDER NAME
ABC PROVIDER ⑰

CCN
0170626097022

CLAIM TYPE

PAGE
1 OF

PAGES
1

CORRECT INFORMATION

PATIENT MEDI-CAL ID NO.
1234567899 ⑱

SUBMITTED INFORMATION
A1123456789

ERROR CODE
0012

LINE
01

FIELD
012

LABEL
□ 1 ㉑ 11234567899

PATIENT NAME
SMITH, MIKE ⑲

㉒

□ 2

⑳

□ 3

This is to certify that the correct information is true, accurate and complete and that the provider has read, understands, and agrees to be bound by and comply with the statements and conditions contained on the back of this form.

Signature of provider or person authorized by provider to bind provider by above signature to statements and conditions contained on this form.

DATE

□ 4

□ 5

□ 6

IF SPECIFICALLY REQUESTED, PLACE LABEL IN THE BOX INDICATED BELOW. THIS SPACE MAY ALSO BE USED FOR COMMENTS.

1	2 ㉓	3
4	5	6

Figure C–9. Example of a completed Medi-Cal Resubmission Turnaround Document (RTD) Form 65-1.

22. Signature. All RTDs must be signed and dated by the provider or an authorized representative.
23. Blocks 1 through 6 are no longer used.

Claims Inquiry Form

A **Claims Inquiry Form (CIF)** 60-1 is used for tracing a claim, resubmitting a claim after a denial, or when requesting an adjustment for underpaid or overpaid claims (Fig. C–10). This form may also be used to request SOC reimbursement for a previously paid claim, but such cases must be submitted separately. CIFs should be submitted within six months of the date of the RAD and mailed in a black and white envelope provided by the EDS.

Providers wishing to refund an incorrect payment may complete a CIF, noting the overpayment, and forward the refund to the fiscal intermediary. Attach a photocopy of the RAD. It should be mentioned that if an overpayment is received and an insurer presses the provider of service for a refund, the insurance plan can always recoup the money requested from the next check. This happens frequently with refunds due Medicare, Medicaid, and other government payers.

For denial and adjustment requests, complete a CIF and attach a legible copy of the corrected claim form, a copy of the RAD on which the claim is listed, and any other pertinent information.

A CIF may be used to trace claims submitted to the fiscal intermediary more than 45 days previously that have not appeared on the RAD as approved or denied and that are not indicated on the most recent RAD as suspended. When submitting a tracer, leave the CCN box blank.

As many as eight claims may be listed on a single CIF when tracing. Do not attach claim copies or any other documentation to a tracer. The CIF request for tracing a claim will automatically review the recipient's history and generate a response letter showing the results of the review. Based on the information in the letter, a CIF may be resubmitted for denial reconsideration, adjustment, or proof of previous timely submission.

PROCEDURE: Completing the Claims Inquiry Form

Each line on the CIF corresponds to a single line on the HCFA-1500 claim form. Complete the lines on the CIF according to the type of inquiry you wish to make. Adjustment and denial reconsideration requests may be combined on one CIF. Tracer requests must be submitted separately.

It is important that the correct number of characters be entered in the spaces provided on the form. Any time a reference is made to a claim previously adjudicated, be certain to indicate the previous CCN and attach a copy of the corrected claim and RAD. *Do not* submit CIFs for claims that are listed under the Suspends heading on the RAD. Each numbered item refers to the numbers on the CIF (see Fig. C–10).

1. Correspondence reference number: Leave blank. The fiscal intermediary will assign a number.
2. Document number: A preimprinted number identifying the CIF.
3. Provider's name/address: Enter provider's name, street address, city, state, and ZIP code.
4. Provider's number: Enter the nine-character provider identification number, plus optional check digit, assigned by the Department of Health Services.
5. Claim type: Enter an "X" in the box indicating the claim type. Check only one box.
6. Delete: Enter an "X" to delete the entire line. Enter the correct billing information on another line.
7. Patient's name or medical record number: Enter up to the first 10 letters of the patient's last name or the first 10 characters of the patient's medical record number.
8. Patient's Medi-Cal identification number: Enter the recipient's identification number that appears on the RAD showing adjudication of that claim.
9. CCN: Enter the 13-digit number assigned by the fiscal intermediary to the claim line in question. This may be found on the RAD. If this line is blank, the inquiry will be considered a tracer request.
10. Date of service: Enter the date in six-digit format (i.e., 0606XX), on which the service was rendered. For consecutive date ranges (block-billed claims), enter the "From" date of service.
11. NDC/UPC or procedure code: Enter the appropriate procedure code, modifier, and drug or supply code if applicable. Codes of less than 11 digits should be left-justified. *Long-term care and inpatient providers may leave this box blank.*
12. Amount billed: Enter the amount originally billed, using the two boxes to the right of the decimal point to reflect cents.
13. Attachment: Enter an "X" when attaching documentation and when resubmitting a denied claim. All CIFs should have attachments except when submitting a tracer.

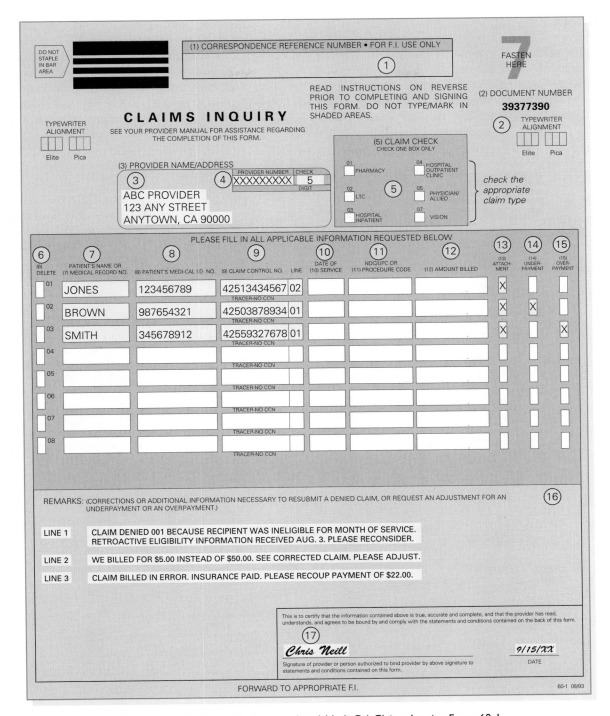

Figure C–10. Example of a completed Medi-Cal Claims Inquiry Form 60-1.

14. Underpayment: Enter an "X" for an underpayment adjustment of a paid claim. *Do not* mark if the claim was denied.

15. Overpayment: Enter an "X" if all or part of the claim was overpaid. *Do not* mark if the claim was denied.

16. Remarks: Use this area to state the reason for submitting a CIF and include the corresponding line number if listing multiple claim lines on the CIF.

17. Signature: The provider or an authorized representative must sign the CIF.

Appeal Process

A provider with a grievance or complaint regarding payment of claims must direct this grievance or complaint to the fiscal intermediary *within 90 days* of the action causing the grievance or complaint. If the 90-day limit is not met, the appeal is subject to automatic denial. Appeals must be submitted using the Appeal Form 90-1 (Fig. C–11) and should include legible copies of supporting documentation (e.g., claim forms, RADs, CIFs, TARs). Appeals are sent in a lavender envelope provided by the EDS. The fiscal intermediary will send an acknowledgment within 15 days

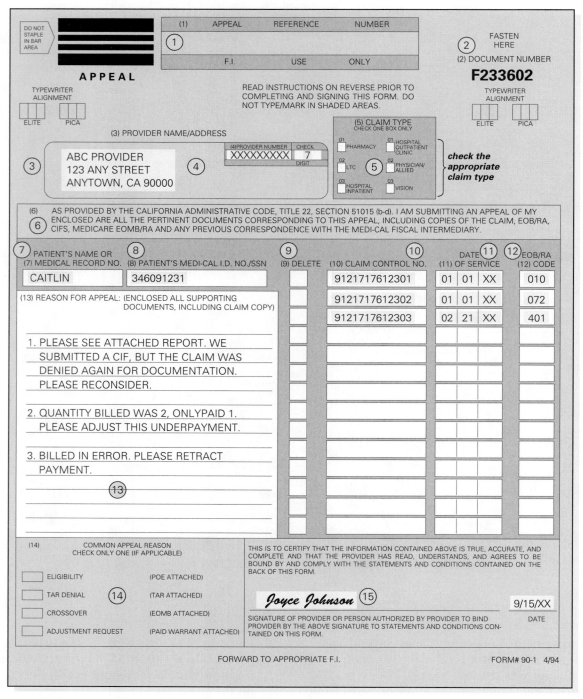

Figure C–11. Example of a completed Medi-Cal Appeal Form 90-1 to be used for denial resubmmissions, underpayment reconsiderations, and overpayment returns.

of receipt and make a decision within 30 days from the date of the acknowledgment. If the appealed claim is approved for reprocessing, it will appear on a RAD. If the provider is not satisfied with the decision, a subsequent appeal may be made. If the provider is still not satisfied with the decision, then judicial remedy no later than 1 year after receipt of the decision may be undertaken.

PROCEDURE: Completing an Appeal Form

Each numbered item refers to the numbers on the Appeal Form shown in Figure C–11.

1. Appeal reference number: Leave blank. The fiscal intermediary will assign a number.
2. Document number: A preimprinted number is used when requesting information about the status of an appeal.
3. Provider's name/address: Enter the provider's name, street address, city, state, and ZIP code.
4. Provider's number: Enter the nine-character provider's identification number, plus check digit, assigned by the Department of Health Services. Without the correct provider number, appeal acknowledgment may be delayed.
5. Claim type: Enter an X in the box indicating the claim type. Check only one box.
6. Statement of appeal: This is for information purposes only.
7. Patient's name or medical record number: Enter up to the first 10 letters of the patient's last name or the first 10 characters of the patient's medical record number.
8. Patient's Medi-Cal identification number/Social Security Number (SSN): Enter the recipient's identification number that appears on the plastic BIC or paper Medi-Cal card.
9. Delete: Enter an "X" to delete the corresponding line. Enter correct billing information on another line.
10. CCN: For adjudicated claims, enter the 13-digit number assigned by the fiscal intermediary to the claim line in question. This number appears on the RAD. When appealing a nonadjudicated claim (i.e., a traced claim that could not be located), the CCN field is not required.
11. Date of service: Enter the date the service was rendered in six-digit format (0102XX). For claims billed in a "From-Through" format, enter the "From" date of service.
12. RAD code or EOB/RA code: When appealing an adjudicated claim, enter the RAD message code for the claim line (e.g., 010, 072, 401).
13. Reason for appeal: Indicate the specific reason for filing an appeal. Remember to attach all supporting documentation.
14. Common appeal reason: Check one of the boxes if applicable. Include a copy of the claim and supporting documents (e.g., TAR, RAD). Box 13 may be left blank if this box is used.
15. Signature: The provider or an authorized representative must sign

---

STUDENT ASSIGNMENT LIST

✔ Study Chapter 12 and Appendix C.
✔ Answer the self-study review questions in the *Workbook* to reinforce the theory learned in these portions of the text and to help prepare you for a future test.
✔ Complete the assignments in the *Workbook* to give you experience abstracting from case histories, posting to ledger cards, and completing forms pertinent to the Medi-Cal program.
✔ Turn to the Glossary at the end of this textbook for a further understanding of the Key Terms used in this chapter.

Student Software Challenge is a software program designed to be used with the seventh edition of the W.B. Saunders textbook *Insurance Handbook for the Medical Office* by Marilyn T. Fordney, CMA-AC.

MINIMUM SYSTEM REQUIREMENTS

Operating System:	Windows 95 or 98 only
Computer:	IBM and compatible PCs with 80486/66 or Pentium CPU
	MS-DOS 5.0 or 6.0
Optimal Screen Requirements:	sVGA or higher graphics adapter operating in 640 × 480, 256-color mode
	CD-ROM drive
	Mouse
Memory:	16 MB RAM

SITE LICENSE

To order a site license for this program contact your local sales representative, or Harcourt faculty support at (800) 222-9570; technical support (800) 692-9010.

INSTALLING THE PROGRAM

The software may be installed on individual computers and is network compatible with most networks, including Novell Netware 4.1 and Windows NT Server 4.0.

Before you can use the software, you must install it on your hard disk. The installer decompresses and copies files from the *Student Software Challenge* CD-ROM onto your hard disk or network and creates a Medical Insurance folder.

Steps to install the *Student Software Challenge* on a computer running Windows 95 or 98.

- Turn off virus protection, disk-security, and other open programs prior to installing *Student Software Challenge*.
- Insert the *Student Software Challenge* CD-ROM into the CD-ROM drive.
- Launch the *Student Software Challenge* installer by double-clicking the file called "install.exe" on the CD-ROM. Launch the installer by selecting **Run** from the Start menu type d:\install.exe in the Command Line (where "d" represents your CD-ROM drive), and press **Enter.** If necessary, substitute the appropriate drive letter for your CD-ROM drive.
- Follow the installation instructions that appear on your screen. There are several options during installation.
  - *Minimum (partial) or full installation may be selected. The default installation option is used to install only those files needed to run the program from the CD-ROM. This is done by choosing the **Run from CD-ROM** option. Installing the CD-ROM runtime version requires approximately 1 MB of free hard-disk space. The entire program may also be installed to a hard disk by choosing the **Full installation** option. Installing the entire program requires approximately 23 MB of free hard-disk space and will enhance the software's performance.*
  - *Location where the program will be installed may be selected. The default location is C:\MI7. Use the Browse feature to change the drive or directory in which the software will be installed. The installation program automatically detects whether there is adequate free space available on the hard disk. If there is not enough space available,*

627

a prompt appears directing you to select another location. Note: To install the software to a network hard disk, use the Browse feature to locate the network drive.

▶ ***Location where student data will be saved may be selected.*** *The program saves log-on information and the results of completed HCFA-1500 forms for each student. The default location for storage of student data is the* `A:\drive` ***(Save student data on the A drive).*** *This option allows the student to save his or her data on a diskette. To save student data in the directory on the hard drive where the* Student Software Challenge *program is installed, choose the* ***Save student data with the program on the hard disk*** *option. Note: If the data diskette option is chosen, the student must have his or her data diskette to log-on and use the program.*

▶ ***Locate and open the Medical Insurance program group to start the program.*** *Then double-click the icon for the Medical Insurance program (MI2.EXE).*

LOGGING ON TO *STUDENT SOFTWARE CHALLENGE*

The student log-on screen will include the following information:

▶ **First Name**. This required field can contain up to 20 characters and is case sensitive. The first name field can include spaces, allowing students to register their first name and middle initial (e.g., Marcia B. or C. David).

▶ **Last Name**. This required field can contain up to 20 characters and is case sensitive.

▶ **Class**. This optional field may be used to enter the name of the class and is limited to a maximum of 30 characters. It is case sensitive.

▶ **Password**. The password field is required and can include a password up to 10 characters. It is case insensitive. There is a prompt to verify the password when entered for the first time.

First-Time Log-on Steps

▶ If the installation is configured to store student data on data diskettes, the data diskette must be inserted in the diskette drive before logging on. If no diskette is detected, the program will prompt for it. *Note*: The program will accept blank, formatted data diskettes as student data diskettes.

▶ The program will begin with a list of students. The class list is organized alphabetically, last name first, from A to Z. There are two buttons available: [OK] and [New].

▶ If your name does not appear in the student list, click **New** to self-register. The program will branch to the log-on registration screen, at which point you will be prompted to enter your first and last names (required), the class (optional), and a password (required). After entering

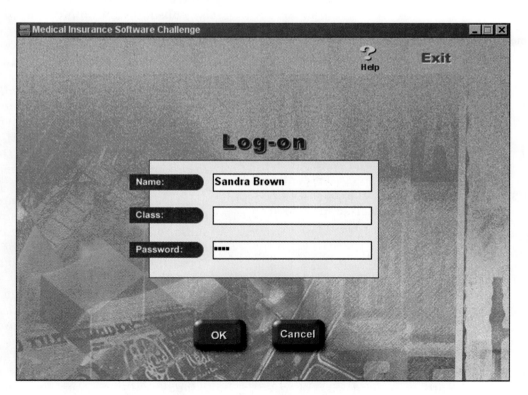

Figure D–1. Log-on screen

the password, a prompt will display, asking you to verify your password by typing it a second time.

▶ After completing the self-registration, a data file with your unique information will be created in the drive and directory specified at installation.

Subsequent Log-on Steps

▶ If the installation is configured to store student data on data diskettes, the data diskette must be inserted in the diskette drive before logging on. If no diskette is detected, the program will prompt for it.

▶ When starting the program in subsequent sessions, select (highlight) your name from the list and click **OK.** A log-on screen will appear; enter your password in the field provided and click **OK.**

USING THE *STUDENT SOFTWARE CHALLENGE*

After logging onto the software, the Patient Cases menu will display. If this is the first time you are using the software, a brief introduction and instructions will display in a dialog on top of the Patient Cases menu. Print or close the instructions after reading them. If you have used the software before and were in the middle of an exercise when you last worked with the program, a bookmark screen will display after logging on. The bookmark allows you to bypass the Patient Cases menu. Click **Continue where you left off** to return to the case on which you were last working. Click **Restart from be-**

ginning of case to restart the case. Click **Cancel** to go to the Patient Cases menu.

The Patient Cases menu includes 10 patient case folders organized alphabetically by the patient's last name.

The case numbers indicate the order of difficulty and coincide with the patient's account numbers. The menu also includes an eleventh file folder labeled "Other Patients." This feature is described in detail on page 632.

Button Bar

The software includes the following buttons on the button bar:

▶ Click the **Patients** button to go to the Patient Cases menu.

▶ Click the **Glossary** button to go to the Glossary to define an abbreviation or look up a word.

▶ Click the **Report** button to access a report listing the cases completed and the scores of your work.

▶ Click the **Print** button to print a hard copy of the information forms or an HCFA-1500 form.

▶ Click the **Help** button to obtain program-software information on the currently displayed screen.

▶ Click the **Exit** button to quit the program. A prompt to confirm your selection will appear.

Working with Patient Cases

▶ Select a patient case. A screen with four folders will display.

  ▶ *The 1st folder contains patient information needed to complete the top portion of the HCFA-1500 insurance claim form.*

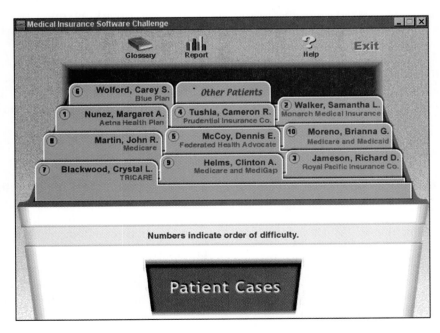

Figure D-2. Patient Cases menu

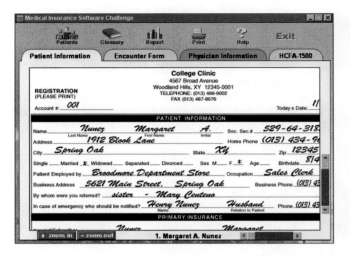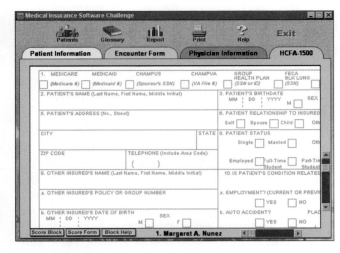

Figure D–3. Patient Information screen and HCFA-1500 form

▶ *The 2nd folder contains either the encounter form or the medical record needed to complete the bottom portion of the HCFA-1500 insurance claim form.*

▶ *The 3rd folder contains physician and clinic information needed to complete the HCFA-1500 insurance claim form.*

▶ *The 4th folder contains a blank HCFA-1500 insurance claim form.*

▶ Click on the folder tabs to display the contents of the folder.

▶ View a different part of the information forms by placing your cursor on the form, clicking and holding down the mouse button (a hand will appear), and dragging the form until the part you are looking for is in view.

OR

▶ Use the scroll bar at the right and bottom sides of the form to scroll horizontally and vertically to locate different sections of the form. The information forms may be enlarged or decreased in size by using the "+200 m in" and "−200 m out" features.

▶ On the HCFA-1500 form you may click in a field to enter information and/or tab from one field to the next to enter information. Use the information provided in the first three folders to complete the HCFA-1500 insurance claim form. You can return to the information forms at any time while completing the HCFA-1500 form for the selected case. It is preferable to print information forms if a printer is connected to your computer.

▶ Check your work on a specific block by placing your cursor in the block and clicking the **Score Block** button. The software will score the selected block and provide feedback on your performance. You have two chances to complete the block correctly.

▶ Click the **Score Form** button when you have completed the form. The software will score the form and display feedback on your performance.

▶ After scoring the form, blocks containing errors will appear in blue. You have two chances to look for and correct errors and score the form. Individual blocks that have been previously scored may be changed, but will only *reflect the score after the 2nd change.*

▶ Print the form for a hard copy of information as it was input.

▶ Click **Report** and choose (highlight) the case you were working on. Click **HCFA-1500 Form** at the bottom of the screen to go to the Print Preview screen and view or print the corrected form. Blocks completed incorrectly will display the correct answer as follows:

An error on the *first attempt* that was corrected on the second attempt will be displayed in **blue bold text.**

An error on the *second attempt* or first attempt errors that were never corrected will be displayed in ***blue, bold italic.***

▶ When using a black and white printer, compare the printout with this screen and highlight all errors (bold and italic blue print) so they are easily distinguished.

Block Help

If you are unsure of what type of information goes in a block, click on the **Block Help** button. This button will display a dialog with information on the selected block. The dialog will contain three buttons labeled Private, Medicare, and TRICARE, for selecting the type of insurance for which you need Block

Help. The default is Private. You can change the default by clicking on one of the other selections.

Scoring and Reporting

The first two attempts on a patient case will be scored; performance data will be stored in the Report. You will receive

> **full credit** (1 point) for completing a field on the *first try,* **half credit** ($^1/_2$ point) for completing a field on the *second try,* **no credit** for incorrect entries *after the second attempt.* **Penalty** of $^1/_2$ point for filling in fields that are not required on either 1st or 2nd attempt.

▶ Access a Report by clicking the **Report** button on the button bar. The Report screen displays the student's name and the current date in the header field. The Report includes a one-line entry for each partially or fully completed case. The Report also stores the HCFA-1500 forms for patients that you created in the Other Patients section of the software. Although these forms are not scored, they are included in the report so that you can access the data even if you have deleted the patient. For these forms, only the Work Date and Patient Name columns are completed. Each entry includes the following information:

▶ **Work date.** *This is the date the case was worked on. In the case of bookmarked cases that were started on one day and completed on another, the work date is the date on which the case was started. If you continue a case on a subsequent date, the Work Date will appear on the HCFA-1500 form as well as "Today's Date."*

▶ **Case number.** *The number that appears on the patient folder in the Patient Cases menu.*

▶ **Patient name.** *The patient name that appears on the patient folder in the Patient Cases menu.*

▶ **Insurance carrier.** *The name of the insurance carrier that appears on the patient folder in the Patient Cases menu.*

▶ **Score.** *The score shows the percentage of fields of the total form that you completed correctly on the first try (1 point) and second try ($^1/_2$ point).*

▶ **Completed.** *This column displays a checkmark for those cases 1 through 10 that have been completed.*

▶ Display a partially or fully completed form from the Report by selecting an entry and clicking on the **HCFA-1500 Form** button. When you display a form from the Report, the software will display the correct answers. Blocks completed incorrectly will display the correct answer marked in **blue, bold text** (first-try errors that were corrected on second attempt) or **blue, bold italic text** (second-try errors or first-try errors that were never corrected).

▶ Zoom in on the HCFA-1500 form when it is displayed from the Report by clicking the **Zoom In** button. To zoom out click the **Zoom Out** button.

▶ To print the form, click the **Print** button on the button bar. The printout from the Report will include a header that says *Printed from Report* with the Student's name, Today's date, Work date, Patient name, and score. If you print the form from

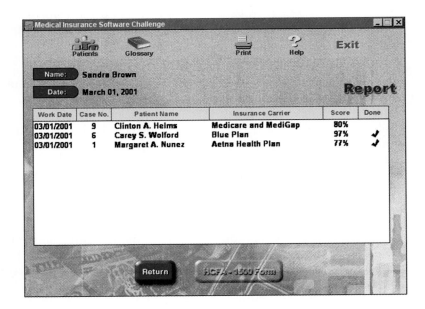

Figure D–4. Report screen

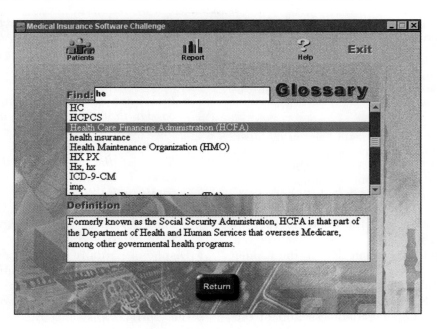

Figure D–5. Glossary screen

the patient case screen, you will have one form that shows your errors as you entered them and one form that shows the correct answers.

▶ Click the **Return** button to return to the input screen viewed before clicking on the **Report** button.

Printing the HCFA-1500 Form

Print the HCFA-1500 form from the patient case screen by clicking on the Print button on the button bar. If you print the form from the Patient Cases screen, your entries will appear as you typed them and errors will be displayed in bold blue. Your performance on the HCFA-1500 form will be recorded in the Report (see Scoring and Reporting).

Other Patients

▶ **Add other patients** by clicking the *"Other Patients"* folder tab on the Patient Cases menu. A list of the Other Patients will display. The *Other Patients* file folder tab on the Patient Cases menu allows you to add up to 50 patients and complete HCFA-1500 forms for them. These patients may be chosen from the *Workbook* or may be cases created by the instructor. The first time you use this feature, the list will be empty.

▶ **Add a new patient** by clicking on the **New Patient** button. The New Patient Registration screen will display. Enter the first name and then the last name of the new patient and click **OK.** The patient's name will be added to the Other Patients' list. Select (highlight) a patient, click **OK,** and a blank HCFA-1500 form will dis-

play. If you leave the HCFA-1500 form in progress, your work will be saved.

▶ **Delete patients** by selecting a name in the list and clicking the **Delete Patient** button. A prompt to confirm the deletion will appear. If you delete a patient from the Other Patients list, you can still display the form for that patient from the Report (see Scoring and Reporting). Remember you can add up to 50 patients to the Other Patients list. Once the limit is reached, you will be prompted to delete patients from the list before adding new ones. To return to the Patient Cases menu, click the **Cancel** button. To return to the Patient Cases menu, click the **Patients** button on the button bar.

Using the Glossary

▶ Click on the **Glossary** button bar to access the Glossary. The Glossary is accessible from all screens in the software except the log-on sequence. It includes a Find text entry field that searches on multiple characters.

▶ Type the first few characters of the word in the Find field to search for a word. The Glossary will automatically scroll to the first term beginning with those characters and display its definition.

▶ Click on a term or abbreviation that is displayed in green in the Patient's Medical Record to automatically go to the Glossary and read the definition.

▶ Click the **Return** button on the Glossary screen to return to the previous screen.

Glossary

Chapter number(s) is shown in parentheses after each term.

Abuse (1): Incidents or practices, not usually considered fraudulent, that are inconsistent with accepted sound medical business or fiscal practices.

Accident (14): An unexpected happening causing injury traceable to a definite time and place.

Accidental death and dismemberment (15): Insurance policy provision that protects the insured if he or she suffers loss of sight or loss of limb(s) or death by accident.

Accounts receivable (9): Total amount of money owed for professional services rendered.

Accounts receivable (A/R) transaction (C): Miscellaneous Medi-Cal accounting transactions as a result of cost settlements, state audits, or refund checks received by the fiscal intermediary.

Active duty service member (ADSM) (13): Active member of the government armed, naval, or air forces.

Actual charge (5): Physician's actual fee for his or her service at the time the insurance claim is submitted to the insurance company or government payer.

Acute (3): Refers to a medical condition that runs a short but relatively severe course.

Adjudication (14): Final determination of the issues in an action according to which judgment is rendered.

Admission review (16): Review for appropriateness and necessity of admissions.

Adverse effect (4): Adverse or pathologic reaction to a drug that occurs when appropriate doses are given to humans for prophylaxis, diagnosis, and therapy.

Age analysis (9): Procedure of systematically arranging the accounts receivable, by age, from the date of service.

Aid to the Blind (AB) (C): A group that is entitled to benefits under the Medi-Cal program.

Aid to Families with Dependent Children (AFDC) (C): A group that is entitled to benefits under the Medi-Cal program.

Aid to the (permanently) Disabled (ATD) (C): A group that is entitled to benefits under the Medi-Cal program.

Alien (17): An individual belonging to another country or people; a foreigner.

Allowable charge (13): Amount on which TRICARE figures the patient's cost-share for covered care. This is based on 75% to 80% of the *allowable* charge.

Ambulatory payment classifications (APCs) (16): System of outpatient hospital reimbursement based on procedures rather than on diagnoses.

American Health Information Management Association (AHIMA) (1): National professional organization for promoting the art and science of medical record management and improving the quality of comprehensive health information for the welfare of the public.

American Medical Association (AMA) (1): National professional society of physicians.

Ancillary services (10): Supportive services other than routine hospital services provided by the facility, such as x-ray films and laboratory tests.

Appeal (8): Request for more payment made by asking for a review of an insurance claim that has been paid or denied by an insurance company.

Applicant (2): Person applying for insurance coverage.

Application form (17): Request form to be completed with pertinent data when applying for employment.

Appropriateness evaluation protocol (AEP) (16): Nineteen criteria for admission under the prospective payment system, separated into two categories: severity of illness and intensity of illness. To allow a patient admission to an acute care facility, one criterion from each category must be met.

Approved charges (11): Fee that Medicare decides the medical service is worth, which may or may not be the same as the actual amount billed. The patient may or may not be responsible for the difference.

Armed Services Disability (15): Disability occurring or aggravated while the patient is in military service.

Assignment (2, 11): Transfer, after an event insured against, of an individual's legal right to collect an amount payable under an insurance contract. For Medicare, an agreement in which a patient assigns to the physician the right to receive payment from the fiscal intermediary. Under this agreement, the physician must agree to accept the program payment as payment in full except for 20% or the *reasonable (allowed or approved) charge* and the deductible. For TRICARE, providers who accept assignment agree to accept 75% or 80% of the TRICARE allowable charge as the full fee, collecting the deductible and 20% or 25% of the allowable charge from the patient.

Attending physician (3): Medical staff member who is legally responsible for the care and treatment given to a patient.

Audit trail (7): Path left by a transaction when it is processed.

Authorized provider (13): Physician or other individual authorized provider of care or a hospital or supplier approved by TRICARE to provide medical care and supplies.

Automated eligibility verification system (AEVS) (C): An interactive voice-response system in the Medi-Cal program that allows providers to access recipient eligibility, clear share of cost, and/or reserve a Medi-Service.

Automatic stay (9): Court order that goes into effect once a bankruptcy petition is filed; all other legal actions are halted, such as attachments and foreclosures.

Back up (7): Duplicate data file; equipment designed to complete or redo the operation if the primary equipment fails.

Balance (9): Amount owed on a credit transaction; also known as the outstanding or unpaid balance.

Bankruptcy (9): Condition under which a person or corporation is declared unable to pay debts.

Batch (7): Group of claims for different patients from one office submitted in one computer transmission.

Beneficiaries (13): Individuals entitled to receive insurance policy or government program health care benefits. Also known as *participants, subscribers, dependents, enrollees,* or *members.*

Benefit period (11, 15): Period of time for which payments for Medicare inpatient hospital benefits are available. A benefit period begins the first day an enrollee is given inpatient hospital care (nursing care or rehabilitation services) by a qualified provider and ends when the enrollee has not been an inpatient for 60 consecutive days. For disability insurance, it is the maximum amount of time that benefits will be paid to the injured or ill person for a disability.

Benefits identification card (BIC) (C): Medi-Cal identification card.

Benign tumor (4): Abnormal growth that does not have the properties of invasion and metastasis and is usually surrounded by a fibrous capsule.

Bilateral (5): When coding surgical procedures, this term refers to both sides of the body.

Bit (7): Binary digit, either a 1 or 0.

Blanket contract (2): Comprehensive group insurance coverage through plans sponsored by professional associations for their members.

Blanket position bond (1): Insurance that provides coverage for all employees regardless of job title.

Blind mailing (17): To send resume with cover letter to possible prospects that the individual does not know personally and who have not advertised for a job opening.

Bonding (1): An insurance contract by which, in return for a stated fee, a bonding agency guarantees payment of a certain sum to an employer in the event of a financial loss to the employer by the act of a specified employee or by some contingency over which the employer has no control.

Breach of confidential communication (3): "Breach" means breaking or violation of a law or agreement. In the context of the medical office it means the unauthorized release of information about the patient.

Buffing (10): Physicians justifying the transference of sick, high-cost patients to other physicians in a managed care plan.

Bug (7): An error in a program.

Bundled codes (5): To group codes together that are related to a procedure.

By report (BR) (14): A report must be submitted with the claim when the notation BR follows the procedure code description. This term is sometimes seen in workers' compensation fee schedules.

Byte (7): The number of bits used to represent one character.

California Children's Services (CCS) (C): A state program for disabled children.

Capitation (2, 10, 16): System of payment used by managed care plans in which physicians and hospitals are paid a fixed, per capita amount for each patient enrolled over a stated period of time, regardless of the type and number of services provided; reimbursement to the hospital on a per-member/per-month basis to cover costs for the members of the plan.

Carrier-direct system (7): Direct electronic transmission of insurance claims from the physician to the insurance company.

Carve outs (10): Medical services not included within the capitation rate as benefits of a managed care contract and may be contracted for separately.

Case rate (16): An averaging after a flat rate is given to certain categories of procedures.

Cash flow (1, 9): In a medical practice, the amount of *actual* cash generated by the medical practice within a given period of time.

Catastrophic cap (13): Upper limit that an active-duty family has to pay under TRICARE Standard-covered medical bills in any fiscal year.

Categorically needy (12): Aged, blind, or disabled individuals or families and children who meet financial eligibility requirements for Aid to Families with Dependent Children, Supplemental Security Income, or an optional state supplement.

Central processing unit (CPU) (7): Brains of a computing device controlling the internal memory that directs the flow and processing of information.

Certification (17): Statement issued by a board or association verifying that a person meets professional standards.

Certified Claims Assistance Professional (CCAP) (17): Certification awarded to a person after appropriate training and by passing a certification examination administered by the Alliance of Claims Assistance Professionals, Inc.

Certified Coding Specialist (CCS) (17): Title received by a person after appropriate training and by passing a certification examination administered by the American Health Information Management Association for hospital based coding.

Certified Coding Specialist-Physician (CCS-P) (17): Title received by a person after appropriate training and by passing a certification examination administered by the American Health Information Management Association for physician based coding.

Certified Electronic Claims Professional (CECP) (17): Certification awarded to a person after appropriate training and by passing a certification examination administered by the Alliance of Claims Assistance Professionals, Inc.

Certified Medical Assistant (CMA) (17): A title received by a person after appropriate training and by passing a certification examination administered by the American Association of Medical Assistants, Inc.

Certified Professional Coder (CPC) (17): Title received by a person after appropriate training and by passing a certification examination administered by the American Academy of Professional Coders.

CHAMPVA (2, 13): The Civilian Health and Medical Program of the Department of Veterans Affairs, a program for veterans with total, permanent, service-connected disabilities or surviving spouses and dependents of veterans who died of service-connected disabilities.

Charge description master (CDM) (16): Computer program that is linked to various hospital departments and includes procedure codes, procedure descriptions, service descriptions, fees, and revenue codes; also known as *charge master.*

Charges (16): The dollar amount a hospital bills an outlier case based on the itemized bill.

Chief complaint (CC) (3, 4): Patient's statement describing symptoms, problems, or conditions as the reason for seeking health care services from a physician.

Child Health and Disability Prevention Program (CHDP) (C): A state health and disability prevention program for children.

Chronic (3): Medical condition persisting over a long period of time.

Chronologic resume (17): A data sheet that outlines experience and education by dates.

Churning (1, 10): Physicians' seeing a high volume of patients—more than medically necessary—to increase revenue. May be seen in fee-for-service or managed care environments.

Civil Service Retirement System (CSRS) (15): Program for federal employees hired before 1984.

Claim (2): A billing sent to an insurance carrier. Also known as *encounter record.*

Claim control number (CCN) (C): A number assigned by the Medi-Cal fiscal intermediary on a Treatment Authorization Request and used for reference when processing the request.

Claims assistance professional (CAP) (1, 17): A practitioner who works for the consumer and helps patients organize, complete, file, and negotiate health insurance claims of all types to obtain maximum benefits as well as tell patients what checks to write to providers to eliminate overpayment.

Claims and eligibility real-time software (CERTS) (C): Computer software that allows Medi-Cal providers to electronically verify recipient eligibility, clear share of cost liability, reserve Medi-Services, perform Family PACT (planning, access, care, treatment) client eligibility transactions, and submit pharmacy or HCFA-1500 claims using a personal computer.

Claims examiner (14): In industrial cases, a representative of the insurer who authorizes treatment and investigates, evaluates, and negotiates the patient's insurance claim and acts for the company in the settlement of claims; also known as *claims adjuster, claim representative, claims administrator.*

Claims Inquiry Form (CIF) (C): A Medi-Cal form used for tracing a claim, resubmitting a claim after a denial, or when requesting an adjustment for underpaid or overpaid claims.

Claims-review type of foundation (10): A type of foundation that provides peer review by physicians to the numerous fiscal agents or carriers involved in its area.

Clean claim (6): A completed insurance claim form that contains all the necessary information without deficiencies so it can be processed and paid promptly.

Clearinghouse (7): Third party administrator (TPA) by which insurance claims are transmitted and who redistributes the claims electronically to various insurance carriers.

Clinical outliers (16): Cases that cannot adequately be assigned to an appropriate DRG owing to unique combinations of diagnoses and surgeries, very rare conditions, or other unique clinical reasons. Such cases are grouped together into clinical outlier DRGs and, therefore, are considered *outliers.*

Closed panel program (10): A form of HMO that limits the patient's choice of personal physicians to those doctors practicing in the HMO group practice within the geographic location and/or facility. A physician must meet very narrow criteria to join a closed panel.

Coding specialist (17): An individual whose expertise is in procedural and/or diagnostic coding.

Coinsurance (2): A cost-sharing requirement under a health insurance policy providing that the insured will assume a percentage of the costs for covered services; for Medicare, after application of the yearly cash deductible, the portion of the reasonable charges (20%) for which the beneficiary is responsible.

Collateral (9): Any possession, such as an automobile, furniture, stocks, or bonds, that secures or guarantees the discharge of an obligation.

Collection ratio (9): Relationship between the amount of money owed and the amount of money collected in reference to the doctor's accounts receivable.

Combination code (4): Single five-digit code used to identify etiology and secondary process (manifestation) or complication of a disease.

Combination resume (17): Data sheet that combines specific dates or work experience with educational skills.

Comorbidity (3, 16): An ongoing condition that exists along with the condition for which the patient is receiving treatment; in regard to DRGs, a preexisting condition that, because of its presence with a certain principal diagnosis, will cause an increase in length of stay by at least 1 day in approximately 75% of cases. Also known as *substantial comorbidity.*

Competitive Medical Plan (CMP) (2): A type of managed care organization created by the 1982 TEFRA legislation for enrollment of Medicare beneficiaries into managed care plans.

Compliance program (3): A management plan composed of policies and procedures to accomplish uniformity, consistency, and conformity in medical record keeping that fulfills official requirements.

Complication (4): Disease or condition arising during the course of, or as a result of, another disease modifying medical care requirements; for DRGs, a condition that arises during the hospital stay that prolongs the length of stay by at least 1 day in approximately 75% of cases. Also known as *substantial complication.*

Comprehensive (C) (3): A term used to describe a level of history and/or physical examination.

Comprehensive code (5): A single code that describes or covers two or more component codes that are bundled together as one unit.

Comprehensive Perinatal Services Program (CPSP) (C): A program that offers a wide range of services to pregnant Medi-Cal recipients.

Comprehensive type of foundation (10): A type of foundation that designs and sponsors prepaid health programs or sets minimum benefits of coverage.

Compromise and release (C and R) (14): An agreement arrived at, whether in or out of court, for settling a workers' compensation case after the patient has been declared permanent and stationary.

Computer billing (9): Producing statements via a computer system.

Computer media claims (CMC) (C): A system that permits submission of Medi-Cal claims via telecommunication through magnetic tape or diskette and modem.

Concurrent care (3): Provision of similar services (e.g., hospital visits) to the same patient by more than one physician on the same day.

Conditionally renewable (2): Insurance policy renewal provision that grants the insurer a limited right to refuse to renew a health insurance policy at the end of a premium payment period.

Confidential communication (1): Privileged communication that may be disclosed only with the patient's permission.

Confidentiality (1): The state of treating privately or secretly, and not disclosing to other individuals or for public knowledge, the patient's conversations or medical records.

Consultation (3): Services rendered by a physician whose opinion or advice is requested by another physician or agency in the evaluation or treatment of a patient's illness or a suspected problem.

Consultative examiner (CE) (15): A physician who is paid a fee to examine and/or test a person for disability under either the SSDI or SSI program.

Consulting physician (3): Provider whose opinion or advice regarding evaluation and/or management of a specific problem is requested by another physician.

Continuing education (CE) (17): Formal education pursued by a working professional and intended to improve or maintain professional competence.

Continuity of care (3): When a physician sees a patient who has received treatment for a condition and is referred by the previous doctor for treatment of the same condition.

Contract (2): A legally enforceable agreement when relating to an insurance policy; for workers' compensation cases, an agreement involving two or more parties in which each is obligated to the other to fulfill promises made. (The contract exists between the physician and the insurance carrier.)

Conversion factor (5): The dollars and cents amount that is established for one unit as applied to a service rendered. This unit is then used to convert various procedures into fee-schedule payment amounts by multiplying the relative value unit by the conversion factor.

Cooperative care (13): Term used when a patient is seen by a civilian physician or hospital for services cost-shared by TRICARE.

Coordination of benefits (13): The coordination of the payment of TRICARE benefits with the payment of benefits made by the double coverage plan, so that there is no duplication of benefits paid between the double coverage plan and TRICARE. Likewise applied to disability programs.

Copayment (copay) (10): Patient's payment (i.e., 20% of a bill or flat fee of $10 per visit) of a portion of the cost at the time the service is rendered. Also referred to as *coinsurance.*

Cost-of-living adjustment (15): Disability insurance provision to increase monthly benefits.

Cost outlier (16): Typical case that has an extraordinarily high cost when compared with most discharges classified to the same DRG.

Cost outlier review (16): Review by a Professional Review Organization (PRO) for the necessity of a patient's hospital admission and to determine whether all services rendered were medically necessary. Cost outlier cases are recognized only if the case is not eligible for day outlier status.

Cost-share (13): The portion of the allowable charges for care on each claim that the patient pays and the portion that TRICARE pays.

Counseling (3): Discussion with a patient, family, or both concerning the diagnosis, recommended studies or tests, prognosis, risks, and benefits of treatment, treatment options, patient and family education, and so on.

County Medical Services Program (CMSP) (C): A county program for medical services.

Cover letter (17): Letter of introduction prepared to accompany a resume when seeking a job.

Covered services (12): Specific services and supplies for which Medicaid will provide reimbursement; these consist of a combination of mandatory and optional services within each state.

Credit (9): 1. From the Latin *credere,* meaning "to believe" or "to trust"; trust in regard to financial obligation. 2. Accounting; entry reflecting payment by a debtor (patient) of a sum received on his or her account.

Credit card (9): Card issued by an organization and devised for the purpose of obtaining money, property, labor, or services on credit.

Creditor (9): Person to whom money is owed.

Critical care (3): In reference to coding professional services, this phrase relates to intensive care provided in a variety of acute life-threatening conditions requiring constant bedside attention by a physician.

Crossover claim (11): Bill for services rendered to a patient receiving benefits simultaneously from Medicare and Medicaid. Medicare pays first and then determines the amounts of unmet Medicare deductible and coinsurance to be paid by Medicaid.

***Current Procedural Terminology* (CPT) (5):** A reference procedural code book using a numerical system for procedures, established by the American Medical Association.

Customary fee (5): The amount that a physician usually charges the majority of her or his patients.

Cycle billing (9): System of billing accounts at spaced intervals during the month based on breakdown of accounts by alphabet, account number, insurance type, or date of first service.

Day outlier review (16): Review of potential day outliers (short or unusually long length of hospital stay) to determine the necessity of admission and number of days before the day outlier threshold is reached as well as the number of days beyond the threshold. The PRO determines the certification of additional days.

Day sheet (2): Register for recording daily business transactions; also known as *daybook* or *daily record sheet.*

Debit card (9): Card permitting bank customers to withdraw from any affiliated automated teller machine (ATM) and to make cashless purchases from funds on deposit without incurring revolving finance charges for credit.

Debt (9): Legal obligation to pay money.

Debtor (9): Person owing money.

Debug (7): To remove errors from a software program or the computer itself.

Deductible (2, 10): Specific dollar amount that must be paid by the insured before a medical insurance plan or government program begins covering health care costs.

Defense Enrollment Eligibility Reporting System (DEERS) (13): An electronic database used to verify beneficiary eligibility for those individuals in the TRICARE programs.

Delinquent claim (8): Insurance claim submitted to an insurance company, for which payment is overdue.

Denied claim (8): Insurance claim submitted to an insurance company in which payment has been rejected owing to a technical error or because of medical coverage policy issues.

Department of Health Services (DHS) (C): Medi-Cal is administered by this state department, which is a department of the California State Human Relations Agency.

Deposition (14): The process of taking sworn testimony from a witness out of court. This is usually done by an attorney.

Detailed (D) (3): A term used to describe a level of history and/or physical examination.

Diagnosis-related groups (DRGs) (16): A patient classification system that categorizes patients who are medically related with respect to diagnosis and treatment and statistically similar in length of hospital stay. Medicare hospital insurance payments are based on fixed dollar amounts for a principal diagnosis as listed in DRGs.

Diagnostic cost groups (DCGs) (11): A system of Medicare reimbursement for HMOs with risk contracts in which enrollees are classified into various DCGs on the basis of each beneficiary's prior 12-month hospitalization history.

Diagnostic creep (16): Coding that is inappropriately altered to obtain a higher payment rate. Also known as *coding creep, DRG creep* or *upcoding.*

Digital fax claim (6): Insurance claim sent to the insurance carrier via facsimile but never printed on paper. The fax is encoded while in electronic form via an optical code reader and electronically entered into the claims processing system.

Dingy claim (6): Dingy claims happen when the Medicare contractor cannot process a claim for a particular service or bill type. The claims are held until the necessary system changes are implemented to pay the claim correctly.

Direct referral (10): Certain services in a managed care plan may not require preauthorization. The authorization request form is completed and signed by the physician and handed to the patient (e.g., obstetrical care, dermatology) to be done directly.

Dirty claim (6): Claim submitted with errors or requiring manual processing for resolving problems or rejection for payment.

Disability Determination Services (DDS) (15): A state Social Security division office that assesses a case for disability benefits.

Disability income insurance (2, 15): A form of health insurance that provides periodic payments to replace income when the insured is unable to work as a result of illness, injury, or disease.

Disabled (11): For purposes of enrollment under Medicare, individuals younger than 65 years of age who have been entitled to disability benefits under the Social Security Act or the railroad retirement system for at least 24 months are considered disabled and are entitled to Medicare.

Discount (9): Reduction of a normal charge based on a specific amount of money or a percentage of the charge.

Disenrollment (10): Member's voluntary cancellation of HMO membership.

Documentation (3): Chronologic detailed recording of pertinent facts and observations about a patient's health as seen in chart notes and medical reports. For computer software, a user's guide to a program or piece of equipment.

Double indemnity (15): A feature in some life and disability insurance policies that provides for twice the face amount of the policy to be paid if death results to the insured from accidental causes.

Downcoding (5): Occurs when the coding system used on a claim does not match that used by the insurance company receiving the claim.

Down time (7): The period during which a computer is malfunctioning or not operating correctly.

DRG creep (16): See *Diagnostic creep.*

Dun message (9): Message or phrase to remind a patient about a delinquent account.

Durable medical equipment (DME) (C): A billing phrase used to specify medical supplies, devices, and equipment to Medicare and Medi-Cal fiscal intermediaries for reimbursement.

Durable medical equipment (DME) number (6): A group or individual provider number used when submitting bills for specific medical supplies, devices, and equipment to the Medicare fiscal intermediary for reimbursement.

E codes (4): A classification of ICD-9-CM coding for external causes of injury rather than disease. E codes are also used in coding adverse reactions to medications.

Early and Periodic Screening, Diagnosis, and Treatment (EPSDT) (12): The EPSDT program covers screening and diagnostic services to determine physical or mental defects in recipients younger than age 21 years and health care, treatment, and other measures to correct or ameliorate any defects and chronic conditions discovered. In New York, this is called the Child Health Assurance Program (CHAP).

Elective surgery (16): Surgical procedure that may be scheduled in advance, is not an emergency, and is discretionary on the part of the physician and patient.

Electronic claim (6): Insurance claim submitted to the insurance carrier via a central processing unit (CPU), tape diskette, direct data entry, direct wire, dial-in telephone, digital fax, or personal computer download or upload.

Electronic claims processor (ECP) (7, 17): Individual who converts insurance claims to standardized electronic format and transmits electronic insurance claims data to the insurance carrier or clearinghouse to help the physician receive payment. Sometimes referred to as *electronic claims professional.*

Electronic claim submission (ECS) (7): Insurance claims prepared on a computer and submitted via modem (telephone lines) to the insurance carrier's computer system. Also called *electronic media claims (EMC).*

Electronic data interchange (EDI) (7): Process by which understandable data items are sent back and forth via computer linkages between two or more entities that function alternatively as sender and receiver.

Electronic Data Systems (EDS) Corporation (C): The Medi-Cal fiscal intermediary in the state of California.

Electronic funds transfer (EFT) (C): A paperless computerized system enabling funds to be debited, credited, or transferred, eliminating the need for personal handling of checks.

Electronic mail (e-mail) (7): Transmitting, receiving, storing, and forwarding of text, voice messages, attachments, or images by computer from one person to another.

Electronic signature (2): Individualized computer access and identification system (i.e., a series of numbers, letters, electronic writing, voice, computer key, and fingerprint transmission [biometric system]).

Eligibility (2): Qualifying factors that must be met before a patient receives benefits (medical services) under a specified insurance plan, government program, or managed care plan.

Eligibility verification confirmation (EVC) (C): A reference number on a printout from the Medi-Cal point-of-service device that verifies that an inquiry was received and eligibility information was transmitted.

Emancipated minor (2): Person younger than 18 years of age who lives independently, is totally self-supporting, and possesses decision-making rights.

Embezzlement (1): Willful act by an employee of taking possession of an employer's money.

Emergency (13): Sudden and unexpected medical condition, or the worsening of a condition, that poses a threat to life, limb, or sight and requires immediate treatment to alleviate suffering (e.g., shortness of breath, chest pain, drug overdose).

Emergency care (3): Health care services provided on an emergency basis or care given in a hospital; emergency department.

Employer identification number (EIN) (6): An individual's federal tax identification number issued by the Internal Revenue Service for income tax purposes.

Employment agency (17): Business organization that refers job applicants to potential employers.

Encounter form (2, 7): See *Multipurpose billing form.*

Encryption (7): To assign a code to represent data. This is done for the purpose of security.

End-stage renal disease (ESRD) (11): Individuals who have chronic kidney disease requiring dialysis or kidney transplant are considered to have ESRD. To qualify for Medicare coverage, an individual must be fully or currently insured under Social Security or the railroad retirement system or be the dependent of an insured person. Eligibility for Medicare coverage begins with the third month after the beginning of a course of renal dialysis. Coverage may begin sooner if the patient participates in a self-care dialysis training program or receives a kidney transplant without dialysis.

Eponym (3): A condition or procedure named after a person or place.

Ergonomic (14): Science and technology that seeks to fit the anatomic and physical needs of the worker to the workplace.

Established patient (3): An individual who has received professional health care services from the physician or another physician of the same specialty who belongs to the same group practice within the past 3 years.

Estate administrator (9): One who takes possession of the assets of a decedent, pays the expenses of administration and the claims of creditors, and disposes of the balance of an estate in accordance with the statutes governing the distribution of decedents' estates.

Estate executor (9): One who takes possession of the assets of a decedent, pays the expenses of administration and the claims of creditors, and disposes of the balance of an estate in accordance with the decedent's will.

Ethics (1): Moral principles and standards in the ideal relationships between the physician and patient and also between physicians.

Etiology (4): The cause of disease.

Etiquette (1): Customs, rules of conduct, courtesy, and manners of the medical profession.

Exclusion(s) (2, 15): Limitations for certain conditions or circumstances for which the health insurance policy will not provide benefits.

Exclusive provider organization (EPO) (2, 10): Type of managed health care plan in which subscriber members are eligible for benefits only when they use the services of a limited network of providers. EPOs are regulated under state health insurance laws. Such plans are for large clinics to participate in and combine fee-for-service PPO and HMO benefits.

Expanded problem focused (EPF) (3): A phrase used to describe a level of history and/or physical examination.

Explanation of benefits (EOB) (8): An explanation of services periodically issued to recipients or providers on whose behalf claims have been paid. Also known in Medicare, Medicaid, and some other programs as a *remittance advice.* In the TRICARE program, it is called a *summary payment voucher.*

Explanation of Medicare benefits (EOMB): See *Remittance advice.*

Expressed contract (2): Verbal or written contract.

Extend (2): To carry forward the balance of an individual ledger.

External audit (3): A retrospective review of medical and financial records by an insurance company or Medicare representative to investigate suspected fraud or abusive billing practices.

Extraterritorial (14): When benefits under the state law apply to a compensable injury to an employee hired in one state but injured outside of that state.

Facility provider number (6): A facility's (hospital, laboratory, radiology office, nursing facility) provider number to be used by the performing physician to report services done at the location.

Facsimile (3): An electronic process for transmitting graphic and written communications.

Family history (FH) (3): Review of medical events in the patient's family, including diseases that may be hereditary or place the patient at risk.

Federal Employees' Compensation Act (FECA) (14): Act instituted in 1908 providing benefits for on-the-job injuries to all federal employees.

Federal Employees Retirement System (FERS) (15): Program for federal employees hired after 1984 or those hired before 1984 who switched from CSRS to FERS.

Fee for service (10): Method of payment in which the patient pays the physician for each professional service performed from an established schedule of fees.

Fee schedule (5, 9, 14): List of charges or established allowances for specific medical services and procedures. See also *Relative value studies (RVS).*

File (7): A collection of related data stored under a single title.

Fiscal agent (12): An organization under contract to the state to process claims for a state Medicaid program; insurance carrier handling claims from physicians and other suppliers of service for Medicare Part B; sometimes also referred to as *fiscal intermediary.*

Fiscal intermediary (FI) (11, 13): An organization under contract to the government that handles claims under Medicare Part A from hospitals, skilled nursing facilities, and home health agencies. For TRICARE and CHAMPVA, the insurance company that handles the claims for care received within a particular state or country. Also known as *fiscal agent, fiscal carrier,* and *claims processor.*

Formal referral (10): Authorization request (telephone, fax, or completed form) required by the managed care organization contract to determine medical necessity.

Format (7): The organization or appearance of data.

Foundation for medical care (FMC) (2, 10): An organization of physicians sponsored by a state or local medical association concerned with the development and delivery of medical services and the cost of health care.

Fraud (1): An intentional misrepresentation of the facts to deceive or mislead another.

Freelance (17): To work for several clients as an independent self-employed individual.

Functional resume (17): Data sheet that highlights qualifications and skills.

Future purchase option (15): *See Cost-of-living adjustment.*

Garnishment (9): Court order attaching a debtor's property or wages to pay off a debt.

Gatekeeper (10): In the managed care system, this is the physician who controls patient access to specialists.

Genetically Handicapped Persons Program (GHPP) (C): A state program for genetically disabled children.

Gigabyte (7): Computer storage capacity that holds approximately 1 billion bytes or characters.

Global surgery policy (5): Medicare phrase relating to patients who have had major operations in which preoperative and postoperative visits, intraoperative services that are a usual part of the surgery, and complications not requiring additional trips to the operating room are packaged together for the fee.

Group provider number (6): A provider number used instead of the individual's physician's number (PIN) for the performing provider who is a member of a group practice that submits claims to insurance companies under the group name.

Grouper (16): The computer software program that assigns DRGs of discharged patients using the following information: patient's age, sex, principal diagnosis, complications/comorbid conditions, principal procedure, and discharge status.

Guaranteed renewable (2, 15): A clause in an insurance policy that means the insurance company must renew the policy as long as premium payments are made. However, the premium may be increased when it is renewed. These policies may have age limits of 60, 65, or 70 years or may be renewable for life.

Guarantor (2): Individual who promises to pay the medical bill by signing a form agreeing to pay or who accepts treatment, which constitutes an expressed promise.

Hard copy (7): A printout from a printer via computer.

Hardware (7): The physical components of a computer system (e.g., display screen, hard disk).

Health benefits advisor (HBA) (13): An individual at military hospitals or clinics who is there to help TRICARE beneficiaries obtain medical care through the military and through TRICARE.

Health Care Financing Administration (HCFA) (11): Formerly known as the Social Security Administration, HCFA is that part of the Department of Health and Human Services that oversees Medicare, among other governmental health programs.

Health Care Financing Administration Common Procedure Coding System (HCPCS) (5): HCFA's Common Procedure Coding System. A national uniform coding structure for reporting physician/supplier services under the Medicare program. A coding system that includes CPT-4, national, and local codes. Pronounced "hick-picks."

Health Care Finder (HCF) (13): Health care professionals, generally registered nurses, who are located at TRICARE Service Centers and help the patient find needed care.

Health insurance (2): A generic term applying to all types of insurance indemnifying or reimbursing for hospital and medical care costs or lost income arising from illness or injury. Also known as *accident and health insurance* or *disability income insurance.*

Health Insurance Claim Form (HCFA-1500) (6): Universal insurance claim form developed and approved by the American Medical Association Council on Medical Service and the Health Care Financing Administration. It is used by physicians and other professionals to bill outpatient services and supplies to TRICARE, Medicare, and some Medicaid programs as well as some private insurance carriers and managed care plans.

Health maintenance organization (HMO) (2, 10): A type of health care program in which enrollees receive benefits when they obtain services that are provided or authorized by selected providers, usually with a primary care physician "gatekeeper." In general, enrollees do not receive coverage for the services or providers who are not in the HMO network, except for emergency services.

Hearing (15): Second level of the appeal process for an individual applying for SSDI or SSI. This is a hearing before an administrative law judge who had no part in the initial or reconsideration disability determination.

High complexity (HC) (3): Phrase used to describe a type of medical decision making when a patient is seen for an E/M service.

High risk (2): A high chance of loss.

History of present illness (HPI) (3): Chronologic description of the development of the patient's present illness from the first sign and/or symptom or from the previous encounter to the present.

Hospice (11): A public agency or private organization primarily engaged in providing pain relief, symptom management, and supportive services to terminally ill patients and their families.

Hospital insurance (11): Known as Medicare Part A. A program providing basic protection against the costs of hospital and related post-hospital services for individuals eligible under the Medicare program.

Implied contract (2): Contract between physician and patient not manifested by direct words but implied or deduced from the circumstance, general language, or conduct of the patient.

In-area (10): Within the geographic boundaries defined by an HMO as the area in which it will provide medical services to its members.

Incomplete claim (6): Any Medicare claim missing required information; such claims are identified to the provider so they may be resubmitted.

Indemnity (2): Benefits paid to an insured while disabled.

Independent medical evaluator (IME) (14): Physicians who make examinations of individuals, independent of the attending physician, and render an unbiased opinion regarding the degree of disability of a worker. IMEs are appointed by the referee or appeals board at state expense.

Independent (or Individual) Practice Association (IPA) (2, 10): A type of HMO in which a program administrator contracts with a number of physicians who agree to provide treatment to subscribers in their own offices for a fixed capitation payment per month. Also referred to as a *medical capitation plan.*

Injury (14): In a workers' compensation policy, this term signifies any injury or disease sustained, arising out of, and in the course of employment, including injury to artificial members and medical braces of all types.

Inpatient (16): Term used when a patient is admitted to the hospital for overnight stay.

Input (7): That which goes into a computer memory bank.

Inquiry (8): See *Tracer.*

In situ (4): Description applied to a malignant growth confined to the site of origin without invasion of neighboring tissues.

Insurance adjuster (14): Individual at the workers' compensation insurance carrier overseeing an industrial case and communicating with the provider of medical care.

Insurance balance billing (9): Statement requesting the difference between the actual charge and an insurance carrier—approved amount.

Insurance billing specialist (1): A practitioner who carriers out claims completion, coding, and billing responsibilities and may or may not perform managerial and supervisory functions; also known as an *insurance claims processor* or *reimbursement specialist.*

Insured (2): Individual or organization protected in case of loss under the terms of an insurance policy.

Intelligent character recognition (ICR) (6): Same as *Optical character recognition.*

Interactive transaction (7): Back and forth communication between user and computer.

Interface (7): The point at which two different systems are linked (e.g., computer to printer or modem).

Intermediate care facilities (ICFs) (11): Institutions furnishing health-related care and services to individuals who do not require the degree of care provided by hospitals or nursing facilities.

Internal review (3): The process of going over financial documents before and after billing to insurance carriers to determine documentation deficiencies or errors.

International Classification of Diseases, Ninth Revision, Clinical Modification **(ICD-9-CM) (4, 16):** A system for classifying diseases and operations to facilitate collection of uniform and comparable health information. This code book will be replaced by ICD-10.

Internet (7): Large interconnected message-forwarding system linking academic, commercial, government, and military computer networks all over the world.

Interview (17): Meeting an individual face to face for evaluating and questioning a job applicant.

Intoxication (4): Diagnostic coding term that relates to an adverse effect rather than a poisoning when drugs such as digitalis, steroid agents, and so on are involved.

Invalid claim (6): Any Medicare claim that contains complete, necessary information but is illogical or incorrect (e.g., listing an incorrect provider number for a referring physician). Invalid claims are identified to the provider and may be resubmitted.

Italicized code (4): Diagnostic code in ICD-9-CM, Volume 1 Tabular list, that may never be sequenced as the principal diagnosis.

Itemized statement (9): Detailed summary of all transactions of a creditor's account.

Keypad (7): A device, separate or part of the keyboard, that contains keys to control mathematical functions.

Kilobyte (7): An expression for standard quantity measurement of disk or computer storage capacity.

Late effect (4): Inactive residual effect or condition produced after the acute phase of an illness or injury has ended.

Ledger card (2, 9): Individual record indicating charges, payments, adjustments, and balances owed for services rendered.

Lien (9, 14): A claim on the property of another as security for a debt. In litigation cases, it is a legal promise to satisfy a debt owed by the patient to the physician out of any proceeds received on the case.

Limiting charge (11): A percentage limit on fees, specified by legislation, that nonparticipating physicians may bill Medicare beneficiaries above the fee schedule amount.

List service (listserv) (1): An online computer service run from a web site where questions may be posted by subscribers.

Local area network (LAN) (7): Interlink of multiple computers that allows sharing of files and devices such as printers.

Long-term disability insurance (15): A provision to pay benefits to a covered disabled person as long as he or she remains disabled, up to a specified period exceeding 2 years.

Looping (16): The automated grouper (computer software program that assigns DRGs) process of searching all listed diagnoses for the presence of any comorbid condition or complication, or searching all procedures for operating room procedures or other specific procedures.

Lost claim (8): Insurance claim that cannot be located after sending it to an insurer.

Low complexity (LC) (3): Phrase used to describe a type of medical decision making when a patient is seen for an E/M service.

Major diagnostic categories (MDCs) (16): Broad classifications of diagnoses. There are 83 coding system–oriented MDCs in the original DRGs and 23 body system–oriented MDCs in the revised set of DRGs.

Major medical (2): Health insurance policy designed to offset heavy medical expenses resulting from catastrophic or prolonged illness or injury.

Malignant tumor (4): Abnormal growth that has the properties of invasion and metastasis (i.e., transfer of diseases from one organ to another).

Managed care organizations (MCOs) (10): A generic term applied to a managed care plan. May apply to EPO, HMO, PPO, integrated delivery system, or other weird arrangement.

Manual billing (9): Processing statements by hand; usually involves photocopying the patient's ledger and placing it in a window envelope, which then becomes the statement.

Maternal and Child Health Program (MCHP) (2, 12): A state service organization to assist children younger than 21 years of age who have conditions leading to health problems.

Medicaid (MCD) (2, 12): A federally aided, state-operated and administered program that provides medical benefits for certain low-income persons in need of health and medical care. California's Medicaid program is known as *Medi-Cal.*

Medi-Cal (12): California's version of the nationwide program known as Medicaid. See *Medicaid.*

Medical necessity (3, 11): Criteria used by insurance companies when making decisions to limit or deny payment in which medical services or procedures must be justified by the patient's symptoms and diagnosis.

Medical record (3): Written or graphic information documenting facts and events during the rendering of patient care.

Medical report (3): A permanent, legal document (letter or report format) that formally states the consequences of the patient's examination or treatment.

Medical service order (14): An authorization given to

the physician, either written or verbal, to treat the injured employee.

Medically indigent (MI) (C): See *Medically needy*.

Medically (or psychologically) necessary (13): Medical or psychologic services considered appropriate care and generally accepted by qualified professionals to be reasonable and adequate for the diagnosis and treatment of illness, injury, pregnancy, and mental disorders, or that are reasonable and adequate for well-baby care.

Medically needy (MN) (12, C): Persons in need of financial assistance and/or whose income and resources will not allow them to pay for the costs of medical care. Also called *Medically indigent* in some states.

Medicare (M) (2, 11): A nationwide health insurance program for persons age 65 years and older and certain disabled or blind persons regardless of income, administered by HCFA. Local Social Security offices take applications and supply information about the program.

Medicare/Medicaid (Medi-Medi) (2, 11): Refers to an individual who receives medical and/or disability benefits from both Medicare and Medicaid programs. Sometimes referred to as a *Medi-Medi case*.

Medicare Secondary Payer (MSP) (11): Primary insurance plan of a Medicare beneficiary that must pay for any medical care or services first before Medicare is sent a claim.

Medicare Summary Notice (MSN) (11): Document received by the patient explaining amount charged, Medicare approved, deductible, and coinsurance for medical services rendered.

Medigap (MG) (11): A specialized insurance policy devised for the Medicare beneficiary that covers the deductible and copayment amounts typically not covered under the main Medicare policy written by a nongovernmental third party payer. Also known as *Medifill*.

Megabyte (7): Computer storage capacity in which one megabyte is equal to 1,000 kilobytes (1,024 characters).

Member (2): Person covered under an insurance program's contract, including (1) the subscriber or contract holder who is the person named on the membership identification card and (2) in the case of (a) two-person coverage, (b) one adult—one child coverage, or (c) family coverage (eligible family dependents enrolled under the subscriber's contract).

Memory (7): Storage in computer.

Mentor (17): Guide or teacher who offers advice, criticism, wisdom, guidance, and perspective to an inexperienced but promising protégé to help reach a life goal.

Military treatment facility (MTF) (13): All uniformed service hospitals. Also known as *military hospitals* or *uniformed service hospitals*.

Modem (7): MOdulator DEModulator unit, a device that converts data into signals for telephone transmission and then (at the receiving end) back again into data.

Moderate complexity (MC) (3): Phrase used to describe a type of medical decision making when a patient is seen for an E/M service.

Modifier (5): In CPT coding, a two-digit add-on or five-digit number (representing the modifier) placed after the usual procedure code number to indicate a proce-

dure or service has been altered by specific circumstances. The two-digit modifier may be separated by a hyphen. In HCPCS Level II coding, one-digit or two-digit add-on alpha characters, placed after the usual procedure code number (see Example G-1).

EXAMPLE G–1

27372-51 (typed on one line)
OR
27372
09951 (typed on two lines)

Mouse (7): A device used to input computer data.

Multipurpose billing form (7): All-encompassing billing form personalized to the practice of the physician, it may be used when a patient submits an insurance billing; also called *charge slip, communicator, encounter form, fee ticket, patient service slip, routing form, superbill,* and *transaction slip*.

Multiskilled health practitioner (MSHP) (1): Individual cross trained to provide more than one function, often in more than one discipline. These combined functions can be found in a broad spectrum of health-related jobs, ranging in complexity including both clinical and management functions. The additional skills added to the original health care worker's job may be of a higher, lower, or parallel level. The terms *multiskilled, multicompetent,* and *cross trained* can be used interchangeably.

National alphanumeric codes (11): Alphanumeric codes developed by HCFA. See *Health Care Financing Administration Common Procedure Coding System (HCPCS)*.

Nationally Certified Insurance Coding Specialist (NCICS) (17): Insurance and coding certification that is awarded by an independent testing agency, the National Center for Competency Testing (NCCT).

National provider identifier (NPI) (6): A Medicare lifetime 10-digit number issued to providers. When adopted, it will be recognized by Medicaid, Medicare, TRICARE, and CHAMPVA programs and may eventually be used by private insurance carriers.

Netback (9): Evaluating a collection agency's performance by taking the amount of monies collected and subtracting the agency's fees.

Networking (17): Exchanging information or services among individuals, groups, or institutions and making use of professional contacts.

New patient (NP) (3): Individual who has not received any professional services from the physician or another physician of the same specialty who belongs to the same group practice within the past 3 years.

No charge (NC) (9): Waiving of the entire fee owed for professional care.

Nonavailability Statement (13): When the uniformed services hospital cannot provide the inpatient care and the patient lives in a certain ZIP code near a military hospital, the patient must obtain this statement, signed by the commanding officer, before getting nonemergency inpatient care at a civilian hospital. INAS means inpatient nonavailability statement.

Noncancellable clause or policy (2, 15): An insurance policy clause that means the insurance company cannot increase premium rates and must renew the policy until the insured reaches the age stated in the contract. Some disability income policies have noncancellable terms.

Nondisability (ND) claim (14): An on-the-job injury that requires medical care but does not result in loss of working time or income.

Nonexempt assets (9): One's total property (in bankruptcy cases) not falling in the exemption category; including money, automobile equity, and property, over a specified amount, depending on the state in which the person lives.

Nonparticipating physician (nonpar) (11): A provider who does not have a signed agreement with Medicare and has an option regarding assignment. The physician may not accept assignment for all services or has the option of accepting assignment for some services and collecting from the patient for other services performed at the same time and place.

Nonparticipating provider (nonpar) (2, 13): A provider who decides not to accept the determined allowable charge from an insurance plan as the full fee for care. Payment goes directly to the patient in this case, and the patient is usually responsible to pay the bill in full.

Nonprivileged information (1): Information unrelated to the treatment of the patient. The patient's authorization is not required to disclose the data unless the record is in a specialty hospital or in a special service unit of a general hospital, such as the psychiatric unit.

Not elsewhere classifiable (NEC) (4): This term is used in the ICD-9-CM diagnostic coding system when the code lacks the information necessary to code the term in a more specific category.

Not otherwise specified (NOS) (4): Unspecified. Used in ICD-9-CM numeric code system for coding diagnoses.

Nursing facility (NF) (11, C): A specially qualified facility that has the staff and equipment to provide skilled nursing care and related services for patients who need medical or nursing care or rehabilitation services. Formerly known as *skilled nursing facility.*

Occupational illness (or disease) (14): One that is produced by hazards peculiar to the occupation of the employee.

Occupational Safety and Health Administration (OSHA) (14): A federal agency that regulates and investigates safety and health standards of jobs.

Old Age Survivors, Health and Disability Insurance (OASHDI) Program (C): A group that is entitled to benefits under the Medi-Cal program.

Optical character recognition (OCR) (6): A device that can read typed characters at very high speed and convert them to digitized files that can be saved on disk. Also known as *intelligent character recognition* (ICR).

Optionally renewable (2): An insurance policy renewal provision in which the insurer has the right to

refuse to renew the policy on a date and may add coverage limitations or increase premium rates.

Ordering physician (3): The physician ordering nonphysician services for a patient (e.g., diagnostic laboratory tests, pharmaceutical services, or durable medical equipment) when an insurance claim is submitted by a nonphysician supplier of services.

"Other" claims (6): Medicare claims not considered "clean" claims that require investigation or development on a prepayment basis (developed for Medicare secondary payer information).

Other health insurance (OHI) (13): Health care coverage for TRICARE beneficiaries through an employer, an association, or a private insurer. A student in the family may have a health care plan through school.

Outpatient (16): Term used when an individual receives medical service from the hospital and goes home the same day.

Output (7): Information transferred from internal memory storage to external storage.

Overpayment (8): More than the due amount paid by the insurer or paid by the patient.

Paper claim (6): An insurance claim submitted on paper, including those optically scanned and converted to an electronic form by the insurance carrier.

Partial disability (15): When an illness or injury prevents an insured person from performing one or more of the functions of his or her regular job.

Participating physician (10): 1. A physician who contracts with an HMO or other insurance company to provide services. 2. A physician who has agreed to accept a plan's payments for services to subscribers (e.g., some Blue plans). Eighty percent of practicing American physicians are participating physicians.

Participating physician (par) (11): Physician agrees to accept payment from Medicare (80% of the approved charges) plus payment from the patient (20% of approved charges) after the $100 deductible has been met.

Participating provider (par) (2, 13): One who accepts TRICARE assignment. Payment in this case goes directly to the provider. The patient must still pay the cost-share outpatient deductible and the cost of care not covered by TRICARE. See *Assignment.*

Partnership program (13): A program that lets TRICARE-eligible individuals receive inpatient or outpatient treatment from civilian providers of care in a military hospital or from uniformed services providers of care in civilian facilities.

Password (7): A combination of letters and numbers that each individual is assigned to access computer data.

Past history (PH) (3): Patient's past experiences with illnesses, operations, injuries, and treatments.

Patient registration form (2): Questionnaire designed to provide identifying data for each patient seen for professional services.

Peer review (8): Review of a patient's case done by a group of unbiased practicing physicians to judge the effectiveness and efficiency of professional care rendered. This is done to discover over-utilization or misutilization of a plan's benefits.

Peer review organization (PRO) (11): A group of practicing physicians paid by the federal government to review hospital care of Medicare patients regarding effectiveness and efficiency.

Pending claim (6): Insurance claim held in suspense due to review or other reason. These claims may be cleared for payment or denied.

Per capita (10): See *Capitation*

Percentage of revenue (16): Fixed percentage of the collected premium rate that is paid to the hospital to cover services.

Per diem (16): Single charge for a day in the hospital regardless of any actual charges or costs incurred.

Permanent and stationary (P & S) (14): A phrase used when a patient's condition has become stabilized and no improvement is expected. It is only after this declaration that a case can be rated for a compromise and release.

Permanent disability (PD) (14): An illness or injury that prevents a person from performing the functions of his or her regular job.

Personal bond (1): Insurance that provides coverage for those who handle large sums of money during business transactions.

Personal insurance (2): Insurance plan issued to an individual (and/or his or her dependents). Also known as *individual contract*.

Petition (14): Commonly used to indicate an appeal; also means any request for relief other than an application.

Phantom billing (1): Billing for services not performed.

Physical examination (PE) (3): Objective inspection and/or testing of a patient by a physician.

Physically clean claim (6): Insurance claims with no staples or highlighted areas. The bar code area has not been deformed.

Physician provider group (PPG) (10): A physician-owned business that has the flexibility to deal with all forms of contract medicine and still offer its own packages to business groups, unions, and the general public.

Physician's fee profile (4): A compilation of each physician's charges and the payments made to him or her over a given period of time for each specific professional service rendered to a patient.

Ping-ponging (1): Excessive referrals to other providers for unnecessary services.

Point-of-service (POS) device or network (C): A piece of equipment interfaced with an analog telephone line used to identify Medi-Cal recipient eligibility, obtain share of cost liability status, key in share of cost payment toward balance, reserve Medi-Services, perform Family PACT (planning, access, care, and treatment) client eligibility transactions, and submit pharmacy or HCFA-1500 insurance claims.

Point-of-service (POS) option (13): Individuals under the TRICARE program can choose to get TRICARE-covered nonemergency services outside the prime network of providers without a referral from the primary care manager and without authorization from a health care finder.

Point-of-service (POS) plan (2, 10): An HMO consisting of a network of physicians and hospitals that provides an insurance company or an employer with discounts on its services. Sometimes referred to as *managed choice*.

Poisoning (4): Condition resulting from an overdose of drugs or chemical substances or from the wrong drug or agent given or taken in error.

Portfolio (17): A compilation of items that represents a job applicant's skills.

Position-schedule bond (1): Insurance that provides coverage for a designated job title rather than a named individual.

Post (2): Record or transfer financial entries, debit or credit, to an account (e.g., day sheet, ledger, bank deposit slip, chest register, or journal).

Preadmission testing (PAT) (16): Treatment, tests, and procedures done 48 to 72 hours before admission of a patient into the hospital. This is done to eliminate extra hospital days.

Preauthorization (2, 13): Requirement in some health insurance plans to obtain permission for a service or procedure before it is done and to see whether the insurance program agrees it is medically necessary.

Precertification (2): To find out whether treatment (surgery, tests, hospitalization) is covered under a patient's health insurance policy.

Predetermination (2): To determine before treatment the maximum dollar amount the insurance company will pay for surgery, consultations, postoperative care, and so forth.

Preferred provider organization (PPO) (2, 10): A type of health benefit program in which enrollees receive the highest level of benefits when they obtain services from a physician, hospital, or other health care provider designated by their program as a "preferred provider." Enrollees may receive substantial, although reduced, benefits when they obtain care from a provider of their own choosing who is not designated as a "preferred provider" by their program.

Premium (2, 11): A monthly fee that enrollees pay for Medicare Part B medical insurance. This fee is updated annually to reflect changes in program costs.

Prepaid group practice model (10): A plan under which specified health services are rendered by participating physicians to an enrolled group of persons, with fixed periodic payments made in advance, by or on behalf of each person or family. If a health insurance carrier is involved, it contracts to pay in advance for the full range of health services to which the insured is entitled under the terms of the health insurance contract. Such a plan is one form of a *health maintenance organization*.

Presumptive eligibility (PE) (C): A federal/state program designed to ease access to prenatal care offering immediate temporary coverage to low-income women pending a formal Medi-Cal application.

Prevailing charge (5): Fee that is most frequently charged in an area by a specialty group of physicians. The top of this range establishes an overall limitation on the charges that a carrier, which considers prevailing charges in reimbursement, will accept as reasonable for a given service without special justification.

Primary care manager (PCM) (13): Physician who is responsible for coordinating and managing all the beneficiary's health care unless there is an emergency.

Primary care physician (PCP) (10): A physician (e.g., family practitioner, general practitioner, pediatrician, obstetrician/gynecologist, or general internist) who oversees the care of patients in a managed health care plan (HMO or PPO) and refers patients to see specialists (e.g., cardiologists, oncologists, surgeons) for services as needed. Also known as a *gatekeeper.*

Primary diagnosis (4): Initial identification of the condition or chief complaint for which the patient is treated for outpatient medical care.

Principal diagnosis (4, 16): A condition established after study that is chiefly responsible for the admission of the patient to the hospital.

Prior approval (12): The evaluation of a provider request for a specific service to determine the medical necessity and appropriateness of the care requested for a patient. Also called *prior authorization* in some states.

Privileged information (1): Data related to the treatment and progress of the patient that can be released only when written authorization of the patient or guardian is obtained.

Problem focused (PF) (3): Phrase used to describe a type of medical decision making when a patient is seen for an E/M service.

Procedure code numbers (5): Five-digit numeric codes that describe each service the physician renders to a patient.

Procedure review (16): Review of diagnostic and therapeutic procedures to determine appropriateness.

Professional Association of Health Care Office Managers (PAHCOM) (17): A nationwide organization dedicated to providing a strong professional network for health care office managers.

Professional component (PC) (5): That portion of a test or procedure (containing both a professional and technical component) which the physician performs, i.e., interpreting an electrocardiogram (ECG), reading an x-ray, or making an observation and determination using a microscope.

Professional courtesy (9): Discount or exemption from charges given to certain people at the discretion of the physician rendering the service.

Professional review organizations (PROs) (16): Groups of licensed physicians and osteopaths engaged in the practice of medicine or surgery in a particular area, formed to ensure adequate review of the services provided by the various medical specialties and subspecialties in the area, as well as providing DRG validation, a group of physicians working with the government to review cases for hospital admission and discharge under government guidelines. Also known as *peer review.*

Program (7): See *Software.*

Prompt (7): A list of items displayed on a CRT from which the typist can choose the function to be performed. Also known as *menu.*

Prospective payment system (PPS) (11): A method of payment for Medicare hospital insurance based on DRGs (a fixed dollar amount for a principal diagnosis).

Prospective review (3): Process of going over financial documents before billing is submitted to the insurance company to determine documentation deficiencies and errors.

Provider identification number (PIN) (6): A carrier-assigned number that every physician uses who renders services to patients when submitting insurance claims.

Provider Telecommunications Network (PTN) (C): Automated voice-response system that allows the provider to use the telephone to obtain checkwrite, claim, and prior authorization information for services rendered through the Medi-Cal program and several other state programs.

Quality assurance program (13): Plan that continually assesses the effectiveness of inpatient and outpatient care in the TRICARE and CHAMPVA programs.

Qui tam **action (11):** An action to recover a penalty, brought by an informer in a situation in which one portion of the recovery goes to the informer and the other portion to the state or government.

Random access memory (RAM) (7): Allows data to be stored randomly and retrieved directly by specifying the address location.

Read-only memory (ROM) (7): Data stored in ROM can be read but not changed. It usually contains a permanent program.

Readmission review (16): Review of patients readmitted to a hospital within 7 days with problems related to the first admission, to determine whether the first discharge was premature and/or the second admission is medically necessary.

Reasonable fee (5, 11): A charge is considered reasonable if it is deemed acceptable after peer review even though it does not meet the *customary* or *prevailing* criteria. This would include unusual circumstances or complications requiring additional time, skill, or experience in connection with a particular service or procedure.

Rebill (8): To send another request for payment for an overdue bill to either the insurance company or patients.

Recertification (17): Renewal of certification after a specified time.

Recipient (12): A person certified by the local welfare department to receive the benefits of Medicaid under one of the specific aid categories; an individual certified to receive Medicare benefits.

Reconsideration (15): First level of appeal process for an individual applying for SSDI or SSI. It is a complete review of the claim by a medical or psychologic consultant/disability examiner team who did not take part in the original disability determination.

Referral (3): Transfer of the total or specific care of a patient from one physician to another.

Referring physician (3): A physician requesting service for a patient when the insurance claim is submitted by the physician performing the service.

Regional office (RO) (15): Social Security state office.

Registered Medical Assistant (RMA) (17): A title earned by completing appropriate training and by passing a registry examination administered by the American Medical Technologists (AMT).

Registered Medical Coder (RMC) (17): A registered title awarded after completion of coursework given by the Medical Management Institute (MMI) with recertification requirements.

Registration (17): Entry in an official registry or record that lists names of persons in an occupation who have satisfied specific requirements or by attaining a certain level of education and paying a registration fee.

Reimbursement (9): Repayment.

Reimbursement specialist (1): See *Insurance Billing Specialist*.

Rejected claim (6, 8): Insurance claim submitted to insurance carrier that is discarded by the system due to a technical error (omission or erroneous information) or because it does not follow Medicare instructions. It is returned to the provider for correction or change so that it may be processed properly for payment.

Relative value studies (RVS) (5): List of procedure codes for professional services and procedures with unit values that indicate the relative value of one procedure over another.

Relative value unit (RVU) (11): Individual building block of RBRVS (resource-based relative value scale). For each service, there are three RVUs: for work, practice expenses, and the cost of professional liability insurance.

Remittance advice (RA) (8, 11): An explanation of services periodically issued to recipients or providers on whose behalf claims have been paid by the Medicare or Medicaid program. Also known in some programs as an *Explanation of Benefits*.

Remittance Advice Details (RAD) (C): Document that accompanies all Medi-Cal payment vouchers (checks) sent to providers of medical services.

Residual benefits (15): Term used in disability income insurance for disability that is not work related. It is the payment of partial benefits when the insured is not totally disabled.

Resource-based relative value scale (RBRVS) (11): A system that ranks physician services by units; a Medicare fee schedule.

Respite care (11): Short-term hospice inpatient stay that may be necessary to give temporary relief to the person who regularly assists with home care of a patient.

Respondent superior (1): "Let the master answer." A physician is liable in certain cases for the wrongful acts of his or her assistant or employees.

Resubmission Turnaround Document (RTD) (C): Document that the Medi-Cal fiscal intermediary sends to providers when a claim form has questionable or missing information.

Resume (17): Summary of education, skills, and work experience, usually in outline form.

Retrospective review (3): Process of going over financial documents after billing an insurance carrier to determine documentation deficiencies and errors.

Review (8): To look over a claim to assess how much payment should be made.

Review of systems (ROS) (3): An inventory of body systems obtained through a series of questions that is used to identify signs and/or symptoms that the patient might be experiencing or has experienced.

Running balance (2): Amount owed on a credit transaction; also known as *outstanding* or *unpaid balance*.

Second-injury fund (14): See *Subsequent injury fund*.

Secondary diagnosis (4): A second reason for an office or hospital encounter that may contribute to the condition or defines the need for a higher level of care but is not the underlying cause.

Secured debt (9): Debt (an amount owed) in which a debtor pledges certain property (collateral), in a written security agreement, to the repayment of the debt.

Self-employment (17): Working for oneself, with direct control over work, services, and fees.

Self-referral (10): Patient in a managed care plan that refers himself or herself to a specialist. The patient may be required to inform the primary care physician.

Sequelae (14): Diseased conditions following, and usually resulting from, a previous disease.

Service area (10): The geographic area defined by an HMO as the locale in which it will provide health care services to its members directly through its own resources or through arrangements with other providers in the area.

Service benefit program (13): Because there are no premiums, TRICARE Standard is considered a service benefit program.

Service-connected injury (13): Injury incurred by a service member while on active duty.

Service retiree (13): Individual who is retired from a career in the armed forces; also known as *military retiree*.

Share of cost (12, C): The amount the patient must pay each month before he or she can be eligible for Medicaid. Also known as *liability* or *spend down*.

Short-term disability insurance (15): A provision to pay benefits to a covered disabled person as long as he or she remains disabled, up to a specified period not exceeding 2 years.

Skip (9): Debtor who has moved and neglected to give a forwarding address.

Slanted brackets (4): Symbol used with a diagnostic code in ICD-9-CM, Volume 2, Alphabetic Index, indicating the code may never be sequenced as the principal diagnosis.

Social history (SH) (3): Age-appropriate review of a patient's past and current activities.

Social Security Administration (SSA) (15): Administers SSDI and SSI programs for disabled persons.

Social Security Disability Insurance (SSDI) (15): Entitlement program for disabled workers or self-employed individuals.

Social Security number (SSN) (6): An individual's tax identification number.

Soft copy (7): That which is displayed on a CRT screen.

Software (7): Instructions (programs) required to make hardware perform a specific task.

Sponsor (13): For the TRICARE program, the service person, either active duty, retired, or deceased, whose relationship makes the patient eligible for TRICARE.

Staff model (10): A type of HMO similar to the group model.

Star symbol (5): Symbol (*) that appears next to certain procedure code numbers indicating special guidelines to be followed when using those surgical codes.

State Disability Insurance (SDI) (2, 15): See *Unemployment Compensation Disability*.

State license number (6): A number issued to a physician that gives him or her the right to practice medicine in the state where issued.

Statute of limitations (9): A time limit established for filing lawsuits.

Stop loss (10, 16): An agreement between a managed care company and a reinsurer in which absorption of prepaid patient expenses is limited; or limiting losses on an individual expensive hospital claim or professional services claim; form of reinsurance by which the managed care program limits the losses of an individual expensive hospital claim.

***Subpoena* (3):** "Under penalty." A writ that commands a witness to appear at a trial or other proceeding and give testimony.

***Subpoena duces tecum* (3):** "In his possession." A subpoena that requires the appearance of a witness with his or her records. Sometimes the judge permits the mailing of records and the physician is not required to appear in court.

Sub rosa films (14): Videotapes made without the knowledge of the subject.

Subscriber (2): The contract holder covered by an insurance program or managed care plan, who either has coverage through his or her place of employment or has purchased coverage directly from the plan.

Subsequent injury fund (SIF) (14): A special fund that assumes all or part of the liability for benefits provided to a worker because of the combined effect of a work-related impairment and a preexisting condition.

Summary payment voucher (13): The document the fiscal agent sends to the provider and/or beneficiary, showing the service or supplies received, allowable charges, amount billed, the amount TRICARE paid, how much deductible has been paid, and the patient's cost-share.

Supplemental benefits (15): Disability insurance provisions that allow benefits to the insured to increase the monthly indemnity or to receive a percentage of the policy premiums if an individual keeps a policy in force for 5 or 10 years or does not file any claims.

Supplemental Security Income (SSI) (11, 12): A program of income support for low-income aged, blind, and disabled persons established by Title XVI of the Social Security Act.

Supplementary medical insurance (SMI) (11): Part B—medical benefits of Medicare program.

Surgical package (5): Unstarred surgical procedure code numbers include the operation; local infiltration, digital block, or topical anesthesia; and normal, uncomplicated postoperative care. This is referred to as a "package," and one fee covers the whole package.

Suspense (8): A processed insurance claim held as pending either due to an error or the need for additional information.

Technical component (5): That portion of a test or procedure (containing both a technical and a professional component) which pertains to the use of the equipment and the operator who performs it, i.e., ECG machine and technician, radiography machine and technician, and microscope and technician.

Temporary disability (TD) (14, 15): The recovery period following a work-related injury during which the employee is unable to work and the condition has not stabilized; a schedule of benefits payable for the temporary disability.

Temporary disability insurance (TDI) (15): See *Unemployment Compensation Disability*.

Tertiary care (10): Services provided by specialists (e.g., neurosurgeons, thoracic surgeons, and intensive care units).

Third party liability (14): Third party liability exists if an entity is liable to pay the medical cost for injury, disease, or disability of a person hurt during the performance of his or her occupation and the injury is caused by an entity not connected with the employer.

Third party subrogation (14): The legal process by which an insurance company seeks from a third party, who has caused a loss, recovery of the amount paid to the policyholder.

Total disability (15): A term that varies in meaning from one disability insurance policy to another. An example of a liberal definition might read, "The insured must be unable to perform the major duties of his or her specific occupation."

Total, permanent service-connected disability (13): Total permanent disability incurred by a service member while on active duty.

Tracer (8): An inquiry made to an insurance company to locate the status of an insurance claim (i.e., claim in review, claim never received, and so forth).

Transfer review (16): Review of transfers to different areas of the same hospital that are exempted from prospective payment.

Treating or performing physician (3): Provider that renders a service to a patient.

Treatment Authorization Request (TAR) form (C): Medi-Cal form that must be completed by a provider for certain procedures and services that require prior approval.

TRICARE (2): Three-option managed health care program offered to spouses and dependents of service personnel with uniform benefits and fees implemented nationwide by the federal government.

TRICARE Extra (13): PPO type of TRICARE option in which the individual does not have to enroll or pay an annual fee. On a visit-by-visit basis, the individual may seek care from an authorized network provider and receive a discount on services and reduced cost-share (co-payment).

TRICARE Prime (13): Voluntary HMO-type option for TRICARE beneficiaries.

TRICARE Service Center (13): Office staffed by TRICARE Health Care Finders and beneficiary service representatives.

Turfing (10): Transferring the sickest, high-cost patients to other physicians so the provider appears as a low-utilizer in a managed care setting.

Two-party check (8): Check that is made out to the physician and the patient by the maker.

Unbundling (5): The practice of using numerous CPT codes to identify procedures normally covered by a single code; also known as *itemizing, fragmented billing, exploding*, or *à la carte medicine*; billing under Medicare Part B for nonphysician services to hospital inpatients furnished to the hospital by an outside supplier or another provider. Under the new law, unbundling is prohibited, and all nonphysician services provided in an inpatient setting will be paid as hospital services.

Unemployment Compensation Disability (UCD) (2, 15): Insurance that covers off-the-job injury or sickness and is paid for by deductions from a person's paycheck. This program is administered by a state agency and is sometimes also known as *State Disability Insurance (SDI)*.

Uniform Bill (UB-92) claim form (16): Uniform Bill insurance claim form developed by the National Uniform Billing Committee for hospital inpatient billing and payment transactions.

Unique provider identification number (UPIN) (6): A number issued by the Medicare fiscal intermediary to each physician who renders medical services to Medicare recipients.

Unsecured debt (9): Any debt (amount owed) that is not secured or backed by any form of collateral.

Upcoding (5): Deliberate manipulation of CPT codes for increased payment.

Urgent care (13): Medically necessary treatment that is required for illness or injury that would result in further disability or death if not treated immediately.

Usual, customary, and reasonable (UCR) (5): A method used by insurance companies to establish their fee schedules. UCR uses the conversion factor method of establishing maximums; the method of reimbursement used under Medicaid by which state Medicaid programs set reimbursement rates using the Medicare method or a fee schedule, whichever is lower.

Utilization review (UR) (10, 16): A process, based on established criteria, of reviewing and controlling the medical necessity for services and providers' use of medical care resources. Reviews are carried out by allied health personnel at predetermined times during the hospital stay to assess the need for the full facilities of an acute care hospital. In managed care systems, such as an HMO, reviews are done to establish medical necessity, thus curbing costs. Also called *utilization* or *management control*.

V codes (4): A classification of ICD-9-CM coding to identify health care encounters for reasons other than illness or injury and to identify patients whose injury or illness is influenced by special circumstances or problems.

Verbal referral (10): Primary care physician informs the patient and telephones to the referring physician that the patient is being referred for an appointment.

Veteran (13): Any person who has served in the armed forces of the United States, especially in time of war; is no longer in the service; and has received an honorable discharge.

Veterans Affairs (VA) disability program (15): Program for honorably discharged veterans who file claim for a service-connected disability.

Veterans Affairs (VA) outpatient clinic (2, 15): A clinic where medical and dental services are rendered to veterans who have service-related disabilities.

Video display terminal (VDT) (7): A television-like screen attached to a computer or word processing terminal; also known as a *cathode ray tube (CRT)*.

Virus (7): A destructive program that attaches and copies itself to other programs in a computer system. Some viruses destroy programs and data after a precise lapse of time.

Voice Drug TAR System (VDTS) (C): A Medi-Cal telecommunication system for processing urgent and initial drug Treatment Authorization Requests, to inquire about the status of previously entered drug TARs, or to inquire whether a patient is receiving continual care with a drug.

Volume performance standard (VPS) (11): Desired growth rate for spending on Medicare Part B physician services, set each year by Congress.

Voluntary disability insurance (15): A majority of employees of an employer voluntarily consent to be covered by an insured or self-insured disability insurance plan instead of a state plan.

Waiting period (WP) (14, 15): For disability insurance, the initial period of time when a disabled individual is not eligible to receive benefits even though unable to work; for workers' compensation, the days that must elapse before workers' compensation weekly benefits become payable.

Waiver of premium (15): A disability insurance policy provision that an employee does not have to pay any premiums while disabled. Also known as *elimination period*.

Withhold (10): A portion of the monthly capitation payment to physicians retained by the HMO until the end of the year to create an incentive for efficient care. If the physician exceeds utilization norms, he or she will not receive it.

Work hardening (14): Individualized program of therapy using simulated or real job duties to build up strength and improve the worker's endurance to be able to work up to 8 hours per day. Sometimes work site modifications are instituted to get the employee back to gainful employment.

Workers' Compensation Appeals Board (WCAB) (14): Board that handles workers' compensation liens and appeals.

Workers' compensation (WC) insurance (2, 14): A contract that insures a person against on-the-job injury or illness. The employer pays the premium for his or her employees.

Write-off (9): Assets or debts that have been determined to be uncollectable and are therefore adjusted off the accounting books as a loss.

Yo-yoing (1): Calling patients back for repeated and unnecessary follow-up visits.

Index

Note: Page numbers followed by f refer to figures; page numbers followed by t refer to tables.

Multimedia CD-ROM
Single-User License Agreement

1. NOTICE. READ THE TERMS AND CONDITIONS OF THIS LICENSE AGREEMENT CAREFULLY BEFORE OPENING THE SEALED PACKAGE CONTAINING THE MULTIMEDIA CD-ROM AND THE COMPUTER SOFTWARE THEREIN (ENTITLED "CD-ROM TO ACCOMPANY INSURANCE HANDBOOK FOR THE MEDICAL OFFICE, 7TH EDITION"), AND THE ACCOMPANYING USER DOCUMENTATION (THE SOFTWARE IS REFERRED TO AS THE "SOFTWARE," THE USER DOCUMENTATION IS REFERRED TO AS THE "USER DOCUMENTATION," AND THESE ARE ALL COLLECTIVELY REFERRED TO AS THE "MULTIMEDIA PRODUCT"). THE MULTIMEDIA PRODUCT IS COPYRIGHTED AND LICENSED (NOT SOLD). WE ARE WILLING TO LICENSE THE MULTIMEDIA PRODUCT TO YOU ONLY ON THE CONDITION THAT YOU ACCEPT ALL OF THE TERMS CONTAINED IN THIS LICENSE AGREEMENT. BY OPENING THIS PACKAGE YOU ARE AGREEING TO BE BOUND BY ALL OF THE TERMS OF THIS AGREEMENT. IF YOU DO NOT AGREE TO THESE TERMS WE ARE UNWILLING TO LICENSE THE MULTIMEDIA PRODUCT TO YOU, AND YOU SHOULD NOT OPEN THE SEALED PACKAGE. IN SUCH CASE, PROMPTLY RETURN THE UNOPENED PACKAGE WITH ALL ACCOMPANYING MATERIAL, ALONG WITH PROOF OF PAYMENT, TO THE AUTHORIZED DEALER FROM WHOM YOU OBTAINED IT FOR A FULL REFUND OF THE PRICE YOU PAID.

THIS LICENSE AGREEMENT SUPERSEDES ALL PRIOR AGREEMENTS, REPRESENTATIONS, OR UNDERSTANDINGS BETWEEN THE PARTIES CONCERNING THE MULTIMEDIA PRODUCT.

"WE," "US," "OUR," AND SIMILAR PRONOUNS REFER TO THE W.B. SAUNDERS COMPANY.

2. **Ownership and License.** Upon all of the terms and conditions herein, we hereby grant to you, and you accept, a non-exclusive limited license to use the Multimedia Product. The Software contained therein is licensed to you in machine-readable, object code form only. This is a license agreement and NOT an agreement for sale. Except as is otherwise specifically provided herein, this license permits you to install and/or use one copy of the Software on a single personal computer that is owned, leased, or otherwise controlled by you. You may change such computers from time to time, so long as the Software is not installed or used on more than a single computer at a time. The Multimedia Product is owned by us or our licensors, and is protected by U.S. and international copyright laws. Your rights to use the Multimedia Product are specified in this Agreement, and we retain all rights not expressly granted to you in this Agreement.

3. **Transfer and Other Restrictions.** You may not rent, lend, or lease the Multimedia Product. You may not and you may not cause or allow others to (a) disassemble, decompile, or otherwise derive source code from the Software), (b) reverse engineer the Software, (c) modify or prepare derivative works of the Multimedia Product or any portion thereof, (d) use the Software in an on-line or Internet system, or (e) use the Multimedia Product in any manner that infringes on the intellectual property rights or other rights of another party.

Notwithstanding the foregoing, you may transfer this license to use the Multimedia Product to another party on a permanent basis by transferring this copy of the license agreement, the Multimedia Product, and all documentation, provided that you provide us with written notification of the transfer and the transferee agrees to be bound by the terms of this license agreement. Such transfer of possession terminates your license with us. Such other party shall be licensed under the terms of this Agreement upon its acceptance of this agreement by its clear written assent (acceptable to us) and initial use of the Multimedia Product. If you transfer the Multimedia Product, you must remove any and all installation files from your computers, hard disks, etc., and you may not retain any copies of those files for your own use.

4. **Limited Warranty and Limitation of Liability.** For a period of sixty (60) days from the date you acquired the Multimedia Product from us or our authorized dealer, we warrant to you, for your benefit alone, that the media containing the Software will be free from defects that prevent you from installing and/or using the Software on your computer. If the Multimedia CD-ROM fails to conform to this warranty, you may, as your sole and exclusive remedy, obtain a replacement free of charge if you return the defective disk to us with a dated proof of purchase. Otherwise, the Multimedia Product is licensed to you on an "AS IS" basis without any warranty of any nature.

WE DO NOT WARRANT THAT THE MULTIMEDIA PRODUCT WILL MEET YOUR REQUIREMENTS OR THAT ITS OPERATION WILL BE UNINTERRUPTED OR ERROR-FREE. WE EXCLUDE AND EXPRESSLY DISCLAIM ALL EXPRESS AND IMPLIED WARRANTIES NOT STATED HEREIN, INCLUDING THE IMPLIED WARRANTIES OF MERCHANTABILITY AND FITNESS FOR A PARTICULAR PURPOSE.

WE SHALL NOT BE LIABLE FOR ANY DAMAGE OR LOSS OF ANY KIND ARISING OUT OF OR RESULTING FROM YOUR POSSESSION OR USE OF THE MULTIMEDIA PRODUCT (INCLUDING DATA LOSS OR CORRUPTION), REGARDLESS OF WHETHER SUCH LIABILITY IS BASED IN TORT, CONTRACT OR OTHERWISE AND INCLUDING, BUT NOT LIMITED TO, ACTUAL, SPECIAL, INDIRECT, INCIDENTAL, EXEMPLARY, AND/OR CONSEQUENTIAL DAMAGES OR ANY LOST PROFITS OR LOST DATA. IF THE FOREGOING LIMITATION IS HELD TO BE UNENFORCEABLE, OUR MAXIMUM LIABILITY TO YOU SHALL NOT EXCEED THE AMOUNT OF THE LICENSE FEE PAID BY YOU FOR THE MULTIMEDIA PRODUCT. THE REMEDIES AVAILABLE TO YOU AGAINST US AND THE LICENSORS OF MATERIALS INCLUDED IN THE MULTIMEDIA PRODUCT ARE EXCLUSIVE.

Some states do not allow the limitation or exclusion of implied warranties or liability for incidental or consequential damages, so the above limitations or exclusions may not apply to you.

The terms of this Section 4 shall survive termination of this license agreement for any reason.

5. **United States Government Restricted Rights.** The Multimedia Product and documentation are provided with Restricted Rights. Use, duplication, or disclosure by the U.S. Government or any agency or instrumentality thereof is subject to the restrictions in F.A.R. 52.227-14 (June 1987) Alternate III (June 1987), F.A.R. 52.227-19 (June 1987), or D.F.A.R.S. 252.227-7013 (b)(3) (November 1995), or applicable successor clauses, and/or similar provisions of the Federal Acquisition Regulations, as applicable. Manufacturer is the W.B. Saunders Company, the Curtis Center, Suite 300, Independence Square West, Philadelphia, PA 19106.

6. **Term and Termination.** This license is effective upon your opening of the sealed package and continues until terminated. This license and your right to use this Multimedia Product automatically terminate if you fail to comply with any provisions of this Agreement, destroy the copy of the Multimedia Product in your possession, or voluntarily return the Multimedia Product to us. Upon termination you will destroy any and all authorized copies of the Multimedia Product and all related documentation and any and all authorized copies thereof.

7. **Miscellaneous Provisions.** This Agreement will be governed by and construed in accordance with the substantive laws of the State of Missouri, and the parties will submit to and will not oppose venue in Missouri state or federal court. This is the entire agreement between us relating to the Multimedia Product, and supersedes any purchase order, communications, advertising or representations concerning the contents of this package. No change or modification of this Agreement will be valid unless it is in writing and is signed by us.

The license fee paid by you is paid in consideration of the license granted under this license agreement.

Should any term of this license agreement be declared void or unenforceable by any court or tribunal of competent jurisdiction, such declaration shall have no effect on the remaining terms hereof. The failure of either party to enforce any rights granted hereunder or to take action against the other party in the event of any breach hereunder shall not be deemed a waiver by that party as to the subsequent enforcement of rights or subsequent actions in the event of future breaches.